£2

KV-553-893

Nerves and the Gastrointestinal Tract

B/WI 102 SIN

FALK SYMPOSIUM 50

Nerves and the Gastrointestinal Tract

EDITED BY

M. V. Singer   **H. Goebell**
Department of Internal Medicine,
University of Essen, Federal Republic of Germany

Proceedings of the 50th Falk Symposium held in Titisee, Federal Republic of Germany, June 2–4, 1988

 MTP PRESS LIMITED
a member of the KLUWER ACADEMIC PUBLISHERS GROUP
LANCASTER / BOSTON / THE HAGUE / DORDRECHT

1989

Distributors

for the United States and Canada: Kluwer Academic Publishers, PO Box 358, Accord
Station, Hingham, MA 02018-0358, USA
for all other countries: Kluwer Academic Publishers Group, Distribution Center, PO Box 322,
3300 AH Dordrecht, The Netherlands

British Library Cataloguing in Publication Data

Falk Symposium (*50th; 1988; Titisee, Germany*)
  Nerves and the gastrointestinal tract.
  1. Gastrointestinal tract – Manuals
  I. Title II. Singer, Manfred V. III. Goebell. H. (Harald)
  599'.0188

  ISBN 0–7462–0114–1

Contents

CONTENTS

CONTENTS

ix

CONTENTS

xi

CONTENTS

SECTION V   PSYCHOVISCERAL AND BEHAVIOURAL ASPECTS OF GUT FUNCTION AND DYSFUNCTION

Preface

From June 2 to 4, 1988, an international symposium about "Nerves and the Gastrointestinal Tract" took place in Titisee. More than 200 scientists and clinicians of various specialities, e.g. neurophysiologists, clinicians and surgeons attended this interdisciplinary meeting. The goal of the symposium was to review our present knowledge relating to the nervous control of gastrointestinal function, especially the influence of the brain on gut function and to improve interdisciplinary communication and stimulate new research. This book presents the proceedings of this international meeting in which the current knowledge of neural control of gastrointestinal function is summarized by scientists whose range of expertise covers comprehensively the influences of the brain and the autonomic nervous system on the gut and the pancreas.

As editors we appreciate the time and effort of the individual authors. We are most grateful to all the contributors and discussants. Especially we would like to thank Dr. H. Falk who gave the necessary financial support and Barbara Beutling who was of great help in organizing the meeting and in preparing this book.

Manfred V. Singer, M.D.
Harald Goebell, M.D.

List of Contributors

K. O. Anderson
Division of Medical Psychology
Department of Psychiatry and Behavioral
  Medicine
Bowman Gray Medical School
Winston-Salem, NC 27104
USA

R. Arnold
Department of Internal Medicine
Philipps University
Baldingerstrasse
D-3550 Marburg
Federal Republic of Germany

J. S. Ball
Department of Biomedical Sciences
University of Sheffield
Sheffield
S10 2TN
UK

K. B????
Zentrum für Innere Medizin
Philipps University
Baldingerstrasse
D-3550 Marburg
Federal Republic of Germany

L. A. Blackshaw
Department of Biomedical Sciences
University of Sheffield
Western Bank
Sheffield S10 2TN
UK

J. C. Bornstein
Department of Human Physiology
Medical School
Flinders University
Bedford Park
South Australia 5042
Australia

L. A. Bradley
Division of Medical Psychology
Department of Psychiatry and Behavioral
  Medicine
Bowman Gray Medical School
Winston-Salem, NC 27104
USA

F. P. Brooks
Department of Medicine and Physiology
University of Pennsylvania School of
  Medicine
3400 Spruce Street
Philadelphia, PA 19104-4283
USA

L. Bueno
Department of Pharmacology
INRA
180 chemin de Tournefeuille
31300 Toulouse
France

T. F. Burks
Department of Pharmacology
University of Arizona
1501 North Campbell Avenue, 5103
Tucson, AZ 85724
USA

G. A. Castro
Department of Physiology and Cell
  Biology
University of Texas Medical School
PO Box 20708
Houston, TX 77225
USA

R. G. Clarke
Department of Surgery
Northern General Hospital
Sheffield
UK

H. J. Cooke
Department of Physiology
The Ohio State University
333 West Tenth Avenue
Columbus, OH 43210
USA

T. Craig
Department of Psychiatry
Rawnsley Building
Manchester Royal Infirmary
Oxford Road
Manchester M13 9WL
UK

F. Creed
Department of Psychiatry
Rawnsley Building
Manchester Royal Infirmary
Oxford Road
Manchester M13 9WL
UK

C. B. Dalton
Division of Gastroenterology
Department of Medicine
Bowman Gray Medical School
Winston-Salem, NC 27104
USA

N. E. Diamant
Department of Medicine
  (Gastroenterology)
Toronto Western Hospital
12–419 McLaughlin Pavilion
399 Bathurst Street
Toronto, Ontario M5T 2S8
Canada

E. P. Dimagno
Mayo Clinic and Foundation
Rochester
Minnesota 55905
USA

R. Dimaline
Department of Physiology
MRC Secretory Control Research Group
University of Liverpool
PO Box 147
Liverpool L69 3BX
UK

G. J. Dockray
Department of Physiology
MRC Secretory Control Research Group
University of Liverpool
PO Box 147
Liverpool L69 3BX
UK

D. A. Drossman
Division of Digestive Diseases
University of North Carolina
420 Burnett-Womack CB #7080
Chapel Hill, NC 27599-7080
USA

J. A. Duenes
Gastroenterology Research Unit
Mayo Clinic
200 First Street S.W.
Rochester, MN 55905
USA

E. Ekblad
Department of Medical Cell Research
University of Lund
Biskopsgatan 5
S-22362 Lund
Sweden

J. F. Erckenbrecht
Department of Internal Medicine
Division of Gastroenterology
Heinrich-Heine-Universität
Moorenstrasse 5
D-4000 Düsseldorf
Federal Republic of Germany

P. Euck
Department of Internal Medicine
Division of Gastroenterology
Heinrich-Heine-Universität
Moorenstrasse 5
D-4000 Düsseldorf
Federal Republic of Germany

W. R. Ewart
Gastrointestinal Science Research Unit
  and Department of Physiology
The London Hospital Medical College
26 Ashfield Street
London E1 2AJ
UK

R. Farmer
Department of Psychiatry
Rawnsley Building
Manchester Royal Infirmary
Oxford Road
Manchester M13 9WL
UK

H.-S. Feng
Department of Medicine and Physiology
University of Pennsylvania School of
  Medicine
A.N. Richards Building
Philadelphia, PA 19104-6085
USA

G. Flemström
Department of Physiology and Medical
  Biophysics
Uppsala University Biomedical Centre
PO Box 572
S-751 23 Uppsala
Sweden

D. A. Fox
ALZA Corporation
950 Page Mill Road
PO Box 10950
Palo Alto, CA 94303-0802
USA

J. B. Furness
Department of Anatomy and Histology
Medical School
Flinders University
Bedford Park
South Australia 5042
Australia

J. R. Garrett
Department of Oral Pathology
The Rayne Institute
King's College Medical and Dental
  School
123 Coldharbour Lane
London SE5 9NU
UK

M. D. Gershon
Department of Anatomy and Cell
  Biology
Columbia University
New York, NY 10032
USA

H. Goebell
Department of Internal Medicine
Division of Gastroenterology
University of Essen
Hufelandstrasse 55
D-4300 Essen 1
Federal Republic of Germany

T. Green
Department of Physiology
MRC Secretory Control Research Group
University of Liverpool
PO Box 147
Liverpool L69 3BX
UK

D. Grundy
Department of Biomedical Science
Alfred Denny Building
University of Sheffield
Western Bank
Sheffield, S10 2TN
UK

M. Gue
Department of Pharmacology
INRA
180 chemin de Tournefeuille
31300 Toulouse
France

N. S. Hakim
Department of Surgery
Guy's Hospital
St Thomas Street
London SE1 9RT
UK

R. Hendriks
Medical School
Flinders University
Bedford Park
South Australia 5042
Australia

G. E. Hermann
Physiology Dept – 4196 Graves Hall
College of Medicine
Ohio State Univ, 333 W. 10th Ave
Columbus, OH 43210
USA

B. I. Hirschowitz
Division of Gastroenterology
University of Alabama at Birmingham
School of Medicine
University Station
Birmingham, AL 35294
USA

C. Hoeren
Department of Internal Medicine
Division of Gastroenterology
Heinrich-Heine-Universität
Moorenstrasse 5
D-4000 Düsseldorf
Federal Republic of Germany

G. Holtman
Division of Gastroenterology
Department of Medicine
University of Essen
Hufelandstrasse 55
D-4300 Essen 1
Federal Republic of Germany

W. Janig
Physiologisches Institut
Christian-Albrechts-Universität
Oeshausenstrasse 40
D-2300 Kiel
Federal Republic of Germany

J. B. M. J. Jansen
Department of Gastroenterology
University Hospital, Building 1 C4-P
PO Box 9600
2300 RC Leiden
The Netherlands

G. Jedstedt
Department of Physiology and Medical
  Biophysics
Uppsala University Biomedical Centre
PO Box 572
S-751 23 Uppsala
Sweden

M. Kirschgessner
College of Physicians and Surgeons
Columbia University
630 West 168th Street
New York, NY 10032
USA

M. Koltzenburg
Physiologisches Institut
Christian-Albrechts-Universität
Oeshausenstrasse 40
D-2300 Kiel
Federal Republic of Germany

L. Knutson
Department of Surgery
Uppsala University Hospital
S-751 85 Uppsala
Sweden

R. Kriebel
Institute of Medical Psychology
University of Essen
Hufelandstrasse 55
D-4300 Essen 1
Federal Repubic of Germany

C. B. H. Lamers
Department of Gastroenterology
University Hospital, Building 1 C4-P
PO Box 9600
2300 RC Leiden
The Netherlands

P. Layer
Medizinische Klinik und Poliklinik
Abteilung Gastroenterologie
Hufelandstrasse 55
D-4300 Essen 1
Federal Republic of Germany

G. M. Lees
Department of Pharmacology
University of Aberdeen
Marischal College
Aberdeen AB9 1AS
UK

O. Lundgren
Department of Physiology
University of Göteborg
Box 33031
S-400 33 Göteborg
Sweden

R. B. Lynn
Department of Medicine
Hospital of the University of Pennsylvania
Dulles 3
3400 Spruce Street
Philadelphia, PA 19104-4283
USA

G. M. Mawe
Department of Anatomy and
  Neurobiology
The University of Vermont
Burlington
VT 05405
USA

S. M. McHugh
Departments of Psychiatry and Medicine
12–419 McLaughlin Pavilion
Toronto Western Hospital
399 Bathurst Street
Toronto
Ontario M5T 2S8
Canada

R. Murphy
Medical School
Flinders University
Bedford Park
South Australia 5042
Australia

W. Niebel
Division of Surgery
University of Essen
Hufelandstrasse 55
D-4300 Essen 1
Federal Republic of Germany

R. Norgren
Department of Behavioral Science
College of Medicine
The Pennsylvania State University
Hershey, PA 17033
USA

S. Pompolo
Departmento de Morfologia
Faculdade de Medicina de Ribeirão Preto
São Paulo
Brasil

F. Porreca
Department of Pharmacology
University of Arizona
1501 North Campbell Avenue, 5111
Tucson, Arizona 85724
USA

J. E. Richter
Division of Gastroenterology
Department of Medicine
Bowman Grey Medical School
Winston-Salem, NC 27104
USA

L. Rudge
Department of Biomedical Sciences
University of Sheffield
Alfred Denny Building
Sheffield S10 2TN
UK

M. G. Sarr
Department of Surgery
Mayo Medical School
200 First Street S.W.
Rochester, MN 55905
USA

M. Schemann
Institut fur Zoophysiologie
Universität Hohenheim
Garbenstrasse 30
D-7000 Stuttgart 70
Federal Republic of Germany

G. Schuster
Department of Internal Medicine
Philipps University
Baldingerstrasse
D-3550 Marburg
Federal Republic of Germany

T. Scratcherd
Department of Physiological Sciences
University of Newcastle upon Tyne
The Medical School
Framlington Place
Newcastle upon Tyne NE2 4HH
UK

J. E. Shook
Duke University Medical Center
PO Box 3094
Durham, NC 27710
USA

M. V. Singer
Medizinische Klinik und Poliklinik
Abteilung für Gastroenterologie
Hufelandstrasse 55
D-4300 Essen 1
Federal Republic of Germany

G. Skoda
Department of Internal Medicine
Division of Gastroenterology
Heinrich-Heine-Universität
Moorenstrasse 5
D-4000 Düsseldorf
Federal Republic of Germany

T. K. Smith
Medical School
Flinders University
Bedford Park
South Australia 5042
Australia

M. P. Spencer
Department of Surgery
Mayo Medical School
200 First Street S.W.
Rochester, MN 55905
USA

W. Stach
Institut für Anatomie der
  Wilhelm-Pieck-Universität
Gertrudenstrasse 9
DDR-2500 Rostock
German Democratic Republic

A. Surprenant
Vollum Institute
Oregon Health Sciences University
3181 S.W. Sam Jackson Park Road
Portland, OR 97201
USA

J. H. Szurszewski
Department of Physiology & Biophysics
Mayo Clinic and Foundation
200 First Street S.W.
Rochester, MN 55905
USA

Y. Tache
VA Wadsworth Medical Center
Centre for Ulcer Research and Education
Building 115, Room 203
Los Angeles, CA 90073
USA

W. G. Thompson
Division of Gastroenterology
Ottawa Civic Hospital
1053 Carling Avenue
Ottawa, Ontario K1Y 4E9
Canada

D. C. Trussell
Medical School
Flinders University
Bedford Park
South Australia 5042
Australia

J. A. Van Lier Ribbink
Department of Surgery
Mayo Medical School
200 First Street S.W.
Rochester, MN 55905
USA

A. Varro
Department of Physiology
MRC Secretory Control Research Group
University of Liverpool
PO Box 147
Liverpool L69 3BX
UK

J. H. Walsh
Director, CURE, UCLA
VA Wadsworth Medical Center
Bldg 115, Rm 115
Los Angeles CA 90073
USA

W. E. Whitehead
Division of Digestive Diseases
Francis Scott Key Medical Center
4940 Eastern Avenue
Baltimore, MD 21224
USA

C. L. Williams
Laboratory for Neuroendocrinology
University of Texas Medical School
6431 Fannin Street, Room 7128 MSMB
Houston, TX 77030
USA

D. L. Wingate
Gastrointestinal Science Research Unit
The London Hospital Medical College
26 Ashfield Street
London E1 2AJ
UK

J. D. Wood
Department of Physiology
The Ohio State University
4084 Graves Hall
333 West 10th Avenue
Columbus, OH 43210-1239
USA

A. R. Zinsmeister
Department of Health Sciences Research
Mayo Clinic
200 First Street S.W.
Rochester, MN 55905
USA

Section I
The enteric nervous system: circuits and development

1
Neuronal circuits in the enteric nervous system

J. B. FURNESS, J. C. BORNSTEIN, T. K. SMITH, R. MURPHY and S. POMPOLO

INTRODUCTION

From the first studies in the 1860s by Auerbach[1] there have been many attempts to trace the connections made within the enteric nervous system. Auerbach was able, for example, to trace nerve fibres between myenteric ganglia and from myenteric ganglia to the circular muscle. Other early studies of projections of enteric neurons include the work of Drasch[2] and Muller[3], who traced fibres from the submucosa to the mucosa, and of Dogiel[4] who followed the processes of some myenteric neurons (Dogiel type I cells). Other physiological studies from last century also had implications for pathways: Lister[5] and Lüderitz[6] considered that the enteric nerve plexuses must contain the neuronal circuits for the control of peristalsis; Pye-Smith et al.[7] deduced that neurons controlling secretion probably have their cell bodies in the submucous ganglia. None the less, it can be fairly said that deductions made about enteric neural circuitry rested on very uncertain grounds indeed until the end of the 1970s. Microscopic studies in particular were fraught with almost insurmountable problems of following barely resolvable neuronal processes through a maze of similar structures in the neuropil.

Application of modern histochemical techniques, particularly immuno-histochemistry, and the discovery of distinguishing chemical features (notably neuropeptides) in subsets of enteric neurons has dramatically improved our knowledge of microscopical anatomy of the enteric nervous system in the last decade (see for review references 8, 9, 10). In the guinea-pig small intestine, the projections of neurons revealed by the presence of some 12 different compounds have been determined (for the compounds mapped up to 1987, see references 9 and this volume Chapter 3; for two later compounds, galanin and the calcium-binding protein, calbindin D 28K, see 11 and 12).

A further stage in the histochemical analysis of enteric circuitry was reached when it was discovered that the same enteric neuron commonly contains several marker substances, for example several neuropeptides or neuropeptides plus an amine[13,14]. Recent studies in which the co-localization of substances in enteric neurons has been correlated with neuronal projections provide a much more complete account of neuronal projections. For example, projections have now been determined for all the nerve cell bodies in submucous ganglia of the guinea-pig small intestine[15].

While physiological studies had provided some general ideas about the circuits that would be predicted for control of movement and, to a lesser extent, secretion, these studies had not been done at a sufficiently detailed level to correlate with recent structural studies. For this reason, experiments using recording via intracellular microelectrodes have been undertaken in recent years to determine accurately the projections of motor neurons to the muscle[16,17] and the types of input to chemically defined neurons have been assessed, again using intracellular microelectrodes[18-23]. The chemistry of the neurons from which recordings were made in these experiments was determined by injecting them with the fluorescent dye, Lucifer yellow, so that they could be relocated, and then processing the tissue for the immunohistochemical demonstration of neuropeptides or other histochemically detectable marker substances.

A simplified partial circuitry for the enteric nervous system in the guinea-pig small intestine is presented in Figure 1.

REPETITIVE NATURE AND OVERLAP OF ENTERIC CIRCUITS

Anatomical studies show that enteric ganglia are embedded in a network of nerve strands that is continuous along and around the intestine. The ganglia are separated by quite small intervals, generally less than 0.5 mm in the guinea-pig small intestine. This arrangement is consistent with physiological observations that motility and secretion reflexes can be elicited by stimulation of sensory receptors at any point along the intestine and that the necessary area for stimulation to give a response can be restricted to only a few millimetres of intestine. Conversely, both the muscle and mucosa at all points along the intestine are innervated by enteric motor neurons. Furthermore, responses at any point in the muscle can be evoked by stimulation of sensory receptors at sites separated by varying distances from the point of recording. Thus it can be deduced that the enteric nervous system contains a series of repeating and overlapping neural circuits. For this reason, the relative uniformity of appearance of enteric ganglia, when studied for the presence of any one of a variety of neuronal markers, is to be expected. It can be anticipated that in a single ganglion of moderate size there will be the cell bodies of sensory neurons, interneurons and final motor neurons. Furthermore, circuits concerned with motility, secretion and blood flow are intertwined at all points along the intestine.

CIRCUITS OF SECRETOMOTOR REFLEXES

Most work on enteric secretomotor reflexes is relatively recent and has involved studies *in vivo*, primarily in cats and rats (see Lundgren, this volume,

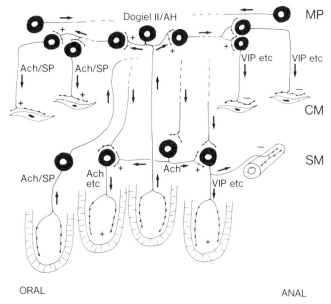

Figure 1 In this simplified schematic diagram of the guinea-pig small intestine, some of the known correlations of enteric circuitry from structural, neurochemical, physiological and pharmacological studies have been depicted. It has been deduced that motor neurons for motility are in the myenteric plexus (MP) and are of two types: excitatory neurons in which acetylcholine (ACh) and substance P (SP) are co-transmitters and inhibitory neurons utilizing VIP and probably another substance or substances as transmitters. Secretomotor neurons are in ganglia of the submucosa (SM). The non-cholinergic, VIP-containing, secretomotor neurons send collaterals to arterioles which they dilate. Two groups of sensory neurons have been tentatively identified: multipolar ACh/SP neurons in the submucous ganglia and Dogiel type II/AH neurons in the myenteric ganglia. Integrating centres for enteric reflexes appear to be primarily located in the myenteric plexus. These centres receive influences from further afield, both orally and anally in the intestine, and from sympathetic ganglia

Chapter 23), studies of secretomotor effects in isolated preparations of mucosa and submucosa in flux chambers in several species (Cooke, this volume, Chapter 22) and analysis of relevant neural pathways in guinea-pigs using intracellular microelectrodes and immunohistochemical techniques[15]. There is a good concordance between these different approaches. They all point to there being cholinergic and non-cholinergic secretomotor neurons in the gut wall and studies with isolated tissues indicate that the cell bodies of these neurons are in submucous ganglia. Secretomotor reflexes can be activated by a variety of intraluminal stimuli and result in the secretion of chloride, accompanied by cations, mainly sodium, and water into the lumen. Sympathetic, noradrenergic neurons inhibit the effectiveness of the reflexes primarily by acting on the final secretomotor neurons. The sympathetic neurons can be regarded as setting the gain of the reflex, i.e. in determining how effective a given luminal stimulus will be in causing water and electrolyte secretion. The activity in the sympathetic noradrenergic neurons is controlled in turn by baroreceptors and volume receptors (Lundgren, this volume, Chapter 23). Thus the secretomotor reflexes act when nutrients are being digested, and water and electrolytes are being absorbed along with these nutrients, in order to return water and electrolytes to the lumen. Secretomotor reflexes are modified by monitors of whole body water and electrolyte status so that the gain of the reflex is set appropriately.

In the guinea-pig small intestine, four histochemically distinct populations of submucous neurons have been identified; their projections have been determined; their inputs have been analysed electrophysiologically and their functions deduced[15]. There appear to be two groups of secretomotor neurons: cholinergic secretomotor neurons (about 30% of neurons) that also contain immunoreactivity for cholecystokinin, calcitonin gene-related peptide, galanin (in most cases) neuropeptide Y, and somatostatin; and non-cholinergic secretomotor neurons (about 45% of neurons) containing dynorphin, galanin and vasoactive intestinal peptide (VIP) immunoreactivity[11]. The combinations of peptides in secretomotor neurons of other species are likely to be different, but VIP appears to be a non-cholinergic secretomotor transmitter in many mammals[16]. There is also a group of neurons (about 10%) that we deduce to be sensory and to transmit information from the mucosa to the myenteric plexus; these are immunoreactive for substance P and choline acetyltransferase. The final type of submucous neuron is cholinergic, represents about 15% of the population and, from electrophysiological and lesion studies, appears to be an interneuron within the submucosa[15,20].

The secretomotor neurons do not project very far along the intestine; they generally supply the mucosa no more than one millimetre away[19,24]. We therefore propose that they might be involved in quite local reflexes, as well as being influenced from further along the intestine. It is probable that integrating centres for the secretomotor reflexes are in the myenteric plexus as the mucosal sensory neurons appear to project to the myenteric plexus and the other submucous neurons receive substantial inputs from this plexus[15].

CIRCUITS OF MOTILITY REFLEXES

Our analysis of the muscle motor reflexes over the last few years has concentrated on identifying the final motor neurons to the muscle and identifying the primary sensory neurons. There has been relatively little progress in elucidating internal connections of the reflex pathways, other than the physiological and pharmacological proof of the existence of such internal connections and the realization that they involve both cholinergic and non-cholinergic excitatory neuro-neuronal transmission.

The motor neurons to the circular muscle have been identified by a combination of structural, chemical, pharmacological and physiological approaches in the small intestine of the guinea-pig. First, by ultrastructural analysis of the consequences of myectomy operations, it has been shown that the nerve fibres in the circular muscle originate from the myenteric ganglia[28]. In the myenteric ganglia, the nerve cells fall into two electrophysio-

6

logically defined classes (Lees *et al.*, this volume, Chapter 7): after-hyperpolar-izing (AH) neurons and neurons receiving prominent cholinergic synaptic inputs (S neurons). Physiological and pharmacological studies indicate that the motor neurons are S neurons[10]. Furthermore, the AH neurons have a distinctive shape: they are Dogiel type II neurons and there is good evidence that neurons of this shape do not project to the muscle but have projections to the mucosa and to other myenteric neurons (Pompolo *et al.*[3], this volume, Chapter 5). Nerve fibres in the circular muscle show immunoreactivity for a number of neuropeptides, including substance P, VIP, enkephalin, neuropep-tide Y, dynorphin, galanin and gastrin releasing peptide[9]. By using single antisera and mixtures of antisera to enkephalin, substance P and VIP, and analysis of the numbers of immunoreactive fibres at the electron microscope level, we have shown that 95% of nerve fibres in the circular muscle contain VIP or substance P but none contains both peptides[26]. There are about equal numbers of VIP and of substance P containing fibres and about 70% of fibres in each group are immunoreactive for enkephalin. Transmission from excitatory nerve fibres to the muscle has three components: one component is blocked by antagonists of receptors for acetylcholine; one by antagonists of receptors for substance P; and one has not yet been found susceptible to pharmacological blockade by antagonists of receptors for possible enteric neurotransmitters[27]. Our interpretation is that acetylcholine and substance P are co-transmitters from excitatory motor neurons to the muscle and that there may be other active substances (in addition to enkephalin which has little direct action on the muscle) in these motor neurons. VIP is almost everywhere inhibitory to intestinal muscle and there is convincing evidence that it is contained in enteric inhibitory neurons and participates in transmission from these neurons to the muscle[28-30]. The projections of neurons with immunoreactivity for VIP are consistent with this interpretation[31,32].

Electrophysiological analysis of the pathways of enteric inhibitory motor neurons shows that they can be divided into two groups[16]. The majority of the neurons project from myenteric ganglia to the circular muscle that lies underneath or within about 1.0 to 1.5 mm or less in the longitudinal direction. The fibres run for 10 mm or more around the circumference of the intestine. A smaller group of inhibitory motor neurons consists of myenteric nerve cells that send fibres for up to 30 mm anally along the intestine to supply the circular muscle.

A similar analysis of the sources of the excitatory inputs to the circular muscle indicates that the projections of most excitatory fibres along the gut are short, from the myenteric ganglia to the underlying circular muscle, but that there are some longer, orally directed fibres extending for up to about 10 mm from their cell bodies of origin[17]. Like the inhibitory neurons, the excitatory neurons extend around the intestine for about half its circumfer-ence. If we add to this the circumferential projections of the neurons that activate the final motor neurons, it can be seen that there is a basis for the observation that contractions or relaxations of the circular muscle generally involve the full circumference of the intestine. Motor neurons that supply the muscle have a number of inputs: they can be activated by distension, through stimuli applied to receptive endings in the mucosa or through the circuits that direct the migrating myoelectric complex. There is circumstantial evidence that Dogiel type II/AH neurons with cell bodies in myenteric ganglia are sensory (Pompolo *et al.*, this volume, Chapter 5). It seems likely that some Dogiel type II/AH neurons are involved in local motility controlling reflexes, although there could also be cell bodies of sensory neurons in submucous ganglia that participate in motility reflexes. The circuitry that lies between primary sensory neurons and motor neurons to the muscle is not known.

CONCLUDING REMARKS

Considerable progress has been made in recent years in correlating the structural, pharmacological and electrophysiological characteristics of neural circuits in the small intestine of the guinea-pig. In general, the circuits that have been deduced fit with physiological studies made in this and other species. In the case of secretomotor reflex pathways, it has been possible to draw partial circuits that incorporate structural analysis from the guinea-pig with physiological and pharmacological analysis *in vitro* and *in vivo* from other species[15]. A conclusion from this work is that there are both cholinergic and non-cholinergic secretomotor neurons with their cell bodies in submucous ganglia and that integrating centres for secretomotor reflexes are in the myenteric ganglia.

On the other hand, the cell bodies of motor neurons to the muscle are in the myenteric ganglia. These neurons are of the S type electrophysiologically and presumed to have Dogiel type I morphology. It has been deduced, but not proven by direct physiological methods, that Dogiel type II/AH neurons with their cell bodies in the myenteric plexus are sensory neurons. It is presumed that some of these neurons are the primary sensory neurons for muscle motor reflexes. While more progress has been made in the last decade than in over a century since the discovery of the enteric plexuses, there are still a number of important questions to be answered, particularly about the circuits through which sensory information is processed and transmitted to the enteric motor neurons.

References

1. Auerbach, L. (1864). Fernere vorläufige Mitteilung über den Nervenapparat des Darmes. *Arch. Pathol. Anat. Physiol.*, **30**, 457–60
2. Drasch, O. (1881). Beiträge zur Kenntnis des feineran Baues des Dünndarmes, insbesondere über die Nerven desselben. *Sitzber Akad. Wiss. Wien*, **82**, 3rd div., 168–98
3. Muller, L.R. (1911). Die Darminnervation. *Dtches. Arch. Klin. Med.*, **105**, 1–43
4. Dogiel, A.S. (1899). Über den Bau der Ganglien in den Geflechten des Darmes und der Gallenblase des Menschen und der Säugetiere. *Arch. Anat. Physiol. Leipzig. Anat. Abt.*, (Jg. 1899): 130–58
5. Lister, J. (1858). Preliminary account of an inquiry into the functions of the visceral nerves, with special reference to the so-called 'inhibitory system'. *Proc. R. Soc. Lond.*, **9**, 367–80
6. Lüderitz, C. (1889). Experimentelle Untersuchungen über die Entstehung der Darmperistal-

tik. *Virchows Arch. Pathol. Anat.*, **118**, 19–36

7. Pye-Smith, P.H., Brunton, T.L. and West, W.H. (1874). Report of the committee appointed for the purpose of investigating the nature of intestinal secretion. In *British Association for the Advancement of Science* (44th Meeting), pp. 54–71. (London: John Murray)

8. Costa, M., Furness, J.B. and Llewellyn-Smith, I.J. (1987). Histochemistry of the enteric nervous system. In Johnson, L.R. (ed.) *Physiology of the Gastrointestinal Tract*, pp. 1–40. (New York: Raven Press)

9. Furness, J.B. and Costa, M. (1987). *The Enteric Nervous System*, xiii + 290 pp. (London and Edinburgh: Churchill Livingstone)

10. Furness, J.B., Llewellyn-Smith, I.J., Bornstein, J.C. and Costa, M. (1988). Neuronal circuitry in the enteric nervous system. *Handbook of Chemical Neuroanatomy.* **6**, 161–218

11. Furness, J.B., Costa, M., Rokaeus, A., McDonald, T.J. and Brooks, B. (1987). Galanin-immunoreactive neurons in the guinea-pig small intestine: their projections and relationships to other enteric neurons. *Cell Tiss. Res.*, **250**, 607–15

12. Furness, J.B., Keast, J.R., Pompolo, S., Bornstein, J.C., Costa, M., Emson, P.C. and Lawson, D.E.M. (1988). Immunohistochemical evidence for the presence of calcium binding proteins in enteric neurons. *Cell Tiss. Res.*, **252**, 79–87

13. Furness, J.B., Costa, M. and Keast, J.R. (1984). Cholineacetyltransferase and peptide immunoreactivity of submucous neurons of the guinea-pig small intestine. *Cell Tiss. Res.*, **237**, 329–36

14. Costa, M., Furness, J.B. and Gibbins, I.L. (1986). Chemical coding of enteric neurons. *Progress in Brain Res.*, **68**, 217–39

15. Bornstein, J.C. and Furness, J.B. (1988). Correlated electrophysiological and histochemical studies of submucous neurons and their contribution to understanding enteric neural circuits. *J. Autonom. Nerv. System.* **25**, 1–13

16. Bornstein, J.C., Costa, M., Furness, J.B. and Lang, R.J. (1986). Electrophysiological analysis of projections of enteric inhibitory motor neurons in the guinea-pig small intestine. *J. Physiol.*, **370**, 61–74

17. Smith, T.K., Furness, J.B., Costa, M. and Bornstein, J.C. (1988). An electrophysiological study of the projections of motor neurons that mediate non-cholinergic excitation in the circular muscle of the guinea-pig small intestine. *J. Autonom. Nerv. Syst.*, **22**, 115–28

18. Bornstein, J.C., Costa, M., Furness, J.B. and Lees, G.M. (1984). Electrophysiology and enkephalin immunoreactivity of identified myenteric plexus neurones of guinea-pig small intestine. *J. Physiol.*, **351**, 313–25

19. Bornstein, J.C., Costa, M. and Furness, J.B. (1986). Synaptic inputs to immunohistochemically identified neurones in the submucous plexus of the guinea-pig small intestine. *J. Physiol.*, **381**, 465–82

20. Bornstein, J.C., Furness, J.B. and Costa, M. (1987). Sources of excitatory synaptic inputs to neurochemically identified submucous neurons of guinea-pig small intestine. *J. Autonom. Nerv. Syst.*, **18**, 83–91

21. Bornstein, J.C., Costa, M. and Furness, J.B. (1988). Intrinsic and extrinsic inhibitory synaptic inputs to submucous neurons of the guinea-pig small intestine. *J. Physiol.*, **398**, 371–90

22. Katayama, Y., Lees, G.M. and Pearson, G.T. (1986). Electrophysiology and morphology of the guinea-pig ileum. *J. Physiol.*, **378**, 1–11

23. Iyer, V., Bornstein, J.C., Costa, M., Furness, J.B., Takahashi, Y. and Iwanaga, T. (1988). Electrophysiology of guinea-pig myenteric neurons correlated with immunoreactivity for calcium-binding proteins. *J. Autonom. Nerv. Syst.*, **22**, 141–50

24. Furness, J.B., Costa, M., Gibbins, I.L., Llewellyn-Smith, I.J. and Oliver, J.R. (1985). Neurochemically similar myenteric and submucous neurons directly traced to the mucosa of the small intestine. *Cell Tiss. Res.*, **241**, 155–63

25. Wilson, A.J., Llewellyn-Smith, I.J., Furness, J.B. and Costa, M. (1987). The source of the nerve fibres forming the deep muscular and circular muscle plexuses in the small intestine of the guinea-pig. *Cell Tiss. Res.*, **247**, 497–504

26. Llewellyn-Smith, I.J., Furness, J.B., Gibbins, I.L. and Costa, M. (1988). Quantitative ultrastructural analysis of enkephalin-, substance P-, and VIP-immunoreactive nerve fibers in the circular muscle of the guinea-pig small intestine. *J. Comp. Neurol.*, **272**, 139–48

27. Bywater, R.A.R. and Taylor, G.S. (1986). Non-cholinergic excitatory and inhibitory junction potentials in the circular smooth muscle of the guinea-pig ileum. *J. Physiol.*, **374**, 153–64

28. Grider, J.R. and Makhlouf, G.M. (1986). Colonic peristaltic reflex: identification of vasoactive intestinal peptide as mediator of descending relaxation. *Am. J. Physiol.*, **251**, 440–5

29. Sjöqvist, A. and Fahrenkrug, J. (1987). Release of vasoactive intestinal polypeptide anally of a local distension of the feline small intestine. *A. Physiol. Scand.*, **130**, 433–8

30. Furness, J.B. and Costa, M. (1988). Identification of transmitters of functionally defined enteric neurons. In Wood, J.D. (ed.) *Handbook of Physiol.: The Gastrointestinal System.* (Washington: American Physiological Society) (In press)

31. Furness, J.B. and Costa, M. (1979). Projections of intestinal neurons showing immunoreactivity for vasoactive intestinal polypeptide are consistent with these neurons being the enteric inhibitory neurons. *Neuroscience Letts.*, **15**, 199–204

32. Costa, M. and Furness, J.B. (1983). The origins, pathways and terminations of neurons with VIP-like immunoreactivity in the guinea-pig small intestine. *Neuroscience*, **8**, 665–76

2
Colonization of the bowel and development of the enteric nervous system by precursors from the neural crest

M.D. GERSHON

THE ENTERIC NERVOUS SYSTEM IS A SEPARATE AND DISTINCT REGION OF THE PNS

The intrinsic innervation of the gut (the enteric nervous system: ENS) is quite different from that of other peripheral organs. Bayliss and Starling[1,2] were the first to realize that the bowel is able to manifest reflex activity in the absence of input from the brain or spinal cord. They showed that extrinsically denervated loops of canine intestine responded to distension with a descending propulsive wave of oral contraction and anal relaxation that they called the 'law of the intestine' (peristaltic reflex). Bayliss and Starling attributed this response to the 'local nervous mechanism' of the bowel. Trendelenburg[3] later obtained a similar pattern of motility from isolated guinea-pig intestine *in vitro*. Since isolated preparations of gut, naturally, have no intact connections with the CNS, Trendelenburg's experiments showed that the gut must contain all the neurons, including intrinsic primary afferents, that are essential for the peristaltic reflex. The ENS is thus a self-contained nervous system and is not simply made up of parasympathetic relay ganglia. In his classification of the autonomic nervous system (ANS), Langley[4] listed three autonomic divisions: the sympathetic, the parasympathetic, and the enteric. Because the number of neurons in the ENS is very large[5,6,7] in proportion to the number of efferent fibres in the vagus nerves[8], Langley[4] believed that most of the neurons of the enteric plexuses are not directly innervated by the CNS. Since he defined the sympathetic and parasympathetic divisions of the ANS by the location of the preganglionic outflows from the CNS, the ENS, for which these connections are minor, cannot be fitted into either division. Langley therefore considered the ENS a separate part of the ANS that receives input from the others. This input to the ENS is, of course, vital. Although the peristaltic reflex can be elicited in the absence of signals from the CNS, the bowel does not normally function without such signals[9]. The gut does receive both a sympathetic and a parasympathetic innervation[6,10]. Primary afferent neurons located in vagal and dorsal root ganglia send peripheral processes to the bowel and central axons to the CNS[11]. Thus, centrally mediated reflexes, as well as locally mediated reflexes, are important in normal gastrointestinal function. Nevertheless, it is possible for animals to survive if the extrinsic innervation of the intestine is cut, but not if intrinsic neurons are congenitally lacking or are destroyed. For example, both in Hirschsprung's disease[12], in which there is a congenital aganglionosis, and in Chagas disease[13], in which enteric neurons are lost secondary to a protozoan infection, the aganglionic tissue functions as an obstruction to the propulsion of material down the gut. The normal motility of the bowel thus involves an interaction between extrinsic and intrinsic neural elements. Basic motor patterns may be dependent on the activity of intrinsic neurons, but be subject to modification by signals from the CNS acting on command neurons controlling intrinsic enteric circuits[14] (See also Kirchgessner and Gershon, this volume, Chapter 6).

The ENS differs not only in its relative autonomy from the remainder of the PNS, but also chemically and structurally[6,7,15,16] (see also Furness et al., this volume, Chapter 1). In fact, the structure of the ENS is more similar to that of the brain than to other regions of the PNS. For example, the degree of phenotypic diversity exhibited by enteric neurons is unequalled elsewhere in the PNS. Most of the same classes of neurotransmitter, if not all of the individual transmitters, that are present in the CNS are also present in the ENS, including acetylcholine (ACh), biogenic amines, amino acids, neuropeptides, and perhaps ATP[17]. Since neuroactive peptides coexist in single neurons in multiple combinations with each other and with small molecule neurotransmitters[6], it is not yet even certain how many chemically different types of neuron there are in the ENS. In addition to the many classes of enteric neuron that can be defined chemically, still more classes can be discerned when neurons are also classified morphologically (see Stach, this volume, Chapter 3).

Clearly, no matter how enteric neurons are classified, there are many kinds. As is also true of the CNS, the collagenous coats that characterize peripheral nerve outside the gut are missing from the ENS[16,18]. Instead of by an endoneurium, the enteric neural elements are supported by enteric glia that resemble the astrocytes of the CNS[19,20] and contain large amounts of glial fibrillary acidic protein (GFAP)[21-24]. Enteric glia extend many processes that give the cells an astrocytic shape[25], and which do not individually wrap around neurites (with one mesaxon per neurite) as do Schwann cells, but instead form partitions between groups of neural processes, so that enteric neurites abut on one another. Moreover, enteric glia also differ from Schwan cells in that they are not surrounded by a basal lamina[16,18,20].

THE ENTERIC NERVOUS SYSTEM IS DERIVED FROM THE NEURAL CREST

All of the neurons and glia of the ENS are the progeny of immigrants. They are derived from precursors that migrate to the bowel from elsewhere in the embryo. The region of origin of these precursors was originally determined by Yntema and Hammond[26,27] who ablated parts of the neural crest in developing chick embryos. Ablation of the rhombencephalic, or 'vagal', crest led to aganglionosis of the bowel in the operated embryos. These observations have been confirmed and extended more recently through the use of chick–quail interspecies chimeras[28]. Quail cells are stably marked by a recognizable pattern of nucleolar-associated heterochromatin that allows them to be distinguished from chick cells in preparations in which DNA is specifically demonstrated[29]. Thus, when chick crest is replaced by that of a quail before migration has begun in the host embryos, the donor quail cells migrate in the resulting chimeras and colonize appropriate organs. The quail nuclear marker then permits the identification of the crest-derived cells in their final sites of residence. Using this technique, Le Douarin and her colleagues have established that the ENS is derived from cells that leave two levels of the neuraxis. Emigrés from the vagal crest (axial levels of somites 1–7) colonize the entire bowel, while émigrés from the sacral crest (caudal to the 28th somite) join those from the vagal crest in colonizing the post-umbilical gut[28,30]. Loring et al.[31], have recently reported that neuraxial cells that give rise to serotonergic neurons migrate away from the ventral rather than the dorsal aspect of neural tube explants in vitro. Since serotonergic neurons are normal constituents of the ENS[6,32–35] these observations have formed the basis for suggesting the possibility that some of the neuraxial precursor cells that colonize the bowel may be derived from the ventral neural tube, as well as from the crest. This possibility has not been confirmed, but neither has it been ruled out. Quail–chick grafts can be expected to transfer at least some neural tube, as well as crest-derived cells to the host embryos, and it is difficult to be certain that ablations of crest leave the neural tube entirely intact. Nevertheless, it is clear that the ENS is formed by particular regions of the neuraxis if not only neural crest. Questions must now be asked about how the formation of such a large and complex nervous system in a distant organ is brought about.

The observation that crest cells migrate to the alimentary tract only from two axial levels raises the question of whether crest cells that enter the bowel have been programmed to do so while still in the premigratory neural crest, or whether they follow defined pathways that lead to the gut from the vagal and sacral regions of the neuraxis. The phenotypic diversity of enteric neurons and the unique structure of the ENS raise the additional question as to whether the fates of crest-derived émigrés are predetermined or are influenced by the microenvironments these cells encounter as they migrate, or as they develop in the wall of the gut. The precise and reproducible location of enteric ganglia within the bowel brings up the question as to what causes émigrés from the crest to stop migrating in correct locations. Finally, the presence in the ENS of a unique type of glial cell, not found elsewhere in the PNS, raises the question of whether the crest-derived precursors of the enteric glia migrate to the bowel together with the cohort of neural precursors, or whether the glial precursors enter the gut along with the fibres and Schwann cells of the extrinsic innervation.

CREST-DERIVED CELLS MIGRATE TO THE GUT ALONG DEFINED PATHWAYS

Premigratory crest cells are probably not programmed to 'find' the gut[28,36]. In experiments in which donor crest from inappropriate axial levels of quail embryos is grafted to the 'vagal' region of chick embryonic hosts the gut of the chimeras becomes colonized by the quail crest cells[28,37,38]. Thus, the enteric destination of migrating crest cells appears to be determined not by the level of the neuraxis at which they are generated, but by the level from which these cells depart. Guidance, therefore, would appear to be a function of the migratory pathway and not an inherent property of crest-derived cells[39-43]. Moreover, at least some crest-derived cells that have migrated to the gut remain plastic and can migrate again. When segments of foregut that have been colonized by cells from the neural crest are transplanted back into younger host embryos, crest-derived cells leave the grafts and colonize various tissues of the hosts[44]. These colonists can be identified if chimeric back-grafts are studied. The destinations reached by the crest-derived cells leaving the back-transplanted enteric grafts are determined by the site in the host embryo in which the graft is situated. Back-transplants of foregut placed between somites and neural tube in the trunk region donate cells that reach dorsal root and sympathetic ganglia, as well as the adrenal medulla; however, they never enter the bowel of the host embryo. In order for cells of the back-grafts to reach the host's gut, the donor foregut must be grafted to the vagal region of the host. Furthermore, the grafts, even at vagal levels, cannot be placed next to the neural tube but must be inserted into the dorsal tube itself, replacing the host's own crest. These observations indicate that crest-derived cells are not endowed with homing information even by prior migration to the gut, nor are cells that have once successfully migrated to the bowel any more capable of finding the gut a second time than are cells that have never made the journey. Instead, crest-derived cells leaving grafted segments of gut appear to follow the same defined pathways of crest migration that naive crest-derived cells would normally follow; reaching targets appropriate for the trunk if the grafts are in the trunk and reaching the gut only if the grafts are placed so as to provide access to the vagal migratory pathway. The vagal pathway, moreover, seems to be accessible to migrating crest cells only where it begins, dorsal to the neural tube; crest-derived émigrés from grafts placed next to the vagal pathway appear to be unable to follow it to the host's bowel.

THE ENTERIC MICROENVIRONMENT INFLUENCES THE PHENOTYPIC EXPRESSION OF CREST-DERIVED CELLS IN THE GUT

Many different types of experiment suggest that the microenvironment established by the non-neuronal cells of the bowel has a major influence on the pattern of phenotypic expression displayed by crest-derived cells in the enteric wall. Grafts of quail crest cells removed from gut-inappropriate levels

14

of the neuraxis will not only colonize the bowel when placed in the vagal region of host-chick embryos, but give rise to a normal-appearing ENS as well. Thus, the ENS of chimeras constructed with trunk to vagal grafts contains cholinergic[28,45], peptidergic[45,50], and serotonergic neurons[38] all of which are normal constituents of the ENS[6]. However, catecholaminergic neurons, which are not normally found in the intestine[48] are not found in the chimeric intestine either[28,45]. On the other hand, catecholaminergic cells (in sympathetic ganglia and the adrenal medulla) are normally formed from truncal crest cells, while serotonergic neurons are not. Similar patterns of phenotypic expression can be obtained when truncal crest cells are directly inserted into explants of aneuronal bowel and grown as chorioallantoic membrane grafts[45]. The gut itself, therefore, appears to be of greater significance in determining which neurotransmitter is expressed by the crest-derived neurons of the ENS, than are the level of the neuraxis from which these émigrés originate, or the environments they encounter while they migrate to the bowel. The hypothesis that the enteric microenvironment plays a critical role in determining the ultimate phenotypes expressed by crest-derived cells in the gut wall is supported by observations that have been made on cells grown *in vitro*.

In the developing avian intestine, intrinsic neurons contain 5-HT[38] or GABA[49], but not tyrosine hydroxylase, a marker for catecholaminergic cells[6]. The ability of crest-derived cells, obtained from the crest itself, the vagal migratory pathway and from within the bowel, to express these phenotypes *in vitro* has been compared[50]. All three phenotypic markers appear in cultures of cranial, vagal or truncal neural crest when these cultures are grown in enriched medium. Crest-derived cells appear to migrate from the vagal neuraxis to the gut through the caudal branchial arches[51,52]. Unexpectedly, therefore, cells in cultures from the third and fourth branchial arches, which would include crest-derived cells migrating to the alimentary tract, express tyrosine hydroxylase, but not 5-HT or GABA[50]. Nevertheless, precursors with the potential ability to express a serotonergic phenotype must still be present in the branchial arches, because 5-HT-immunoreactive cells appear in the cultures when branchial arches are co-cultured with aneural hindgut. Co-cultured explants of bowel can thus 'rescue' the serotonergic phenotype. Tyrosine hydroxylase, as well as 5-HT and GABA immunoreactivities, are found in cultured cells obtained from chick gut dissociated at seven days of incubation; however, tyrosine hydroxylase immunoreactivity is no longer expressed by cells in cultures derived from the bowel dissociated at later ages. Branchial arch or cardiac explants appear to be able to prevent 5-HT expression in co-cultures with crest-derived cells; nevertheless, the further addition of explants of gut to these co-cultures can bring out the serotonergic phenotype. These observations suggest that precursors with the capacity to express 5-HT, GABA or tyrosine hydroxylase are found at several levels of the neuraxis. However, the expression of these phenotypes may be repressed by contact with other tissues, this repression may occur either while the crest-derived cells are migrating or in their final sites of residence. For example, the microenvironment of the branchial arches may prevent expression of 5-HT or GABA by crest cells migrating through them and the bowel may ultimately (after day eight of development) suppress expression of tyrosine hydroxylase. The repression of some types of phenotypic expression may be transient and reversible by the microenvironment that crest cells encounter when they finish migrating. Thus, the ability to express 5-HT and GABA, which is not displayed by crest-derived cells en route to the gut in the branchial arches, appears to recover when these cells reach the bowel and are exposed to the enteric microenvironment.

Further indications of the importance of the enteric microenvironment in the development of crest-derived cells in the wall of the gut have been obtained from studies of the mammalian bowel. Enteric neurons do not become morphologically recognizable in fetal mice until day E12 when they can be distinguished in the foregut and day E15 when they can be observed in the hindgut[53,54]; nevertheless, crest-derived neural and glial precursor cells are present in the developing alimentary tract much before neural properties are expressed[54-56]. These crest-derived cells can be detected because they give rise to progeny that express clear neural or glial markers. If the fetal bowel is explanted and neurons or glia eventually develop *in vitro*, it can be deduced that crest-derived precursors were present in the fetal gut at the time of its explantation. Cultures thus provide an indirect assay for the presence of crest-derived precursor cells. Through the use of this assay it has been found that these cells reach the fetal mouse gut on days E9–10 and that even the terminal bowel is colonized in fetal mice of more than 33 somites[57]. The development of the ENS from precursors *in vitro* can be exploited not only to study the timing of the colonization of the gut by émigrés from the neural crest, but also to analyse factors that influence colonization and neural development. When uncolonized segments of gut, either from mice or chicks, are co-cultured with various sources of crest-derived cells these cells migrate to the recipient bowel, populate it, and form neurons and glia[60]. This phenomenon will occur even when crest-derived cells and gut are from species as different as chick and mouse. Crest-derived cells can be obtained for these co-culture experiments from explants of chick, mouse or quail neural tube, or even from recently colonized chick or mouse foregut. Crest-derived cells leave such explants of bowel and colonize a recipient explant of gut placed nearby in the same culture dish.

Evidence supporting the hypothesis that phenotypic expression by the crest-derived precursors of enteric neurons and glia is critically influenced by the microenvironment these cells encounter within the gut has been obtained from experiments involving co-cultures of crest-derived cells from quail embryos with explants of developing mouse gut[58]. The effects of the enteric tissue on the expression of several markers of crest cell development were followed. These markers included melanogenesis as well as 5-HT, tyrosine hydroxylase, NC-1[59] and GlN1[60] immunoreactivities. The explants of murine gut were found significantly to enhance the expression of 5-HT and NC-1 immunoreactivities by the quail crest-derived cells and, especially near the gut, to cause increased numbers of 5-HT-, NC-1- and GlN1-immunoreactive cells to assume a neuronal morphology. In contrast, the expression of TH immunoreactivity by the quail cells is reduced rather than enhanced by the murine gut and melanogenesis is unchanged. Explants of murine metanephros do not have an effect similar to that of explants of bowel and actually inhibit expression of 5-HT immunoreactivity and the acquisition of a neuritic contour by NC-1-immunoreactive cells. The effect of enteric explants on crest cell development is thus specific to the bowel and is not a general action of the murine mesenchyme; these experiments therefore demonstrate that the enteric microenvironment affects the pheno-typic expression of subsets of crest-derived cells.

The influence of the enteric microenvironment on developing crest-derived cells could be instructive or selective. Uncommitted crest cells could be induced by factors or contact with enteric mesenchymal cells or the matrix they secrete to give rise to gut-specific neuronal phenotypes. Alternatively, appropriate subsets of pre-committed crest-derived cells could be selected by the enteric microenvironment and survive while inappropriate subsets die. Experiments dealing with populations of crest-derived cells cannot differentiate between these two possibilities. In order to do so it will be necessary to follow the development of clones of crest-derived cells in the enteric microenvironment, either by placing a single cell in the enteric mesenchyme or by stably labelling one cell of a population. This has not yet been done. Nevertheless, whether the influence of the enteric microenviron-ment is instructive or selective, it is clear that it plays a vital role in determining the fates of crest-derived cells in the gut.

THE EXTRACELLULAR MATRIX OF THE FETAL BOWEL MAY PROVIDE SIGNALS THAT CAUSE CREST-DERIVED NEURAL PRECURSORS TO CEASE MIGRATING AND EXTEND NEURITES

Enteric ganglia appear to be arranged in an orderly manner in both plexuses[61]. This order implies that crest-derived cells do not stop migrating at random intervals and come to reside wherever they happen to be located at the time. Instead, cessation of migration is more likely to be a response to stop signals. Experiments with the lethal spotted (ls/ls) mutant mouse[62-64] suggest that such stop signals may exist and be materials in the extracellular matrix.

As do human patients with Hirschsprung's disease, ls/ls mice have a congenital megacolon secondary to a segmental aganglionosis of the terminal bowel. Although the affected region contains no neuronal perikarya, the tissue is not denervated. It contains many nerves in the adventitia, between the longitudinal and circular muscle, and in the submucosa[65]. The length of colon in which submucosal ganglia are absent is longer than that which lacks myenteric ganglia[61]. Both myenteric and submucosal plexuses are hypoganglionic orad to the aganglionic zones. The ganglia are irregularly distributed in the hypoganglionic regions, but eventually assume a more regular pattern in the more proximal bowel. The ultrastructure of the nerves in the aganglionic portion of the gut of ls/ls mice is that of non-enteric peripheral nerve[61,65]. Axons are supported by Schwann cells that individually envelop neurites and are each surrounded by a basal lamina and an endoneurial sheath of connective tissue. Atypically for murine intestine, some of the axons in the aganglionic tissue are myelinated. The nerves in the adventitia of the aganglionic regions are connected to small ectopic located outside of the gut. These small ganglia also have the structure of non-enteric peripheral nerve. In the hypoganglionic region of the *ls/ls* colon some of the ectopic ganglia extend through the longidutinal muscle to fuse with ganglia of the myenteric plexus. This observation suggests that the ectopic ganglia may be derived from the same wave of crest-derived émigrés as that which colonizes the gut; however, some of these cells may form ectopic ganglia outside the bowel because they cannot enter the presumptive aganglionic terminal region. The extraenteric structure of the ectopic ganglia would then be an expected consequence of their not having been exposed to the enteric microenvironment during development.

In order to locate the perikarya of the neurons from which the nerves found in the terminal colon of *ls/ls* mice are derived, retrograde tracers, true Blue and wheat germ agglutinin coupled to horseradish peroxidase (WGA-HRP), were injected into the wall of the gut in this region[61]. Injections of the tracers into the terminal bowel of control mice labelled neurons in myenteric ganglia near the injection site, in ganglia oral to the injection site, and in ganglia outside the bowel. Labelled extrinsic neurons were found in hypogastric sympathetic ganglia, dorsal root ganglia (L_6–S_2) and the sacral parasympathetic nucleus (S_2). Similar injections in *ls/ls* mice failed to label any neurons (which are not present) near the injection site. However, neurons were labelled in the hypoganglionic bowel proximal to the aganglionic zone. In addition, all the extrinsic neurons found to be labelled by injections of tracer in control mice were also labelled in *ls/ls* mice, with the exception of the sacral parasympathetic nucleus. These observations indicate that the lesion in the aganglionic segment of the *ls/ls* gut does not interfere with the growth of extrinsic or even intrinsic nerve processes. These observations suggest that neural and glial precursors respond differently to the tissue in the presumptive aganglionic bowel than do the growing neurites of developing neurons.

NEURAL AND GLIAL PRECURSORS FAIL TO COLONIZE THE TERMINAL COLON OF *ls/ls* MICE

Although murine neural precursors cannot be recognized directly by demonstrating any currently known marker, their presence can be detected indirectly by using the explant-culture assay system discussed above[54]. When explants of proximal bowel from fetal *ls/ls* mouse foregut are cultured, neurons and glia develop *in vitro*[66]. In contrast, when similar explants of the terminal 2 mm of fetal *ls/ls* mouse hindgut are cultured, neurons and glia virtually never appear. These observations suggest that viable crest-derived neural and glial precursor cells may be unable to colonize the terminal *ls/ls* bowel. The length of gut from which aneuronal cultures are reproducibly obtained is constant; therefore, the presumptive aganglionic tissue can be identified, as the last 2 mm of *ls/ls* bowel, prior to the development of megacolon. It has been suggested that the terminal bowel of the *ls/ls* mouse does not

18

become colonized by crest-derived precursor cells because these cells migrate so slowly down the gut that they fail to reach the presumptive aganglionic region before it becomes non-receptive to colonizing cells[53]. However, removal of the entire bowel from fetal animals and allowing it to develop in culture, so that migrating crest-derived cells would have more time to reach the terminal zone before an unidentified developmental event intervenes and cuts off migration, fails to result in colonization of the presumptive aganglionic segment[57]. The terminal region remains conspicuously aneuronal. In fact, satellite ganglia can be identified in these cultures developing from neural precursors that evidently migrate out of the proximal colonized portion of the gut in a direction that takes them away from the aganglionic tissue. These observations suggest that crest-derived cells fail to enter the terminal portion of the *ls/ls* gut because they cannot, not because they do not reach it within a critical period of time *in vivo*.

Co-culture experiments were done to determine whether crest-derived cells from non-mutant sources can colonize the presumptive aganglionic region of the *ls/ls* bowel and also to ascertain whether crest-derived cells from *ls/ls* mice are able to colonize control segments of bowel[63]. Crest-derived cells migrating away from explants of chick, quail or mouse or neural tube[67] readily colonize recipient explants of control mouse, chick or quail gut *in vitro*[57]. Likewise, crest-derived cells, will also leave segments of foregut and migrate to, colonize and form ganglia in a recipient explant of aneuronal bowel *in vitro*. For example, the foregut from a fetal mouse will provide cells that form neurons in chick or quail hindgut and chick or quail foregut will provide precursors that give rise to neurons in an explant of aneuronal hindgut from a control mouse fetus. Aneuronal murine hindgut can, as noted earlier, be obtained from mouse fetuses that are 30–33 somites in length. Crest-derived cells migrating out of the foregut of *ls/ls* mice are as effective as their counterparts from control avian or murine foregut in producing neurons in recipient explants of chick or control mouse hindgut. In contrast, however, no source of crest-derived cells ever gives rise to neurons in the presumptive aganglionic bowel of *ls/ls* mice. These experiments clearly demonstrate that it is the presumptive aganglionic bowel of *ls/ls* mice that is abnormal, and not the crest-derived cells themselves or their rate of migration within the proximal portion of the gut. This tissue thus permits neurites to grow into it but appears to be inhospitable for the migration of neural precursors.

OVERABUNDANCE OF COMPONENTS OF BASAL LAMINAE IN THE PRESUMPTIVE AGANGLIONIC REGION OF THE GUT OF *ls/ls* MICE

An extraordinary overabundance and maldistribution of laminin and type IV collagen immunoreactivities has been revealed by immunocytochemically examining the distribution of these components of basal laminae in the developing intestines of control and *ls/ls* mice[68]. A parallel increase in alcian blue staining also occurs, suggesting that glycosaminoglycans also accumulate during development of the mutant bowel. These abnormalities of the extracellular matrix can be detected as early as day E11, a time prior to the earliest appearance of recognizable neurons in the terminal colon in control mice. In control mice, laminin and type IV collagen immunoreactivities are present in formed basal laminae beneath the mucosal and serosal epithelia of the hindgut, as well as around blood vessels in the enteric mesenchyme. Immunoreactivity of these components is also found in the extracellular space of the mesenchyme, suggesting that laminin and type IV collagen, which are not organized into distinct basal laminae, are secreted by mesenchymal cells. In contrast, a broad zone of laminin and type IV collagen immunoreactivities that encompasses the entire width of the mesenchyme where smooth muscle will form, is found in the presumptive aganglionic segments of the bowel of ls/ls mice.

The region where accumulation of laminin and type IV collagen immunoreactivities occurs is restricted in its distribution to the presumptive aganglionic portion of the bowel. In its location in the outer gut mesenchyme, this zone of accumulated matrix materials lies athwart the path that migrating crest-derived cells would have to take to colonize the terminal colon. These observations are consistent with the view that the overproduction (or decreased turnover with consequent accumulation) of several components of the extracellular matrix is causally related to the development of aganglionosis in ls/ls mice. The fact that the accumulated components of the extracellular matrix are all found in basal laminae suggests that the defect may involve a co-ordinate and localized defect in the production or regulation of the production of basal laminae.

BASAL LAMINAE SURROUNDING SMOOTH MUSCLE CELLS OF THE MUSCULARIS MUCOSA ARE ABNORMAL IN THE AGANGLIONIC SEGMENTS OF ADULT ls/ls MICE

Electron microscopic examination of the aganglionic region of the ls/ls bowel in adult mice reveals that the smooth muscle of the muscularis mucosa is highly abnormal[65,68]. The layer itself is much thicker than either the muscularis mucosa of the terminal colon of control mice or that of the more proximal bowel of the same ls/ls animals. The thicker muscularis mucosa in the aganglionic tissue contains approximately the same number of cells per unit length of tissue as in the controls, but the individual muscle cells of the abnormal tissue are hypertrophic and the spaces between cells are widened. The hypertrophic smooth muscle cells appear to be secretory, in that they contain an extensive rough endoplasmic reticulum and a large Golgi apparatus. The wide spaces between the smooth muscle cells is due to a reduplication and thickening of their encircling basal laminae. These abnormalities in mature animals suggest that precursors of smooth muscle, particularly that of the muscularis mucosa, are abnormal early in development and are responsible for the accumulation of components of basal laminae in the presumptive aganglionic tissue. The muscularis mucosa cannot be recognized as a distinct layer until after birth. Nevertheless, a distinct

20

hypertrophy of the innermost layer of the circular muscle can be recognized as early as day E16 in the presumptive aganglionic region of the colon of *ls/ls* mouse fetuses. It is thus possible that these innermost smooth muscle cells and their precursors are the cells in the *ls/ls* mouse fetus that are defective, and that they give rise, in adults, to the abnormal muscularis mucosa.

The accumulation of extracellular matrix materials detected by immunocytochemistry is mirrored by abnormalities in the ultrastructural appearance of the extracellular space in the terminal bowel of fetal *ls/ls* mice. The distribution of one of these components, proteoglycan (PG), can be visualized in preparations that are prepared with a fixative solution containing ruthenium red[69]. Ruthenium red fixation retains PG and causes them to precipitate in the form of granules that can be recognized by electron microscopy[69,70]. Most PG granules in the fetal gut are 20–50 nm in diameter and are connected by thin filaments ~5 nm in diameter[71]. PG granules are also found adherent to collagen fibrils which, however, are much less common than the 5 nm filaments in the fetal bowel at ages E11–16. In addition, many PG granules are embedded in the mucosal basal lamina and are associated with the plasma membranes of mesenchymal cells, especially on microspikes. A smaller PG granule, ~15 nm in diameter, is also seen in both the lamina rara interna and externa of the mucosal basal lamina. Appropriate enzymatic treatments of the tissue reveal that the larger PG granules are probably chondroitin sulfate, the 5 nm filaments are probably hyaluronic acid, and the smaller PG granules heparan sulphate. The aganglionic region of the *ls/ls* colon differs from control at early ages in the length of the 5 nm filaments and in the distribution of the larger PG granules. The 5 nm filaments are longer in the abnormal tissue and are studded with a greater number of PG granules/unit length of filament than in the control bowel. The normal regular-appearing intercellular lattice of these filaments is disrupted in the presumptive aganglionic gut and there are more PG granules associated with microspikes on the surfaces of mesenchymal cells. On the other hand, approximately equal numbers of the larger PG granules can be found in control and presumptive aganglionic tissue. The abnormality in the presumptive aganglionic colon thus is of the distribution, not of the amount of chondroitin sulphate-containing granules. In contrast, the increased alcian blue staining that was detected in the presumptive aganglionic gut, revealing an accumulation of glycosaminoglycans, is reflected in the increased length of the filaments of hyaluronic acid. At day E16 large lakes can be discerned between developing mesenchymal and smooth muscle cells in the aganglionic *ls/ls* bowel. These lakes contain massive accumulations of PG arrayed on hyaluronic acid filaments. These ultrastructural observations confirm that the extracellular matrix is abnormal in the mesenchyme of the presumptive aganglionic region of the gut of *ls/ls* mice.

GROWTH ON RECONSTITUTED BASAL LAMINAE APPEARS TO INHIBIT THE MIGRATION OF CREST-DERIVED NEURAL PRECURSORS OUT OF THE DEVELOPING MURINE GUT *IN VITRO*

As a working hypothesis, it is proposed that migrating crest-derived cells express laminin receptors (or receptors for other components of basal laminae) when they arrive in the bowel that activate neurite extension and cause the cells to cease migrating. These receptors probably correspond to the recently described 110 kDa neural laminin receptor[72,73], which is separate and distinct from the smaller, previously described 67 kDa laminin receptor that promotes the adherence of cells to their substrates[72]. Prior to their arrival in the gut, it is postulated that the crest-derived cells only express the 67 kDa adhesion-promoting laminin receptor. In consequence, premature extension of neurites does not occur even if the crest-derived cells come into contact with laminin, as they undoubtedly do as they migrate. On the other hand, the extension of neurites can be stimulated to occur if the crest-derived cells encounter an accumulation of laminin within the bowel. This hypthesis therefore assumes that neural and glial precursors, under normal conditions, only become responsive as neurons to components of basal laminae at the end of their route of migration. The overabundance of components of basal laminae, including laminin, in the presumptive aganglionic gut of *ls/ls* mice may cause the crest-derived cells to extend neurites and even to withdraw from the cell cycle before they have finished migrating. This premature event would lead the terminal bowel to become aganglionic. The timing of the appearance of the defect, just when crest-derived cells are migrating in the terminal gut, probably results in an absolute aganglionosis that is limited to a small zone in the most terminal part of the bowel; however, the accumulation of components basal laminae continues so that later events are affected even more than earlier events. As a result, the hypoganglionic zone in the immediately more proximal region of the gut is disorganized, which may result from incomplete filling of this region with precursors that normally follow the paths of the early pioneers that make up the front of the crest-derived cell migration. It may also lead to the observed more severe defect of the submucosal plexus than the myenteric. Since the submucosal plexus apparently develops as the result of a second migration of cells from the primordial myenteric ganglia[51,74–76], precursor cells have to migrate through the circular layer of smooth muscle in order to form the submucosal plexus. This second migration makes the submucosal precursors highly susceptible to an accumulation of components of basal laminae. They would also have to cross the innermost layer of circular muscle, the most abnormal of the mesenchymal tissues of the presumptive aganglionic colon. The later migration may thus be related to the particularly extensive aganglionosis of the submucosa in *ls/ls* mice.

Several observations support the hypothesis that the accumulated basal lamina material in the presumptive aganglionic bowel is causally related to the development of the aganglionosis. It is known that laminin promotes neurite extension[77–79] and it has also been demonstrated that a monoclonal antibody that recognizes a complex formed between laminin and heparan sulphate proteoglycan interferes with neurite extension[80]. Moreover, the 110 kDa laminin receptor that has been linked to the promotion of neurite extension[72,73] does not appear on crest-derived cells as they leave the neural crest proper, but can be recognized on these cells within the gut[81]. Finally, the phenomenon discussed above, that crest-derived precursors migrate out of explants of bowel *in vitro* and give rise to satellite ganglia that project back to the original explants, does not occur if the explants are grown on reconstituted basal laminae (Matrigel™) instead of type 1 collagen[81]. Further tests of the hypothesis are underway.

It is by no means clear that the defect in the *ls/ls* mouse that is responsible for the development of aganglionosis is identical to the defect responsible for the pathogensis of Hirschsprung's disease. However, the two conditions are sufficiently similar that it is possible that the *ls/ls* mouse is a model of the human condition. If so, considerable insight may be derived from studying the murine model that will ultimately be of use in understanding the derivation of Hirschsprung's disease and determining means of detecting the aganglionosis early and even of preventing it. Studies of *ls/ls* mice also promise to provide insight into the normal mechanisms responsible for the cessation of migration of neural and glial precursors and for ganglion formation. Components of basal laminae may function as molecular stop signals recognized by migrating enteric crest cells.

SUMMARY

The ENS is a large, complex and unique division of the PNS that is structurally similar to the CNS. It displays a high degree of phenotypic diversity in its component neurons, lacks internal collagen, and contains glial cells that are astrocytic in contour, lack basal laminae and rich in GFAP. The ENS is derived from émigrés from the neural crest. These émigrés appear not to be endowed with 'homing' information, but instead appear to be directed to the gut by migration along defined pathways that lead to the bowel from vagal and sacral regions of the neuraxis. Final determination of neural phentoypes and the pattern of neuronal organization appears to be a function of the enteric microenvironment, although whether the mechanism involved is one of selection or instruction remains to be elucidated. The terminal portion of the bowel is aganglionic in the *ls/ls* mouse. This aganglionosis appears to be caused by a regional abnormality that is intrinsic to this region of the gut. Evidence from co-culture experiments indicates that crest-derived neural and glial precursor cells cannot enter the presumptive aganglionic zone, although it permits the growth of neurites from either intrinsic or extrinsic neurons. An overabundance and maldistribution of components of basal laminae has been found both by immunocytochemistry and electron microscopy in the presumptive aganglionic region of the *ls/ls* mouse gut. Moreover, the smooth muscle cells of the muscularis mucosa in the aganglionic region of the adult *ls/ls* bowel are hypertrophic, secretory in appearance and surrounded by reduplicated layers of basal laminae. The hypothesis has been advanced that components of basal laminae, such as laminin, may activate receptors on migrating crest-derived cells, causing these cells to cease migrating and to extend neuritic processes. Premature activation of these receptors by the accumulated components of basal laminae that occurs in the presumptive aganglionic ls/ls bowel may give rise to aganglionosis. In support of this hypothesis it has recently been observed that 110 kDa neural laminin receptors are expressed by crest-derived cells after they arrive in the gut and migration of neural precursors out of explants of bowel in vitro is inhibited by growth on reconstituted basal lamina material.

Acknowledgements

This work was supported by National Institutes of Health grants NS 12969 and NS 07062.

References

1. Bayliss, W.M. and Starling, E.H. (1899). The movements and innervation of the small intestine. J. Physiol. (Lond.), 24, 99–143
2. Bayliss, W.M. and Starling, E.H. (1900). The movements and innervation of the large intestine. J. Physiol. (Lond.), 26, 107–18
3. Trendelenburg, P. (1917). Physiologische und pharmakolische Versoche uber die Dunndarm peristaltick. Arch. Exp. Pathol. Pharmacol. (Naunyn-Schmiedebergs), 81, 55–129
4. Langley, J.N. (1921). The Autonomic Nervous System, Part 1. (Cambridge: W. Heffer)
5. Furness, J.B. and Costa, M. (1980). Types of nerves in the enteric nervous system. Neuroscience, 5, 1–20
6. Furness, J.B. and Costa, M. (1987). The Enteric Nervous System. (New York: Churchill-Livingstone)
7. Gershon, M.D. (1981). The enteric nervous system. Annu. Rev. Neurosci., 4, 227–71
8. Hoffman, H.H. and Schnitzlein, H.N. (1969). The number of vagus nerves in man. Anat. Rec., 139, 429–35
9. Roman, C. and Gonella, J. (1981). Extrinsic control of digestive tract motility. In Johnson, LR. (ed.) Physiology of the Gastrointestinal Tract, pp. 289–333 (New York: Raven Press)
10. Kuntz, A. (1963). The Autonomic Nervous System, 4th Edn. (Lea and Febiger, Philadelphia)
11. Ewart, W.R. (1985). Sensation in the gastrointestinal tract. Comp. Biochem. Physiol., 82A, 489–93
12. Howard, E.R. (1972). Hirschsprung's disease: a review of the morphology and physiology. Postgrad. Med. J., 48, 471–7
13. Meneghelli, U. (1985). Chagas' disease: a model of denervation in the study of digestive tract motility. Brazilian J. Med. Biol. Res., 18, 255–69
14. Wood, J.D. (1987). Physiology of the enteric nervous system. In Johnson, L.R. (ed.) Physiology of the Gastrointestinal Tract, Vol. 1, 2nd Edn, pp. 67–109. (New York: Raven Press)
15. Gershon, M.D. and Erde, S.M. (1981). The nervous system of the gut. Gastroenterology, 85, 929–37
16. Gabella, G. (1987). Structure of muscles and nerves in the gastrointestinal tract. In Johnson, L.R. (ed.) Physiology of the Gastrointestinal Tract, 2nd Edn., pp. 335–82 (New York: Raven Press)
17. Burnstock, G. (1972). Purinergic nerves. Pharmacol. Rev., 24, 509–81
18. Gabella, G. (1972). Fine structure of the myenteric plexus. J. Anat., 111, 69–97
19. Gabella, G. (1971). Glial cells in the myenteric plexus. Z. Naturforsch., 26B, 244–5
20. Cook, R.D. and Burnstock, G. (1976). The ultrastructure of Auerbach's plexus in the guinea-pig. II. Non-neuronal elements. J. Neurocytol., 5, 195–206

21. Jessen, K.R. and Mirsky, R. (1980). Glial cells in the enteric nervous system contain glial fibrillary acidic protein. *Nature*, **286**, 736–7

22. Jessen, K.R., Thorpe, R. and Mirsky, R. (1984). Molecular identity, distribution and heterogeneity of glial fibrillary acidic protein: an immunoblotting and immunohistochemical study of Schwann cells, satellite cells, enteric glia and astrocytes. *J. Neurocytol.*, **13**, 187–200

23. Björklünd, H., Dahl, D. and Singer, A.M. (1984). Neurofilament and glial fibrillary acidic protein-related immunoreactivity in rodent enteric nervous system. *Neuroscience*, **12**, 277–87

24. Rothman, T.P., Tennyson, V.M. and Gershon, M.D. (1986). Colonization of the bowel by the precursors of enteric glia: Studies of normal and congenitally aganglionic mutant mice. *J. Comp. Neurol.*, **252**, 493–506

25. Erde, S.M., Sherman, D. and Gershon, M.D. (1985). Morphology and serotonergic innervation of physiologically identified cells of the guinea pig's myenteric plexus. *J. Neurosci.*, **5**, 617–33

26. Yntema, C.L. and Hammond, W.S. (1952). Origin of intrinsic autonomic ganglia of trunk viscera in the chick embryo. *Anat. Rec.*, **112**, 404

27. Yntema, C.L. and Hammond, W.S. (1954). The origin of intrinsic ganglia of trunk viscera from vagal neural crest in the chick embryo. *J. Comp. Neurol.*, **101**, 515–41

28. Le Douarin, N.M. (1982). *The Neural Crest*, Developmental and Cell Biology, Series 12. (Cambridge: Cambridge University Press)

29. Le Douarin, N.M. (1974). Cell recognition based on natural morphological nuclear markers. *Med. Biol.*, **52**, 281–319

30. Le Douarin, N.M. and Teillet, M.-A. (1973). The migration of neural crest cells to the wall of the digestive tract in avian embryo. *J. Embryol. Exp. Morphol.*, **30**, 31–48

31. Loring, J.F., Barker, D.L. and Erickson, C.A. (1988). Migration and differentiation of neural crest and ventral neural tube cells *in vitro*: Implications for *in vitro* and *in vivo* studies of the neural crest. *J. Neurosci.*, **8**, 1001–15

32. Gershon, M.D. (1982). Serotonergic neurotransmission in the gut. *Scand. J. Gasteroentol.*, **17**, 27–41

33. Gershon, M.D. (1982). Enteric serotonergic neurones. In Osborne, N. (ed.) *Biology of Serotonergic Transmission*, pp. 363–99. (New York Wiley)

34. Costa, M., Furness, J.B., Cuello, A.C., Verhofstad, A.A.J., Steinbusch, H.W.J. and Elde, R.P. (1982). Neurons with 5-hydroxytryptamine-like immunoreactivity in the enteric nervous system: their visualization and reactions to drug treatment. *Neuroscience*, **7**, 351–64

35. Gershon, M.D., Mawe, G.M. and Branchek, T.A. (1988). 5-Hydroxytryptamine and enteric neurons. In Fozard, J.R. (ed.) *Peripheral Actions of 5-Hydroxytryptamine*. (In press)

36. Thiery, J.P., Duband, J.L. and Delouvée, A. (1982). Pathways and mechanisms of an avian trunk neural crest cell migration and localization. *Dev. Biol.*, **93**, 324–43

37. Le Douarin, N.M. and Teillet, M.-A. (1974). Experimental analysis of the migration and differentiation of neuroblasts of the autonomic nervous system and of neuroectodermal mesenchymal derivatives, using a biological cell marking technique. *Dev. Biol.*, **41**, 162–84

38. Rothman, T.P., Sherman, D., Cochard, P. and Gershon, M.D. (1986). Development of the monoaminergic innervation of the avian gut: Transient and permanent expression of phenotypic markers. *Dev. Biol.*, **116**, 357–80

39. Noden, D.M. (1975). An analysis of the migratory behavior of avian cephalic neural crest cells. *Dev. Biol.*, **42**, 106–30

40. Noden, D.M. (1983). The embryonic origins of avian craniofacial muscles and associated connective tissues. *Am. J. Anat.*, **168**, 257–76

41. Noden, D.M. (1984). Craniofacial development: New views on old problems. *Anat. Rec.*, **208**, 1–13

42. Newgreen, D.F., Ritterman, M. and Peters, E.A. (1979). Morphology and behaviour of neural crest chick embryo *in vitro*. *Cell Tissue Res.*, **203**, 115–40

43. Newgreen, D.F. and Thiery, J.P. (1980). The source and distribution of fibronectin in early avian embryos at the time of neural crest migration. *Cell Tissue Res.*, **211**, 269–92

44. Rothman, T.P., Le Douarin, N.M. and Gershon, M.D. (1986). Pathways followed by crest cells migrating from developing quail gut back-grafted into younger chick embryos: comparison of vagal and truncal grafts. *Neurosci. Abst.*, **12**, 768

45. Smith, J.P., Cochard, P. and Le Douarin, N.M. (1977). Development of choline acetyltransferase and cholinesterase activities in enteric ganglia derived from presumptive adrenergic and

cholinergic levels of neural crest. *Cell Diff.*, **6**, 199–216

46. Fontaine-Pérus, J.C., Chanconie, M. and Le Douarin, N.M. (1982). Differentiation of peptidergic neurones in quail-chick chimeric embryos. *Cell Diff.*, **11**, 183–93

47. cFontaine-Pérus, J.C., Chanconie, M.J., Polak, J.M. and Le Douarin, N.M. (1981). Origin and development of VIP and substance P containing neurons in the embryonic avian gut. *Histochemistry*, **71**, 313–23

48. Furness, J.B., Costa, M. and Freeman, C.G. (1979). Absence of tyrosine hydroxylase activity and dopamine β-hydroxylase in intrinsic nerves of the guinea-pig ileum. *Neuroscience*, **4**, 305–10

49. Baetge, G. and Gershon, M.D. (1986). GABA in the PNS: Demonstration in enteric neurons. *Brain Res. Bull.*, **16**, 421–24

50. Mackey, H.M., Payette, R.F. and Gershon, M.D. (1988). Tissue effects on the expression of serotonin, tyrosine hydroxylase, and GABA in cultures of neurogenic cells from the neuraxis and branchial arches. *Development*. (In press)

51. Payette, R.F., Bennett, G.S. and Gershon, M.D. (1984). Neurofilament expression in vagal neural crest-derived precursors of enteric neurons. *Dev. Biol.*, **105**, 273–87

52. Tucker, G.C., Ciment, G. and Thiery, J.P. (1986). Pathways of avian neural crest cell migration in the developing gut. *Dev. Biol.*, **116**, 439–50

53. Webster, W. (1973). Embryogenesis of the enteric ganglia in normal mice and in mice that develop congenital megacolon. *J. Emb. Exp. Morphol.*, **30**, 573–85

54. Rothman, T.P. and Gershon, M.D. (1982). Phenotypic expression in the developig murine enteric nervous system. *J. Neurosci.*, **2**, 381–93

55. Rothman, T.P., Nilaver, G. and Gershon, M.D. (1984). Colonization of the developing murine enteric nervous system and subsequent phenotypic expression by the precursors of peptidergic neurons. *J. Comp. Neurol.*, **225**, 13–23

56. Rothman, T.P., Tennyson, V.M. and Gershon, M.D. (1986). Colonization of the bowel by the precursors of enteric glia: studies of normal and congenitally aganglionic mutant mice. *J. Comp. Neurol.*, **252**, 493–506

57. Jacobs-Cohen, R.J., Payette, R.F., Gershon, M.D. and Rothman, T.P. (1987). Inability of neural crest cells to colonize the presumptive aganglionic bowel of *ls/ls* mice: requirement for a permissive microenvironment. *J. Comp. Neurol.*, **255**, 425–38

58. Coulter, H.D., Gershon, M.D. and Rothman, T.P. (1988). Neural and glial phenotypic expression by neural crest cells in culture: Effects of control and presumptive aganglionic bowel from *ls/ls* mice. *J. Neurobiol.* (In press)

59. Vincent, M., Duband, J.-L. and Thiery, J.-P. (1983). A cell surface determinant expressed early on migrating avian neural crest cells. *Dev. Brain Res.*, **9**, 235–8

60. Barbu, M., Ziller, C., Rong, P.M. and Le Douarin, N.M. (1986). Heterogeneity in migrating neural crest cells revealed by a monoclonal antibody. *J. Neurosci.*, **6**, 2215–25

61. Payette, R.F., Tennyson, V.M., Pham, T.D., Mawe, G.M., Pomeranz, H.D., Rothman, T.P. and Gershon, M.D. (1987). Origin and morphology of nerve fibers in the aganglionic colon of the lethal spotted (*ls/ls*) mutant mouse. *J. Comp. Neurol.*, **257**, 237–52

62. Lane, P.W. (1966). Association of megacolon with two recessive spotting genes in the mouse. *J. Hered.*, **57**, 29–31

63. Bolande, R.P. (1975). Animal model of human disease. Hirschsprung's disease, aganglionic or hypoganglionic megacolon; animal model: aganglionic megacolon in piebald and spotted mutant strains. *Am. J. Pathol.*, **79**, 189–92

64. Bolande, R.P. and Towler, W.F. (1972). Ultrastructural and histochemical studies of murine megacolon. *Am. J. Pathol.*, **69**, 139–62

65. Tennyson, V.M., Pham, T.D., Rothman, T.P. and Gershon, M.D. (1986). Abnormalities of smooth muscle, basal laminae, and nerves in the aganglionic segments of the bowel of lethal spotted mutant mice. *Anat. Rec.*, **215**, 267–81

66. Rothman, T.P. and Gershon, M.D. (1984). Regionally defective colonization of the terminal bowel by the precursors of enteric neurons in lethal spotted mutant mice. *Neuroscience*, **12**, 1293–1311

67. Cohen, A.M. and Konigsberg, I.R. (1975). A clonal approach to the problem of neural crest determination. *Dev. Biol.*, **46**, 262–80

68. Payette, R.F., Tennyson, V.M., Pomeranz, H.D., Pham, T.D., Rothman, T.P. and Gershon, M.D. (1988). Accumulation of components of basal laminae: Association with the failure of neural crest cells to colonize the presumptive aganglionic bowel of *ls/ls* mutant mice. *Dev.*

Biol., **125**, 341–60
69. Hay, E.D. (1978). Fine structure of embryonic matrices and their relation to the cell surface in ruthenium red-fixed tissues. *Growth*, **42**, 399–423
70. Hunziker, E.B. and Schenk, R.K. (1987). Structural organization of proteoglycans in cartilage. In *Biology of Proteoglycans.* pp. 155–85. (New York: Academic Press)
71. Tennyson, V.M., Payette, R.F., Pomeranz, H.D., Rothman, T.P. and Gershon, M.D. (1988). Ruthenium red staining in the aganglionic segment of the terminal colon of *ls/ls* mouse embryos. *Anat. REc.*, **220**, 96A
72. Kleinman, H.K., Ogle, R.C., Cannon, F.B., Little, C.D., Sweeney, T.M. and Luckenbill-Edds, L. (1988). Laminin receptors for neurite formation. *Proc. Natl. Acad. Sci. USA*, **85**, 1282–86
73. Smalheiser, N. and Schwartz, N. (1987). Cranin: a laminin binding protein of cell membranes. *Proc. Natl. Acad. Sci. USA*, **84**, 6457–461
74. Epstein, M.L., Sherman, D. and Gershon, M.D. (1980). Development of serotonergic neurons in the chick duodenum. *Dev. Biol.*, **77**, 22–40
75. Gershon, M.D., Epstein, M.L. and Hegstrand, L. (1980). Colonization of the chick gut by progenitors of enteric serotonergic neurons: distribution, differentiation, and maturation within the gut. *Dev. Biol.*, **77**, 41–51
76. Tam, P.K.H. and Lister, J. (1986). Developmental profile of neuron-specific enolase in human gut and its implications in Hirschsprung's disease. *Gastroenterology*, **90**, 1902–6
77. Lander, A.D., Tomaselli, K., Calof, A.L. and Recihardt, L.F. (1983). Studies on extracellular matrix components that promote neurite outgrowth. *Cold Spring Harbor Symp. Quant. Biol.*, **48**, 611–23
78. Lander, A.D., Fujii, D.K. and Reichardt, L.F. (1985). Laminin is associated with the 'neurite outgrowth-promoting factors' found in conditioned media. *Proc. Natl. Acad. Sci. USA*, **82**, 2183–7
80. Matthew, W.D. and Patterson, P.H. (1983). The production of a monoclonal antibody that blocks the action of a neurite-outgrowth promoting factor. *Cold Spring Harbor Symp. Quant. Biol.*, **48**, 625–31
81. Pomeranz, H.D., Payette, R.F., Smalheiser, N.R. and Gershon, M.D. (1988). Localization of 3070 immunoreactivity in developing chicks: relationship to neural expression by cells derived from the neural crest. *Neurosci. Abst.* (In press)

3
A revised morphological classification of neurons in the enteric nervous system

W. STACH

INTRODUCTION

Knowledge about the variety of elements of the neuron population of the enteric nervous system is of vital importance for understanding its functional organization. It should be pointed out that, in the era of advanced immunohistochemistry[1,2,3] and electrophysiology[4,5], the morphology can contribute remarkably to this problem. This paper will describe a solution to a kind of deadlock. This deadlock has arisen by the projection of electrophysiological and immunohistochemical results onto only three morphologically defined types of neurons. The method of silver impregnation applied in the present work permits the selective and simultaneous presentation of very different types of neurons in whole mounts of the pig's gastrointestinal tract. The excellent quality of nerve cell visualization in the three large expanded and vertically linked ganglionic nerve plexuses – *Pl. myentericus*[6], *Pl. submucosus externus*[7,8–15], *Pl. submucosus internus*[16] – makes it possible to render a differentiation of neurons according to visible and demonstrable morphological features.

Whereas Dogiel[17] and many other authors who succeeded him, e.g. Lawrentjew[18], Rintoul[19], Gunn[20], Stach[8,10,11] differentiated, in effect, according to shape only, this writer and colleagues have recognized, defined and used further features for differentiation over the past few years[21–33]. The classification has therefore been enlarged by about eight neuron populations and consequently made more reliable. (Investigations concerning two further types of neurons are still under way.) Tables 1 to 8 provide summaries of the types of neurons classified in the enteric ganglia in the form of an 'identity card' listing the features of each neuron.

Except for the dendritic type II neurons the eight neuron populations have been distinguished and defined in the porcine small intestine and especially in *Pl. myentericus* (Auerbach). The tables also give information about occurrence and distribution in the other ganglionic plexuses and in different parts of the small intestine. The fundamental morphological features for the definition of the various neuron populations are specified in item 1 to 8 of each table. The definitions have been expanded by inclusion of data on immunohistochemistry of the neurons and their classification by electrophysiological criteria. Moreover, the terms 'functional classification' (e.g. interneuron) and 'functional role' (e.g. inhibitory vasoactive motor neuron) could be proclaimed as further features.

MATERIALS AND METHODS

The walls of the small and large intestines of one-to-fourteen week-old and adult pigs were dissected into whole mounts (longitudinal muscle layer with the attached *Pl. myentericus*, submucosa with the *Pl. submucosus externus* and *Pl. submucosus internus*).

Nerve cell visualization was realized by the silver impregnation method of Cauna[34].

RESULTS

The results obtained from the morphological investigations concerning the differentiation and classification of neuron populations of the enteric nervous system are summarized in summary form in the following Tables (1–8), partly supplemented by some of our immunohistochemical results and some information from electrophysiological studies in the guinea-pig. A series of micrographs (Figures 1–8) are presented to illustrate the morphological features that are summarized in the tables.

Table 1 Type I neuron identify card (see Figures 1a,b,c; 2a; 3a; 6d; 8a)

1.	*Morphological definition*: radially multidendritic (short, lamellar), uniaxonal, the most frequent of all multidendritic uniaxonal neurons, rarely biaxonal
2.	*Dendrites*: very short lamellar dendrites of coarse shape and/or longer lamellar dendrites with some bizarre branchings, not infrequently some lamellar axon dendrites arise from the axon, a longer main dendrite sometimes present (see 7)
3.	*Neurite projections*: orad (about 85%), aborad (about 15%)
4.	*Cell relationships*: detached and in aggregates, not infrequently in pairs close together, giving rise to neurites that run together
5.	*Topography*: predominantly orad parts of ganglia
6.	*Regional distribution*: only in *Pl. Auerbach*, from duodenum to ileum
7.	*Vascularization*: greater than type II, distinctly less than type III
8.	*Synaptic inputs*: synaptic structures at the soma and the lamellar dendrites[8,10], adrenergic[35], peptidergic[36-38]
9.	*Neurochemistry*: not determined in swine
10.	*Electrophysiological type*: S/type 1[3-5,39-42]

See reference 23 for morphological features

Table 2   Type II neuron identity card (see Figures 1c; 2a,b,c,d; 8b,d,e)

1. *Morphological definition*: principally adendritic, pseudo-uniaxonal multiaxonal, tendency to primary and secondary branching of the neurites close to cell body
2. *Dendrites*: rare or absent, but see dendritic type II neurons (Table 7)
3. *Neurite projections*: predominantly circular (in secondary strands and in the circular musculature), vertical (towards the submucosa and mucosa) and longitudinal (within the Pl. *Auerbach* and in the longitudinal musculature)
4. *Cell relationships*: predominantly in aggregates
5. *Topography*: periphery of ganglia
6. *Regional distribution*: in all plexuses, from duodenum to ileum and colon
7. *Vascularization*: least-vascularization of all types of neurons
8. *Synaptic inputs*: somata, axon initial segments, adrenergic[35,38], peptidergic[36,37,45-50]
9. *Neurochemistry*: CGRP, VIP, SP. (?) SOM[47-51]
10. *Electrophysiological type*: AH/type 2[3-5,39-42]

References 24, 25, 28 and 43 for morphological features

Table 3   Type III neuron identity card (see Figures 1c; 3a,b,c; 8a,b,c)

1. *Morphological definition*: radially multidendritic (*long, some branched, tapering*), uniaxonal
2. *Dendrites*: long, slender, relatively little branched, continual decrease in diameter away from cell body
3. *Neurite projections*: orad (about 15%), aboral (about 85%)
4. *Cell relationships*: predominantly in ganglionic aggregates
5. *Topography*: central and aboral parts of ganglia, Type III neuron areas are all found in Pl. *Schabadasch*
6. *Regional distribution*: Pl. *Auerbach*, Pl. *Schabadasch*, decreasing frequency from duodenum to ileum
7. *Vascularization*: highly vascularized, especially in type III neuron areas in Pl. *Schabadasch*
8. *Synaptic input*: somata, dendrites, adrenergic[35,52]; serotonergic[38,51,53,54]; peptidergic[36,37,45,53]
9. *Neurochemistry*: serotonin, probably bombesin too[54,55]
10. *Electrophysiological type*: S/type 1, AH/type 2, type 3 or type 4[4]

References 22, 23, 25 and 26 for morphological features

Table 4   Type IV neuron identity card (see Figures 4a,b,c,d; 5e

1. *Morphological definition*: from polar to radially multidendritic (short and medium length, tapering), uniaxonal, eccentric nucleus, recognizable axon hillock
2. *Dendrites*: relatively sparse dendrite trimming, frequently polar, slightly branched, frequently short dendrites at the nuclear pole, opposite the axon (head dendrites)
3. *Neurite projections*: vertically, towards the submucosa and mucosa
4. *Cell relationships*: in centralized and decentralized aggregates
5. *Topography*: ganglionic and extra ganglionic, in type II neuron areas
6. *Regional distribution*: in all plexuses, increasing in frequency from duodenum to ileum
7. *Vascularization*: slightly vascularized
8. *Synaptic inputs*: somata, dendrites, chemistry not determined
9. *Neurochemistry*: Not determined in swine
10. *Electrophysiological type*: not known

References 21, 25, 27 and 28 for morphological features

Table 5 Type V neuron identity card (see Figures 5a,b,c,d,e)

1.	*Morphological definition*: polar multidendritic (long, short, tapering, branched), uniaxonal; two forms of existence; isolated and in special aggregates; extremely eccentric nuclei
2.	*Dendrites*: few mostly long and branched dendrites from isolated neurons; many short and long dendrites within pair formations and bigger special aggregates
3.	*Neurite projections*: predominantly aboral
4.	*Cell relationships*: detached and in special aggregates
5.	*Topography*: ganglionic, without order
6.	*Regional distribution*: *Pl. Auerbach* and *Pl. Schabadasch* from the terminal jejunum to the terminal ileum, increasing in frequency
7.	*Vascularization*: not determined
8.	*Synaptic inputs*: somata, dendrites within the aggregates, chemistry not determined
9.	*Neurochemistry*: exact results not known
10.	*Electrophysiological type*: not known

References 25 and 30 for morphological features

Table 6 Type VI neuron identity card (see Figures 6a,b,c,d)

1.	*Morphological definition*: axon – dendritic, long, short, tapering, branched, partly lamellar dendrites arise from the initial part of the axon, uniaxonal
2.	*Dendrites*: besides the characteristic dendrites that arise from the axon and predominantly short soma dendrites, frequently there exists a spear tip-shaped dendrite on the antiaxonal pole
3.	*Neurite projections*: predominantly aboral
4.	*Cell relationships*: detached and in aggregates
5.	*Topography*: ganglia, aboral parts
6.	*Regional distribution*: *Pl. Auerbach* and *Pl. Schabadasch*, increasing in frequency from duodenum to ileum
7.	*Vascularization*: highly vascularized, second only to type III neurons
8.	*Synaptic inputs*: somata, dendrites, chemistry not known
9.	*Neurochemistry*: not known
10.	*Electrophysiological type*: not known

References 29–32 for morphological features

Table 7 Dendritic type II neuron identity card (see Figures 7a–g)

1.	*Morphological definition*: multidendritic, short, long, tapering, pseudo-uniaxonal and multiaxonal, tendency to primary and secondary branching of the neurites close to the cell body
2.	*Dendrites*: from sparse to frequent, sometimes polar, sometimes radially arranged, dendrites do not often branch
3.	*Neurite projections*: not exactly known at present, some are directed to the mucosa
4.	*Cell relationships*: detached and in small aggregates
5.	*Topography*: predominantly ganglionic, without order
6.	*Regional distribution*: *Pl. Meissner*, *Pl. Schabadasch*, characteristic of the colon, less frequent in the small intestine
7.	*Vascularization*: not determined
8.	*Synaptic inputs*: not known
9.	*Neurochemistry*: not known
10.	*Electrophysiological type*: not known

References 24 and 33 for morphological features

Table 8 (VIP) minineuron identity card (see Figures 2a,d; 4b,c; 8a–e)

1.	*Morphological definition*: bizarre multidendritic, uniaxonal, morphologically probably a separate type
2.	*Dendrites*: predominantly radial arrangement, some relatively long with prominent branching
3.	*Neurite projections*: not determined
4.	*Cell relationships*: frequently in aggregates
5.	*Topography*: without order in ganglia and connective strands, frequently in close neighbourhood of type II neurons
6.	*Regional distribution*: in all plexuses, especially in *Pl. Meissner*, from duodenum to ileum
7.	*Vascularization*: not determined
8.	*Synaptic inputs*: somata, dendrites, peptidergic
9.	*Neurochemistry*: VIP, GAL (very probable)[56]
10.	*Electrophysiological type*: not known

Reference 56 for morphological features

DISCUSSION

The specific features, listed in Tables 1–8 and Figures 1–8 allow a conception of the morphology of each of the eight types of neurons. Simultaneously, an impression of the variety and complexity of the neuronal organization of the enteric nervous system is vividly conveyed. It should also be pointed out, that behind each neuron type a whole neuron population is concealed, consisting of hundreds of thousands or millions of nerve cells.

We consider that the morphologically defined neuron classification has direct functional relevance. It is possible to use it sensibly and effectively as a basis for analysis and for correlation with results which have been elaborated by other methods, for example, immunohistochemical studies, electrophysiological studies or pathway tracing studies.

Although numerous aspects of the classification scheme presented here could be discussed, three points should be concentrated upon; the misidentification of neurons as Dogiel type III; the presence of a group of dendritic type II neurons; and the recognition of VIP minineurons.

The first discussion concerns the type III neurons[12–14,17,21–23,25,26,28] and the type IV neurons[21,25,27,28]. In the guinea-pig there have been found and described CGRP, CCK, CHAT, SOM, NPY, GAL – immunoreactive neurons with an exclusively vertically directed neurite course, i.e. towards the submucosa and mucosa. Cell bodies of these neurons occur both in the *Pl. myentericus* (Auerbach) and in the ganglia of the submucosa, and they have been definitely regarded as Dogiel type III neurons[57,58]. It is safe to say that this classification is not correct. This incorrect projection of immunohistochemical results on to Dogiel's type III neurons possibly has historical reasons and is also the consequence of a disregard of our[27] morphologically defined type IV neurons (Table 5; Figures 4a,b,c,d; 5e). The type III neurons, of which Dogiel[17] left a hermaphrodite description and only two drawings, have largely been ignored by morphologists.

Dogiel's postulate could be confirmed[8,21–23,25,26] by giving evidence for a type III neuron population with individual features (see Table 3; Figures 3a,b,c). The features of this real type III neuron population simply do not correspond with the description of the morphological features of the CGRP, CCK, CHAT, SOM, NPV, GAL – immunoreactive neurons[57,58].

The morphological description in the quoted studies completely apply to our type IV neurons. They essentially support our morphologically defined neuron classification that between the neuronal organization of the enteric nervous system of the pig and the guinea-pig there exist no fundamental differences.

Of particular interest is the discovery of a dendritic type II neuron population (Table 8; Figures 7a–g) described by Stach and Radke[33]. Their dendrites are, among other things, evidence for the existence of the adendritic pseudouniaxonal or multiaxonal type II neuron population. In the pig's small intestine approximately 95% of type II neurons are adendritic, in the pig's large intestine about 90%. In *Pl. Schabadasch* and *Pl. Meissner* of the pig's large intestine adendritic and dendritic type II neurons occur together and transitional forms, with one to three short, mostly branchless soma protrusions are also encountered. That means, if we speak of Dogiel's type II neurons, that we are dealing with adendritic, pseudo-uniaxonal or multiaxonal neurons, which electrophysiologically represent AH type 2[59] neurons[3–5,39–42].

As a morphologist, this writer has gained the impression, that the electrophysiological distinction between S type 1 and AH type 2 neurons depends upon the question, whether the neurons in question are dendritic (uniaxonal) or adendritic (pseudo-uniaxonal or multiaxonal). It would be interesting to know, how the dendritic, pseudo-uniaxonal or multiaxonal type II neurons behave in this respect.

The VIP/GAL neurons, e.g. in the submucosa of the pig's duodenum[60,61] and in the submucosa of the guinea-pig's small intestine, possess a strong resemblance to those VIP/(GAL) minineurons (Table 8; Figures 2a,d, 4b,c, 6b, 8a–e) that have been demonstrated[8] in the *Pl. Auerbach, Pl. Schabadasch* and *Pl. Meissner* of the pig's small intestine.

Figures 1–8 Neuron types of the *Pl. myentericus* (Auerbach, Figures 1, 2, 3a, 4, 5, 6, 8a,d), of the *Pl. submucosus externus* (Schabadasch, Figures 2b,c, 8b,c) and of the *Pl. submucosus internus* (Meissner, Figure 8e) of the pig's small intestine. Figures 1a,b,c, 2a,b, 3a,b, 4c, 5c, 6d, 8a,b,c,d,e are from jejunum; Figures 2c,d, 3d, 4a,b,d,e, 6a,b,c, are from ileum. The *Pl submucosus internus* (Meissner) of the porcine colon is illustrated in Figure 7a–g.

Method: silver impregnation according to Cauna[34]

Magnification: x 160–1c; x 200–8b; 240–3c; x 320–2d, 4d, 5e, 8c; x 400–2a,b, 3a,b, 5a, 6, 8a,d; x 480–2c, 4a,b, 5c,d, 6a, 7a–g, 8e; x 500–4c; x 640–6b,d x 800–1a,b, 6c

Abbreviations: I–VI –corresponding neuron types

dII –dendritic type II neuron

mi –minineuron

v –connective strand from *Pl. Auerbach* to the *Pl. Schabadasch*

⟶ –axons

→→ –axon dendrites

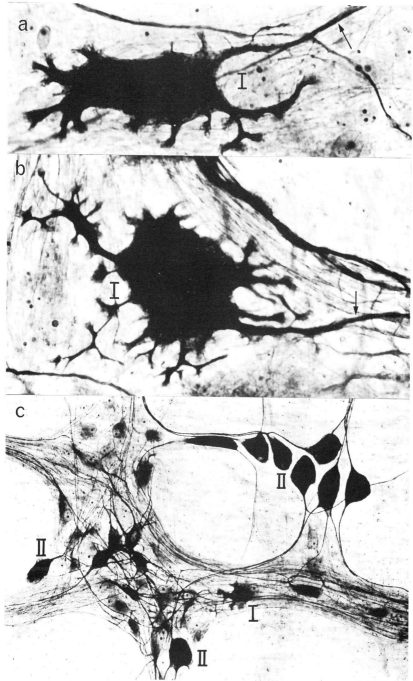

Figure 1

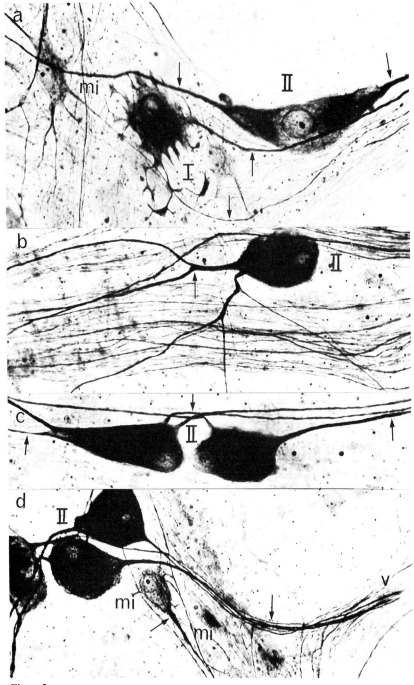

Figure 2

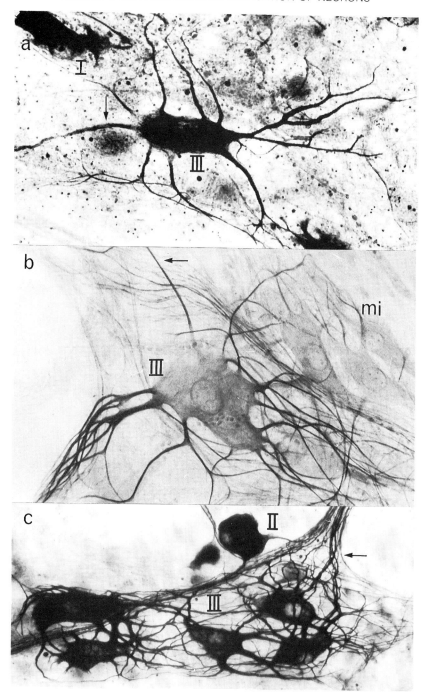

Figure 3

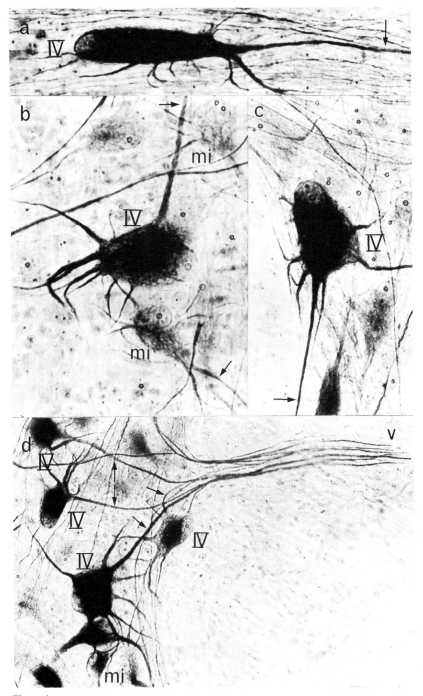

Figure 4

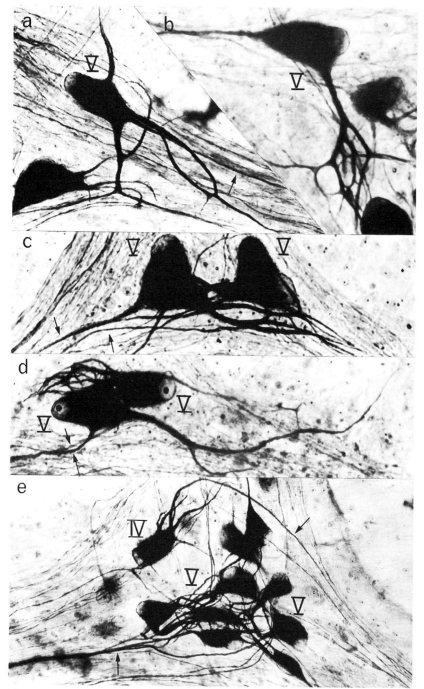

Figure 5

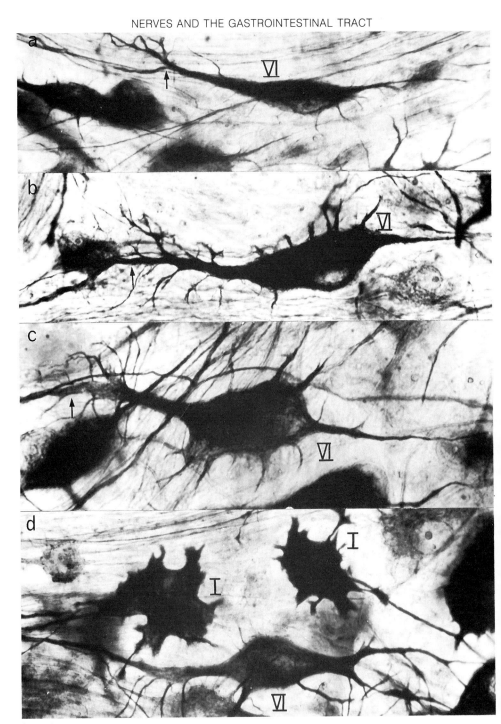

Figure 6

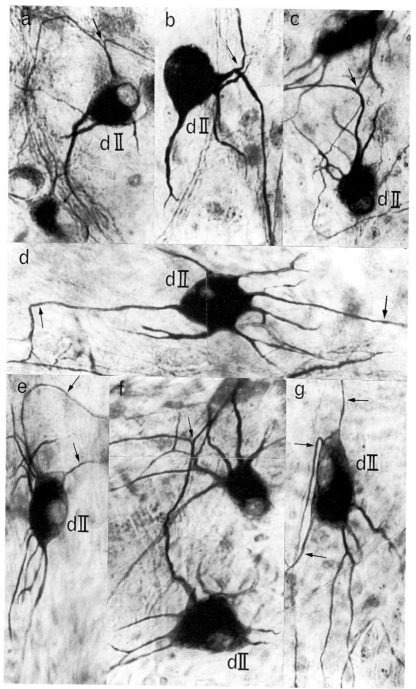

Figure 7

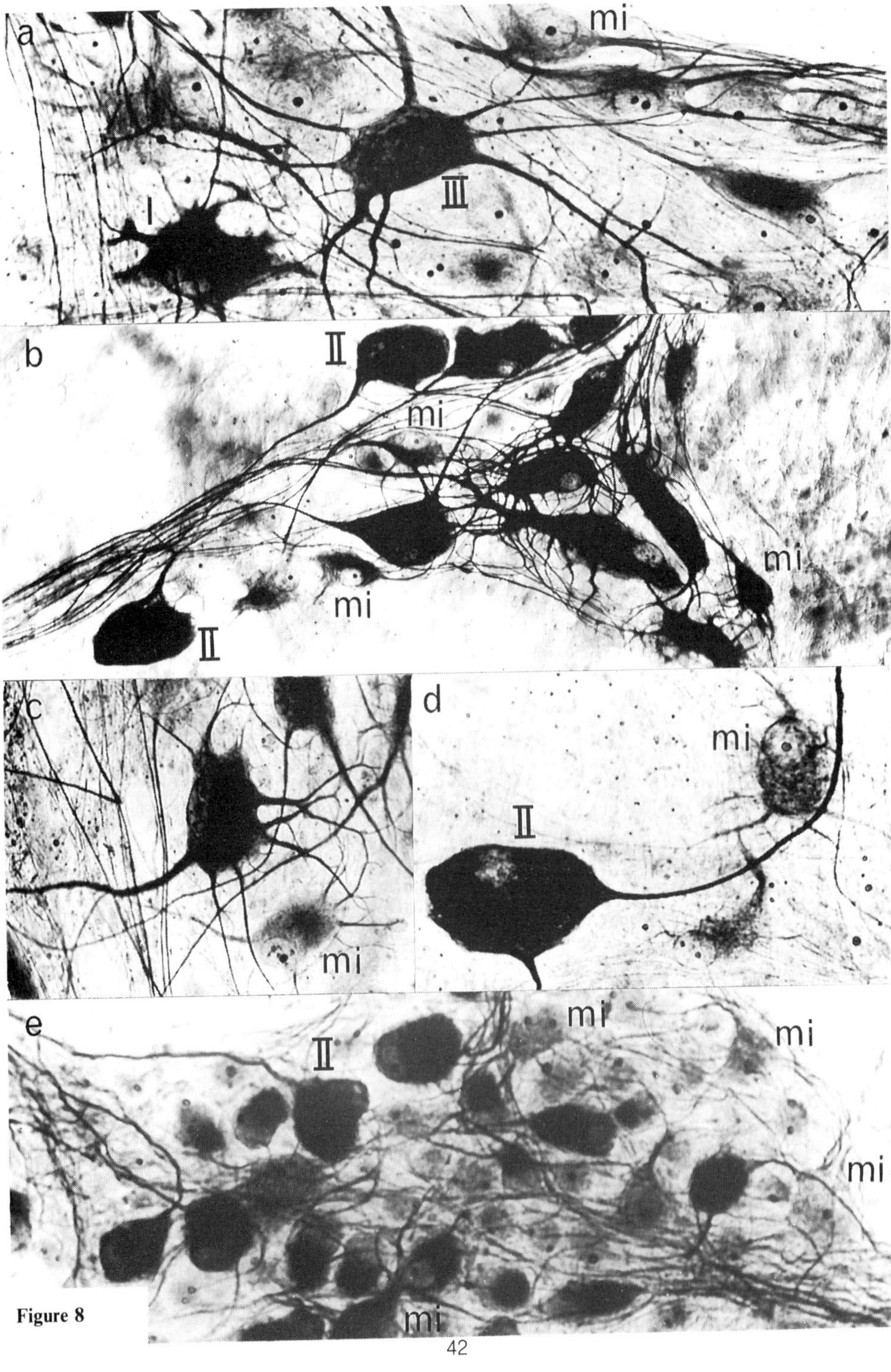

Figure 8

References

1. Costa, M., Furness, J.B. and Gibbins, I.L. (1986). Chemical coding of enteric neurons. *Progr. Brain Res.*, **68**, 217–39
2. Costa, M., Furness, J.B. and Llewellyn-Smith, L.J. (1987). Histochemistry of the enteric nervous system. In Johnson, L.R. (ed.) *Physiology of the Gastrointestinal Tract*, Vol. 1, 2nd Edn., pp. 1–39. (New York: Raven Press)
3. Furness, J.B. and Costa, M. (1987). *The Enteric Nervous System*. (Edinburgh: Churchill Livingstone)
4. Wood, J.D. (1987). Physiology of the enteric nervous system. In Johnson, L.R. (ed.) *Physiology of the gastrointestinal tract*, 2nd Edn., pp. 67–109
5. Wood, J.D. (1987). Neurophysiological theory of intestinal motility. *Jpn. J. Smooth Muscle Res.*, **23**, 143–86
6. Auerbach, L. (1862). *Über einen Plexus myentericus, einen bisher unbekannten ganglio-nervösen Apparat im Darmkanal der Wirbeltiere*. Vorläufige Mitteilung. (Breslau: F. Morgenstern)
7. Schabadasch, A. (1930). Intramurale Nervengeflechte des Darmrohrs. *Z. Zellforsch. Microsk. Anat.*, **10**, 320–85
8. Stach, W. (1969). Neurohistologische Untersuchungen an den Nervengeflechten der Dickdarmwand. Ein Beitrag zur Innervation des Magen-Darmkanals. Med. Habil-Schrift, Rostock
9. Stach, W. (1973). Light and electron-microscopic investigations on the innervation of the musculature of the colon. *Folio Morphol. Warsaw*, **32**, 457–67
10. Stach, W. (1974). Morphologie und Histochemie von Synapsen im Bereich des Magen-Darmkanals. *J. Neural Transmission*, Suppl. **11**, 79–101
11. Stach, W. (1975). Nervengeflechte und Nervenzellen der Dickdarmwand. *Zentralbl. Chir.*, **100**, 75–85
12. Stach, W. (1977). Neuronenstruktur und -architektur im Plexus submucosus externus (Schabadasch) des Duodenums. *Verh. Anat. Ges. Jena*, **71**, 867–71
13. Stach, W. (1977). Die differenzierte Gefäßversorgung der Dogielschen Zelltypen und die bevorzugte Vaskularisation der Typ I-Zellen [after precised definition type III neurons] in den Ganglien des Plexus submucosus externus (Schabadasch) des Schweins. *Z. Mikrosk.-Anat. Forsch.*, **95**, 421–9
14. Stach, W. (1977). Der Plexus submucosus externus (Schabadasch) im Dünndarm des Schweins. I. Form, Struktur und Verbindungen der Ganglien und Nervenzellen. *Z. Mikrosk.-Anat. Forsch.*, **91**, 737–55
15. Stach, W. (1979). In Memoriam ARNOLD LEONOWITSCH SCHABADASCH. *J. Hirnforsch.*, **20**, 453–4
16. Meissner, G. (1857). Über die Nerven der Darmwand. *Z. Rat. Med. NF*, **8**, 364–6
17. Dogiel, A.S. (1899). Ueber den Bau der Ganglien in den Geflechten des Darmes und der Gallenblase des Menschen und der Säugetiere. *Arch. Anat. Physiol. Anat. Abt.*, **1899**, 130–58
18. Lawrentjew, B.J. (1929). Experimentell-morphologische Studien über den feineren Bau des autonomen Nervensystems. II. Über den Aufbau der Ganglien der Speiseröhre nebst einigen Bemerkungen über das Vorkommen und die Verteilung zweier Arten von Nervenzellen in dem autonomen Nervensystem. *Z. Mikrosk-Anat. Forsch.*, **18**, 233–62
19. Rintoul, J.R. (1960). The comparative morphology of the enteric nerve plexuses. *MD Thesis*, University of St. Andrews
20. Gunn, M. (1968). Histological and histochemical observations on the myenteric and submucous plexuses of mammals. *J. Anat.*, **102**, 223–39
21. Stach, W. (1979). Neuronentypen der intramuralen Nervenplexus des Schweinedünndarms. In *Argumenta Communicationum V. Congressus Anatomicus Europensis. XXII. Colloquium scientificum Universitatis Carolinae*, Praga, 10–14 September, p. 397
22. Stach, W. (1979). Die differenzierte Gefäßversorgung der Dogielschen Zelltypen und die bevorzugte Vaskularisation der Typ I/2-Zellen [after precised definition type III neurons] in den Ganglien des Plexus myentericus (Auerbach) des Schweins. *Anat. Anz.*, **145**, 464–73
23. Stach, W. (1980). Zur neuronalen Organisation des Plexus myentericus (Auerbach) im Schweinedünndarm. I. Type I-Neurone. *Z. Mikrosk.-Anat. Forsch.*, **94**, 883–9
24. Stach, W. (1981). Zur neuronalen Organisation des Plexus myentericus (Auerbach) im

Schweinedünndarm. II. Typ II-Neurone. *Z. Mikrosk.-Anat. Forsch.*, **95**, 161–82

25. Stach, W. (1981).)U'ber die Erweiterung der Dogielschen Neuronentypisierung innerhalb des Darmwandnervensystems. *Verh. Anat. Ges. Jena*, **75**, 945–7

26. Stach, W. (1982). Zur neuronalen Organisation des Plexus myentericus (Auerbach) im Schweinedünndarm. III. Typ III-Neuron. *Z. Mikrosk.-Anat. Forsch.*, **96**, 497–516

27. Stach, W. (1982). Zur neuronalen Organisation des Plexus myentericus (Auerbach) im Schweinedünndarm. IV Typ IV-Neurone. *Z. Mikrosk.-Anat. Forsch.*, **96**, 972–94

28. Stach, W. (1983). Über morphologisch definierte vertikale Verbindungen innerhalb des Darmwandnervensystems im Schweinedünndarm. *Verh. Anat. Ges. Jena*, **77**, 577–8

29. Stach, W. (1984). Six morphologically defined neuron types in the myentericus plexus (Auerbach) of the porcine small intestine. *Acta Anat. Basel*, **120**, 69–70

30. Stach, W. (1985). Zur neuronalen Organisation des Plexus myentericus (Auerbach) im Schweinedünndarm. V. Typ V-Neurone. *Z. Mikrosk.-Anat. Forsch.*, **99**, 562–82

31. Stach, W. (1987). Morphologisch definierte Neuronen-typisierung im Darmwandnervsystem des Schweinedünndarms, speziell im Plexus myentericus (Auerbach). *Verh. Anat. Ges. Jena*, **81**, 735–6

32. Stach, W. (1987). Conditions, principles and criteria of the morphologically based classification of neurons in the porcine small intestine. *Acta Anat. Basel*, **130**, 87–8

33. Stach, W. and Radke, R. (1987). Dendritic pseudouni- and multiaxonal type II neurons of the enteric nervous system in the porcine small intestine. *Acta Anat. Basel*, **130**, 88

34. Cauna, N. (1959). The mode of termination of the sensory nerves and its significance. *J. Comp. Neurol.*, **113**, 169–210

35. Scheuermann, D.W. and Stach, W. (1983). External adrenergic innervation of the three neuron types of Dogiel in the plexus myentericus and the plexus submucosus externus of the porcine small intestine. *Histochemistry*, **77**, 303–11

36. Scheuermann, D.W. and Stach, W. (1985). A simultaneous demonstration of particular enteric neuronal cell types with the NADH: Nitro BT-dehydrogenase reaction and of nerve fibres containing enkephalin-like immunoreactivity in the myenteric plexus of the porcine small intestine. *Histochemistry*, **82**, 269–73

37. Scheuermann, D.W. and Stach, W. (1985). NADH-dehydrogenase reaction in combination with immunoperoxidase (PAP) staining for light microscopic observation on the interneuronal relations of the enteric nervous system of the pig. *Acta Anat. Basel*, **124**, 31–4

38. Stach, W. and Scheuermann, D.W. (1986). Kombination der NADH-Dehydrogenasereaktion mit der Glyoxylsäurefluoreszenz, der indirekten Immunfluoreszenz und der PAP-Technik zur Darstellung interneuronalerBeziehungen im Darmwandnervensystem. *Verh. Anat. Ges. Jena*, **80**, 683–4

39. Hodgkiss, J.P. and Lees, G.M. (1983). Morphological studies of electrophysiologically-identified myenteric plexus neurons of the guinea-pig ileum. *Neuroscience*, **8**, 593–608

40. Bornstein, J.C., Costa, M., Furness, J.B. and Lees, G.M. (1984). Electrophysiology and enkephalin immunoreactivity of identified myenteric plexus neurons of guinea-pig small intestine. *J. Physiol.*, London, **351**, 313–25

41. Erde, S.M., Shermann, D. and Gershon, M.D. (1985). Morphology and serotonergic innervation of physiologically identified cells of the guinea pig's myenteric plexus. *J. Neurosci.*, **5**, 617–36

42. Katayama, Y., Lees, G.M. and Pearson, G.T. (1986). Electrophysiology and morphology of vasoactive-intestinal-peptide-immunoreactive neurons of the guinea-pig ileum. *J. Physiol. Lond.*, **378**, 1–11

43. Schulz, F., Thierbach, Th. and Stach, W. (1986). Form, Topographie und Neuritenverlauf der Typ II-Neurone im Plexus Auerbach des Schweinedünndarms. *Verh. Anat. Ges. Jena*, **80**, 685–6

45. Stach, W. and Scheuermann, D.W. (1984). Distribution of enkephalinergic axons in relation to well-defined neuron types of the myenteric plexus (Auerbach) and the plexus submucosus externus (Schabadasch) of the porcine small intestine. *Acta Anat. Basel*, **120**, 70

46. Scheuermann, D.W. and Stach, W. (1987). Histochemische und immunhistochemische Nachweise von klassischen Neurotransmittern und Peptidhormonen im Darmwandnervensystem des Schweinedünndarms. *Verh. Anat. Ges. Jena*, **81**, 731–2

47. Scheuermann, D.W., Stach, W. and Timmermans, J.-P. (1987). CGPR (calcitonin generelated peptide) in Neuronen und Axonen des Darmwandnervensystems im Schweinedünndarm. *Verh. Anat. Ges. Jena*, **82**. (In press)

48. Stach, W. Scheuermann, D.W. and Timmermans, J.-P. (1987). Substanz P in Neuronen und Axonen des Darmwandnervensystems im Schweinedünndarm. *Verh. Anat. Ges. Jena*, **82**. (In press)
49. Stach, W., Scheuermann, D.W. and Timmermans, J.-P. (1988). Struktur und Funktion der Dogielschen Typ II-Neurone im Darmwandnervensystem des Schweinedünndarms. *Verh. Anat. Ges. Jena*, **83**. (In press)
50. Scheuermann, D.W., Stach, W., De Groodt-Lasseel, M.H.A. and Timmermans, J.-P. (1987). Calcitonin gene-related peptide in morphologically well-defined Type II neurons of the enteric nervous system in the porcine small intestine. *Acta Anat. Basel*, **129**, 325–8
51. Scheuermann, D.W. and Stach, W. (1984). Distribution of somatostatin-like immunoreactive nerves and ganglion cells in the myenteric plexus of the porcine small intestine. *Acta Anat. Basel*, **120**, 64
52. Stach, W. and Scheuermann, D.W. (1985). Konzentrationen externer noradrenerger Axongeflechte im Bereich von Typ III-Neuronenaggregaten und dichten Kapillargeflechten des Plexus submucosus externus (Schabadasch) im Schweinedünndarm. *Z. Mikrosk.-Anat. Forsch.*, **99**, 617–26
53. Stach, W. and Scheuermann, D.W. (1987). Spezifische Charakteristika der Typ III-Neurone im Darmwandnervensystem des Schweinedünndarms. *Verh. Anat. Ges. Jena*, **81**, 737–8
54. Scheuermann, D.W., Stach, W. and Timmermans, J.-P. (1988). Serotonin-immunoreactivity in the wall of the porcine small intestine. *Verh. Anat. Ges. Jena*, **83**. (In press)
55. Scheuermann, D.W., Stach, W. and Timmermans, J.-P. (1987). Bombesin - immunoreactivity in the nervous system of the wall of the porcine small intestine. *Acta Anat. Basel*, **130**, 82
56. Stach, W., Scheuermann, D.W. and Timmermans, J.-P. (1987). VIP–immunorreactive minieurons in the nervous system of the wall of the porcine small intestine. *Acta Anat.*, *Basel*, **130**, 88
57. Furness, J.B., Costa, M., Gibbins, I.L., Llewellyn-Smith, I.J. and Oliver, J.R. (1985). Neurochemically similar myenteric and submucous neurons directly traced to the mucosa of the small intestine. *Cell Tissue Res.*, **241**, 155–63
58. Furness, J.B., Costa, M., Rökaeus, Å, McDonald, T.J. and Brooks, B. (1987). Galanin-immunoreactive neurons in the guinea-pig small intestine: their projections and relationships to other enteric neurons. *Cell Tissue Res.*, **250**, 607–15
59. Nishi, S. and North, R.A. (1973). Intracellular recording from the myenteric plexus of the guinea-pig ileum. *J. Physiol. Lond.*, **231**, 471–91
60. Melander, T., Hökfelt, T., Rökaeus, Å, Fahrenkrug, J., Tatemoto, K. and Mutt, V. (1985). Distribution of galanin-like immunoreactivity in the gastrointestinal tract of several mammalian species. *Cell Tissue Res.*, **239**, 253–70
61. Bishop, A.E., Polak, J.M., Bauer, F.E., Christofides, N.D., Carlei, F. and Bloom, S.R. (1986). Occurrence and distribution of a newly discovered peptide, galanin, in the mammalian enteric nervous system. *Gut*, **27**, 849–57

4
Projections of enteric peptide-containing neurons in the rat

E. EKBLAD, R. HÅKANSON AND F. SUNDLER

INTRODUCTION

The nervous control of visceral functions is exerted by extrinsic (parasympathetic, sympathetic and sensory) neurons as well as by intrinsic neurons (for reviews see 1 and 2). The digestive tract is rich in intrinsic neurons traditionally referred to as the enteric nervous system. The enteric neurons are organized as small ganglia situated either in the submucosa (submucous ganglia or Meissner's plexus) or between the two muscle layers (myenteric ganglia or Auerbach's plexus). These ganglia and their interconnecting nerve strands form a continuous meshwork with nerve cell bodies accumulated at the nodes of the meshwork. The enteric nervous system is rich in regulatory peptides[3-5]. In fact, the digestive tract seems to be richer in neuropeptides than any other tissue outside the brain. Among recognized gut neuropeptides are: substance P (SP); neurokinin A (NKA); vasoactive intestinal peptide (VIP); peptide histidine isoleucine (PHI); gastrin-releasing peptide (GRP); calcitonin gene-related peptide (CGRP); neuropeptide Y (NPY); galanin; enkephalin; and somatostatin.

Processes such as absorption, secretion and co-ordinated peristaltic activity are to a great extent regulated by intramural nerve reflexes[6-8]. Analysis of the functional role of the enteric peptide-containing neurons in these processes would be facilitated by knowledge of the polarities and projections of each individual neuronal system. One way of studying neuronal projections in the gut is to make local lesions of nerve pathways. Lesions in the form of, for example, myectomy or myotomy were first described by Furness and Costa[9]. As a result of studies using such lesions they were able to outline the projections of several neuronal populations in the guinea-pig small intestine (for a review see 5). The present report summarizes our findings on the distribution, origin and projections of enteric peptide-containing neurons in the small and large intestine of the rat.

MATERIALS AND METHODS

Animals. Adult female Sprague–Dawley rats (150–200 g) were used.

Denervation procedures

Severing extrinsic nerves:

(1) Bilateral subdiaphragmatic truncal vagotomy and pyloroplasty.

(2) Chemical sympathectomy by 6-hydroxy-dopamine.

(3) Nerve crush by clamping the mesenteric blood vessels and the surrounding mesentery of an intestinal loop approximately 10 cm in length.

Severing intrinsic nervous pathways (Figure 1):

(1) Circumferential myectomy, i.e. removal of the outer longitudinal smooth muscle layer with adherent myenteric ganglia from a 10 mm segment of the gut.

(2) Transection with end-to-end anastomosis.

(3) Nerve crush by circumferential clamping with a pair of forceps.

The animals were killed 8–10 days later. The projection patterns of the various peptide-containing neurons were deduced by examination of the subsequent axonal degeneration (Figure 2). The nerve fibre length was established by measuring the distances from the lesion to the region showing a normal supply of nerve terminals. This distance includes one region lacking immunoreactive terminals and one region showing a gradual increase in the number of nerve terminals. Distances were measured using a micrometer scale inserted in the visual field.

Immunocytochemistry

Tissue specimens from the mid-jejunum and the transverse colon of operated and unoperated rates were fixed overnight in Stefanini's fixative, rinsed in Tyrode solution containing 10% sucrose and processed for immunocyto-chemistry either as whole mounts or as cryostat sections. The indirect immunofluorescence method was used for the demonstration of the following neuropeptides: VIP, NPY, SP, GRP, CGRP, galanin, enkephalin and somatostatin. For controls, antisera that had been inactivated by the addition of excess amounts of antigen (10–100 μg of synthetic peptide/ml diluted antiserum) was used. Coexistence of neuropeptides was studied by sequential (VIP/NPY) or double (CGRP/SP, CGRP/VIP and CGRP/somatostatin) immunostaining. (For further details see references 10–13.)

Myectomy

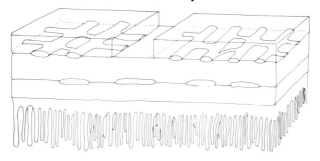

Transection

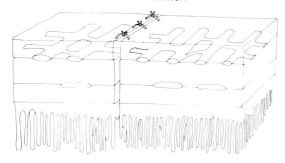

Clamping

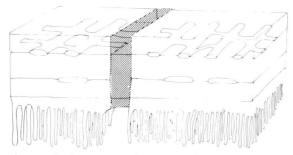

Figure 1 Procedures used to interrupt enteric nervous pathways. Myectomy involves circumferential removal of 10 mm of the outer longitudinal muscle layer with adherent myenteric ganglia, thus severing the nervous pathways emanating from these ganglia. Transection is followed by suturing the severed ends. Clamping interrupts enteric nervous pathways by crushing the nerves for 3 to 4 mm with a pair of forceps. The two latter procedures severed nervous pathways in both myenteric and submucous ganglia.

Intact enteric nervous pathways

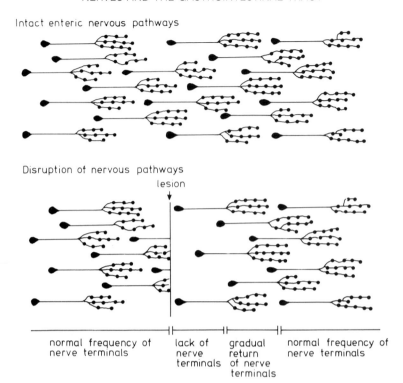

Disruption of nervous pathways

lesion
↓

| normal frequency of nerve terminals | lack of nerve terminals | gradual return of nerve terminals | normal frequency of nerve terminals |

Figure 2 Diagram illustrating the unidirectional projections of a hypothetical population of enteric neurons and the proposed consequences of local disruption of the pathways. In the diagram it is assumed (perhaps erroneously) that all projections of this hypothetical neuronal population are of the same length. Cell bodies and preterminals have a low neuropeptide content. The nerve terminals are rich in the neuropeptide

RESULTS

General distribution

Numerous peptide-containing nerve fibres and nerve cell bodies were found throughout the intestines. The occurrence and topographic distribution of the various neuronal populations are illustrated in Figure 3. NPY was found in the entire population of intramural VIP neurons in the small intestine. In the large intestine only a small population of the VIP-containing neurons harboured NPY. In addition, NPY occurred in noradrenergic fibres which were distributed mainly around blood vessels. SP and CGRP occurred in separate nerve fibre populations in the smooth muscle and mucosa, while coexisting in a population of perivascular fibres. In the large intestine a subpopulation of submucous CGRP-containing neurons stored also somatostatin.

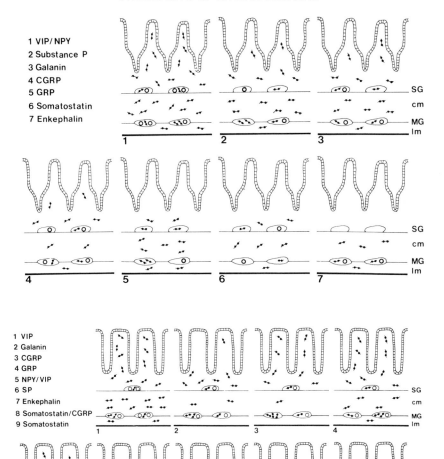

Figure 3 Schematic outline of the topography and relative density of peptide-containing nerve fibres (–●–●–) and nerve cell bodies (○) in the rat small (upper panel) and large (lower panel) intestine. SG, Submucous ganglia; cm, circular muscle; MG, myenteric ganglia; lm, longitudinal muscle

Extrinsic denervation

Mesenteric clamping or sympathectomy eliminated perivascular NPY- (and noradrenaline-)containing fibres. Mesenteric clamping eliminated perivascular SP/CGRP-(small and large intestine) and CGRP-(large intestine) containing fibres. Other types of peptide-containing nerve fibres were not overtly affected by extrinsic denervation.

Projections of enteric neurons

Myenteric neurons
The myenteric neurons were found to project to other myenteric ganglia and to the smooth muscle layers. Except for GRP-containing neurons in the large intestine, which to some extent projected to the mucosa and submucosa, there was no evidence of projections of myenteric neurons to the mucosa or submucosa. Myenteric neurons containing VIP/NPY (Figure 4), VIP (large intestine), GRP, galanin or somatostatin issued descending projections. CGRP-containing neurons issued descending projections in the large intestine, while they projected in both oral and anal directions in the small intestine. SP-containing neurons issued descending projections in the small intestine, whereas they were ascending in the large intestine. Enkephalin-containing neurons gave off ascending projections in both small and large intestine. The projection distances for myenteric neurons were in the range 2–7 mm, except for the galanin-containing and the GRP-containing neurons which issued approximately 15 and 20 mm long projections respectively.

Submucous neurons
Generally, the submucous neurons projected to other submucous ganglia and to the mucosa and submucosa. However, since some scattered nerve fibres containing VIP/NPY, CGRP (small intestine) or VIP (large intestine) remained in the circular muscle underlying the myectomy, these submucous neurons seemed also to issue projections to subjacent circular muscle. Most of the submucous neurons, i.e. those storing galanin, GRP, somatostatin or SP (small intestine) (Figure 5) or CGRP, somatostatin/CGRP or GRP (large intestine) issued both ascending and descending projections. Those storing CGRP, VIP/NPY (small intestine) and VIP (large intestine) issued ascending projections only. No oro-anal projections could be detected for those submucous neurons storing VIP/NPY or galanin in the large intestine. Submucous SP-containing neurons were too few in the large intestine to allow any conclusion as to the projection pattern. Projection distances in the mucosa and submucosa ranged from 2 to 8 mm, the longest projections being those issued by CGRP-containing neurons in the small intestine. The results are summarized in Figure 6.

DISCUSSION

The list of neuropeptides in the gut is steadily growing[4,5]. Many (perhaps all) enteric neurons harbour more than one neurotransmitter candidate[14,15]. The functional significance of the diverse and complex chemical coding of the enteric neurons is unknown. An outline of the polarities and projections of different subpopulations of enteric neurons based on their peptide content

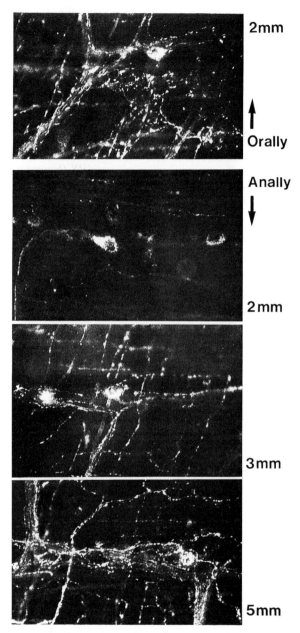

2mm

↑
Orally

Anally
↓

2mm

3mm

5mm

Figure 4 VIP nerve fibres and cell bodies in rat jejunum, 10 days after myectomy. Whole mounts of longitudinal smooth muscle with adherent myenteric ganglia. No loss of VIP fibres orally to the lesion. Up to 2 mm anally to the lesion the number of VIP fibres was markedly reduced. Further distally the nerve fibre density returned to normal. The occurrence and distribution of VIP nerve cell bodies were not affected by the lesion (x135)

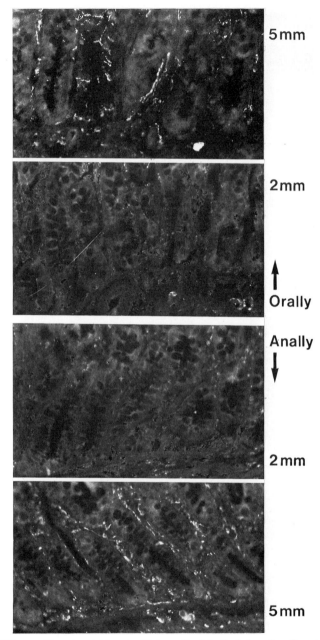

5mm

2mm

↑
Orally

Anally
↓

2mm

5mm

Figure 5 SP nerve fibres in rat jejunum, 10 days after intestinal clamping. Cryostat sections, mucosa and submucosa visible. Both orally and anally there was a loss of SP fibres for approximately 4 mm. At 5 mm in both directions the innervation was back to normal (x105)

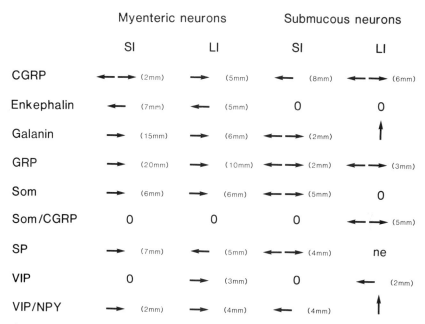

Figure 6 Polarities (marked with arrows) and projection distances (in mm) of peptide-containing neuronal populations in the rat small (SI) and large (LI) intestine. → indicates descending projections, ← indicates ascending projections and ↑ indicates that no oro-anal projections can be demonstrated, 0 means absence of nerve fibres, ne stands for not examined

is given in Figure 6. In order to meet the demands for precise regulation and co-ordination of complex processes such as peristalsis, absorption and secretion, the enteric neurons have to interact in a highly ordered fashion. This is reflected in the finding that each population of neurons shows a well-defined distribution and projection pattern, as revealed by the lesion experiments. So far this type of study has been performed in a limited number of species: guinea-pig (for review see 5), rat[10-13] and dog[16].

It seems that there are considerable species variations concerning the chemical coding, distribution and projections of individual enteric neuronal populations. To illustrate this the myenteric NPY- and/or VIP-containing neurons in the small intestine may serve as an example. In the rat the two peptides are colocalized in the same neurons with descending pathways[12]. In the guinea-pig[5] and dog[16], VIP and NPY seem to be stored in different neuronal populations. In the guinea-pig both VIP- and NPY-containing neurons are descending[5], but in the dog VIP-containing neurons are descending while NPY-containing neurons are ascending[16]. Further, the structural organization and chemical coding of the enteric nervous system is not identical in all segments of the gut, as revealed here in the rat (see also refs. 10–13). There is a tendency for shorter neuronal projections in the large intestine than in the small intestine. It is remarkable that there are neuronal projections in the large intestine that project in the opposite direction from those in the small intestine. Thus, for instance the processes of myenteric SP neurons are descending in the small intestine while ascending in the large intestine.

The basic organization, however, seems to be uniform and the differences are probably to be considered as minor in the overall organization. None the less, regional differences as well as species differences highlight the necessity to secure a precise mapping of each enteric nerve population as a basis for the understanding of the neuronal circuits involved in the regulation of gut functions.

Acknowledgements

The study was supported by the Swedish Medical Research Council (project nos. 1007, 4499 and 6944), the Påohlsson Foundation, the Swedish Society of Medicine and Magnus Bergvalli Foundation.

References

1. Schofield, G.C. (1968). Anatomy of muscular and neuronal tissues in the alimentary canal. In Code, C.F. (ed.) *Handbook of Physiology*, Vol. IV, The Alimentary Canal, pp. 1579–1628. (Maryland: Waverly Press)
2. Gabella, G. (1979). Innervation of the gastrointestinal tract. *Int. Rev. Cytol.*, **59**, 129–93
3. Makhlouf, G.M. (1985). Enteric neuropeptides: Role in neuromuscular activity of the gut. *Trends Pharm. Sci.*, **6**, 214–18
4. Håkanson, R. and Sundler, F. (1986). The role of peptide messengers in the neuroendocrine system: Hormones, neurotransmitters or neuromodulators. In Schou, J.S., Geisler, A. and Norn, S. (eds.) *Drug Receptors and Dynamic Processes in Cells*. Alfred Benzon Symp. 22, pp. 62–77. (Copenhagen, Munksgaard)
5. Costa, M., Furness, J.B. and Llewellyn-Smith, I.J. (1987). Histochemistry of the enteric nervous system. In Johnson, L.R. (ed.) *Physiology of the Gastrointestinal Tract*, pp. 1–40. (New York: Raven Press)
6. Costa, M. and Furness, J.B. (1982). Nervous control of intestinal motility. In Bertaccini, G. (ed.) *Handbook of Experimental Pharmacology*, Vol. 59, pp. 279–82. (Berlin: Springer-Verlag)
7. Cooke, H.J. (1986). Neurobiology of the intestinal mucosa. *Gastroenterology*, **90**, 1057–81
8. Wood, J.D. (1987). Physiology of the enteric nervous system. In Johnson, L.R. (ed.) *Physiology of the Gastrointestinal Tract*, pp. 67–109 (New York: Raven Press)
9. Furness, J.B. and Costa, M. (1979). Projections of intestinal neurons showing immunoreactivity for vasoactive intestinal peptide are consistent with these neurons being the enteric inhibitory neurons. *Neurosci. Lett.*, **15**, 199–204
10. Ekblad, E., Ekman, R., Håkanson, R. and Sundler, F. (1984). GRP neurones in the rat small intestine issue long anal projections. *Regul. Peptides*, **9**, 279–87
11. Ekblad, E. Rökaeus, Å, Håkanson, R. and Sundler, F. (1985). Galanin nerve fibers in the rat gut: Distribution, origin and projections. *Neuroscience*, **16**, 355–63
12. Ekblad, E., Winther, C., Ekman, R., Håkanson, R. and Sundler, F. (1987). Projections of peptide-containing neurons in rat small intestine. *Neuroscience*, **20**, 169–88
13. Ekblad, E., Ekman, R., Håkanson, R. and Sundler, F. (1988). Projections of peptide-containing neurons in rat large intestine. *Neuroscience*, **27**, 655–74
14. Sundler, F., Alumets, J., Ekblad, E., Böttcher, G. and Håkanson, R. (1985). Coexistence of peptides in the neuroendocrine system. In Håkanson, R. and Thorell, J. (eds.) *Biogenetics of Neurohormonal Peptides*, pp. 213–43 (London: Academic Press)
15. Costa, M., Furness, J.B. and Gibbins, I.L. (1986). Chemical coding of enteric neurons. In Hökfelt, T., Fuxe, K. and Pernow, B. (eds.) *Coexistence of Neuronal Messengers: A new principle in chemical transmission*, *Progr. Brain Res.*, Vol. 68, pp. 217–40. (Amsterdam: Elsevier)
16. Daniel, E.E., Furness, J., Costa, M. and Belbeck, L. (1987). The projections of chemically identified nerve fibers in canine ileum. *Cell Tissue Res.*, **247**, 377–84

5
Dogiel type II neurons in the guinea-pig small intestine: ultrastructure in relation to other characteristics

S. POMPOLO, J. B. FURNESS, J. C. BORNSTEIN, R. HENDRIKS
AND D. C. TRUSSELL

INTRODUCTION

The ways that neuronal shapes in the enteric nervous system are commonly referred to derive from the work of Dogiel[1,2]. The neurons that he referred to as type II are multipolar with cell bodies that are round or ovoid when viewed in whole-mount preparations. In the myenteric plexus of the guinea-pig small intestine, most of the processes of these neurons run circumferentially[3,4]. Electrophysiological studies, also made in the myenteric plexus of this species, have shown the Dogiel type II cells to exhibit longlasting after-hyperpolarizations, that is, to be AH neurons[5,6]. It is intriguing that Dogiel[2] proposed that the type II neurons were sensory and that, before the correlation between shape and electrophysiology was known, Nishi and North[7] and Hirst et al.[8] suggested that AH neurons were sensory. We have recently found that a majority (85%) of the Dogiel type II neurons in the guinea-pig small intestine are reactive for certain calcium-binding proteins (calbindins)[9,10]. This has allowed us to identify and study specifically the ultrastructure of Dogiel type II neurons for the first time[11]. In this paper, we comment on those ultrastructural observations and their relations to morphological and physiological studies of the Dogiel type II neurons, with particular reference to the suggestions of Dogiel[2], Nishi and North[7] and Hirst et al.[8] that they might be sensory.

NEURONAL SHAPE

Dogiel[1,2] examined the shapes of neurons in whole mounts stained with methylene blue; the majority of subsequent studies in which cell shapes have been described have used either histological stains or immunohistochemical means to reveal the neurons. While these methods are generally quite useful, they are deficient when cell bodies lie close to one another or their processes overlap, as is the case for the Dogiel type II cells in the guinea-pig small intestine. This drawback can be overcome if individual cells are filled with dye, injected via a microelectrode, and the dye used to reveal the shape of the neuron[3-7,12].

Intracellular dye injection has confirmed the existence of cells in the myenteric plexus of the guinea-pig small intestine conforming to Dogiel's description of type II neurons (Figure 1). The somata are ovoid, about 45 μm long and about 22 μm wide. They have from one to seven long processes. If there is only one process this divides soon after leaving the cell body and may divide further. Thus the Dogiel type II neurons are either multipolar or pseudo-unipolar. Most of the processes of the neurons run circumferenti-ally[3,4,13], and some seem to end in relation to other myenteric neurons[10]; a conclusion that is sustained by the ultrastructural studies discussed below. Dogiel[2], Erde et al.[13] and Furness et al.[4] all examined these cells in the guinea-pig small intestine. Dogiel was able to trace processes from them to the mucosa and the other authors, who injected cells after removal of the circular muscle and mucosa, found processes broken off where they had entered the circular muscle coat. About 85% of Dogiel type II cells in this plexus are reactive for calbindins (Iyer et al.[10]). We have found by direct tracing and by analysis of the consequences of surgical removal of sections of myenteric plexus (myectomy) that calbindin-reactive Dogiel type II cells provide a dense fibre network in the mucosa (see Figure 2) but do not provide terminals to the muscle.

In conclusion, light microscope studies indicate that Dogiel type II neurons with cell bodies in myenteric ganglia have several processes that run circumferentially to other myenteric ganglia and that many of them also have a process that projects to the underlying mucosa.

ELECTROPHYSIOLOGY

Two types of myenteric neuron can be distinguished electrophysiologically, S neurons and AH neurons[7,8,14,15]. S neurons have synaptic inputs through which prominent fast excitatory potentials can be elicited. They rarely show prolonged after-hyperpolarizations following soma action potentials, whereas AH neurons have longlasting after-hyperpolarizations that lower cell excit-ability but lack the prominent fast potentials of S neurons. Electrophysiolog-ical analysis combined with dye filling to reveal cell shape has shown that Dogiel type II neurons are almost all AH neurons[3,4,6,10].

Other properties of these neurons are that they have tetrodotoxin-resistant soma action potentials, carried in part by an inward calcium current, and that the after-hyperpolarization is due to an opening of potassium channels activated by an increase in intracellular free calcium. For several seconds after a soma action potential, action potentials reaching the cell body via a process fail to evoke further action potentials in the soma[16]. We have recently

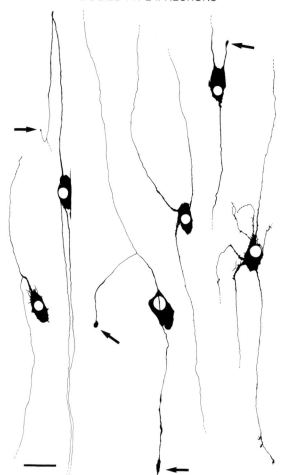

Figure 1 Shapes of type II neurons in the myenteric plexus of the guinea-pig ileum. These neurons were impaled with glass microelectrodes containing the dye Lucifer yellow CH that was used to fill the cells. The dye deposit was made permanent by an immunohistochemical method and the neurons were drawn with the aid of a camera lucida[4]. The Dogiel type II neurons are multipolar or pseudo-unipolar, with the majority of their processes running circumferentially in the myenteric plexus (vertically in this figure). In addition, one or two processes from some of these neurons pass into the circular muscle layer and are recognized by the expansion bulbs formed where they were broken off prior to impalements being made (arrows). Calibration: 40 μm

confirmed the observation of Nishi and North[7] that more than one process of an AH neuron can conduct an action potential. This means that an action potential reaching the cell body through one process could, if it invades the soma, travel away from the cell via another process. The state of excitability of the soma, influenced in part by the presence of a post-spike after-hyperpolarization, will determine whether an action potential arriving via one process will in fact initiate action potentials in other processes leaving

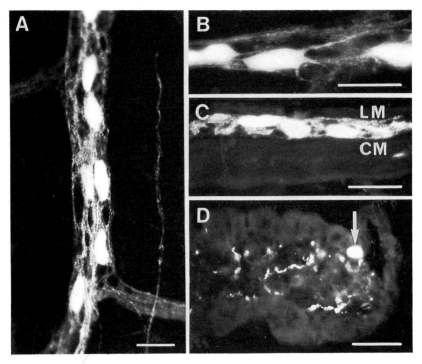

Figure 2 Calcium binding protein (calbindin D 28K) immunoreactivity in neurons of the small intestine. A. Reactivity in nerve cell bodies and fibres in a myenteric ganglion. All reactive cell bodies are similarly large and of ovoid appearance. B. This micrograph shows processes emerging from a calbindin reactive nerve cell body which, like other reactive cell bodies, had Dogiel type II morphology. C. Section through the outer musculature. Cell bodies and fibres can be seen in a myenteric ganglion, but the adjacent muscle layers (LM and CM) are not innervated, although nerve trunks carrying reactive fibres pass through the circular muscle to the submucosa and mucosa. D. Reactive fibres in a villus. The fibres form a rich subepithelial plexus. A reactive endocrine cell is also seen (arrow). Calibration: $50\,\mu$m (all micrographs)

the cell[17,18]. Thus, the cell body can have a gating function. AH neurons receive slow excitatory synaptic inputs which would be predicted to facilitate the passage of impulses across the soma[18].

ULTRASTRUCTURE

We have studied the ultrastructure of Dogiel type II neurons by exploiting the observation that many of these neurons and only neurons of this shape, are immunoreactive for calbindins in the myenteric plexus of the guinea-pig small intestine. Under the electron microscope, neurons immunoreactive for calbindins are large with generally smooth surfaces, confirming their appearance in the light microscope. Cytoplasmic features that distinguish these neurons are numerous elongated, electron-dense mitochondria (Figures 3–6), frequent peripherally placed secondary lysosomes (Figure 5), and

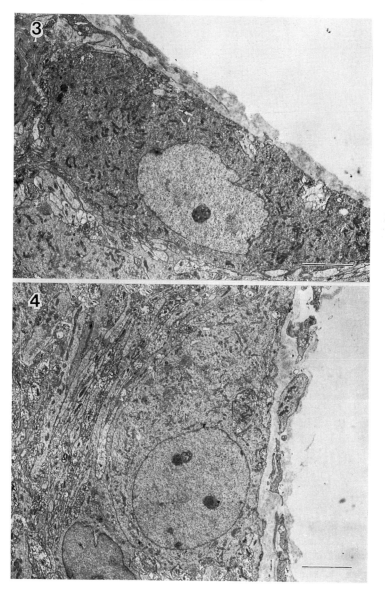

Figures 3 and 4 Low power electron micrographs from myenteric ganglia reacted for the immunocytochemical demonstration of calbindin D 28K. A reactive cell body, with its typical prominent electron dense mitochondria, is shown in Figure 3 and a non-reactive cell is shown in Figure 4. Cytoplasmic details of these two cells are shown in Figures 5 and 6. Calibrations: 4 μm

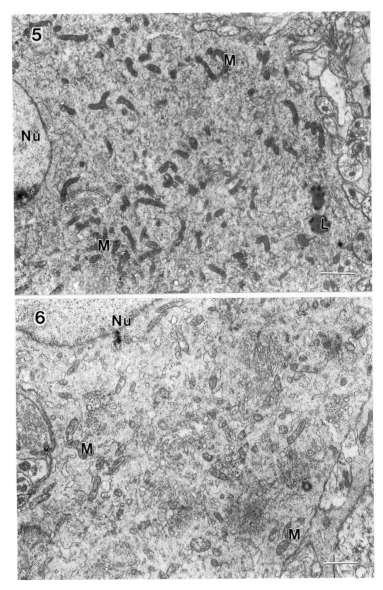

Figures 5 and 6 The appearance of the cytoplasm in a calbindin reactive neuron (Figure 5) and a typical non-reactive neuron (Figure 6). These same neurons are shown at lower power in Figures 3 and 4. The reactive neurons contain numerous elongated electron dense mitochondria (M) and frequent secondary lysosomes (C), whereas the mitochondria in most non-reactive cells are fewer and less electron-dense and secondary lysosomes are rarer. Nu: nucleus. Calibrations: 1 μm

dispersed Golgi apparatus. The majority of non-immunoreactive neurons do not share these features (e.g. Figures 4 and 6). Some neurons do have similar numbers of electron-dense mitochondria, but these neurons are smaller than the immunoreactive neurons. In the present work, about 30% of cell bodies were reactive, about 60% were unreactive and ultrastructurally dissimilar, and about 10%, despite being unreactive, had similar cytoplasmic features to the reactive neurons. Having studied the calbindin-immunoreactive neurons, we are able to recognize the same neurons in conventionally fixed and stained tissue; their ultrastructural features correspond to those of neurons classified as type 6 by Cook and Burnstock[19]. Long processes of these neurons, bearing occasional short spines, run into the neuropil. Also in the neuropil are numerous immunoreactive fibre profiles, some of which are varicose.

An important part of the analysis was to determine the synaptic relations of the calbindin reactive neurons. We have used three features to identify synapses ultrastructurally: presynaptic accumulations of small vesicles, close apposition between adjacent membranes, and post-synaptic densities (Figures 7 and 8). In addition to these defined synapses, many close appositions between vesicle containing varicosities and cell bodies were seen; these may well function as sites of transmission. Nevertheless, we have confined our quantitation of synapses to those relationships showing post-synaptic densities.

Sections were taken through ganglia in the plane of the myenteric plexus and synapses on sections of neurons passing through their nuclei were counted. An average of 0.2 reactive and 1.0 unreactive presynaptic elements were encountered in single sections through calbindin immunoreactive neurons; non-reactive, dissimilar neurons received an average of 1.8 reactive and 2.8 non-reactive inputs and non-reactive, but similar, neurons received averages of 1.8 and 4.1 reactive and non-reactive synapses, respectively. Seventy per cent of dissimilar, non-reactive neurons received at least one reactive synapse whereas 80% of calbindin-reactive neurons received no reactive synapses in sections passing through the nucleus. There were few synaptic relationships between fibres in the neuropil. The majority of these were reactive synapses on non-reactive fibres or both pre- and postsynaptic elements were non-reactive; it was rare to find either reactive or non-reactive fibres synapsing on calbindin-positive nerve fibres.

Calbindin-reactive neurons receive few synapses, but they provide a high proportion of the synapses that are on other myenteric neurons. The cell bodies of calbindin-reactive neurons have distinguishing features that allow them to be recognized even in conventionally fixed tissue.

IMPLICATIONS

A considerable body of evidence indicates that reflex changes in circular muscle activity can be evoked by mechanical or chemical stimuli applied to the mucosa[18,20,21]. In the guinea-pig small intestine, the cell bodies of motor neurons that supply the muscle are in the myenteric plexus[22]. It follows that

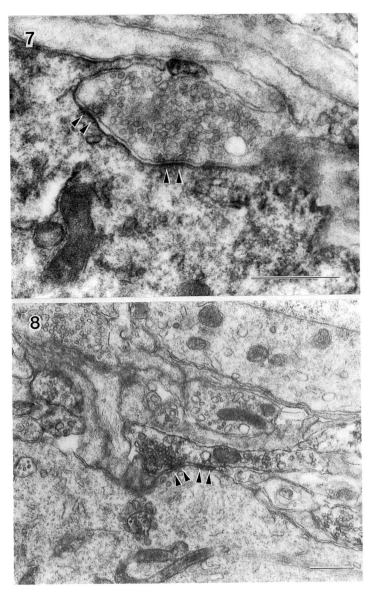

Figures 7 and 8 Examples of synapses encountered in preparations reacted for calbindin localization: in Figure 7 a non-reactive synapse occurs on a reactive neuron and in Figure 8 a synapse made by a reactive nerve fibre on a non-reactive cell body is shown. Calibrations: 0.4 μm

there must be pathways through which mucosal stimuli pass to the myenteric plexus. In the myenteric plexus the only neurons with suitable morphology to be the sensory neurons of this pathway are the Dogiel type II neurons, because all other neurons in the myenteric plexus, with very rare exceptions, appear to have only one long, axon-like process[4]. There are many Dogiel type II neurons with a process that extends to the mucosa and other processes that run circumferentially within the myenteric plexus. Our ultrastructural investigations indicate that the processes of Dogiel type II neurons make synapses on the majority of other neurons in the myenteric plexus, which in turn implies that these neurons influence the excitability of most other neurons. Some of the neurons on which the type II neurons synapse are probably interneurons, via which reflexes are transmitted orally and aborally, while others might be motor neurons to the muscle if there are local monosynaptic reflexes[18].

Nishi and North[7] and Hirst et al.[8] suggested that the AH (Dogiel type II neurons) are sensory because in the initial electrophysiological studies they appeared not to receive synaptic inputs. However, Wood and Mayer[23] discovered that groups of stimulus pulses could evoke slow synaptic potentials in these neurons and it is now agreed that this is so. Thus the present structural studies confirm that the Dogiel type II neurons, apparently in common with all other myenteric neurons, receive synaptic inputs. The presumed sensory neurons of the myenteric plexus therefore differ from the sensory neurons of spinal ganglia, which have no synapses on their cell bodies. For the spinal sensory neurons, modulation of sensory input can be at or close to their endings in the dorsal horns; for the myenteric sensory neurons a site of modulation is probably the cell body. It is interesting that synaptic inputs to the cell bodies of sensory neurons can be found in invertebrates[24]. Excitatory synaptic inputs to Dogiel type II/AH neurons act by the closure of calcium-dependent potassium channels. This has the effect of dramatically increasing the excitability of the cells and in particular decreasing the refractory period caused by the slow after-hyperpolarization. Thus the AH neurons are able to discharge action potentials at a greater rate when influenced by excitatory transmitter, and action potentials that would not otherwise traverse the cell body from an incoming process to an output process can do so[18]. The origins of the inputs that may modify the excitability of the Dogiel type II neurons remain to be determined, though many of them appear to come from local neurons in the myenteric plexus[25].

In conclusion, current evidence is consistent with earlier suggestions that the Dogiel type II neurons are sensory. Some of these neurons are probably involved in reflexes that arise from the mucosa and pass via the myenteric plexus to the muscle. The sensory neurons appear to be gated by their intrinsic properties, but this gating can be reduced by activity in excitatory inputs to the neurons.

Acknowledgements

This work was supported by a grant from the N.H. and M.R.C. (Australia) and a Fellowship to Sueli Pompolo from F.A.P.E.S.P. (Sao Paulo, Brazil).

We thank Michele Hoffman for help in typing the manuscript. We are grateful to Dr D.E.M. Lawson who kindly supplied the antiserum to calbindin used in this work.

References

1. Dogiel, A.S. (1986). Zwei Arten sympathischer Nervenzellen. *Anat. Anz.*, **11**, 679–89
2. Dogiel, A.S. (1899). Über den Bau der Ganglien in den Geflechten des Darmes und der Gallenblase des Menschen und der Saugetiere. *Arch. Anat. Physiol.*, Leipzig, Anat. Abteil., Jahrgang 1899, 130–58
3. Hodgkiss, J.P. and Lees, G.M. (1983). Morphological studies of electrophysiologically identified myenteric plexus neurons of the guinea-pig ileum. *Neuroscience*, **8**, 593–608
4. Furness, J.B., Bornstein, J.C. and Trussell, D.C. (1988). Shapes of nerve cells in the myenteric plexus of the guinea-pig small intestine revealed by the intracellular injection of dye. *Cell Tiss. Res.* **254**, 561–71
5. Bornstein, J.C., Costa, M., Furness, J.B. and Lees, G.M. (1984). Electrophysiology and enkephalin immunoreactivity of identified myenteric neurons of guinea-pig small intestine. *J. Physiol. (Lond.)*, **351**, 313–25
6. Katayama, Y., Lees, G.M. and Pearson, G.T. (1986). Electrophysiology and morphology of vasoactive intestinal peptide-immunoreactive neurones of the guinea-pig ileum. *J. Physiol. (Lond.)*, **378**, 1–11
7. Nishi, S. and North, R.A. (1973). Intracellular recording from the myenteric plexus of the guinea-pig ileum. *J. Physiol. (Lond.)*, **231**, 471–91
8. Hirst, G.D.S., Holman, M.E. and Spence, I. (1974). Two types of neuron in the myenteric plexus of the guinea-pig duodenum. *J. Physiol. (Lond.)*, **236**, 303–26
9. Furness, J.B., Keast, J.R., Pompolo, S., Bornstein, J.C., Costa, M., Emson, P.C. and Lawson, D.E.M. (1988). Immunocytochemical evidence for the presence of calcium-binding proteins in enteric neurons. *Cell Tiss. Res.*, **252**, 79–87
10. Iyer, V., Bornstein, J.C., Costa, M., Furness, J.B., Takahashi, Y. and Iwanaga, T. (1988). Electrophysiology of myenteric neurons immunoreactive for calcium binding proteins in the guinea-pig. *J. Autonom. Nerv. Syst.*, **22**, 141–50
11. Pompolo, S. and Furness, J.B. (1988). Ultrastructure and synaptic relationships of calbindin-reactive, Dogiel type II neurons, in myenteric ganglia of guinea-pig small intestine. *J. Neurocytol.* **17**, 771–82
12. Bornstein, J.C., Furness, J.B. and Costa, M. (1987). Sources of excitatory synaptic inputs to neurochemically identified submucous neurons of guinea-pig small intestine. *J. Autonom. Nerv. Syst.*, **18**, 83–91
13. Erde, S.M., Sherman, D. and Gershon, M.D. (1985). Morphology and serotonergic innervation of physiologically identified cells of guinea pig's myenteric plexus. *J. Neurosci.*, **5**, 617–33
14. North, R.A. (1982). Electrophysiology of the enteric neurons. In Bertacini, G. (ed.) *Mediators and Drugs in Gastrointestinal Motility I.* pp. 145–79. (Berlin: Springer)
15. Wood, J.D. (1981). Physiology of the enteric nervous system. In Johnson, L.R. (ed.) *Physiology of the Gastrointestinal Tract*, pp. 1–38. (New York: Raven Press)
16. North, R.A. and Nishi, S. (1974). Properties of the ganglion cells of the myenteric plexus of the guinea-pig ileum determined by intracellular recording. In Daniel, E.E. (ed.) *Proc. 4th Int. Symp. on Gastrointestinal Motility*, pp. 667–76. (Vancouver: Mitchell Press)
17. Wood, J.D. and Mayer, C.J. (1979). Serotonergic activation of tonic type enteric neurons in guinea pig small intestine. *J. Neurophysiol.*, **42**, 594–693
18. Furness, J.B. and Costa, M. (1987). *The Enteric Nervous System.* (Edinburgh: Churchill Livingstone)
19. Cook, R.D. and Burnstock, G. (1976). The ultrastructure of Auerbach's plexus in the guinea-pig. I. Neuronal elements. *J. Neurocytol.*, **5**, 171–94
20. Hukuhara, T., Yamagani, M. and Nakayama, S. (1958). On the intestinal intrinsic reflexes. *Jpn. J. Physiol.*, **8**, 9–20
21. Thomas, J.E. and Baldwin, M.V. (1971). The intestinal mucosal reflex in the unanaesthetized

dog. *Am. J. Dig. Dis.*, **16**, 642–7
22. Wilson, A.J., Llewellyn-Smith, I.J., Furness, J.B. and Costa, M. (1987). The source of nerve fibres forming the deep muscular and circular muscle plexuses in the small intestine of the guinea-pig. *Cell Tiss. Res.*, **247**, 497–504
23. Wood, J.D. and Mayer, C.J. (1978). Intracellular study of electrical activity in Auerbach's plexus in guinea-pig small intestine. *Pflüg. Archiv., Europ. J. Physiol.*, **374**, 265–75
24. Elekes, K. and Florey, E. (1987). New types of synaptic connections in crayfish stretch receptor organs: an electron microscopic study. *J. Neurocytol.*, **16**, 613–26
25. Bornstein, J.C., North, R.A., Costa, M. and Furness, J.B. (1984). Excitatory synaptic potentials due to activation of neurons with short projections in the myenteric plexus. *Neuroscience*, **11**, 723–31

6

Identification of vagal and submucosal inputs to the myenteric plexus by retrograde and anterograde transport

A. L. KIRCHGESSNER AND M. D. GERSHON

Uniquely among regions of the PNS, the enteric nervous system (ENS) can mediate reflex activity in the absence of input from the CNS[1,2]. In fact, the number of efferent axons in the subdiaphragmatic vagus nerves is known to be extremely small and is much smaller than the number of neurons in the bowel[3,4]. It is thus clear that the ENS must contain intrinsic primary afferent neurons that are responsible for its autonomy. These neurons evidently link sensory receptors, which have been demonstrated to lie in the mucosa, with motor neurons that reside in the myenteric plexus and are responsible for excitation or inhibition of the smooth muscle of the muscularis externa[5,6,7]. Nevertheless, despite the relative independence of the ENS, the CNS is able to affect gastrointestinal motility. It has been postulated that it does so by vagal activation of command neurons[8]. These putative cells are thought to activate preprogrammed enteric circuits that are responsible for the response of the bowel to vagal stimulation. Through the activation of command neurons, therefore, the small number of vagal axons could have a profound effect on the output of the gut. Neither the intrinsic primary afferent neurons nor the vagal terminals on the putative command neurons have been identified. The submucosal plexus is known to innervate the mucosa[2], where enteric sensory receptors are located, and pseudo-unipolar and bipolar submucosal neurons that resemble DRG neurons and neurons in organs of special sense have been described[5,9]. It has thus been proposed that at least some of the intrinsic enteric primary afferent neurons of the bowel are located in the submucosal plexus. Nevertheless, no submucosal to myenteric projections, which are critical to the supposition that there are submucosal primary afferent neurons, have been found. In order to determine whether such projections exist, the submucosal plexus was examined following the microinjection of a retrograde tracer (Fluoro-Gold[10,11] or 4-acetoamido, 4'-

isothiocyanostilbene-2,2'-disulphonic acid[11,12]) into single myenteric ganglia. In addition, the myenteric plexus was studied following the iontophoretic injection of an anterograde tracer (*Phaseolus vulgaris* leucoagglutinin[11,13,14]; PHA-L) into single submucosal ganglia.

MATERIALS AND METHODS

Male guinea-pigs ($\sim$500 g) were stunned and exsanguinated. The small intestine was removed, the lumen was washed with Krebs solution and the tissue was transferred to a beaker containing fresh oxygenated Krebs solution. A piece of ileum (10 cm long) was opened and pinned flat. For the injections of tracers, the mucosa was removed and the tissue was superfused in a chamber on the stage of an inverted microscope with nifedipine-containing Krebs solution at 37°C. Ganglia were visualized using differential interference contrast optics and were injected from the bevel/led tip of a glass micropipette[11]; 2.5–3.0 h were allotted for retrograde, and 20–24 h (under culture conditions) for anterograde, transport. Fluoro-Gold and SITS were ejected from the micropipettes with pressure, but PHA-L was injected iontophoretically using a 5 μA positive (cathodal) current for 5 min. Preparations were then fixed, dissected into layers containing the enteric plexuses, and examined as whole mounts by fluorescence microscopy or, for PHA-L, by immunocytochemistry.

PHA-L was injected iontophoretically (7 μA for 45 min) into the dorsal motor nuclei of the vagus (DMX) of 15 female rats (200–250 g). PHA-L (2.5%) was injected uni- or bilaterally using a micropipette with a tip diameter of 30–50 μm. The injections were made at the level of the caudal tip of the area postrema, 0.3 mm lateral to the midline at a depth of 0.8–0.6 mm below the dorsal surface of the medulla. The muscle layers and skin were approximated and closed with silk sutures. The animals were allowed to survive for 10–21 days postoperatively to allow time for anterograde transport. Rats were killed with an overdose of sodium pentobarbital (100–mg/kg) and perfused transcardially with 100 ml of 0.9% saline followed by 300 ml of a fixative solution consisting of 4% (w/v) formaldehyde (from paraformaldehyde) in 0.1 M phosphate buffer (pH 7.4). The subdiaphragmatic oesophagus, stomach and small intestine were removed and placed immediately into a beaker of oxygenated Krebs solution at 37°C. Some animals were injected with colchicine (5 mg/kg; ip) the day before they were killed in order to enhance the immunocytochemical detection of neuropeptides in nerve cell bodies. Vibratome sections (50 μm) of the brainstem were cut in the coronal plane and collected in phosphate-buffered saline (PBS).

For immunocytochemistry, whole mounts of tissue were first incubated with 4% (v/v) normal goat serum in phosphate-buffered saline (PBS) for 30 min (to reduce non-specific background staining). Normal goat serum (4%) and 1.0% Triton-X 100 (to enhance penetration of the immunoreagents) were added to all subsequent solutions containing antisera. The preparations were then exposed to goat anti-PHA-L serum (Vector Laboratories) for 24–48 h at 4°C. After washing with PBS, the whole mounts were incubated for

3 h with biotinylated rabbit anti-goat IgG (Kirkegaard and Perry; diluted 1:400). The whole mounts were then incubated for 1 h with avidin conjugated to fluorescein isothiocyanate (FITC; diluted 1:200; Vector Labs.), washed and mounted in buffered 50% glycerol (pH 9.0), containing 0.4 mg/ml of p-phenylenediamine[15]. Sites of immunoreactivity were visualized by vertical fluorescence microscopy using a Leitz 'L$_2$' filter cube (exciting filter BP 450-490; dichroic mirror RKP 510, barrier filter BP 525/20). Biotinylated secondary antibodies were also localized with alkaline phosphatase-labelled avidin (diluted 1:400, incubated for 24 h at 4°C; Vector Labs.). The alkaline phosphatase-labelled avidin was visualized in tissues by using an alkaline phosphatase substrate kit (Vector Labs.; Kit III) in the presence of 10 mM MgCl$_2$ and 1 mM levamisole (Sigma Chemical Co.). To identify the neurons apparently contacted by PHA-L-labelled fibres, neuropeptides or 5-HT were simultaneously examined by immunocytochemistry along with PHA-L. The two antigens were sequentially immunostained using primary antisera raised in different species in combination with species-specific secondary antisera. Whole mounts were incubated for the immunohistochemical demonstration of transported PHA-L using FITC-labelled avidin as described above, followed by incubation overnight (at 4°C) with antisera raised in rabbits against vasoactive intestinal polypeptide (VIP; diluted 1:800; kindly supplied by Dr Gajanan Nilaver), galanin (GAL; diluted 1:1000; Milab, Sweden), tyrosine hydroxylase (TH; diluted 1:500; Eugene Tech), 5-HT (diluted 1:100; Amac) or enkephalin (ENK; diluted 1:250; Milab, Sweden [this antiserum does not distinguish between leucine and methionine enkephalins]). Affinity-purified tetramethylrhodamine isothiocyanate (TRITC)-labelled anti-rabbit secondary antibody (diluted 1:100; Jackson Immuno Research Labs.) was then applied for 3 h at room temperature. A Leitz 'N$_2$' filter/dichroic mirror cube (exciting filter BP 530-560; dichroic mirror RKP 580; barrier filter LP 580) was used to detect TRITC fluorescence. There was no cross detection between the FITC ('L$_2$') and TRITC ('N$_2$') selective dichroic mirror-filter cubes.

RESULTS AND DISCUSSION

In the myenteric plexus, Fluoro-Gold injection sites (Figure 1) were found to be restricted to a portion of a single ganglion, although some spread of the tracer beyond the confines of the injected ganglion occurred. A small number of the neurons of the injected ganglion were fluorescent and additional neurons in distant myenteric ganglia (predominantly orad) were also retrogradely labelled. About 5–6 submucosal neurons deep to, but not directly underneath, the injected myenteric ganglion contained Fluoro-Gold and only rarely was there more than one labelled neuron in a submucosal ganglion (Figure 2). When control injections of Fluoro-Gold were placed into the muscle instead of a ganglion, some myenteric neurons near the injection site became fluorescent; however, there was no labelling of neurons in the submucosal plexus. These observations suggest that the circular muscle of the guinea-pig intestine is innervated by myenteric, but not submucosal

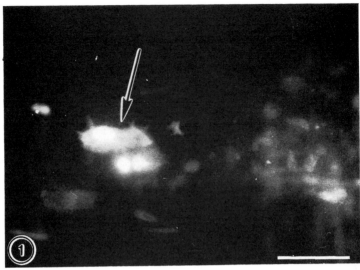

Figure 1 Fluoro-Gold injected into a single ganglion of the myenteric plexus of the small intestine. Note that neurons at some distance from the site of injection (→) have become fluorescent and that there are no fluorescent neurons between these cells and the injection site. Some smooth muscle cells outside the injected ganglion fluoresce and glial fluorescence can also be discerned within the injected ganglion. Note that Fluoro-Gold fluorescence can be seen in both the cytoplasm and the nucleus of the labelled cells. Scale bar = 50 μm. (From Kirchessner and Gershon, 1989)

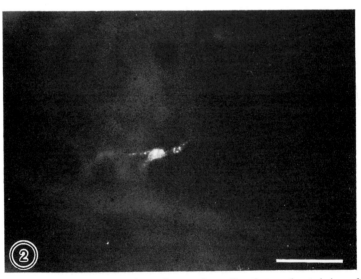

Figure 2 Fluorescence of a neuron in a submucosal ganglion that was located circumferential to the myenteric ganglion injected with Fluoro-Gold. Note the punctate cytoplasmic fluorescence. Scale bar = 50 μm. (From Kirchgessner and Gershon, 1989)

ganglion cells. A further control showed that, if connections between the myenteric and submucosal plexuses were severed by dissection before injecting Fluoro-Gold into myenteric ganglia, no submucosal neurons became labelled. Similar results were obtained following the microinjection of SITS into individual myenteric ganglia and when Fluoro-Gold injections were made in the proximal colon. The results of retrograde labelling thus support the hypothesis that submucosal ganglia project to the myenteric plexus.

Confirmation that submucosal to myenteric projections exist was achieved by injecting individual submucosal ganglia with the anterograde tracer, PHA-L. Following injection of PHA-L into a single submucosal ganglion all of the neurons of that ganglion were filled by the tracer (Figure 3). Anterograde movement of PHA-L was made evident by its accumulation proximal to the points of transection of axons damaged during the dissection (Figure 4). In addition, small-diameter boutons were labelled in ~ 2 myenteric ganglia (Figures 5 and 6), as well as in several distant submucosal ganglia (intrasubmucosal projections were bidirectional, but predominantly descending). Additional labelled fibres travelled with blood vessels or surrounded mucosal crypts.

The neurons of the DMX that project to the gut were located by retrograde transport following the injection of Fluoro-Gold into the rat's stomach. To localize the enteric terminals of the vagi, PHA-L was injected bilaterally by iontophoresis into the DMX of the rat. The region injected with PHA-L corresponded to that found to be labelled by retrograde transport of Fluoro-Gold. In the DMX PHA-L filled neurons; these cells sent axonal projections (Figure 7) out of the brain in the roots of the vagus nerves. Vagal terminal axons, labelled with PHA-L could be followed for very long distances in the stomach and small intestine (Figure 8). The fibres were more numerous in the stomach than in the small intestine, although labelled vagal axons could be visualized as far distally as the terminal ileum. Vagal efferent axons were extremely few in number (Figures 8 and 9), entered a minority of ganglia (Figure 9) and contacted a minority of the neurons within these ganglia (Figure 10). The fibres tended to travel in bundles and to send off individual varicose terminal axons that entwined around unlabelled ganglion cells (Figure 11). No PHA-L-labelled vagal efferent fibres were found in the submucosal plexus in the muscular layers of the gut or in the mucosa.

Preliminary data obtained with double label immunocytochemical techniques suggest that neurons in the myenteric plexus that are contacted by vagal efferents are more likely to contain VIP or 5-HT, than enkephalin or galanin, because vagal efferent terminals were identified that appeared to contact VIP- and 5-HT-, but not enkephalin- or galanin-immunoreactive neurons. Nevertheless, by light microscopy it is not possible to establish with certainty whether or not apparent contacts are actually synapses; therefore, until vagal efferent terminals are identified by electron microscopy in material in which peptides or other neurotransmitters are simultaneously demonstrated, it will be impossible to be certain about the identity of the neurons upon which vagal efferent fibres synapse. Some, but not all, of the vagal preganglionic fibres contained galanin immunoreactivity, although none appeared to be TH-immunoreactive. The TH-immunoreactive axons

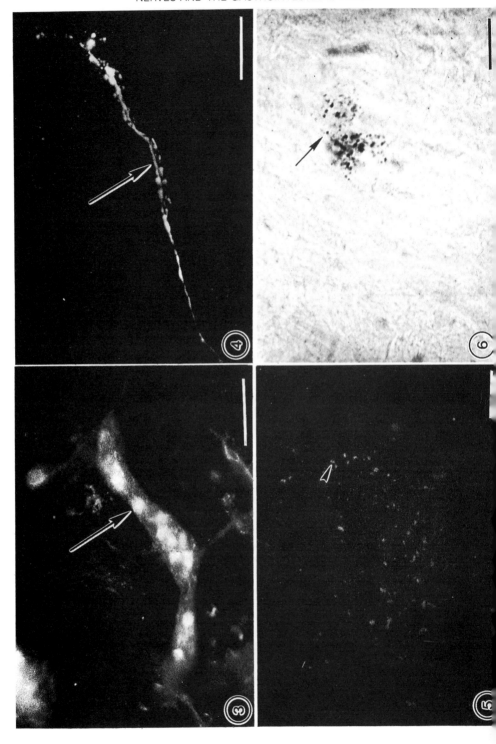

Figures 3–6 Anterograde labelling and filling of neurons following injection of PHA-L into a single ganglion of the submucosal plexus. **Figure 3**: Note that some neurons (→) within the ganglion are completely filled with PHA-L. **Figure 4**: A single varicose axon in the submucosal plexus filled with PHA-L (→) can be followed to its end, which was severed during the dissection. Note the accumulation of PHA-L at the cut end, indicative of anterograde transport of PHA-L. Scale bars = 50 μm. **Figure 5**: Anterograde labelling in the myenteric plexus following injection of PHA-L into a single ganglion of the submucosal plexus. Scattered small fluorescent terminal varicosities surround non-labelled neurons in a myenteric ganglion. **Figure 6**: PHA-L immunoreactivity visualized with a biotinylated secondary antiserum and avidin-alkaline phosphatase. The appearance of the labelled terminals (→) is similar to that seen with immunofluorescence. Scale bars = 10 μm. (From Kirchgessner and Gershon, 1988)

in the rat's vagus nerves may thus be mainly, if not entirely, derived from the superior cervical ganglion[16–19], even though TH-immunoreactive cells have been found in the DMX[19,20]. The role of galanin in vagal preganglionic axons is unclear; however, it is possible that galanin is co-stored in these fibres with acetylcholine and acts as a co-transmitter or neuromodulator at some vagal synapses with enteric neurons.

The failure to detect vagal preganglionic axons in the submucosal plexus following injection of PHA-L into the DMX may indicate that submucosal ganglion cells receive no direct input from the DMX. Since the DMX does evoke secretomotor responses in the bowel[21] and secretomotor neurons are known to reside in the submucosal plexus[2] (see also Bornstein *et al.*, abstract, this volume) a vagal innervation of submucosal ganglia was expected. Many

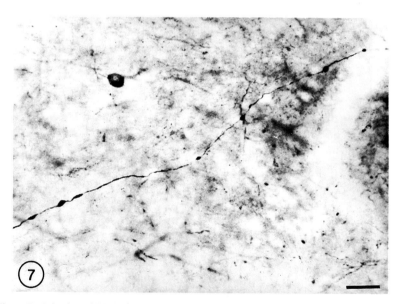

Figure 7 Injection of PHA-L into the DMX. PHA-L immunoreactivity demonstrated with a biotinylated secondary antiserum and avidin-alkaline phosphatase. A single labelled fibre passes from the DMX through the ventrolateral reticular formation to leave the brain in the roots of the vagus nerve. Scale bars = 50 μm

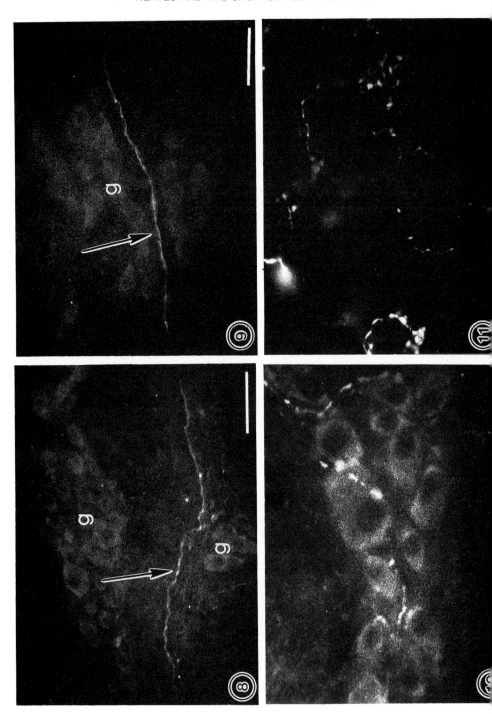

Figures 8–11 Immunofluorescence of vagal terminal axons in the myenteric plexus of the stomach and ileum. **Figure 8**: A vagal fibre ($\rightarrow$) coursing through the myenteric plexus of the rat stomach. The fibre passes between two ganglia (g). **Figure 9**: A vagal fibre ($\leftarrow$) coursing through the myenteric plexus of the rat ileum. The fibre passes along an apparent tract that bifurcates a myenteric ganglion (g). **Figure 10**: Individual PHA-L-labelled vagal fibres have peeled off a bundle and given rise to varicose terminals that contact a minority of the neurons of a gastric myenteric ganglion. **Figure 11**: Individual PHA-L-labelled varicose vagal fibres appear to form rings around unlabelled ganglion cells in a gastric myenteric ganglion. Scale bars = 50 μm

myenteric neurons project to the submucosal plexus[2]; therefore, it is possible that vagal effects on submucosal neurons are relayed via myenteric ganglia. A radioautographic study of the distribution of vagal fibres in the rat gut following the injection of ³H-leucine into the DMX has previously been reported[22]. In this investigation the resolution of the radioautographic technique and use of sectioned material did not permit the numbers of labelled fibres or innervated cells to be discerned. Labelling was reported of myenteric ganglia as far distally as the colon; no mention was made of labelling of submucosal ganglia. The observations that submucosal neurons do, in fact, project to the myenteric plexus are consistent with the hypothesis that at least some of the intrinsic enteric primary afferent neurons of the bowel reside in the submucosal plexus. This hypothesis is further supported by reports that some submucosal neurons receive little or no synaptic input[23] (Bornstein *et al.*, this volume). None of these observations rules out the possibility that there may also be myenteric neurons that function as primary afferents (Pompolo *et al.*, Chapter 5, this volume). The findings that vagal efferent fibres are relatively rare in comparison to intrinsic axons of the enteric plexuses and contact only a small number of neurons in a subset of myenteric ganglia are consistent with the suggestion that the vagi activate command neurons in particular myenteric ganglia.

Acknowledgements

This work was supported by National Institutes of Health grants NS 12969 and NS 07062. During part of the time the work was conducted Annette Kirchgessner was a Pharmacology-Morphology fellow of the Pharmaceutical Manufacturer's Association Foundation.

References

1. Gershon, M.D. (1981). The enteric nervous system. *Annu. Rev. Neurosci.*, **4**, 227–72
2. Furness, J.B. and Costa, M. (1987). *The Enteric Nervous System.* (New York: Churchill Livingstone)
3. Langley, J.N. (1921). *The Autonomic Nervous System. Pt.* 1. (Cambridge: Heffer)
4. Hoffman, H.H. and Schnitzlein, H.N. (1969). The number of vagus nerves in man. *Anat. Rec.*, **139**, 429–35
5. Bülbring, E., Lin, R.C.Y. and Schofield, G. (1958). An investigation of the peristaltic reflex in relation to anatomical observations. *Q. J. Exp. Physiol.*, **43**, 26–37

6. Kosterlitz, H.W. and Lees, G.M. (1964). Pharmacological analysis of intrinsic intestinal reflexes. *Pharmacol. Rev.*, **16**, 301–39

7. Kosterlitz, H.W. (1968). Intrinsic and extrinsic nervous control of motility of the stomach and intestine. In Code, C.F. (ed.) *Handbook of Physiology. Sect. 6, Alimentary Canal, Vol. 4, Motility*, pp. 2147–71. (Washington DC: Am. Physiol. Soc.)

8. Wood, J.D. (1987). Physiology of the enteric nervous system. In Johnson, L.R. (ed.) *Physiology of the Gastrointestinal Tract, Vol.* 1, pp. 67–109. 2nd edn. (New York: Raven Press)

9. Schofield, G. (1968). Anatomy of muscular and neural tissues in the alimentary canal. In Code, E.F. (ed.) *Handbook of Physiology, The Alimentary Canal*, Vol. 4, pp. 1579–1628. (Washington DC: American Physiological Society)

10. Schmued, L.C. and Fallon, J.H. (1986). Fluoro-Gold: a new fluorescent retrograde axonal tracer with numerous unique properties. *Brain Res.*, **377**, 147–54

11. Kirchgessner, A.L. and Gershon, M.D. (1988). Projections of submucosal neurons to the myenteric plexus of the guinea pig intestine: *In vitro* tracing of microcircuits by retrograde and anterograde transport. *J. Comp. Neurol.* **277**, 487–98

12. Takaki, M., Wood, J.D. and Gershon, M.D. (1985). Heterogeneity of ganglia of the guinea pig myenteric plexus: An in vitro study of the origin of terminals within single ganglia using covalently bound fluorescent retrograde tracer. *J. Comp. Neurol.*, **235**, 488–502

13. Gerfen, C.R. and Sawchenko, P.E. (1984). An anterograde neuroanatomical tracing method that shows the detailed morphology of neurons, their axons and terminals: Immunohistochemical localization of an axonally transported plant lectin, *Phaseolus vulgaris* leucoagglutinin (PHA-L). *Brain Res.*, **290**, 219–38

14. Gerfen, C.R. and Sawchenko, P.E. (1985). A method for anterograde axonal tracing of chemically specified circuits in the central nervous system: combined *Phaseolus vulgaris* leucoagglutinin (PHA-L) tract tracing and immunohistochemistry. Brain Res., **343**, 144–50

15. Johnson, G.D. and de C. Nogueira Araujo, G.M. (1981). A simple method of reducing the fading of immunofluorescence during microscopy. *J. Immunol. Meth.*, **43**, 349–50

16. Ahlman, H., Lundberg, J., Dahlström, A. and Kewenter, J. (1976). A possible vagal adrenergic release of serotonin from enterochromaffin cells in the cat. *Acta Physiol. Scand.*, **98**, 366–75

17. Muryobayashi, T., Mori, J., Fujiwara, M. and Shimamoto, K. (1968). Fluorescence histochemical demonstration of adrenergic nerve fibers in the vagus nerve of cats and dogs. *Jpn. J. Pharmacol.*, **18**, 285–93

18. Nielsen, K.C., Owman, C.H. and Santini, M. (1969). Anastomosing adrenergic nerves from the sympathetic trunk to the vagus at the cervical level in the cat. *Brain Res.*, **12**, 1–9

19. Blessing, W.W., Willoughby, J.O. and Joh, T.H. (1985). Evidence that catecholamine-synthesizing perikarya in rat medulla oblongata do not contribute axons to the vagus nerve. *Brain Res.*, **348**, 397–400

20. Kahlia, M., Fuxe, K., Goldstein, A. and Harfstrand, A. (1984). Evidence for the existence of dopamine-, adrenaline-, and noradrenaline-containing vagal motor neurons in the brainstem of the rat. *Neurosci. Lett.*, **50**, 57–62

21. Kerr, F.W.L. and Preshaw, R.M. (1969). Secretomotor function of the dorsal motor nucleus of the vagus. *J. Physiol.*, **205**, 405–15

22. Connors, N.A., Sullivan, J.M. and Kubb, K.S. (1983). An autoradiographic study of the distribution of fiber from the dorsal motor nucleus of the vagus to the digestive tube of the rat. *Acta Anat.*, **115**, 266–71

23. Surprenant, A. (1984). Two types of neurones lacking synaptic input in the submucous plexus of guinea-pig small intestine. *J. Physiol.* (*Lond.*), **351**, 363–78

24. Pompolo, S. and Furness, J.B. (1988). Ultrastructure and synaptic relations of myenteric Dogiel type II neurons revealed by immunoreactivity for calcium binding protein (CaBP) in the guinea pig ileum. *This volume*

7
Electrophysiological characteristics of guinea-pig myenteric plexus neurons immunoreactive for dynorphin A(1–8)

G. M. LEES, D. J. LEISHMAN AND G. T. PEARSON

INTRODUCTION

As their name was intended to convey, the dynorphin series of neuropeptides, derived from prodynorphin, have potent agonist actions at opioid receptors in intestinal preparations *in vitro*[1,2,3]. Furthermore, since dynorphin A(1–8) may act as an endogenous ligand for the κ-subtype of opioid receptor[3], this neuropeptide is likely to be one of the most important members of this family.

Nevertheless, information concerning the origin, location, and pharmacological activities of pro-enkephalin-derived peptides in the gastrointestinal tract has eclipsed that of prodynorphin-derived neuropeptides. Indeed, only a few short reports have been published on the occurrence of dynorphin-like immunoreactivity in enteric nerves and cell bodies of myenteric and submucous plexuses[4–8]. To our knowledge, no detailed information has been published about the types of myenteric plexus neurons (or processes) in which dynorphin A(1–8) is localized. Since the precursor molecules for the enkephalin and dynorphin series need not occur in the same neuron[9,10], we wished to compare and contrast the characteristics of neurons showing dynorphin A(1–8)-like immunoreactivity (Dyn-IR) with those containing pro-enkephalin-derived peptides[11,12,13].

In order to determine the electrophysiological characteristics of Dyn-IR neurones, it was necessary to mark the cells from which recordings were made, so that they could be identified unequivocally after subjecting the tissue to standard immunohistochemical procedures for revealing neuropeptide immunoreactivity[12,14]. Moreover, for successful correlations to be made, certain criteria (Table 1) had to be satisfied. The dye used was Lucifer Yellow, which has previously been shown to be both a reliable fluorescent marker

Table 1 Requisites for reliable cross-correlations

1.	Unequivocal identification of recorded neurone
2.	Adequate staining to reveal soma morphology and location of principal proceses
3.	Unequivocal characterization of properties for electrophysiological classification
4.	Satisfactory immunohistochemical characterization

and a satisfactory agent for demonstrating the morphology of enteric neurons[12,14-16]. In addition, Lucifer Yellow is ionized in aqueous solution and in certain solutions of electrolytes; thus, the dye itself can be used as an electrolyte in the solution filling the intracellular micropipette for the purposes of electrical recording. Furthermore, this dye is compatible with the required fluorescence immunohistochemical methods.

METHODS

Male albino guinea-pigs (weighing 180–310 g) were killed by a blow to the head and bled out. Segments (5–10 cm long) of ileum were isolated from the small intestine, at least 10 cm from the ileocaecal valve and the luminal contents gently flushed out with warmed Krebs solution (35–37°C) of the following composition (mM): NaCl 118, KCl 4.75, $CaCl_2$ 2.54, $MgSO_4$ 1.2, NaH_2PO_4, 1.15, $NaHCO_3$ 25.0, glucose 11.1. This solution was thoroughly gassed with 95% O_2 and 5% CO_2. To reduce spontaneous movements and to prevent stimulus-evoked contractions of the smooth muscle, the solution also contained nifedipine (0.5 μM) and hyoscine (2 μM).

The segments were opened along their mesenteric borders and pinned flat under light tension on a bed of Sylgard, mucosal side uppermost. As previously described[14], the mucosa, submucosa and circular muscle layers were gently stripped off to expose the myenteric plexus, which remained adherent to the underlying longitudinal muscle. Preparations were viewed in transmitted and incident (reflected) light. Neurons were impaled under direct visual control and intracellular recordings were made from myenteric plexus neurons with glass micropipettes filled with a solution of Lucifer Yellow CH (0.5% w/v) dissolved in 0.5 M KCl, as previously described[14]. Signals were displayed on an oscilloscope and a Gould two-channel pen recorder and most were simultaneously stored on tape for subsequent analysis.

Nerve fibres within the myenteric plexus were stimulated transmurally by means of pairs of platinum wire electrodes placed above and below the preparation towards the oral and anal ends of the segment. The preparation could also be stimulated via a movable focal microelectrode (tip dia. 7–12 μm) filled with 0.16 M NaCl. Stimuli were usually 0.5 ms in duration and were delivered either as single shocks or as volleys consisting of 5–30 pulses at 1–10 Hz.

Hyperpolarizing current pulses (0.02–0.2 nA, 100 ms duration at 1 Hz) passed through the recording electrode were usually sufficient to stain the impaled neuron, in addition to providing electrotonic potentials for testing the input impedance of the neuron in question. Once a neuron had been successfully stained and characterized electrophysiologically, its position in the ganglion was noted, as well as the location of that ganglion in relation to others and any landmarks. These checks were necessary in order to reidentify the neuron after fixation and the immunohistochemical procedures[12,14].

The anti-dynorphin antisera were raised in rabbits and were obtained from Peninsula (Europe) Ltd under the numbers IFK-8697, RAS-8697N and 61022. Incubation of these antibodies with pure peptides (1.0–10 μM) showed that the immunoreactivity was lost with dynorphin A(1–8), slightly suppressed with dynorphin A(1–9) but not detectably reduced with dynorphin A(1–11) or longer fragment, nor with the heptadecapeptide, dynorphin A, itself. It was also not inhibited following incubation with either the pro-enkephalin-derived peptides, [Met]- and [Leu]-enkephalin, [Met]-enkephalyl-Arg-Phe and [Met]enkephalyl-Arg-Gly-Leu or the unrelated peptides, vasoactive intestinal peptide and substance P. Thus, the anti-dynorphin A(1–8) antibodies have a very high degree of selectivity. Moreover, they were routinely used at dilutions of 1:800 and colchicine pretreatment was unnecessary for the detection of Dyn-IR in neuron somata or processes. Dyn-IR was never found in preparations that had been exposed to either the second (fluorescently labelled) antibody alone or the second antibody (anti-rabbit) after the latter had been exposed to rabbit serum. Similar checks were made for the anti-enkephalin antibody, NOC 1, a mouse monoclonal antibody which recognizes principally [Leu]enkephalin.

Full details of the methods used to distinguish the fluorescence of Lucifer Yellow from the specific immunoreactivity of a neuropeptide, as revealed by rhodamine fluorescence, have already been published[12,14].

RESULTS

For this investigation, the electrophysiological classification of Hirst, Holman and Spence[17] was adopted. This categorization is based on easily identified events, namely fast excitatory post-synaptic potentials (EPSPs) and membrane hyperpolarization following the firing of a single-action potential. Those neurons that receive fast EPSPs are called S neurons; in such cells there is only a brief undershoot following the soma action potential. In contrast, the hallmark of the other broad class, the AH neuron, is a longlasting after-hyperpolarization (typically 5–20 s) associated with an increase in membrane conductance. According to this classification AH neurons do not show fast EPSPs. Neurons which could not be assigned unequivocally to either of these two types were excluded from the study.

A total of 113 myenteric plexus neurons from 18 preparations were successfully studied for Dyn-IR both electrophysiologically and immuno-histochemically. In 83 of these, transmural or focal electrical stimulation with single pulses elicited one or more fast EPSPs (Figure 1); depolarization of these cells by current passed through the recording electrode resulted in the firing of one or more action potentials, which were not followed by a

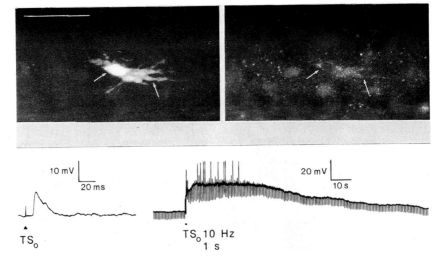

Figure 1 Morphological and electrophysiological properties of a dynorphin-immunoreactive S neuron of guinea-pig myenteric plexus. **Upper panels:** left, fluorescence photomicrograph of neuronal morphology revealed by Lucifer Yellow injected intracellularly; right, rhodamine immunofluorescence in an area corresponding exactly to the soma of the stained neuron. Calibration: 50 μm. **Lower panel:** intracellular electrophysiological records from the same neuron as shown above. Left, fast excitatory post-synaptic potentials evoked in the neuron by transmural electrical stimulation (one pulse) on the oral side of the neuron at a distance of 5 mm (TS_o); right, slow excitatory post-synaptic potential and spontaneous firing of action potentials in the neuron due to transmural electrical stimulation at 10 Hz for 1 s. Downward vertical lines are electrotonic potentials due to the passage of constant current pulses (0.05 nA for 100 ms at 1 Hz) through the recording electrode, across the soma membrane, to test changes in input resistance of the cell. Resting membrane potential was -65 mV. Action potentials limited in amplitude by frequency response of pen recorder

longlasting after-hyperpolarization. Thus, they all had the features of S-neurons. The remainder (30) were indisputably AH neurons.

Dyn-IR was unequivocally detected in 54/83 S neurons (Figure 1). As was found for enkephalin-immunoreactive myenteric plexus neurons[12,13], every Dyn-IR S neuron that was stained adequately to reveal its morphology (53/54 neurons) had a single long process and a soma with numerous stubby

Table 2 Opioid peptide-immunoreactivity of S neurons of the guinea-pig myenteric plexus

Opioid peptide	Antibody	No. of S neurons studied	Percentage immunoreactive	Reference
Dyn A(1–8)	IFK-8697 RAS-8697N	83	65	Lees et al. Titisee, 1988
Enk	NOC 1	56	30	Lees et al. Titisee, 1988
Enk	RM 198 B	102	31	Katayama et al.[13]
Enk	RM 198 B	50	30	Bornstein et al.[12]

processes, i.e. Dogiel type I morphological features[12,14] (Figure 1). AH neurons had smooth somata with several long processes and none showed Dyn-IR (Figure 2).

In contrast, a parallel study of 71 myenteric plexus neurons, 17 S neurons showed enkephalin-like immunoreactivity (Enk-IR). In confirmation of previous observations, Enk-IR was found to be confined to S neurons but

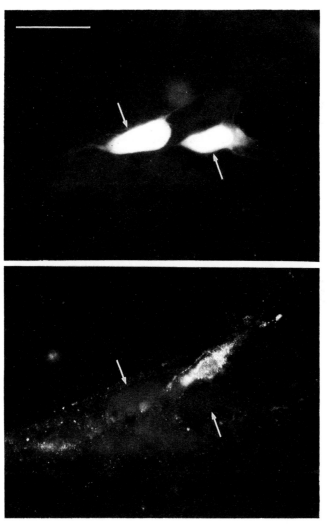

Figure 2 Lack of dynorphin-immunoreactivity of two Dogiel type II neurons stained with Lucifer Yellow. **Upper panel,** Fluorescence photomicrograph of two neurons stained with Lucifer Yellow and showing smooth somata and long processes; these cells were typical of AH neurons of myenteric plexus. **Lower panel,** rhodamine fluorescence indicative of immunoreactivity for dynorphin A(1–8) in a neighbouring neuron. Note the absence of immunoreactivity in the two stained cells. Caibration: 50 μm.

the proportion (17/56 cells; 30%) of all S neurons was lower than that for Dyn-IR (65%) (Table 2).

In 30/36 Dyn-IR neurons and 7/7 Enk-IR neurons tested, non-cholinergic slow EPSPs were elicited in response to transmural or focal volley stimulation. There was no preferred orientation of either the fast or slow EPSPs in Dyn- or Enk-IR neurons (Figure 3).

DISCUSSION

The most striking finding of this study was the very high proportion of S neurons showing Dyn-IR (65%) compared to that containing Enk-IR (Table 2). The proportion of S neurons with Enk-IR has been consistently about 30%, despite the proven excellence of the anti-enkephalin antibodies used for fluorescence immunohistochemistry. The difference could be due to one or other of several factors.

First, if all neurons containing pro-enkephalin-derived peptides also contained pro-dynorphin-derived peptides and vice versa, then one would have to conclude that our observed differences in the proportions of S neurons were spurious. It could be, for example, that enkephalin-immunoreactivity is much more susceptible to distortion or suppression as a result of intracellular recording than is Dyn-IR; alternatively, they might be equally susceptible but dynorphin A(1–8) may be less easily released from the somata under the conditions of stimulation and recording.

On the other hand, the difference may be genuine, since there is no *a priori* reason why pro-dynorphin and pro-enkephalin should coexist in the same neurons[9]. In favour of there being a greater number of Dyn-IR than Enk-IR neurons, are the immunohistochemical observations of Costa, Furness and Cuello[10]. These authors adduced evidence for at least four populations of opioid peptide containing neuron, two of which showed both Dyn- and Enk-IR. From their estimates of the size of these populations, one would

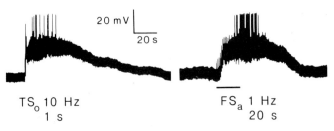

Figure 3 Slow excitatory post-synaptic potentials (intracellular recording) in a myenteric plexus S neuron showing immunoreactivity to dynorphin A(1–8). Left, slow excitatory post-synaptic potential (EPSP) and spontaneous firing of action potentials induced by transmural electrical stimulation at 10 Hz for 1 s at a distance of about 4 mm orally (TS_o). Right, slow EPSP and associated action potentials induced in the same neuron by focal stimulation of an interganglionic connecting strand at 1 Hz for 20 s at a distance of about 70 μm on the anal side of the neuron (FS_a). Resting membrane potential: left -65 mV, right -62 mV. Action potentials limited in amplitude by frequency response of pen recorder

expect to have a considerably greater chance of recording electrophysiologically from a Dyn-IR neuron (S neuron) than from an Enk-IR neuron. Immunohistochemical studies in our laboratory supports the view that the total population of Dyn-IR neurons is probably larger. We have, however, been unable to distinguish neurons with Dyn-IR or Enk-IR on the basis of their electrophysiological properties or their synaptic connections.

As has previously been found[12,13], AH neurons did not show Enk-IR. It is therefore interesting that Dyn-IR could not be detected in AH neurons.

In view of the large numbers of neurons that are likely to contain dynorphin A(1–8) and the richness of their fast and slow excitatory synaptic inputs, it seems likely that Dyn-IR neurons constitute an important population of myenteric plexus neurons.

Acknowledgements

Our thanks to Mrs Margaret J. Gray for invaluable technical support. This investigation was supported by the Medical Research Council and the SmithKline (1982) Foundation. DJL is a Medical Faculty Endowment Scholar of the University of Aberdeen.

References

1. Goldstein, A., Tachibana, S., Lowney, L.T., Hunkapiller, M. and Hood, L. (1979). Dynorphin-(1–13); an extraordinarily potent opioid peptide. *Proc. Natl. Acad. Sci. USA*, **76**, 6666–70
2. James, I.F., Fischi, W. and Goldstein, A. (1984). Opioid receptor selectivity of dynorphin gene products. *J. Pharmacol. Exp. Ther.*, **288**, 88–93
3. Corbett, A.D., Paterson, S.J., McKnight, A.T., Magnan, J. and Kosterlitz, H.W. (1982). Dynorphin 1–8 and dynorphin 1–9 are ligands for the κ subtype of opiate receptor. *Nature*, **299**, 79–81
4. Watson, S.J., Akil, H., Ghazarossian, V.E. and Goldstein, A. (1981). Dynorphin-immunocytochemical localization in brain and peripheral nervous system: Preliminary studies. *Proc. Natl. Acad. Sci. US*, **78**, 1260–68
5. Vincent, S.R., Dalsgaard, C.-J., Schultzberg, M., Hokfelt, T., Christensson, I. and Terenius, L. (1984). Dynorphin-immunoreactive neurons in the autonomic nervous system. *Neuroscience*, **11**, 973–84
6. Furness, J.B. and Costa, M. (1987). *The Enteric Nervous System*, 1st edn, (Edinburgh: Churchill Livingstone)
7. Costa, M., Furness, J.B. and Gibbins, I.L. (1986). Chemical coding of enteric neurons. In Hokfelt, T., Fuxe, K. and Pernow, B. (eds.) *Progress in Brain Research*, **68**, p. 217. (Amsterdam: Elsevier)
8. Lees, G.M., Leishman, D.J. and Pearson, G.T. (1988). Dynorphin A (1–8)-immunoreactivity in the guinea-pig and rat isolated small intestine. *J. Physiol.*, **403**, 65p
9. Khachaturian, H., Lewis, M.E. and Watson, S.J. (1983). Colocalization of pro-enkephalin peptides in rat brain neurones. *Brain Res.*, **279**, 369–73
10. Costa, M., Furness, J.B. and Cuello, A.C. (1985). Separate populations of opioid-containing neurones in the guinea-pig intestine. *Neuropeptides*, **5**, 445–8
11. Furness, J.B., Costa, M. and Miller, R.J. (1983). Distribution and projections of nerves with enkephalin-like immunoreactivity in the guinea-pig small intestine. *Neuroscience*, **8**, 653–64
12. Bornstein, J.C., Costa, M., Furness, J.B. and Lees, G.M. (1984). Electrophysiology and enkephalin immunoreactivity of identified myenteric plexus neurones of guinea-pig small intestine. *J. Physiol.*, **351**, 313–25

13. Katayama, Y., Lees, G.M. and Pearson, G.T. (1986). Electrophysiological and morphological similarities between myenteric plexus neurones showing immunoreactivity to enkephalin (ENK) and vasoactive intestinal peptide (VIP) in guinea-pig isolated ileum. *J. Physiol.*, **378**, 101P

14. Katayama, Y., Lees, G.M. and Pearson, G.T. (1986). Electrophysiology and morphology of vasoactive-intestinal-peptide-immunoreactive neurones of the guinea-pig ileum. *J. Physiol.*, **378**, 1–11

15. Bornstein, J.C., Costa, M. and Furness, J.B. (1986). Synaptic inputs to immunohistochemically identified neurones in the submucous plexus of guinea-pig small intestine. *J. Physiol.*, **381**, 465–82

16. Bornstein, J.C., Costa, M. and Furness, J.B. (1987). Sources of excitatory synaptic inputs to neurochemically identified submucous neurons of guinea-pig small intestine. *J. Autonomic Nerv. Syst.*, **8**, 83–91

17. Hirst, G.D.S., Holman, M.E. and Spence, I. (1974). Two types of neurones in the myenteric plexus of duodenum in the guinea-pig. *J. Physiol.*, **236**, 303–26

8
Relationship of gallbladder ganglia to the enteric nervous system: structure, putative neurotransmitters and direct neural connections

G. M. MAWE AND M. D. GERSHON

The structure and chemistry of the enteric nervous system (ENS) differ from those of the remainder of the peripheral nervous system[9,12]. Like the central nervous system, the ENS is supported by glia, rather than by Schwann cells[2,4,11,16,18], and lacks internal collagen and basal laminae[1,11]. Although the gallbladder originates as an outgrowth of the fetal gut, its innervation differs from that of the bowel in that the guinea-pig gallbladder has one, rather than two ganglionated plexuses[3]; nevertheless, it is not yet clear whether the intrinsic ganglia of the gallbladder are structurally and functionally like those of the ENS or whether, instead, they resemble extraenteric autonomic ganglia. Moreover, the possibility that communication between the gut and the gallbladder may be mediated by nerves, as well as by the endocrine release of hormones, such as cholecystokinin, has not previously been established or eliminated.

The current study of the guinea-pig gallbladder was undertaken in order to determine whether the structure and neurochemical characteristics of the ganglia of the gallbladder are analogous to those of the ganglia of the ENS and whether the gallbladder receives a direct afferent innervation from neurons in the duodenum. To evaluate the structural and neurochemical similarities between the ganglia of the gallbladder and those of the bowel, markers were selected for characteristics of enteric ganglia that are unique to the ENS. These markers included the immunocytochemical demonstration of laminin and 5-HT. Laminin is present in the basal lamina that surrounds enteric ganglia but, like collagen and basal laminae, laminin is not found within the ganglia themselves[1]. In contrast, laminin is abundant inside all other peripheral ganglia. 5-HT, an enteric neurotransmitter[13,15], is found in the cell bodies of neurons of the myenteric pleus[5,8], but not in extraenteric parasympathetic ganglia. In addition several other neuropeptides that are present in the ENS, as well as tyrosine hydroxylase (TH) and dopamine β-hydroxylase (DBH), which are not present in small intestinal ganglia[9] were also studied. To determine whether neurons in the duodenum project to the gallbladder, tracers were injected into the wall of the gallbladder and the duodenum was examined for the presence of neurons labelled by retrograde transport of the markers.

METHODS

Male guinea-pigs were stunned by a blow to the head and exsanguinated. In some experiments chemical sympathectomy was done by injecting animals subcutaneously with 6-hydroxydopamine (6-OHDA; 100 mg/kg). This dose of 6-OHDA destroys extrinsic sympathetic terminal axons in the ENS[14]. Whenever chemical sympathectomy was done, its effectiveness was verified by immunostaining TH (see below) in the bowel. Only rare, non-varicose preterminal sympathetic axons remained on following administration of 6-OHDA, and these could often be traced to swollen retraction bulbs, indicative of destruction of the terminal arborizations of the fibres. For the immunocytochemical examination of the gallbladder, the organ was removed, opened, pinned out (mucosal side up) and fixed for 2 h with a solution containing 4% formaldehyde (from paraformaldehyde) in 0.1 M sodium phosphate buffer at pH 7.4. The fixed tissues were processed as whole mounts or frozen and sectioned (at 10 μm) in a cryostat-microtome. Whole mounts or sections on slides were then permeabilized with 0.2% Triton X-100 for 30 min and incubated with primary antisera at appropriate dilutions in phosphate buffered saline (0.1 M; PBS) containing 4% normal horse serum and Triton X-100 for 24–48 h at 4°C. Controls were exposed to normal serum of the appropriate species and processed with the experimental tissue. After removal of the primary antibody, sections were washed and incubated for 1 h, either with species-specific secondary antibodies labelled with fluorescein isothiocyanate (FITC) or Texas Red, or with biotinylated species-specific secondary antibodies followed by avidin-Texas Red. Sections were mounted with a medium that contained 0.1% p-phenylenediamine in 90% glycerol buffered with 10% sodium bicarbonate (pH 9.0). Texas Red was visualized by fluorescence microscopy using a Leitz 'N$_2$' filter cube (exciting filter BP 530-560; dichroic mirror RKP 580; barrier filter LP 580; no FITC fluorescence is passed by this filter/mirror combination). FITC was visualized with a Leitz 'L$_2$' narrow band filter cube (exciting filter BP 450-490; dichroic mirror RKP 510, barrier filter BP 525/20; no Texas Red fluorescence is visible through this filter/mirror combination). Selection of primary antibodies raised in different species in combination with species-specific secondary antibodies and contrasting fluorophores permitted the simultaneous detection of two antigens in the same tissue sections. Primary immune reagents included: rabbit anti-laminin sera (Collaborative Research, Bedford, MA); rabbit anti-vasoactive intestinal polypeptide (VIP; from Dr. Gajanan Nilaver of the

University of Oregon); rabbit anti-TH sera (Eugene Tech, Allendale, NJ); rabbit anti-DBH serum (Eugene Tech); mouse monoclonal antibodies to microtubule associated protein II (MAP 2; from Dr. Kenneth Kosik); rat monoclonal antibodies to substance P (Seralabs); rabbit anti-calcitonin gene-related peptide (CGRP; Peninsula). For the demonstration of 5-HT immunoreactivity tissue was pretreated *in vitro* with 5,7-dihydroxytrypta-mine[5] (5,7-DHT). When this was to be done, chemical sympathectomy was always performed with 6-OHDA 24 h prior to removal of the gallbladder so that 5,7-DHT would not be taken up non-specifically by sympathetic axons. In some experiments tissue was pretreated *in vitro* with colchicine[10] (1 mg/ml; for 12–24 h) in order to increase the intrasomatic concentration of neuropeptides.

In order to inject the gallbladder with a retrograde tracer, adult male guinea-pigs were anaesthetized with Ketamine (50 mg/kg) and xylazine (5 mg/kg). The abdomen was opened and the gallbladder was exposed. Access to the gallbladder was facilitated by cutting the mesenteries that attach it to the anterior peritoneal lining. Fluoro-Gold (4.0% in isotonic saline; Fluorochrome, Inc., Englewood, CO) or wheatgerm agglutinin coupled to horseradish peroxidase (WGA-HRP; 1.0% in isotonic saline; Sigmal Chemical Co, St. Louis, MO) were injected in a volume of 1.0 μl/injection into the wall of the gallbladder. Ten injections were made in each gallbladder. For controls, in three animals, the cystic duct was ligated prior to injection of tracer, and in three additional cases 10 injections of the tracers were placed on the peritoneal surface of the gallbladder near the duodenum. Cases in which Fluoro-Gold or WGA-HRP were found in the duodenum in a pattern that mimicked that obtained with control injections of the tracers were discarded.

Forty-eight hours after injection of tracer, animals were anesthetized and perfused through the heart with 100 ml of saline. The gallbladder, cystic duct, duodenum, stomach and proximal jejunum were removed and stretched flat prior to fixation with 4% formaldehyde in 0.1 M sodium phosphate buffer (pH 7.4). The remaining carcass of the animals was then perfused with 300 ml of the same fixative and was used for the study of the extraenteric sources of innervation of the gallbladder. Tissues were frozen, sectioned and mounted on glass slides. Tissues from animals injected with Fluoro-Gold were examined by vertical fluorescence microscopy using a Leitz 'A' cube (wide band ultraviolet excitation filter; excitation: 323 nm, emission: 408 nm). Tissues from animals in which WGA-HRP had been injected were processed as described by Mesulam[17] to locate sites of peroxidase activity with tetramethylbenzidine (TMB). In order to visualize unlabelled neurons, the sections were counterstained with 1.0% neutral red before dehydration. The TMB reaction product was visualized with both darkfield and differential interference contrast optics.

RESULTS AND DISCUSSION

Laminin and MAP 2 immunoreactivities were demonstrated simultaneously in the same tissue sections. MAP 2 is limited in its distribution to the cell bodies and dendrites of neurons; therefore, it facilitates the recognition of ganglia and the delineation of ganglionic boundaries in sections examined by fluorescence microscopy. The MAP II-immunostained areas, corresponding to the ganglia of the gallbladder, were devoid of laminin immunoreactivity. However, laminin immunoreactivity was found in a distinct line around the perimeter of the ganglia. These observations imply that, as is true of the myenteric plexus, there are no basal laminae (and thus no connective tissue) within the ganglia of the gallbladder. On the other hand these ganglia, again like those of the myenteric plexus, are probably surrounded by a periganglionic basal lamina that is rich in laminin.

5-HT immunoreactivity was found in whole-mount preparations in a large number of varicose fibres within the confines of gallbladder ganglia and in the interganglionic fibre tracts. Moderate 5-HT immunoreactivity was also seen in small cell bodies that were present in about 30% of the ganglia. 5-HT can be taken up non-specifically by noradrenergic axons in the gut[7]. To determine whether anti-5-HT serum immunostained noradenergic axons that remained following chemical sympathectomy and that had non-specifically taken up 5-HT (or the 5,7-DHT used in the demonstration of 5-HT immunoreactivity[5]), TH and 5-HT immunoreactivities were simultaneously demonstrated in the same whole mounts of the wall of the gallbladder. There was little or no overlap of the two antigens. The 5-HT-immunoreactive gallbladder neurites, therefore, are not noradrenergic axons. Moreover, unlike noradrenergic axons, but like the serotonergic neurons of the bowel, the 5-HT-immunoreactive gallbladder neurites evidently fail to take up 6-OHDA. The gallbladder, therefore, in common with the ENS, contains intrinsic serotonergic elements.

Substance P, CGRP, and VIP immunoreactivities were also found in the ganglionated plexus of the gallbladder. Substance P immunoreactivity was seen in the ganglia and interganglionic connectives and also in paravascular nerve bundles that accompanied large blood vessels (Figure 1). The distribution of CGRP (Figure 2) was very similar to that of substance P. CGRP-immunoreactive fibres were found in ganglia, interganglionic connectives, and the paravascular nerve bundles. When tissue was immunostained to demonstrate substance P and CGRP simultaneously in the same whole mounts, an extensive overlap in the distribution of fibres and varicosities was observed, implying that there is extensive coincident expression of substance P and CGRP in the wall of the gallbladder. In contrast to substance P and CGRP, VIP immunoreactivity was limited in its distribution to the ganglia and interganglionic connectives of the gallbladder and was not seen in association with blood vessels. VIP immunoreactivity was present in intrinsic gallbladder neurons as well as in varicose nerve processes.

NPY immunoreactivity was found in both neuronal perikarya and fibres in the ganglionated plexus of the gallbladder and in many perivascular nerve fibres. Two types of neural plexuses were found external to the large arteries of the gallbladder wall. One, a perivascular plexus, consisted of a dense, surrounding network of apparently interconnecting varicose fibres that completely encircled the vessels. The other, the paravascular nerve bundles mentioned above, did ot fully encircle the vessels but were grouped into

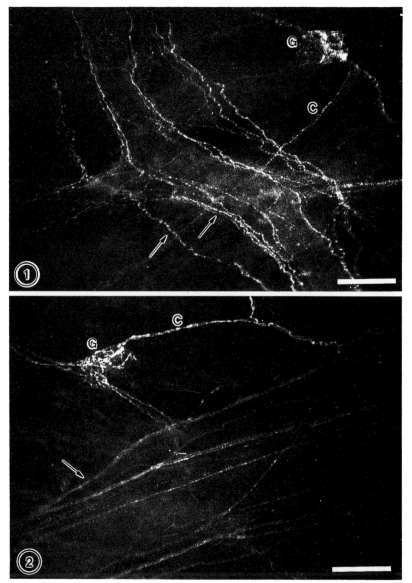

Figures 1 and 2 Substance P and CGRP immunoreactivities in the wall of the gallbladder. **Figure 1**: Substance P immunoreactivity in a gallbladder ganglion (G) and in loose, non-varicose, paravascular bundles of nerves (→) following the path of large arteries. Substance P immunoreactivity is also found in connectives (C) of the ganglionated plexus. The marker = 50 μm. **Figure 2**: CGRP immunoreactivity in a gallbladder ganglion (G) and in loose, non-varicose, paravascular bundles of nerves (→) following the path of large arteries. CGRP immunoreactivity is also found in connectives (C) of the ganglionated plexus. The marker = 50 μm

relatively thick bundles of non-varicose fibres that adjoined the arteries. Interconnections were much less common between paravascular nerve bundles than between fibres participating in the perivascular plexuses. The presence of NPY immunoreactivity in perivascular nerves suggested that these fibres might be sympathetic axons. NPY is known to be present in sympathetic axons in the gut[9]. In order to determine to what extent the NPY innervation of the gallbladder wall was derived from extrinsic sympathetic ganglia chemical sympathectomy was done with 6-OHDA. After administration of 6-OHDA, no NPY immunoreactivity was detectable in perivascular nerves in the gallbladder; therefore, perivascular NPY-immunoreactive nerve fibres in the wall of the gallbladder are probably entirely of sympathetic origin. NPY immunoreactivity persisted in neurons and fibres of the ganglionated plexus of the gallbladder, even after the destruction of sympathetic axons had been accomplished with 6-OHDA; consequently, the bulk of the NPY immunoreactivity in the ganglionated plexus is probably derived from intrinsic NPY-immunoreactive neurons of the plexus itself.

TH immunoreactivity, like that of NPY, was found in the ganglia and interganglionic connectives of the ganglionated plexus, and could also be seen in perivascular nerves. In contrast to either the submucosal or myenteric plexuses of the small intestine, which have no intrinsic TH-immunoreactive neurons, TH immunoreactivity was present in small cell bodies in the ganglionated plexus of the gallbladder. These cells were not numerous; usually there were no more than 1–3 cells per ganglion. After administration of 6-OHDA, TH immunoreactivity was virtually abolished from perivascular nerves and fewer TH-immunoreactive fibres were present in the ganglionated plexus; nevertheless the number of TH-immunoreactive perikarya within the ganglia increased dramatically (to about 5–7 cells per ganglion). These observations confirm that perivascular TH-immunoreactive nerve fibres are of sympathetic origin. However, the presence of intrinsic TH-immunoreactive cells and TH-immunoreactive fibres that are resistant to 6-OHDA in the ganglionated plexus indicates that the guinea-pig gallbladder, unlike the small intestine, contains intrinsic catecholaminergic neurons. In this respect, the ganglionated plexus of the gallbladder resembles the myenteric plexus of the guinea-pig proximal colon, which also contains a small number of intrinsic catecholaminergic neurons[6].

The reason for the increase in the number of TH-immunoreactive neurons in gallbladder ganglia after administration of 6-OHDA is not immediately apparent. At least two possibilities might be envisioned. A failure of axonal transport of TH might occur, leading to accumulation of TH in cell bodies, if the terminal arborizations of intrinsic catecholaminergic neurons were destroyed by 6-OHDA. The accumulation of TH in perikarya might, in turn, cause more of these cells to be detected by immunocytochemistry. Alternatively, the loss of a putative sympathetic neural input to intrinsic gallbladder neurons, as a result of administration of 6-OHDA, might induce an increase in the expression of TH within the denervated cells. Cai and Gabella[3] reported small intensely fluorescent cells in the gallbladder when they treated tissue with glyoxylic acid. The observations of glyoxylic acid-induced histofluorescence and TH immunoreactivity in small cells within gallbladder ganglia indicates that intrinsic catecholaminergic cells are present in the organ. The resistance of at least some of the TH-immunoreactive fibres of the ganglionated plexus to 6-OHDA suggests, but does not prove, that the catecholaminergic cells are neurons and not SIF cells. It remains to be demonstrated what catecholamine these cells contain.

In order to determine whether the TH-immunoreactive cells in gallbladder ganglia have the ability to synthesize norepinephrine (NE), the distribution of DBH immunoreactivity in the gallbladder was analysed. DBH-immunoreactive nerve fibres were found in ganglia, interganglionic connectives and in perivascular nerves. DBH immunoreactivity was also present in neurons in gallbladder ganglia; however, these neurons were more numerous and much larger than the cells of the gallbladder ganglia that displayed TH immunoreactivity. DBH and TH immunoreactivities were simultaneously demonstrated in the same whole-mount preparations in order to ascertain whether they were coexpressed in the same cells. An overlapping distribution of DBH- and TH-immunoreactive fibres and varicosities was observed, but the two antigens were not found in the same perikarya (Figures 3 and 4). The gallbladder ganglia thus contain two distinct populations of cells, one of which expresses TH immunoreactivity and the other of which is DBH-immunoreactive. The lack of DBH in the small intrinsic TH-immunoreactive cells in gallbladder ganglia indicates that the catecholamine responsible for the glyoxylic acid-induced histofluorescence of these cells is probably dopamine. The role of DBH in the larger neurons in gallbladder ganglia is unclear. Since the neurons have never been demonstrated to contain an endogenous catecholamine, it is by no means certain that the enzyme is catalytically active.

The second aim of this study was to determine whether neurons in the duodenum project to the gallbladder. To accomplish this we used the retrograde tracers, WGA-HRP or Fluoro-Gold. When either of these tracers was injected into the wall of the gallbladder neurons were found to be labelled in the myenteric plexus of the duodenum near the ampulla of Vater. In addition, neurons were found to be labelled by retrograde transport in the celiac ganglion as well as bilaterally in the nodose, and thoracic (T_5-T_{11}) dorsal root ganglia and the dorsal motor nuclei of the vagus. Transganglionic labelling by WGA-HRP was also detected in the nucleus of the solitary tract. The extrinsic innervation of the gallbladder ganglia is thus derived from the bowel, in addition to dorsal root and vagal sensory, sympathetic postganglionic and parasympathetic preganglionic neurons. These observations lend further support to the idea that the ganglionated plexus of the gallbladder should be viewed as analogous to, and perhaps an extension of, the ENS.

SUMMARY AND CONCLUSIONS

In their lack of internal basal laminae, and their containing serotonergic neurons, ganglia of the gallbladder are similar to the ganglia of the ENS

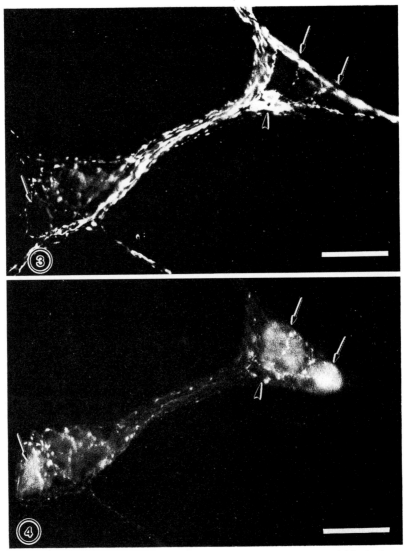

Figures 3 and 4 Simultaneous demonstration of TH and DBH immunoreactivities in the same whole mounts of the wall of the gallbladder. **Figure 3**: TH immunoreactivity (Texas Red immunofluorescence) in two interconnected ganglia of the gallbladder. The ganglia at the upper right contains a cluster of three TH-immunoreactive cells ( ), while the ganglion at the lower left contains none. Varicose TH-immunoreactive fibres are also prominent in the connectives (c) of the ganglionated plexus. The position of cells that contain DBH immunoreactivity (not fluorescent in this illustration; compare with Figure 4) are shown by the (→). The marker = 20 μm. **Figure 4**: DBH immunoreactivity (FITC immunofluorescence) demonstrated simultaneously in the same field as that shown in Figure 3. The same two ganglia are illustrated. Many large neurons can be seen that contain DBH immunoreactivity (→). These neurons are not TH-immunoreactive (compare with Figure 3). The neurons that can be observed in Figure 3 to have TH immunoreactivity are not DBH-immunoreactive (   )

and dissimilar to extraenteric autonomic ganglia. Like enteric ganglia, gallbladder ganglia also contain a variety of intrinsic peptidergic neurons including those demonstrated by antibodies to NPY, VIP, and substance P.

Neurons in ganglia of the myenteric plexus of the duodenum, near the ampulla of Vater, project to the gallbladder. Other extrinsic neural projections are received from the dorsal motor nuclei of the vagus (parasympathetic preganglionic), the celiac (sympathetic postganglionic), nodose (sensory) and thoracic dorsal root (sensory) ganglia.

Gallbladder ganglia are analogous to and perhaps extensions of the ENS.

Gallbladder ganglia differ from ganglia of the small intestine in that they contain intrinsic catecholaminergic cells that display TH immunoreactivity and DBH-immunoreactive neurons that contain neither TH nor a catecholamine. Chemical sympathectomy with 6-OHDA increases the number of detectable TH-immunoreactive cells in gallbladder ganglia, although it destroys sympathetic postganglionic axons in perivascular nerves. The mechanism underlying this response to chemical sympathectomy remains to be determined.

Acknowledgements

The study was supported by NIH grants 12969, NS 07062, NS 26995 and a grant from the PMAF.

References

1. Bannerman, P.G., Mirsky, R., Jessen, K.R., Timpl, R. and Duance, V.C. (1986). Light microscopic immunolocalization of laminin, type IV collagen, nidogen, heparan sulphate proteoglycan and fibronectin in the enteric nervous system of the rat and guinea-pig. *J. Neurocytol.*, **15**, 733–43
2. Björklünd, H., Dahl, D. and Seiger, A. (1984). Neurofilament and glial fibrillary acid protein-related immunoreactivity in rodent enteric nervous system. *Neuroscience*, **12**, 277–87
3. Cai, W. and Gabella, G. (1983). Innervation of the gallbladder and biliary pathways in the guinea-pig. *J. Anat.*, **136**, 97–109
4. Cook, R.D. and Burnstock, G. (1976). The ultrastructure of Auerbach's plexus in the guinea-pig. I. Neuronal elements. *J. Neurocytol.*, **5**, 171–94
5. Costa, M., Furness, J.B., Cuello, A.C., Verhofstad, A.A.J., Steinbusch, H.W.J. and Elde, R.P. (1982). Neurons with 5-hydroxytryptamine-like immunoreactivity in the enteric nervous system: Their visualization and reactions to drug treatment. *Neuroscience*, **7**, 351–63
6. Costa, M. and Furness, J.B. (1971). Storage, uptake and synthesis of catecholamines in the intrinsic adrenergic neurons of the proximal colon of the guinea-pig. *Z. Zellforsch.*, **120**, 364–85
7. Drakontides, A.B. and Gershon, M.D. (1972). Studies of the interaction of 5-hydroxytryptamine (5-HT) and the perivascular innervation of the guinea pig caecum. *Br. J. Pharmacol.*, **45**, 417–34
8. Dreyfus, C.F., Bornstein, M.B. and Gershon, M.D. (1977). Synthesis of serotonin by intrinsic neurons of the myenteric plexus grown in organotypic tissue culture. *Brain Res.*, **128**, 125–39
9. Furness, J.B. and Costa, M. (1987). *The Enteric Nervous System.* (New York: Churchill Livingstone)
10. Furness, J.B., Costa, M. and Keast, J.R. (1984). Choline acetyltransferase and peptide immunoreactivity of submucous neurons in the small intestine of the guinea-pig. *Cell Tissue*

Res., **237**, 329–36

11. Gabella, G. (1987). Structure of muscles and nerves in the gastrointestinal tract. In Johnson, L.R. (ed.) *Physiology of the Gastrointestinal Tract*, 2nd Edn. New York, Raven Press, pp. 335–82

12. Gershon, M.D. (1981). The enteric nervous system. *Annu. Rev. Neurosci.*, **4**, 227–72

13. Gershon, M.D. (1982). Enteric serotonergic neurons. In Osborne, N. (ed.) *Biology of Serotonin Transmission*, pp. 363–99. (Chichester: John Wiley)

14. Gershon, M.D. and Sherman, D.L. (1987). Noradrenergic innervation of serotoninergic neurons in the myenteric plexus. *J. Comp. Neurol.*, **259**, 193–210

15. Gershon, M.D., Mawe, G.M. and Branchek, T.A. (1988). 5-Hydroxytryptamine and enteric neurons. In Fozard, J.R. (ed.) *Peripheral Actions of 5-hydroxytryptamine* (In press)

16. Jessen, K.R., Thorpe, R. and Mirsky, R. (1984). Molecular identity, distribution and heterogeneity of glial fibrillary acidic protein: an immunoblotting and immunohistochemical study of Schwann cells, satellite cells, enteric glia and astrocytes. *J. Neurocytol.*, **13**, 187–200

17. Mesulam, M.-M. (1978). Tetramethylbenzidine for horseradish peroxidase neurohistochemistry: a non-carcinogenic blue reaction product with superior sensitivity for visualizing neural afferents and efferents. *J. Histochem. Cytochem.*, **26**, 106–17

18. Rothman, T.P., Tennyson, V.M. and Gershon, M.D. (1986). Colonization of the bowel by the precursors of enteric glia: studies of normal and congenitally aganglionic mutant mice. *J. Comp. Neurol.*, **252**, 493–506

9
Neurophysiology of the gastric myenteric plexus

M. SCHEMANN AND J. D. WOOD

INTRODUCTION

The intrinsic nervous system of the gut has a primary role in the control of gastrointestinal functions[1,2]. Interconnected neural networks in the myenteric and submucosal plexuses are determinants of organized behaviour of effector systems such as the musculature[1,2] and the mucosal epithelium[3,4]. Electrophysiological investigation of the intrinsic nervous system has led to the emergence of several new concepts relative to the neurophysiology of control of the effector systems. It has become clear that the occurrence of motor patterns of behaviour such as the migrating motor complex and the peristaltic and segmental movements, as well as the co-ordinated spatiotemporal relations of intestinal contractions are dependent upon functional circuits in the intrinsic nervous system.

Patterns of motor and secretory behaviour that are unique to the stomach appear also to reflect operation of intramural neuronal circuits. Nevertheless, unlike the small and large intestines, too little has been known about the cellular neurophysiology of neurons in the stomach to permit development of neurophysiological theories of gastric behaviour. The stomach is a highly specialized region of the gastrointestinal tract, where it is likely that corresponding specialization of neural control will be reflected by neuronal electrical and synaptic properties different from those found in the enteric nervous system of the intestine. This was the motivation for the studies described in this chapter. These studies had the overall aim of determining the electrophysiological behaviour of myenteric neurons of the stomach in order to obtain baseline information for comparison with the better known properties of intestinal myenteric neurons.

GENERAL METHODS

The electrical and synaptic behaviour of myenteric neurons in the corpus of the guinea-pig were investigated with intracellular recording methods. Access to the gastric myenteric plexus was gained by dissecting away the mucosa and overlying muscle layers to expose the plexus on the mucosal side of the longitudinal muscle layer. Conventional methods of intracellular recording and current injection with electronic bridge circuits were used[5]. Focal electrical stimulation of the interganglionic connectives or ganglionic surface was used to evoke synaptic responses in the cell bodies of the ganglion cells. Putative neurotransmitters/neuromodulators were applied either by pressure microejection from fine-tipped pipettes or by addition to the superfusion solution. Other drugs, for example receptor blocking agents, were usually added to the superfusion solution.

MORPHOLOGY

The histoanatomy of the gastric myenteric plexus of the guinea-pig was found to be significantly different from the myenteric plexus of the small intestine. In the small intestine myenteric plexus, the ganglia are elongate and oriented with their long axes around the circumference[6]; whereas, the gastric ganglia were stellate with six to eight connectives projecting from the ganglia in all directions. Impalements were made in cell bodies located within the ganglia.

ELECTRICAL BEHAVIOUR

Three subtypes of ganglion cells were identified and classified as Gastric I, Gastric II and Gastric III neurons based on their electrophysiological behaviour (Figure 1). About 50% of 287 neurons belonged to the Gastric I category, about 30% were Gastric II and about 20% belonged to the Gastric III group.

Gastric I neurons were characterized by repetitive spike discharge throughout intrasomatic injection of depolarizing current pulses of 100 ms duration. Gastric II neurons discharged only one action potential at the onset of the 100 ms depolarizing pulses. Repetitive discharge, as observed in Gastric I neurons, never occurred in the Gastric II cells. Gastric III neurons were the least excitable of the three types and never discharged action potentials to depolarizing current injection regardless of the strength of the pulse. The Gastric III neurons were characterized also by larger resting membrane potentials and lower input resistance than the other two neuronal types (Table 1).

There is also an electrophysiological basis for classification of myenteric ganglion cells in the small intestine of the guinea pig[1,7,8]. (Table 1). S/Type 1 neurons discharge repetitively during longlasting depolarizing current injection. They show anodal-break excitation at the offset of hyperpolarizing current injection and are considered to be the most excitable of the small intestinal neurons. Spikes in these neurons are blocked by tetrodotoxin. The repetitive discharge of Gastric I neurons is similar to this kind of behaviour for the S/Type 1 neurons; however, the Gastric I neurons do not consistently

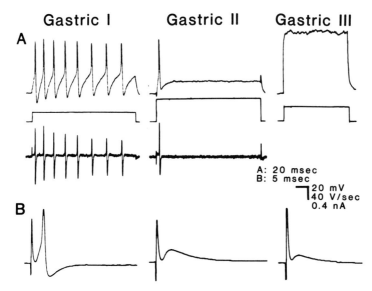

Figure 1 Electrical behaviour of gastric neurons. **A** Gastric I neurons discharged repetitively during depolarizing current pulses. Gastric II neurons discharged a single spike only at the onset of depolarizing current pulses. Gastric III neurons did not discharge spikes in response to depolarizing current. Upper trace is transmembrane voltage, middle trace is injected current and lower trace is dV/dT. **B** Focal electrical stimulation of interganglionic fibre tracts evoked fast EPSPs in all gastric neurons. Highest safety factor for EPSP-evoked spikes was found in Gastric I neurons. Gastric III neurons had smallest amplitude and shortest duration EPSPs. Sharp vertical deflections represent stimulus artefacts

display the property of anodal-break excitation. Synaptic behaviour, as discussed below, does differ between S/Type 1 and Gastric I neurons.

AH/Type 2 small intestinal neurons are characterized by the following properties:

(1) discharge of only a single action potential at the onset of 100 ms duration depolarizing current pulses;

(2) larger resting potentials than S/type 1 neurons;

(3) lower input resistance than S/Type 1 neurons;

(4) absence of anodal-break excitation;

(5) tetrodotoxin-resistant action potentials;

(6) longlasting hyperpolarizing after-potentials of several seconds duration in association with the spikes.

No gastric neurons with this combination of properties were found. Gastric II neurons behaved similarly in discharging only a single spike at the onset of long duration depolarizing pulses. Nevertheless, the Gastric II neurons did not show longlasting hyperpolarizing post-spike potentials (Table 1).

Table 1 Comparative properties of intestinal and gastric myenteric neurons

Property	Small intestine	Stomach
Morphology	Circular orientation	Honeycombed-like meshwork
Cell types	S/Type 1	Gastric I
	AH type 2	Gastric II
	type 3	Gastric III
TTX insensitive spikes	Yes	No
After- hyperpolarization	Yes	No
ACH receptors	Nicotinic	Nicotinic
	Muscarinic	
Fast EPSPs	100% S type 1	100% Gastric I
	20% AH type 2	100% Gastric II
	100% type 3	100% Gastric III
Behaviour of Fast EPSPs		
Nicotinic	Yes	Yes
Run down	Yes	No
Safety factor	Low	High
Multiple inputs	+	+++
Spontaneous	+	+++
Presynaptic inhibition	Yes	No
Autoinhibition	Yes	No
Slow EPSPs	Yes	No
Slow IPSPs	Yes	No

There is a calcium component to the inward current during the rising phase of the action potential in AH/Type 2 intestinal neurons and this accounts for the resistance to blockade of the spikes by tetrodotoxin (Table 1). Elevation of intrasomal calcium during the spike leads to opening of calcium-dependent potassium channels, which account for the longlasting hyperpolarizing after-potentials. Action potentials in both Gastric I and II neurons were blocked by tetrodotoxin (Table 1). It appears that these neurons are like intestinal S/Type 1 neurons in that sodium is the principal inward charge carrier during the action potential. Absence of a calcium component in the currents of the action potential in gastric neurons accounts for absence of longlasting hyperpolarizing after-potentials in these neurons. Whether the gastric neurons possess calcium-dependent potassium channels is unknown.

The hyperpolarizing after-potentials in AH/Type 2 neurons function to prolong the relative refractory period and thereby limit the frequency at which the ganglion cell soma can discharge action potentials. No such mechanism exists in the gastric neurons, and this accounts in part for their ability to discharge spikes reliably to the high frequency fast synaptic input described below.

Intestinal Type III neurons have high resting membrane potentials, low input resistance and do not discharge spikes to injection of depolarizing current irrespective of the strength of the current. Focal electrical stimulation of interganglionic connectives evokes prominent nicotinic cholinergic fast excitatory postsynaptic potentials (EPSPs) in these neurons; although, the EPSPs never evoke spikes. Gastric III neurons behave in similar fashion, with the exception that the fast EPSPs in these neurons are less prominent relative to the fast EPSPs in the other two categories of gastric neurons.

SYNAPTIC BEHAVIOUR

Focal electrical stimulation of interganglionic connectives or focal stimulation applied to the surface of the ganglion, which contained the impaled neuron, evoked fast EPSPs in all gastric neurons (Figure 1; Table 1). The fast EPSPs always evoked spikes in the Gastric I neurons. This occurred with a high safety factor indicated by inability to prevent EPSP-evoked spikes even when the membrane was hyperpolarized to near the potassium equilibrium potential by injected current. The safety factor for EPSP-evoked spikes was intermediate in the Gastric II neurons; that is, all EPSPs did not evoke spikes and it was easier to prevent EPSP-evoked spikes by membrane hyperpolarization. Gastric III neurons did not discharge spikes during fast EPSPs and, therefore, had the lowest safety factor of the three groups of neurons.

Most of the gastric ganglion cells received fast inputs from all of the interganglionic connectives and from multiple axons within each individual connective. These inputs came from the oral, aboral and circumferential directions without any preferential direction for the inputs.

Spontaneously occurring fast EPSPs were observed in 30% of 287 gastric neurons and were of equal prevalence in the three types of cells. This is a much higher frequency of spontaneous inputs than is observed in small intestinal myenteric neurons, but compares with the proportion of neurons with spontaneous fast EPSPs in the large intestinal myenteric plexus of the guinea-pig[9].

Both spontaneous and stimulus-evoked fast EPSPs were blocked by hexamethonium (Figure 2). Application of acetylcholine by microejection evoked depolarizing responses in association with reduced input resistance that were similar to the fast EPSPs (Figure 2). These responses to acetylcholine were also blocked by hexamethonium. This suggests that the fast EPSPs in the gastric neurons, like fast EPSPs elsewhere in the gut's nervous system, are mediated by nicotinic cholinergic receptors.

Stimulus-evoked fast EPSPs in the intestinal myenteric plexus decrease in amplitude when evoked repetitively and this 'run-down' occurs at very low frequencies of stimulation of 0.1 Hz or less[7]. No synaptic 'run-down' resembling that in the intestinal myenteric plexus was ever observed in the gastric neurons (Table 1). The gastric fast EPSPs followed stimulus frequencies up to 80 Hz without any indications of the 'run-down' phenomenon.

The axons of the nicotinic synapses in the intestinal myenteric plexus possess a variety of presynaptic receptors that, when activated, suppress release of acetylcholine and thereby reduce the fast EPSPs. One type of presynaptic receptor on small intestinal axons is an M_2 muscarinic cholinergic receptor[10]. These receptors are involved in a negative feedback loop that results in autoinhibition of acetylcholine release as the neurotransmitter accumulates at the presynaptic receptor[11]. No evidence for presynaptic muscarinic receptors on axons of the gastric myenteric plexus was obtained in our study.

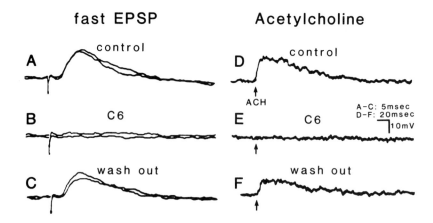

Figure 2 Synaptic behaviour of gastric neurons. **A** Control fast EPSP evoked by focal electrical stimulation of fibre tract. **B** Blockade of fast EPSP by hexamethonium (C_6, 200 μM). **C** Recovery of fast EPSP after washout of C_6. **D** Control microapplication of ACh. **E** Blockade of ACh response by C_6 (200 μM). **F** Recovery of ACh response after washout of C_6. Each record of A–C consists of two superimposed traces. Microejection pipette contained 1 mM ACh; duration of ejection pulse was 4 ms

Slow EPSPs

Focal electrical stimulation of interganglionic connectives in the intestinal myenteric plexus evokes slow synaptic potentials as well as fast EPSPs. These may be slow EPSPs or slow inhibitory postsynaptic potentials (IPSPs).

Slow EPSPs are slowly rising depolarizing responses associated with increased input resistance that last for several seconds or minutes. Dramatic augmentation of membrane excitability, together with suppression of hyper-polarizing after-potentials, often result in spike discharge at high frequency in trains that last for several seconds[1,2]. The functional significance of slow EPSPs appears to be a mechanism for longlasting activation or inhibition of effector responses. No slow EPSPs were evoked by focal electrical stimulation of the interganglionic connectives in the stomach.

Slow IPSPs in intestinal neurons are the inverse of slow EPSPs. They are prolonged hyperpolarizing potentials in association with decreased input resistance and suppression of excitability. No slow IPSPs were observed in response to focal stimulation of the interganglionic connections in the stomach.

CONCLUSION

The results of our initial study of the cellular neurophysiology of ganglion cells in the myenteric plexus of the gastric corpus of the guinea-pig revealed pronounced differences compared with the intestinal myenteric plexus of the same animal. This was not unexpected because the neural networks of the stomach must control and co-ordinate the behaviour of motor and secretory systems that are entirely different from the intestine. The differences between the neurophysiological behaviour of the gastric and intestinal myenteric plexuses undoubtedly reflect different adaptations for the specialized functions that are performed in each organ.

Acknowledgements

We thank our colleagues J. M. Palmer, K. Tamura and P. R. Wade for many fruitful discussions during the course of the study. They simultaneously conducted electrophysiological studies on the intestinal myenteric plexuses from the same guinea-pigs and their day-to-day results were important controls for the on the gastric neurons. The research was supported by National Institutes of Health Grant 5 RO1 DK37238 to J. D. Wood and Deutsche Forschungsgemeinschaft Fellowship Sche 267/1-1 and 267/1-2 to M. Schemann.

References

1. Wood, J. D. (1987). Physiology of the enteric nervous system. In Johnson, L.R. (ed.) *Physiology of the Gastrointestinal Tract*, 2nd Edn, pp. 67–109. (New York: Raven Press)
2. Wood, J.D. (1987). Neurophysiological theory of intestinal motility. *Jpn. J. Smooth Muscle Res.*, **23**, 143–86
3. Cooke, H.J. (1986). Neurobiology of the intestinal mucosa. *Gastroenterology*, **90**, 1057–81
4. Cooke, H.J. (1987). Neural and humoral regulation of small intestinal electrolyte transport. In Johnson, L.R. (ed.) *Physiology of the Gastrointestinal Tract*, 2nd Edn, pp. 1307–50. (New York: Raven Press)
5. Wood, J.D. and Mayer, C.J. (1978). Intracellular study of electrical activity of Auerbach's plexus in guinea-pig small intestine. *Pflug. Arch.*, **374**, 265–75
6. Gabella, G. (1987). Structure of muscles and nerves in the gastrointestinal tract. In Johnson, L.R. (ed.) *Physiology of the Gastrointestinal Tract*, 2nd Edn, pp. 335–81. (New York: Raven Press)
7. Nishi, S. and North, R.A. (1973). Intracellular recording from the myenteric plexus of the guinea-pig ileum. *J. Physiol. (Lond.)*, **231**, 471–91
8. Hirst, G.D.S., Holman, M.E. and Spence, I. (1974). Two types of neurons in the myenteric plexus of duodenum in the guinea-pig. *J. Physiol. (Lond.)*, **236**, 303–26
9. Wade, P.R. and Wood, J.D. (1988). Synaptic behaviour of myenteric neurons in the guinea-pig distal colon. *American J. Physiol. (Gastrointest. Liver Physiol.)* (18), **25**. (In press)
10. North, R.A., Slack, B.E. and Surprenant, A. (1985). Muscarinic M_1 and M_2 receptors mediate depolarization and presynaptic inhibition in guinea-pig enteric nervous system. *J. Physiol. (Lond.)*, **368**, 435–52
11. Wood, J.D. (ed.) (1988). Electrical and synaptic behavior of enteric neurons. In Wood, J.D. (ed.) *Handbook of Physiology, Gastrointestinal Motility and Blood Flow*, (Bethesda, Maryland: American Physiological Society). (In press)

10
The afferent peptidergic innervation of the upper gastrointestinal tract

G. J. DOCKRAY, T. GREEN and A. VARRO

INTRODUCTION

Visceral afferent neurons have been studied by electrophysiological methods for many years, but it is only recently that attention has been given to the possible transmitters they might employ. It is now plain that, along with other small-diameter primary afferents, those serving the alimentary tract make and secrete a number of biologically active peptides which are potential transmitter candidates. There are good reasons to think that, as in somatic afferents, peptides are synthesized in nerve cell bodies of the sensory ganglia and transported not only to central nerve terminals, but also to peripheral terminals in the gut. In addition, there is a rapidly increasing body of evidence to indicate that the peptides released at the peripheral terminals of visceral afferents mediate a variety of biological effects. Together the evidence suggests that this system participates in the normal control of digestion, including for example the protection of gastric mucosa from acid-peptic attack. In the present account we propose to discuss the organization of the afferent peptidergic innervation of the gastrointestinal tract, and the possible physiological roles of peptides that might be released at peripheral terminals of these neurons. A review of the recent literature can also be found in Dockray and Sharkey[1].

EXPERIMENTAL APPROACHES

We have studied the neurochemical organization of visceral afferent systems using immunohistochemistry, retrograde tracing, radioimmunoassay, and nerve lesioning by chemical or surgical methods[2-7]. Together these approaches have made it possible to: identify different peptides in afferent neurons projecting to the gut; quantify different populations of chemically identified neurons; determine peripheral patterns of distribution; and quantify rates of axonal transport. Most of the data considered below have been obtained by the use of retrograde tracing and immunohistochemistry. Thus markers such as True Blue have been injected into afferent terminal regions in the gut, where they are taken up by nerve fibres and transported to nerve cell bodies. The latter can be visualized in extrinsic ganglia by fluorescence microscopy. We have so far studied oesophagus, stomach and pancreas in detail. This approach gives information on both the afferent and efferent innervation, although we shall be concerned here only with the former. It is usually necessary to establish that positive results are not a consequence of non-specific spread or leakage of the tracer dye. By coupling retrograde tracing with immunohistochemistry it has been possible to define different types of chemically identified neurons that project to a particular tissue. We have so far used for these studies polyclonal antibodies to substance P, calcitonin gene related peptide (CGRP), somatostatin, morphine modulating peptide (MMP), bombesin and VIP, and monoclonal antibodies to the CCK-related peptide caerulein.

Quantitative studies of the rates of transport of peptide in rat visceral afferents have been made following nerve ligation and radioimmunoassay of nerve trunk extracts to measure accumulation and depletion of immunoreactive peptides on either side of the ligatures. Nerve lesion studies have also been used to quantify the amount of peptide in terminal areas. In addition to surgical approaches to visceral afferent lesioning, e.g. coeliac ganglionectomy (which removes spinal afferents that pass through the coeliac ganglion) and splanchnic section, the neurotoxin capsaicin has also been of great value. When given to new-born rats capsaicin selectively lesions small diameter afferents[8] which are the major population of visceral afferent fibres[9-11].

RETROGRADE TRACING AND IMMUNOHISTOCHEMISTRY

Spinal afferents

Following administration of True Blue to the ventral face of the stomach in rat, mouse or guinea-pig, numerous fluorescent-labelled True Blue cells may be seen in the nodose ganglia, spinal ganglia, coeliac superior mesenteric ganglion complex, and dorsal motor nucleus of the vagus (a few cells may also be seen in the n. ambiguus)[4,6]. The spinal ganglia are labelled in roughly equal numbers on both sides but the left nodose ganglion contains about 10 times more fluorescent neurons than that on the right side. Previous section of the splanchnic nerve or removal of the coeliac ganglion through which spinal afferents pass, abolishes the staining in dorsal root ganglia providing direct evidence that there is specific uptake from the stomach. The spinal ganglia labelled are at levels T5 to L2 with T9 to T11 containing the most labelled cells (Figures 1 and 2).

Combined immunohistochemistry and retrograde tracing indicates that approximately 80% of spinal afferents to the stomach contain immunoreactive GCRP in the rat[4,6,12]. There is, however, some segmental variability since in T6 to T8, CGRP occurs in only 30–40% of True-Blue-labelled cells (Figure 2). In the mouse and guinea-pig CGRP also occurs in a high

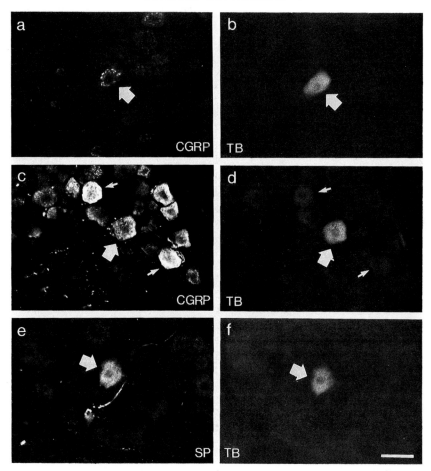

Figure 1 Immunohistochemical localization of CGRP (a,c) and substance P, (e) in neurons labelled with True Blue (b,d,f) retrogradely transported from the stomach in rat (a,b), mouse (c,d) and guinea-pig (e,f). Large arrows indicate same cells labelled with True Blue and by immunohistochemistry; small arrows indicate immunoreactive cells without True Blue. Note a and b from same sections, as are c and d, e and f. Scale bar 50 μm

proportion of gastric spinal afferents, and there seems to be no difference between the pyloric antral part of the stomach and the acid secreting part in this respect (Figure 3). The spinal afferents projecting to the pancreas are also rich in CGRP[13]. In the case of oesophageal innervation, there is a supply of spinal afferents that are mainly CGRP-immunoreactive, although in general the oesophagus is served by more vagal than spinal afferents[5]. It is worth noting that in the oesophagus, unlike the stomach, CGRP is also present in motoneuron terminals[14].

Substance P-immunoreactive cells are also abundant in the spinal afferent innervation of the stomach, pancreas and oesophagus[4,15]. In the rat and mouse this population of neurons makes a rather smaller contribution to

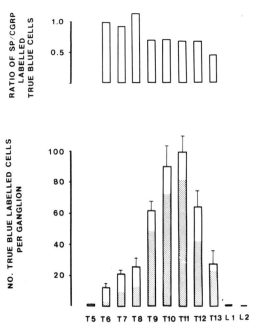

Figure 2 Lower panel: spinal distribution of True-Blue-labelled cells projecting to the rat stomach; the stippled areas indicate the fraction of True-Blue-labelled cells that are immunoreactive for CGRP. Note that about 35% of cells in T6 are CGRP-immunoreactive compared with 80% in T11. Upper panel: ratio of substance P to CGRP immunoreactive True-Blue-labelled cells. In T6 the ratio is close to 1, but in L1 there are roughly twice as many CGRP-immunoreactive neurons compared with substance P-immunoreactive cells

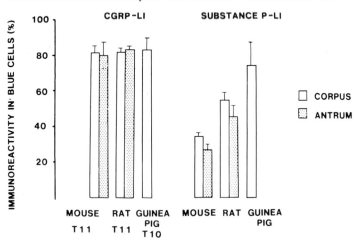

Figure 3 The contribution of CGRP and substance P immunoreactive dorsal root ganglia neurons to the gastric innervation in the rat, guinea-pig and mouse. Note that in all three species, CGRP accounts for about 80% of the afferent innervation of the gastric corpus and antrum, whereas there are species differences in the contribution of substance P

the total spinal gastric innervation compared with CGRP immunoreactive neurons (Figure 3); in guinea-pig substance P and CGRP immunoreactive neurons make an approximately equal contribution to the total gastric spinal innervation. These results can be related to co-localization studies which indicate that, in the rat, substance P occurs in a sub-population of CGRP dorsal root ganglia cell bodies, while in the guinea-pig, it is found in over 90% of all CGRP spinal afferents[16-18]. In the rat, the diameter of CGRP immunoreactive cells that project to the stomach ranged from 15 to 60 μm, and the median was 30–35 μm. The diameter of substance P immunoreactive gastric afferent neurons was for the most part less than 35 μm, so that while about a third of CGRP-immunoreactive neurons had a diameter greater than 35 μm, less than 10% of substance P immunoreactive cells were in this range. Evidently, gastric spinal afferents containing both substance P and CGRP are likely to be smaller diameter than those containing CGRP alone (Figure 4). There may also be a segmental variation in the distribution of gastric afferents containing these two peptides; in rat dorsal root ganglia from T6 to T9 the ratio of substance P to CGRP-immunoreactive gastric afferent neurons was about 1 whereas in L1 it was about 0.5 (Figure 2). These results suggest neurochemical differences between dorsal root ganglia

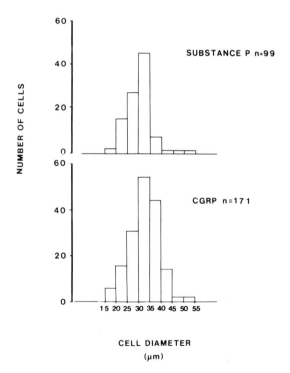

Figure 4 Frequency distribution of the neuronal cell body diameter of substance P (top) and CGRP (bottom)-immunoreactive cells in rat dorsal root ganglia projecting to the stomach. Approximately 35% of CGRP-immunoreactive neurons have diameters greater than 35 μm compared with about 10% of substance P-immunoreactive neurons

in their contributions to the gastric afferent innervation.

In guinea-pig (but not in rat) there is CCK in some CGRP-containing afferents[18]; our retrograde tracing data suggest that this population of afferent neurons accounts for about 9% of the projection to the stomach. In this context it is worth emphasizing that care is needed in the interpretation of immunohistochemical studies of CCK in afferent neurons, since certain C-terminal specific CCK antibodies cross-react in immunohistochemistry with CGRP (presumably due to the common Phe-amide in the two peptides)[19]. We have used for immunohistochemical studies of CCK in afferents a mouse monoclonal antibody to caerulein which does not cross-react with CGRP[20]. In the rat, this antibody does not react with primary sensory neurons.

In the rat somatostatin occurs in a population of CGRP-containing spinal afferent neurons[17]. The retrograde tracing data suggest, however, that there is little or no somatostatin-immunoreactivity in visceral afferents (Figure 5). Several other peptides have been reported to occur in spinal afferents. These include VIP which increases in somatic afferents after section of the nerve trunk[21]; in the cat, VIP-immunoreactive afferents have been described in the sacral nerve[22,23]. However, in our hands a range of antibodies to VIP and other peptides derived from the VIP-PHI precursor fail to reveal afferents to the upper gut either in intact animals, or following section of the splanchnic nerve. Dynorphin- and Leu-enkephalin immunoreactivities have also been reported in sacral afferents in the cat[24], and in some cutaneous and airway afferents in the guinea-pig[18]. We have recently shown that antibodies to MMP[25], react with a population of gastric spinal afferents in the rat[6]; radioimmunoassay studies indicate the presence of true MMP-immunoreactivity in rat spinal cord extracts (Holmes and Dockray, unpublished studies). Some of the material localized by immunohistochemistry may indeed be the authentic peptide; however, in absorption experiments CGRP (which shares a C-terminal Phe-amide with MMP) inhibited immunostaining, so that we cannot be sure of the specificity of this localization. The main conclusion to arise from the evidence available so far is that CGRP and substance P are the major peptides present in spinal afferents to the upper gastrointestinal tract; other peptides are produced in dorsal root ganglia cells but these appear to be either distributed to different terminal regions or to exhibit species variation in distribution.

Vagal afferents

Fluorescent True-Blue-labelled cells are readily found in vagal sensory ganglia following injection of tracer into the stomach or pancreas. The ventral face of the stomach and the duodenal lobe of the pancreas tend to be served by the left nodose and the dorsal surface of the stomach and the splenic lobe of the pancreas by the right nodose. In the rat there are abundant cells in the nodose ganglia that are immunoreactive for substance P and CGRP[4,6,26], but these tend to be concentrated at the rostral pole of the ganglion whereas the True-Blue-labelled cells are in the midpart and the caudal pole. Not surprisingly, therefore, there is a relatively low proportion of True-Blue-labelled cells containing substance P or CGRP-immunoreactivity (Figures 5 and 6). Essentially similar results have been obtained in guinea-pig and mouse. It seems probable that vagal afferent peptidergic neurons make a relatively minor contribution to the subdiaphragmatic projection; they are, however, likely to be an important component of the innervation of thoracic structures. In the guinea-pig, there are also somatostatin and VIP-immunoreactive vagal afferent neurons, which probably supply the airways; whether or not they also supply the gut is uncertain[26]. In humans, substance P, VIP and enkephalin immunoreactivities have been identified in the subdiaphragmatic vagal branches; the latter may be in vagal efferents, but the former are in afferents[27].

Distribution of peripheral terminals

Within the stomach, immunoreactive CGRP fibres have been localized to the myenteric plexus, circular smooth muscle, mucosa and submucosal especially around blood vessels (Figure 7)[6,28,29]. Pretreatment of neonatal rats with capsaicin, section of the splanchnic nerve or removal of the coeliac/superior mesenteric ganglion complex produces a near-total depletion of immunoreactive CGRP in the stomach, indicating that this material is of spinal afferent origin. This accords with the observation that immunoreactive nerve cell bodies are absent from the stomach so that gastric CGRP originates more or less exclusively from extrinsic neurons. In contrast, there are abundant substance P immunoreactive nerve cell bodies in the myenteric

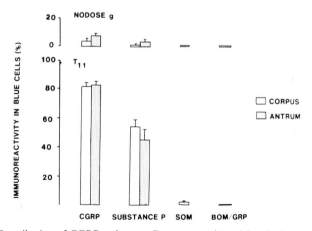

Figure 5 Contribution of CGRP, substance P, somatostatin and bombesin/gastrin releasing peptide (GRP)-like immunoreactivities to the gastric afferent innervation in the rat. Note that CGRP makes the largest contribution to the gastric spinal innervation; less than 10% of vagal gastric afferents are peptidergic. In the guinea-pig 10–15% of CGRP-immunoreactive gastric afferents also contain CCK immunoreactivity

111

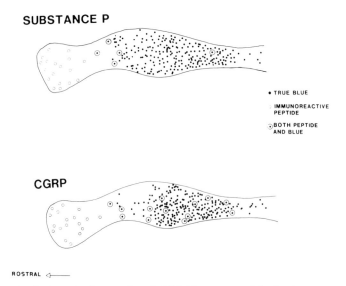

SUBSTANCE P

• TRUE BLUE

IMMUNOREACTIVE
PEPTIDE

BOTH PEPTIDE
AND BLUE

CGRP

ROSTRAL

Figure 6 Distribution of substance P and CGRP-immunoreactivity in the vagus compared with the distribution of True-Blue-labelled cells retrogradely labelled from the stomach. Note that while most peptidergic neurons are at the rostral end (left) most True-Blue-labelled cells are in the middle or caudal pole (right)

plexus and there are striking populations of nerve fibres in all the major layers. In rats pretreated with capsaicin there is a loss of substance P from the mucosa and from gastric submucosal blood vessels[4], but it is more difficult to discern differences elsewhere in the stomach compared with controls. It appears then, that substance P in the mucosa and submucosal blood vessels is largely afferent in origin, but that in the stomach muscle and myenteric plexus is probably mainly of intrinsic origin. The finding that CGRP (whether or not co-localized with other peptides) is present in a high proportion of spinal afferents, and that it is absent from intrinsic gastric neurons makes this peptide an important marker for the distribution of peripheral terminals of spinal afferents in the stomach.

In the pancreas, substance P and CGRP immunoreactive nerve fibres are found around the islets and passing through the parenchyma[4,13,18,29]. There are also some CGRP immunoreactive cells in the islets. In capsaicin-treated rats the immunoreactive nerve fibres are lost, indicating that they are of afferent origin.

A rich population of CGRP immunoreactive fibres occurs in the prevertebral ganglia, and these too are lost in capsaicin-pretreated rats[6]. It would appear that these fibres are collaterals of afferents passing through the ganglia en route from terminal regions in the gut to the spinal cord. It has been known for some time that there are also substance P-containing afferent collaterals in the prevertebral ganglia[30].

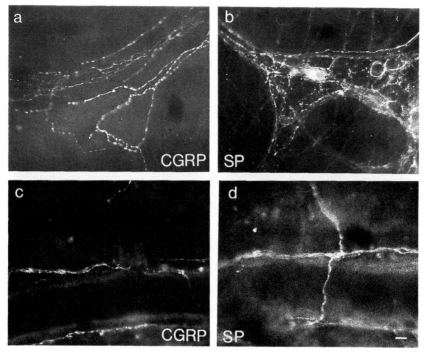

Figure 7 Immunohistochemical localization of CGRP (a,c) and substance P (b,d) in whole mounts of rat stomach. The myenteric plexus is shown in a and b, and submucosal blood vessels in c and d. Note CGRP immunoreactive fibres, but not cell bodies, whereas immunoreactive substance P cell bodies can be seen in myenteric plexus. Scale bar 10 μm

RADIOIMMUNOASSAY STUDIES

Tissue distribution

Radioimmunoassay of CGRP in extracts of stomach and coeliac ganglia from control, capsaicin-treated and surgically lesioned rats, has provided direct quantitative support for the idea that all gastric CGRP is of afferent origin. In rats that have been coeliac ganglionectomized, gastric CGRP was reduced by about 80%, but in capsaicin-treated rats it was reduced to below the limit of detection (Table 1)[7,29]. These observations are consistent with the retrograde tracing data described above that indicate most gastric CGRP

Table 1 Concentrations (pmol.g^{-1}) of CGRP in tissue extracts of control, capsaicin-treated and coeliac ganglionectomized rats

Tissue	Control	Capsaicin	Coeliac ganglionectomized
Gastric corpus	5.2 ± 0.8	<0.1	0.9 ± 0.2
Antrum	8.0 ± 1.3	<0.1	0.8 ± 0.1
Duodenum	4.8 ± 1.3	<0.1	0.6 ± 0.2
Coeliac ganglion	51.3 ± 7.6	4.1 ± 2.4	—

is of spinal afferent origin (and that the remainder is of vagal afferent origin). In extracts of the coeliac ganglion from capsaicin-treated rats we have found low, but significant, amounts of CGRP immunoreactivity. The origins of this material are unknown; it could conceivably come from capsaicin-resistant afferents, or more likely it might originate from fibres projecting to the prevertebral ganglia from distal regions of the gut (which, unlike stomach, contain intrinsic CGRP neurons). For comparison in these studies we have also assayed the same extracts for opioid peptides (Leu-enkephalin and Met-enkephalin Arg[6] Gly[7] Leu[8]) which are found in intrinsic gastric neurons, and in prevertebral ganglion nerve fibres, but on current evidence are not present in primary afferents. The results indicate that these peptides do not change in concentration in cirumstances where CGRP is depleted, suggesting that there are not non-specific effects of afferent nerve lesions on neuropeptides produced by intrinsic gut neurons[7]. HPLC and gel chromatography of gastric extracts shows a major peak of immunoreactivity that has the properties of intact 37-residue CGRP. We and others[29] have, however, also found immunoreactive material that appears to correspond to C-terminal CGRP fragments; the significance of this material is presently unknown.

Rates of axonal transport

The availability of a sensitive CGRP assay has made it possible to directly measure the transport velocity of CGRP in splanchnic and vagal nerve trunks. Following ligation of the splanchnic nerve for 24 or 72 h there was a marked accumulation of immunoreactive material on the proximal side; there was also a depletion on the distal side (Figure 8). The calculated mean transport rates are 0.7 mm h^{-1} in the splanchnic nerve, and 1.6 mm h^{-1} in the vagus nerve[7]. The latter rate is in good agreement with previous estimates of the axonal transport rates of substance P in the rat vagus[1,31,32]. Other peptides, including CCK8 and somatostatin, are transported at broadly similar rates in a variety of different species[1,2,31,32]. The concentrations of CGRP in control sections of splanchnic nerve trunk were 85 fmol mm^{-1}, this compares with concentrations in the vagus of 7–20 fmol mm^{-1} for substance P, 0.4–2.9 fmol mm^{-1} for somatostatin and 0.7 fmol mm^{-1} for VIP; CGRP in rat vagus occurs in similar concentrations to SP. Evidently CGRP concentrations in the rat splanchnic nerve are high compared with those of peptides in the vagus.

PERIPHERAL ACTIONS OF NEUROPEPTIDES FROM GUT AFFERENTS

Several experimental approaches have recently provided insight into the possible roles of peptides released at the peripheral endings of afferents in stomach and small intestine. Three of these are worth mentioning. First, administration of the neurotoxin capsaicin has been used either to stimulate visceral afferents or (in rats treated when young with high doses) selectively

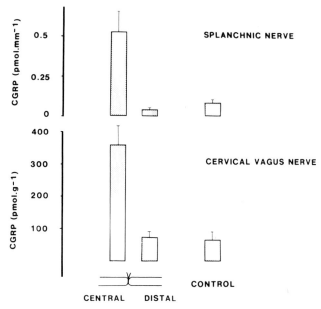

Figure 8 Axonal transport of CGRP in rat vagus and splanchnic nerve trunks. Ligation of the splanchnic nerve and cervical vagus was performed in pentobarbitone anaesthetized rats. After 24 h segments of nerve trunks (vagus 7 mm, splanchnic 3 mm) were taken on either side of the ligature. The results for the vagus are expressed as $pmol.g^{-1}$ but since it proved difficult to weigh splanchnic samples accurately these results are expressed as $pmol.mm^{-1}$. Note accumulation on the proximal side of the ligatures, indicating axonal transport towards the gut. In the splanchnic, there is also a significant ($p < 0.05$, t test) depletion on the distal side. In the vagus a depletion was found only after 72 h (results not shown)

to lesion the afferent fibres prior to studies of gut function. Secondly, electrical stimulation of extrinsic nerve trunks has given information on antidromically released peptides. Since autonomic efferents are also stimulated by this approach it is usually necessary to employ pharmacological blockade (atropine, hexamethonium, guanethidine and adrenergic antagonists) of the main autonomic transmitters. Thirdly, the action of peptides known to occur in afferents has been examined; interpretation of the results of this approach is complicated by the fact that the relevant peptides are also found elsewhere and are not exclusively localized in visceral afferents.

Blood flow
Close arterial injection of low doses of capsaicin evokes a reproducible increase in superior mesenteric artery blood flow in the anaesthetized dog[33]. This response is decreased by prior administration of antibodies to substance P or CGRP, suggesting a role for these peptides in mediating this effect. Small additional decreases in the blood flow response to capsaicin are also obtained with antibodies to CCK and to VIP.

Motility

In the guinea-pig small intestine, capsaicin or antidromic stimulation of the extrinsic nerve pedicle produces a contraction of longitudinal smooth muscle *in vitro*. The response can be blocked by desensitization to substance P and appears to involve both direct effects of substance P on the longitudinal smooth muscle and indirect effects secondary to the release of acetylcholine from myenteric neurons[34]. In the cat, antidromic activation of vagal and splanchnic afferents has been associated with a contractile response of the stomach that could be due to release of substance P[35,36]. In the rat duodenum, capsaicin produces a relaxation which depends on the integrity of the splanchnic innervation and is said to be mimicked by CGRP[37]. In part, this may be due to release of a non-adrenergic, non-cholinergic inhibitor from myenteric neurons since (at least in guinea-pig ileum) CGRP is excitatory to myenteric neurons[38].

Gastric mucosal function

Exogeneous CGRP is a powerful inhibitor of gastric acid secretion in a variety of species[39-41]. There is some evidence that CGRP selectively releases gastrointestinal somatostatin, which might account for its acid inhibitory actions[42]. Other evidence suggests the gastric afferent innervation may well play a part in protecting the mucosa from acid-peptic damage. Thus, rats that have been pretreated with capsaicin are more prone to develop haemorrhagic lesions of the gastric mucosa in response to any of several ulcerogenic challenges, suggesting that visceral afferents mediate mucosal defence mechanisms[43]. It has been suggested that these effects might be mediated via an increase in mucosal blood flow; this notion is attractive because both substance P and CGRP are potent vasodilators, although recent results suggest that CGRP might have no effect on mucosal blood flow in the dog[44]. In the cat, antidromic stimulation of afferents is associated with mucosa bicarbonate secretion and this would be compatible with a protective effect on the mucosa[45].

Pancreas

Both substance P and CGRP act directly on guinea-pig pancreatic acinar cells to evoke amylase release[46-48]. The physiological importance of these actions is not clear; we have been unable to produce similar effects with these peptides in dispersed rat pancreatic acinar cells *in vitro*, and in conscious dogs, CGRP does not influence pancreatic responses to feeding[40]. In capsaicin-pretreated rats, the acinar cell response to CCK appears to be the same as in control rats (S. Hackett, D. Thwaites and G. J. Dockray, unpublished observations). At least with regard to the exocrine pancreas, then, the role of these neuropeptides at the periphery is uncertain. It has been suggested that CGRP might inhibit basal and glucose or carbachol-stimulated insulin secretion in the mouse[49].

Prevertebral ganglia

At the inferior mesenteric ganglion in the guinea-pig, substance P produces a long, slow depolarization of ganglion cell bodies that mimics the response to stimulation of nerve trunks[50]. The effects of nerve stimulation are seen after cholinergic blockade and are produced by both efferent and afferent nerve trunk stimulation, which is consistent with the idea that the transmitter is released from the collaterals of afferents passing through the ganglion. Capsaicin reduced the substance P content of the ganglion and abolished the slow EPSP. These results together provide strong evidence for a neuromodulatory role for substance P released at afferent collaterals around sympathetic nerve cell bodies[50].

PHYSIOLOGICAL SIGNIFICANCE

The data reviewed above suggest that a high proportion of spinal afferents to the upper gut contain biologically active peptides, notably CGRP and substance P, that are transported towards the periphery. There is also clear evidence for the transport of these peptides to the central endings of visceral afferents; there are terminals in laminae I and II in spinal cord, as well as baskets of fibre terminals in laminae V[51]. Peptidergic afferent fibres are found at several levels in the gut including mucosa, submucosa, smooth muscle, blood vessels and nerve cell bodies of the myenteric and prevertebral ganglia (Figure 9). Spinal afferents have long been thought to play a part in mediating the transmission of visceral sensations, especially pain, from the gut to the CNS[52]. Electrophysiological studies suggest that some spinal afferents mediate the discharge of slowly adapting mechanoreceptors and respond to distension or contraction of the gut; they have punctate receptive fields on the serosal surface of the gut and surrounding mesentery, as well as in the muscle layers[10,11]. It remains unknown whether or not different neurochemically identified subpopulations of afferents can be distinguished electrophysiologically. Either way, stimulation of peptidergic afferents should release peptides at any or all of several different levels in the gut. In the case of cutaneous afferents which are well studied in this respect, the peptides released at peripheral endings increase local blood flow and capillary permeability[53]. The latter effect cannot be demonstrated in the gut, where capillary permeability is already much higher than in many other tissues. Instead, however, there is an elaborate network of other possible actions.

Stimulation of gut spinal afferents might be expected to release peptides that activate a hierarchical series of reflexes that influence mucosal and smooth muscle function, and blood flow. In the first instance these effects could be exerted by direct actions, but they could also be evoked indirectly by actions on myenteric and prevertebral ganglion cells. The continuous turnover of CGRP at the ends of splanchnic afferents suggests that this system plays a part in the normal control of gut function; it should therefore be seen as an additional component to the endocrine, paracrine and intrinsic nervous mechanisms controlling secretion, blood flow and motility. In addition, of course, visceral peptidergic afferents may have an important part to play in activation of a full autonomic reflex mediated at the level of the CNS autonomic outflow. In this context it is important to note that central administration of CGRP increases plasma noradrenaline, inhibits

A.

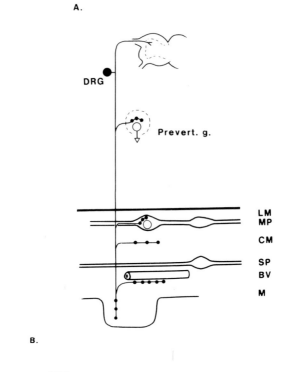

B.

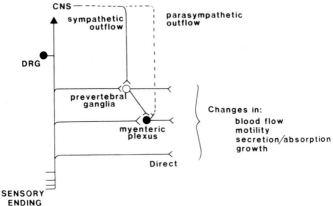

Figure 9 **A** top, schematic representation of the distribution of CGRP-containing afferent fibres in the stomach, and **B** below, the possible hierarchial organization of reflexes that would be generated by stimulation of afferent nerve endings. Electrophysiological studies suggest there are slowly adapting mechanoreceptor endings in the muscle as well as serosa. The mucosal afferents could be rapidly adapting mechanoreceptors that are also chemoreceptors. Activation could evoke: (i) axon reflexes that directly influence blood flow, motility, secretion or trophic changes; (ii) indirect effects via actions at (a) myenteric nerve cell bodies and (b) prevertebral ganglion nerve cell bodies; and (iii) classical autonomic reflexes via modulation of the sympathetic or parasympathetic outflow

acid secretion (by a vagal pathway), and stimulates the fasting pattern of intestinal motility in the rat[54-58]. Finally, it should be noted that in other systems inflammatory responses have in part a neurogenic afferent component: the position of the peptidergic afferents of the gut as the first level in the pathway mediating the transfer of noxious information from the gut to the CNS, means that they are also potential modulators of gastrointestinal inflammatory reactions.

Acknowledgements

We are grateful to the University of Liverpool for a research studentship and to the MRC for financial support. The help of Christine Carter in preparing this manuscript is also gratefully acknowledged.

References

1. Dockray, G.J. and Sharkey, K.A. (1986). Neurochemistry of visceral afferent neurones. *Prog. Brain Res.*, **67**, 133–48
2. Dockray, G.J., Gregory, R.A., Tracy, H.J. and Zhu, W.-Y. (1981). Transport of cholecystokin-in-octapeptide-like immunoreactivity toward the gut in afferent vagal fibres in cat and dog. *J. Physiol.*, **314**, 501–11
3. Sharkey, K.A., Williams, R.G., Schultzberg, M. and Dockray, G.J. (1983). Sensory substance P-innervation of the urinary bladder: possible site of action in capsaicin in causing urine retention in rats. *Neuroscience*, **10**, 861–68
4. Sharkey, K.A., Williams, R.G. and Dockray, G.J. (1984). Sensory substance P innervation of the stomach and pancreas: Demonstration of capsaicin-sensitive sensory neurones in the rat by combined immunohistochemistry and retrograde tracing. *Gastroenterology*, **87**, 914–21
5. Green, T. and Dockray, G.J. (1987). Calcitonin gene-related peptide and substance P in afferents to the upper gastrointestinal tract in the rat. *Neurosci. Lett.*, **76**, 151–56
6. Green, T. and Dockray, G.J. (1988). Characterization of the peptidergic afferent innervation of the stomach in the rat, mouse and guinea-pig. *Neuroscience*, **25**, 181–93
7. Varro, A., Green, T., Holmes, S. and Dockray, G.J. (1988). Calcitonin gene-related peptide in visceral afferent nerve fibres: quantification by radioimmunoassay and determination of axonal transport rates. *Neuroscience*. **26**, 927–32
8. Buck, S.H. and Burks, T.F. (1986). The neuropharmacology of capsaicin: review of some recent observations. *Pharmacol. Rev.*, **38**, 179–226
9. Andrews, P.L.R. (1986). Vagal afferent innervation of the gastrointestinal tract. *Prog. Brain Res.*, **67**, 65–86
10. Morrison, J.F.B. (1977). The afferent innervation of the gastrointestinal tract. In Brooks, F.P. and Evers, P. (eds.), *Nerves and the Gut*, pp. 297–326. (Thorofare, NT: Charles Slack)
11. Janig, W. and Morrison, J.F.B. (1986). Functional properties of spinal visceral afferents supplying abdominal and pelvic organs, with special emphasis on visceral nociception. *Prog. Brain Res.*, **67**, 87–114
12. Su, H.C., Bishop, A.E., Power, R.F., Hamada, Y. and Polak, J.M. (1987). Dual intrinsic and extrinsic origins of CGRP- and NPY-immunoreactive nerves of rat gut and pancreas. *J. Neuroscience*, **7**, 2674–87
13. Sternini, C. and Brecha, N. (1986). Immunocytochemical identification of islet cells and nerve fibers containing calcitonin gene-related peptide-like immunoreactivity in the rat pancreas. *Gastroenterology*, **90**, 1155–63
14. Rodrigo, J., Polak, J.M., Fernandez, L., Ghatei, M.A., Mulderry, P. and Bloom, S.R. (1985). Calcitonin gene-related peptide immunoreactive sensory and motor nerves of the rat, cat and monkey esophagus. *Gastroenterology*, **88**, 444–51

15. Lindh, B., Dalsgaard, C.-J., Elfvin, L.-G., Hokfelt, T. and Cuello, A.C. (1983). Evidence of substance P-immunoreactive neurons in dorsal root ganglia and vagal ganglia projecting to the guinea pig pylorus. *Brain Res.*, **269**, 365–69

16. Gibson, S.J., Polak, J.M., Bloom, S.R., Sabat, I.M., Mulderry, P.M., Ghatei, M.A., McGregory, G.P., Morrison, J.F.B., Kelly, J.S., Evans, R.M. and Rosenfeld, M.G. (1984). Calcitonin gene-related peptide immunoreactivity in the spinal cord of man and of eight other species. *Neuroscience*, **4**, 3101–11

17. Ju, G., Hokfelt, T., Brodin, E., Fahrenkrug, J., Fischer, J.A., Frey, P., Elde, R.P. and Brown, J.C. (1987). Primary sensory neurons of the rat showing calcitonin gene-related peptide (CGRP) immunoreactivity and their relation to substance P-, somatostatin-, galanin-, vasoactive intestinal polypeptide- and cholecystokinin-immunoreactive ganglion cells. *Cell Tissue Res.*, **247**, 417–31

18. Gibbins, I.L., Furness, J.B. and Costa, M. (1987). Pathway-specific patterns of the co-existence of substance P, calcitonin gene-related peptide, cholecystokinin and dynorphin in neurons of the dorsal root ganglia of the guinea pig. *Cell Tissue Res.*, **248**, 417–37

19. Ju, G., Hokfelt, T., Fischer, J.A., Frey, P., Rehfeld, J.F. and Dockray, G.J. (1986). Does cholescystokinin-like immunoreactivity in rat primary sensory neurons represent calcitonin gene-related peptide? *Neurosci. Lett.*, **68**, 305–10

20. Williams, R.G., Dimaline, R., Varro, A., Isetta, A.M., Trizio, D. and Dockray, G.J. (1987). Cholecystokinin octapeptide in rat central nervous system: Immunocytochemical studies using a monoclonal antibody that does not react with CGRP. *Neurochem. Int.*, **4**, 433–42

21. Shehab, S.A.S. and Atkinson, M.E. (1986). Vasoactive intestinal polypeptide increases in areas of the dorsal horn of the spinal cord from which other neuropeptides are depleted following peripheral axotomy. *Exp. Brain Res.*, **62**, 422–30

22. Kawatani, M., Low, I.P., Nadelhaft, I., Morgan, C. and De Groat, W.C. (1983). Vasoactive intestinal polypeptide in visceral afferent pathways to the sacral spinal cord of the cat. *Neurosci. Lett.*, **42**, 311–16

23. Kawatani, M., Nagel, J. and De Groat, W.C. (1986). Identification of neuropeptides in pelvic and pudendal nerve afferent pathways to the sacral spinal cord of the cat. *J. Comp. Neurol.*, **249**, 117–32

24. Basbaum, A.J., Cruz, L. and Weber, E. (1986). Immunoreactive dynorphin B in sacral primary afferent fibers of the cat. *J. Neurosci.*, **6**, 127–33

25. Tang, J., H-Y., Yang, T. and Costa, E. (1984). Inhibition of spontaneous and opiate-modified nociception by an endogenous neuropeptide with Phe-Met-Arg-Phe-NH$_2$-like immunoreactivity. *Proc. Natl. Acad. Sci. USA.*, **81**, 5002–05

26. Lundberg, J.M., Hokfelt, T., Nilsson, G., Terenius, L., Rehfeld, J., Elde, R. and Said, S. (1978). Peptide neurons in the vagus, splanchnic and sciatic nerves. *Acta Physiol. Scand.*, **104**, 499–501

27. Lundberg, J.M., Hokfelt, T., Kewenter, J., Pettersson, G., Ahlman, H., Edin, R., Dahlstrom, A., Nilsson, G., Terenius, L., Uvnas-Wallensten, K. and Said, S. (1979). Substance P-, VIP-, and enkephalin-like immunoreactivity in the human vagus nerve. *Gastroenterology*, **77**, 468–71

28. Clague, J.R., Sternini, C. and Brecha, N.C. (1985). Localization of calcitonin gene-related peptide-like immunoreactivity in neurons of the rat gastrointestinal tract. *Neurosci. Lett.*, **56**, 63–8

29. Sternini, C., Reeve, J.R. Jr. and Brecha, N. (1987). Distribution and characterization of calcitonin gene-related peptide immunoreactivity in the digestive system of normal and capsaicin-treated rats. *Gastroenterology*, **93**, 852–62

30. Matthews, M.R. and Cuello, A.C. (1982). Substance P-immunoreactive peripheral branches of sensory neurons innervate guinea pig sympathetic neurons. *Proc. Natl. Acad. Sci. USA*, **79**, 1668–72

31. Gilbert, R.F.T., Emson, P.C., Fahrenkrug, J., Lee, C.M., Penman, E. and Wass, J. (1980). Axonal transport of neuropeptides in cervical vagus nerve of the rat. *J. Neurochem.*, **34**, 105–13

32. MacLean, D.B. and Lewis, S.F. (1984). Axoplasmic transport of somatostatin and substance P in the vagus nerve of the rat, guinea pig, and cat. *Brain Res.*, **307**, 135–45

33. Rozsa, Z., Varro, A. and Jancso, G. (1985). Use of immunoblockade to study the involvement of peptidergic afferent nerves in the intestinal vasodilatory response to capsaicin in the dog. *Eur. J. Pharmacol.*, **115**, 59–64

34. Bartho, L., Holzer, P., Lembeck, F. and Szolcsanyi, J. (1982). Evidence that the contractile response of the guinea-pig ileum to capsaicin is due to release of substance P. *J. Physiol.*, **332**, 157–67

35. Delbro, D., Fandriks, L., Lisander, B. and Andersson, S.A. (1982). Gastric atropine-sensitive excitation by peripheral vagal stimulation after hexamethonium antidromic activation of afferents. *Acta Physiol. Scand.*, **114**, 433–40

36. Delbro, D., Fandriks, L., Rosell, S. and Folkers, K. (1983). Inhibition of antidromically induced stimulation of gastric motility by substance P receptor blockade. *Acta Physiol. Scand.*, **118**, 309–16

37. Maggi, C.A., Manzini, S., Giuliani, S., Santicioli, P. and Meli, A. (1986). Extrinsic origin of the capsaicin-sensitive innervation of rat duodenum: possible involvement of calcitonin gene-related peptide (CGRP) in the capsaicin-induced activation of intramural non-adrenergic non-cholinergic neurons. *Naunyn-Schmiedeberg's Arch. Pharmacol.*, **334**, 172–80

38. Palmer, J.M., Schemann, M., Tamura, K. and Wood, J.D. (1986). Calcitonin gene-related peptide excites myenteric neurons. *Eur. J. Pharmacol.*, **132**, 163–70

39. Tache, Y., Pappas, T., Laufenburger, M., Goto, Y., Walsh, J.H. and Debas, H. (1984). Calcitonin gene-related peptide: potent peripheral inhibitor of gastric acid secretion in rats and dogs. *Gastroenterology*, **87**, 344–49

40. Pappas, T., Debas, H.T., Walsh, J.H., Rivier, J. and Tache, Y. (1986). Calcitonin gene-related peptide-induced selective inhibition of gastric acid secretion in dogs. *Am. J. Physiol.*, **250**, G127–G133

41. Tache, Y., Pappas, T., Lauffenburger, M., Goto, Y., Walsh, J.H. and Debas, H.T. (1984). Calcitonin gene-related peptide: potent peripheral inhibitor of gastric acid secretion in rats and dogs. *Gastroenterology*, **87**, 344–49

42. Dunning, B.E. and Taborsky, G.J. Jr. (1987). Calcitonin gene-related peptide: a potent and selective stimulator of gastrointestinal somatostatin secretion. *Endocrinology*, **120**, 1774–81

43. Holzer, P. and Sametz, W. (1986). Gastric mucosal protection against ulcerogenic factors in the rat mediated by capsaicin-sensitive afferent neurons. *Gastroenterology*, **91**, 975–81

44. Leung, F.W., Tallos, E.G., Tache, Y.F. and Guth, P.H. (1987). Calcitonin gene-related peptide inhibits acid secretion without modifying blood flow. *Am. J. Physiol.*, **252**, G215–G218

45. Fandriks, L. and Delbro, D. (1983). Neural stimulation of gastric bicarbonate secretion in the cat. An involvement of vagal axon-reflexes and substance P? *Acta Physiol. Scand.*, **118**, 301–4

46. Gardner, J.D. and Jensen, R.T. (1987). Secretagogue receptors on pancreatic acinar cells. In Johnson, L.R. (ed.) *Physiology of the Gastrointestinal Tract*, 2nd Edn, pp. 1109–27. (New York: Raven Press)

47. Zhou, X-C., Villanueva, M.L., Noguchi, M., Jones, S.W., Gardner, J.D. and Jensen, R.T. (1986). Mechanism of action of calcitonin gene-related peptide in stimulating pancreatic enzyme secretion. *Am. J. Physiol.*, **251**, G391–G397

48. Seifert, H., Sawchenko, P., Chesnut, J., Rivier, J., Vale, W. and Pandol, S.J. (1985). Receptor for calcitonin gene-related peptide: binding to exocrine pancreas mediates biological actions. *Am. J. Physiol.*, G147–G151

49. Petersson, M., Ahren, B., Bottcher, G. and Sundler, F. (1986). Calcitonin gene-related peptide: occurrence in pancreatic islets in the mouse and the rat, and inhibition of insulin secretion in the mouse. *Endocrinology*, **119**, 865–9

50. Otsuka, M., Konishi, S., Yanagisawa, M., Tsunoo, A. and Akagi, H. (1982). Role of substance P as a sensory transmitter in spinal cord and sympathetic ganglia. *Ciba Foundation Symposium*, **91**, 13–34

51. Sharkey, K.A., Sobrino, J.A. and Cervero, F. (1988). Evidence for a visceral afferent origin of substance P-like immunoreactivity in lamina V of the rat thoracic spinal cord. *Neuroscience.* (In press)

52. Hertz, A.F. (1911). *The Sensibility of the Alimentary Canal.* (London: Oxford University Press, Hodder and Stoughton)

53. Lembeck, F. and Gamse, R. (1982). Substance P in peripheral sensory processes. *Ciba Foundation Symposium*, **91**, 35–54

54. Fisher, L.A., Kikkawa, D.O., Rivier, J.E., Amara, S.G., Evans, R.M., Rosenfeld, M.G., Vale, W.W. and Brown, M.R. (1983). Stimulation of noradrenergic sympathetic outflow by calcitonin gene-related peptide. *Nature*, **305**, 534–6

55. Tache, Y., Gunion, M., Lauffenberger, M. and Goto, Y. (1984). Inhibition of gastric acid secretion by intracerebral injection of calcitonin gene-related peptide in rats. *Life Sci.*, **35**, 871–8

56. Lenz, H.J., Mortrud, M.T., Rivier, J.E. and Brown, M.R. (1985). Central nervous system actions of calcitonin gene-related peptide on gastric acid secretion in the rat. *Gastroenterology*, **88**, 539–44

57. Lenz, H.J., Hester, S.E., Saik, R.P. and Brown, M.R. (1986). CNS actions of calcitonin gene-related peptide on gastric acid secretion in conscious dogs. *Am. J. Physiol.*, **250**, G742–G748

58. Fargeas, M.J., Fioramonit, J. and Bueno, L. (1985). Calcitonon gene-related peptide: Brain and spinal action on intestinal motility. *Peptides*, **6**, 1167–71

Summary
The enteric nervous system: circuits and development

J. B. FURNESS

The session highlighted the substantial progress made in the last ten years in analysis of enteric neural circuits and their development. It continued that progress and pointed to new directions. The major theme of the session was the attempts being made to correlate neurochemistry, morphology, projections and connections, ultrastructure and functions of individual neurons. It is anticipated that such correlations will allow enteric neural circuits to be fully described. Shapes of nerve cell bodies were discussed by Dr Stach. He built on the original descriptions in the 1890s by Dogiel of types I, II and III cells by identifying additional categories (IV, V, VI and small neurons). He pointed out that the cells differed in their chemistry and supported the claim by Dogiel that cell shape and function are related. This theme was taken up by Dr Lees who summarized experiments in which electrophysiological properties, cell shape and chemistry have been correlated. This has been achieved by recording from intracellular microelectrodes containing marker dyes that are injected into the neurons. In the myenteric plexus of the guinea-pig small intestine there are two electrophysiological neuron types, AH and S neurons. The studies with dye-filled electrodes indicate that Dogiel type II neurons are AH neurons. Dr Lees reported that dynorphin and enkephalin immunoreactivity was only in S neurons and that many of these had Dogiel type I morphology. The ultrastructure of the Dogiel type II neurons was described by Dr Pompolo. This is the first time that enteric neurons of known electrophysiological type and known morphology have been characterized ultrastructurally. The correlation was made possible by the discovery that immunoreactivity for calbindin is exclusively in type II/AH neurons. Type II/AH neurons are large cells that contain characteristic numerous, elongated, electron-dense mitochondria. They have multiple long processes, some going to the mucosa and others forming synapses on other myenteric neurons. It was proposed that the Dogiel type II/AH neurons are sensory. The chemistry and projections of intestinal neurons were discussed by Drs Ekblad, Kirschgessner, Mawe and Dockray. An important conclusion from Dr Ekblad's work was that, although the projections and organization of enteric circuits shows a high degree of order that can be analysed with immunohistochemical methods, the chemistries of neurons differ between species. Dr Ekblad successfully used lesions to analyse enteric pathways, but these methods are not appropriate in all cases, for example in examining projections from submucous neurons. Dr Kirschgessner has made a breakthrough in such studies by showing that restricted injections of the tracers Fluoro-Gold and *Phaseolus vulgaris* lectins can be used to trace local connections. An important observation was that submucous neurons projecting to the myenteric plexus were demonstrated. Such neurons had been hypothesized before, but never revealed directly. Tracing studies described by Dr Mawe demonstrated that duodenal neurons project to the gallbladder. Most of the electrophysiological studies of enteric neurons have been on the guinea-pig small intestine. It is therefore important that studies of other areas are now being made. Dr. Schemann described his studies of neurons in the guinea-pig stomach. All the neurons received fast synaptic inputs, but varied in their responsiveness to intracellular current injections; some being tonically activated; some phasically; and some being refractory to excitation in this manner. No neurons like the intestinal AH neurons were found. This is a tantalizing finding, given the prominence of such neurons in the small intestine.

In conclusion, the session emphasized the progress being made in correlated studies of enteric neurons. Structure, chemistry and function certainly seem to be correlated and it appears that an adequate structural and functional analysis of enteric neural circuits is within sight.

Section II
Nerves and the upper gastrointestinal tract

11
Central and peripheral nervous control of gastric secretion

B. I. HIRSCHOWITZ

Gastric secretion is part of a complex integrated system by which higher organisms feed, digest and regulate their nutrition. The system controls and integrates feeding behaviour; swallowing; salivary, gastric, pancreatic and biliary secretion; gastrointestinal motility, blood flow, and absorption; and, ultimately, blood sugar and caloric homeostasis. Gastric function is controlled and integrated at several hierarchical levels that share or overlap many components of the digestive complex. For convenience the topic will be divided into central and peripheral controls.

CENTRAL CONTROLS

Central vagal complex

The central nervous system (CNS) controls secretion and motility of the stomach via the vagus nerves[1] through fibres originating in the medulla from neurons of the dorsomotor nucleus of the vagus (DMNV), as well as the nucleus ambigus (NA) and the nucleus tractus solitarius (NTS). The vagi are mixed brachiomeric nerves comprising both afferent and efferent fibres. Visceral efferents comprise only about 3% of the nearly 60 000 fibres that constitute the abdominal vagi in humans[2]. Neurons of gastric vagal efferents have been localized by selective retrograde tracing techniques[3-5] to the DMNV and the NTS[4,5]. Pancreatic, cardiovascular and lung efferents coexist[6]. Gastric efferents from the NA appear to be largely motor[7].

Primary visceral sensory information is relayed to the DMNV via the tractus solitarius and the NTS that surrounds it. General somatic afferent fibres of the vagus nerve arise from cells of the superior ganglion of the vagus nerve, whereas both general and special visceral afferent fibres originate in the larger inferior ganglion (nodose ganglion). The fibres entering the solitary tract bifurcate into short-ascending and longer-descending components. Descending vagal components in the tractus solitarius gradually diminish in number as collaterals and terminals are given off to the NTS. Some vagal visceral fibres descend caudal to the obex, where the NTS of the two sides merge to form the commissural vagal nucleus.

The rostral or lateral part of the NTS receives mainly taste fibres and is also known as the gustatory nucleus; the caudal or medial NTS receives mainly general visceral afferents. Gastrointestinal afferents end in the parvocellular subnucleus[4,5]. The NTS connects with the NA, the thalamic ventral posteromedial nucleus concerned with gustatory sensations, the hypoglossal and salivary nuclei, the DMNV, and the paraventricular parvocellular nucleus of the hypothalamus.[8] The NTS is also closely linked with the respiratory and vasomotor control centres.

A cross-section of the medulla (Figure 1A) shows the relative location of the nuclei comprising the central vagal complex. Major connections are illustrated in Figure 1B.

Functional anatomy of the central vagal complex

Electrical stimulation of the DMNV in cats leads to vigorous, prolonged gastric secretion[9,10]. The DMNV is the critical relay for stimulation of gastric secretion due to hypoglycaemia[11]. While the DMNV neurons are not directly stimulated by a lack of glucose,[12] there are a number of sites from which the DMNV can be stimulated indirectly either electrically or by glucose deprivation. The DMNV is activated by electrical stimulation of the lateral hypothalamus (LH)[9] or by glucose deprivation of the LH by local application of 2-deoxy-D-glucose (2-DG)[13-15] or of pentagastrin[16]. Local destruction of the lateral hypothalamus blocks both feeding behaviour and stimulation of secretion resulting from systemically injected 3-O-methylglucose (3-O-MG)[13] or insulin hypoglycaemia[15,17], confirming the importance of the lateral hypothalamus in control of gastric secretion. The connections between the hypothalamus and the vagal nuclei have been traced by ter Horst et al.[6] and by Sawchenko and Swanson[18] and apparently involve transfer via neurons in the globus pallidus with probable relay in the brainstem reticular formation[19].

Destruction of the ventromedian hypothalamus (VMH) causes an increase in basal acid and pepsin secretion in rats[20], suggesting that the VMH restrains the lateral hypothalamus, one major site from which both feeding[21] and gastric secretion are stimulated by glucoprivation. Ishikawa et al.[22] found that in most but not all rats tested, electrical stimulation of the VMH partly inhibited 2-DG-stimulated acid secretion. Other sites that may originate signals stimulating gastric secretion via DMNV are median forebrain bundle (MFB)[14]. and the medial and lateral components of NTS, especially the rostral ends[12,23]. Injection of 2-DG into the liver circulation also stimulates gastric secretion, probably via the NTS.[12,15,24]

Glucose-dependent trigger sites identified by surgical or local anesthetic ablation during systemic hypoglycaemia (insulin or the glucoprivic analogues 2-DG and 3-O-MG), and by localized application of 2-DG were further identified by [^{14}C]-2-DG uptake in brains of hypoglycaemic rats and mice.[25]

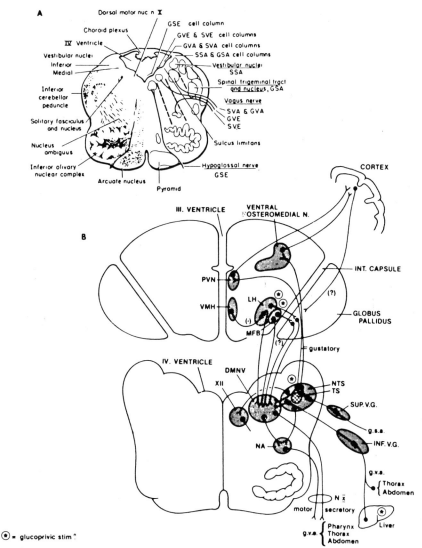

Figure 1 **A** Schematic transverse section of the medulla showing its basic features. Cell columns related to functional components of the cranial nerve are indicated on the right. Functional components of cranial nerves are both general and special. Functional components of the vagus nerve are shown in relation to particular nuclei. Heavy dashes separate the nuclei of the various cell columns on the right side. SSA, special somatic afferents; SUP VG, superior vagal ganglion; SVA, special visceral afferent; SVE, special visceral efferents; TS, tractus solitarius; VMH, ventromedian hypothalamus. Sites stimulated by glucoprivation: LH, MFB, NTS, NA (from *Core Text of Neuroanatomy*[19])

B Schematic illustration of the connections of the central vagal complex. DMNV = dorsomotor nucleus of the vagus; gsa, general somatic afferents; gva, general visceral afferents; gve, general vagal efferents; INF VG, inferior vagal ganglion; LH, lateral hypothalamus; MFB, median forebrain bundle; NA, nucleus ambiguus; NTS, nucleus tractus solitarius; NX, vagus nerve; PVN, paraventricular nucleus;

Vagal excitation by glucoprivation

Simici, Popesco and Diculesco[26] first reported stimulation of gastric secretion during insulin-induced hypoglycaemia 60 years ago. La Barre and de Cespedes[27] showed stimulation of gastric acid secretion by cross-circulating hypoglycaemic blood into the head of a recipient dog connected to its stomach by only the vagus nerves. The effects of hypoglycaemia can be blocked irreversibly by bilateral vagotomy and reversibly by cooling the vagal trunks to 4–8°C[28] by injection of local anaesthetic into the nerve trunks[29] and by systemically given atropine[1,21].

Glucose analogues: 2-deoxy-D-glucose and 3-O-methylglucose

The brain can also be deprived of glucose by intravenous administration of non-metabolized glucose analogues (2-DG) and 3-O-MG[30–34]. Unlike insulin[35,36], these agents do not inhibit acid secretion[34]. The glucose analogue 2-DG is a competitive inhibitor of glucose transport and phosphohexose isomerase activity, forming 2-DG-6-phosphate and blocking the further uptake and metabolism of glucose, thus effectively causing cytoglucopenia (Figure 2)[34,37]. Threshold doses of 2-DG in most species exceed 25 mg/kg, and maximal stimulation of gastric secretion is seen at 100–200 mg/kg. Rather than inhibiting phosphohexose isomerase activity, 3-O-MG competes for cellular glucose transport. Thus much larger doses (~ 1 g/kg) of 3-O-MG than of 2-DG are required to activate glucose-dependent neural centres[34,38]. The gastric response to a single dose of 2-DG is prolonged (often >4 h) and not readily reversed by subsequent injection of glucose[31,34,38]. Gastric secretion can be sustained without fading for 24 h or more by continuous 2-DG infusion[39]. Effects of systemically injected 2-DG or 3-O-MG have been shown, among others, in humans[31], dogs[34,39], cats[40], rats[30,32,38], chickens[41], and sheep[35], whereas insulin hypoglycaemia does not stimulate

CEREBRAL GLUCOPRIVATION

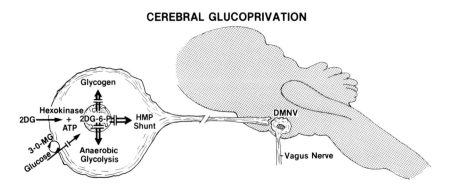

Figure 2 Diagram of mechanism of action of glucose analogs in causing cerebral glucoprivation at sites that act via the DMNV. 2-DG, 2-deoxy-D-glucose. 2DG-6-P, 2-deoxy-D-glucose-6-phosphate; 3-O-methylglucose; HMP, hexose monophosphate

the vagus in sheep[42] and goats[43] at glucose levels as low as 10 mg/100 ml. In sheep brains, the high levels of hexokinase[44] may explain the tolerance of hypoglycaemia and intolerance to 2-DG, manifested by convulsions[45].

Vagal excitation stimulates equally acid, pepsin (Figure 3) and gastric antral motility[46], and all are equally and rapidly inhibited by atropine or interruption of vagal trunk transmission[28,47]. Glucoprivation stimulates not only gastric secretion via cholinergic pathways and the release of gastrin[48,49] but also causes the pancreas to secrete[40] and the stomach, gallbladder and gut to contract; produces hunger and thirst[31,37]; and stimulates sympathetic adrenomedullary discharge[32,37], anterior pituitary hormones (especially growth hormones and renin and vasopressin release[37], and directly and indirectly the many homeostatic responses required to restore the glucose equilibrium. Serum $[K^+]$ falls and $[Na^+]$ rises[31,34]. With 2-DG, serum glucose[31] and plasma free fatty acids increase because of adrenergic activation[32,37,50]. Insulin secretion fails to rise[37], presumably because, after 2-DG injection, the β-cells recognize and respond to the cellular glucoprivation rather than to the secondary hyperglycaemia.

Vagal effects with various stimuli can be shown to be graded. Thus gastrin release and the gastric secretory[49] and motor[46] responses to 2-DG are dose dependent[51]. Electrical stimulation of the vagus can produce graded responses by varying either the voltage[52] or the stimulus frequency[53]. Thus the vagus does not act as an all-or-none switch but more like a tuning device. However,

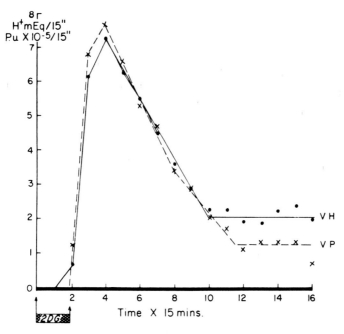

Figure 3   Acid and pepsin outputs in gastric fistula dogs with intact vagi given 2-DG 100 μg/kg iv over a period of 30 min (reprinted by permission of the *American Journal of Physiology*[34])

it is not normal for blood glucose concentrations to fall to levels generally associated with experimental maximal activation of the vagus. It is not known how physiological changes of glucose content or metabolism in glucose-dependent neurons normally modulate the gastric and other mechanisms invoked by other stimuli of the DMNV and feeding centres.

By contrast with 2-DG, the glucose analogues 5-thioglucose and gold thioglucose preferentially localize in and destroy the ventromedian hypothalamus,[54] producing the same effects as electrical destruction of the VMH[20], i.e. hyperphagia, polydipsia, obesity and increased basal secretion[54]. The VMH is thought to modulate or restrain the stimulatory centre of the lateral hypothalamus thereby affecting appetite and thirst as well as gastric secretion.

Non-glucose-related chemical stimuli of the central vagus

Most non-glucose-related compounds that stimulate the secretory vagus are also neural inhibitors. These include systemically injected 5($\gamma\gamma$-dimethylallyl)-5-ethylbarbituric acid, alcohol (eliminated by bilateral vagotomy[55],) and GABA (γ-aminobutyric acid) through either GABA A or B receptors[56-58]. The exact location of the central action of the GABA agonists is not known. Although GABA stimulates gastric secretion, application of the GABA antagonist bicuculline to previously identified neurons in the DMNV stimulates antral motility[59]. This suggests that gastric secretion and antral motility are affected oppositely by GABA, whereas glucoprivation stimulates both together.

Mechanism of nerve cell stimulation

The cellular mechanism that might excite neuronal activity through deprivation of an essential energy substrate, such as glucose, is unknown. Possibly the neurons of the sites sensitive to the lack of glucose exist in a suppressed state that is depolarized by ACh in ACh-sensitive cells, maintained by energy- or substrate-dependent, endogenous ionic (e.g. K^+) currents, analogous to the M-current described by Brown[60,61]. If the analogy holds, glucose deprivation would activate the cell by altering the frequency and pattern of cell firing. The mechanisms remain to be studied.

The prolonged reponse to baclofen[56,57] and to glucoprivation and the difficulty of reversing the vagal stimulation by elevating blood sugar after insulin hypoglycemia[62] or 2-DG injection[32,34] indicate that the mechanism of stimulation may not depend directly on glucose concentration but on the presence of a slowly cleared metabolite or a slowly corrected cell deficit accumulated as a result of glucose lack. It is unlikely that central vagal stimulation is entirely glucose related, since many other apparently unrelated compounds also stimulate the gastric vagus.

Brain peptides
Of the more than two dozen peptides that have been identified in brain[63,64] by immunostaining none has been specifically identified with the DMNV

complex. TRH occurs in the DMNV, the NTS and the NA[65], and TRH, as well as sulphated CCK intracerebroventricularly (ICV) stimulates gastric secretion via the vagus[66]. For inhibitory effects of centrally active peptides see below.

Cortical and cephalic stimulation of gastric secretion

The central vagus can also be stimulated by more distant signals from the cerebral cortex, and by conditions requiring additional caloric intake such as cold or lactation[1]. Olfactory and visual signals[67,68], suggestion of eating under hypnosis[69] and intense discussion of food[67] can all stimulate human gastric secretion. The additional gustatory input from chewing tasty food (sham feeding) further increases the response to about 50% of maximum obtainable with gastrin or histamine[7,70-74] and to 60–80% of that obtainable with insulin hypoglycemia[75]. The various afferent gustatory signals are summated and integrated probably in the limbic system[23,76], converging on the DMNV and the NA via the MFB and descending reticular pathways.

Sham feeding acts via the vagus and is completely atropine sensitive[7,73,77]. Sham feeding in humans stimulates secretion of acid and pepsin, as well as bicarbonate[78] and pancreatic secretion and gastric motility. The duration of response long outlasts the duration of chewing by 60–90 min and is independent of the amount chewed[7]. In dogs secretion may be stimulated for hours by sham feeding. The prolonged after-response indicates that a complex central mechanism is entrained and sustained without external reinforcement. No definitive studies have been done to truncate the response centrally. Elevation of blood sugar does not inhibit sham feeding responses[79]; peripheral vagal trunk interruption[1,80] or atropine inhibit within seconds. Prolonged responses are not due to gastrin since gastrin release in humans is stimulated little or none ($< 5-10$ pg/ml) by sham feeding; whereas stronger stimulation by 2-DG or hypoglycaemia does release gastrin in humans and animals.

Because it is simple to perform and safer than insulin hypoglycaemia[35] sham feeling has been used as a test for vagal intactness after surgery[71,81-83]. However, by the same token, the magnitude and duration of response do not represent any measure of vagal tone or capacity.

Inhibition of gastric secretion
Antagonists of central vagal stimulation include the following.

(1) Pretreatment with glucose or mannose, which are energy substrates for brain, but not fructose, galactose or xylose which are not, will prevent glucoprivic stimulation by 2-DG, 3-O-MG or insulin[34];
(2) Bromocriptine reduced 2-DG stimulated gastric secretion[84], in either conscious or anaesthetized rats. Dopamine antagonists, e.g. haloperidol, prevented inhibition. The site of this dopamine action is unknown.
(3) Local anaesthetics, e.g. lignocaine, applied to the LH blocked gastric effects of systemic 2-DG or 3-O-MG.[13] General anaesthesia with pento-barbital[85] markedly inhibited (> 90%) the gastric responses to 2-DG or

insulin hypoglycaemia. Studies of central vagal stimulation in anaesthetized animals should therefore be interpreted with extreme caution.

(4) Gastric secretion is inhibited by ICV epinephrine, norepinephrine, opioids and much more potently by bombesin[86,87] even after bilateral vagotomy[66]. The pathways for this action are not clear, but ICV bombesin and other peptides have some or all of the following profound additional effects:

   (a) epinephrine release is stimulated, causing an increase in circulating glucagon and glucose,
   (b) body temperature is lowered,
   (c) behaviour is altered,
   (d) feeding is depressed.

   It is thus evident that ICV injection may produce a number of non-specific effects, since all structures surrounding the ventricles are equally accessible to the compound being injected. More critical studies will require targeted microinjections of putative peptide agents to localize effects; a physiologic role for any effects found will require even more sophisticated experiments.

(5) Antimuscarinics acting peripherally, e.g. pirenzepine[88], inhibit vagal stimulation by 2-DG of acid and pepsin secretion. Atropine blocked $GABA_B$ vagal stimulation of secretion but not the vagal trunk spike activity[57], i.e. the effect of atropine was not central.

Electrical stimulation of vagal trunks

If the nerve is not damaged, secretion of acid may be maintained for hours by electrical stimulation of the distal vagal trunk. Graded responses of acid and pepsin may be obtained by varying the frequency (0.5–8 Hz, 4–5 V, 4–5 ms per impulse)[53,89]; and, in chickens, by varying voltage (20–50 V, 1 ms, 10 Hz)[90]. Electrical stimulation of brainstem produces bilateral vagal impulses of 0.5–5 Hz, suggesting that the optimal frequency most commonly reported, 4–10 Hz, may be appropriate for efferent vagal trunk stimulation, compared to the rate of 30–50 Hz measured for afferent impulses and for motor stimulation from central nuclei[91]. At lower frequencies only mucin is stimulated; acid and pepsin are stimulated at higher frequencies[53] while above 30 and up to 120 Hz acid secretion was inhibited[92]. These data may be species-dependent as, in the rat stimulated by a GABA agonist, frequencies of 250 Hz have been recorded in the efferent vagi[58]. These results suggest a possible additional discriminatory mechanism, other than anatomical, for separate control of various intestinal functions. Much remains to be discovered about anatomic and signal discrimination in the vagal control of gastric secretomotor function.

Vagal afferents

The more than 95% of the fibres in the abdominal vagal trunks that are afferent may be preferentially devoted to processing signals for intestinal motor reflexes[93,94]. From recordings of single vagal fibres, the sensory system is activated by both chemical[95,96] and mechanical stimuli. These signals can also be detected in the DMNV[97-99]. Mechanoreceptors are divided into slow (i.e. steady-state or tone sensors) and rapid, representing rate of change that presumably determines anticipatory motor changes. Slowly adapting mucosal chemoreceptors, especially abundant in the antral mucosa, activate another set of C-fibre afferents when stimulated by 0.1 N NaOH or 0.1 N HCl, threshold $pH > 8.0$ or < 3.0. Individual fibres responded to acid or alkali but never to both[95,100].

Macromolecules in afferent neurons

Visceral afferents involve both vagal and spinal neurons[101]. Identification by immunohistochemistry, radioimmunoassay, nerve ligature and toxin block of axonal transport, retrograde marker tracing, and more sophisticated measurements of physiological functions have shown that visceral afferents synthesize and transport a number of biologically active peptides, all of which also occur as well in the brain, in nerves and in endocrine cells elsewhere in the body[102]. Each belongs to a family of related peptides with similar patterns of biological activity[101,103,104]. Moreover, as with many transmitters, each peptide may have a wide spectrum of biological activity, depending on its site of release[105]. Physiological interpretations of topo-graphic location should thus be made with appropriate caution.

Nerve cell bodies in the nodose ganglion of the vagus contain peptides that stain with antibodies to substance P, CCK-gastrin, somatostatin, VIP, and possibly calcitonin gene-related peptide. These are transported distally in afferent fibres[106], since they accumulate central to vagal trunk ligatures. Substance P, somatostatin-14, G-17 and CCK-8 have also been found in vagal nerve extracts[90,103,104,107]. Substance P is the most abundant (50–250 pmol/g). Most of the substance-P-containing afferent neurons of the nodose ganglion of the vagus involve the thoracic organs rather than the upper gastrointestinal tract, though a few substance-P-containing fibres can be traced by double labelling from the anterior wall of the rat stomach to the ventral end of the nodose ganglion[101]. Peptides and proteins synthesized by cell bodies of afferent neurons are also transported to the NTS as well as to the periphery. Because axonal flow is bidirectional, transported substances accumulate on both sides of a ligature on the vagus nerve trunk; double ligature and immobilization of axonal flow (including axonal flow of the dye True Blue) by colchicine or capsaicin[108] suggest that $\sim 70\%$ of peptides or proteins are stationary.

Small-diameter vagal axons also contain and transport several important receptors, three of which have been studied in some detail: muscarinic ACh receptors[109]; opioid receptors[110]; and CCK receptors[111]. A proportion of these receptors, like the various messenger peptides, is transported in both directions at rates roughly two times faster in the centrifugal than the centripetal direction[109,111].

Different biologically active mobile peptides and receptors may coexist in afferent neurons with conventional transmitter substances[102,112]. Although the flow of signals in the afferent neurons is toward the CNS, the bulk of peptides are transported to the periphery, where they are released and may contribute to axonal reflexes. Moreover, peptides released distally may produce responses in secretion, circulation, smooth muscle and gut mucosa, either directly or indirectly through action on ganglia or release of active intermediates (e.g. histamine)[101]. From these data it would appear that afferent neurons of the vagus may also be effectors. The afferent vagal neurons may represent yet another level of integration and control of gastric function between the ENS and CNS.

Vagovagal reflexes

Distension of the innervated stomach produces secretion from the fundus as well as gastrin release via long-loop reflexes[80]. After mechanically stimulating vagal afferents, Davison and Grundy[113] recorded activity from efferent vagal fibres in chloralose-anaesthetized rats. Distension of the stomach increased the rate of firing in one group of fibres, while another group responded in a reciprocal manner with a decreased spontaneous rate of firing. Vagotomy eliminated the reflexes. The destination of the efferent signals (excitatory or inhibitory) could not be determined, nor were the physiological responses recorded. It is probable that the reflexes involve motor rather than secretory efferents[93].

Electrical stimulation (5 V, 1 ms, 10 Hz; 10 s on/10 s off) of the proximal end of the cut left cervical vagus caused about half as much gastric secretion as unilateral right efferent vagus stimulation in pentobarbital-anaesthetized rats[114]. The response was diminished by about 40–50% after electrolytic lesions of the ipsilateral hypothalamus. The results were interpreted as being due to the interruption of the predominantly excitatory influence of the paraventricular nucleus on the NTS and hence on the DMNV. These results and those of Harper et al.[115], using the central cut end of one abdominal vagus rather than the cervical vagus, describe long-loop vagovagal contralateral secretory reflexes, as well as contralateral reflexes.

PERIPHERAL CONTROLS

Both the traditional gastric and intestinal phases of gastric secretion fall largely under the heading of peripheral controls.

The gastric phase describes gastric secretion resulting from the presence of food in the stomach. Responses result from distension, which activates antrofundal and local neuronal reflexes and long-loop vagovagal mechanisms. Other responses depend on chemical stimuli: food products after digestion stimulate gastrin and probably other peptides; secreted acid completes the feedback loop by inhibiting gastrin release. The intestinal phase comprising stimulation of gastric secretion by amino acids and inhibition by fat and acid in the intestine is much less well defined.

Enteric nervous system

The notion that the stomach is 'denervated' by surgical vagotomy in the treatment of peptic (duodenal) ulcer has obscured the fact that the ENS is not only interposed between the CNS and the gut as a relay station but is an independent integrating neural network, with structural, chemical and functional properties analogous to those of the CNS. The ganglia of the gut are even more developed than the autonomic prevertebral ganglia[99] and more closely resemble CNS organization in the compact organization of neurons and glial cells. A blood–ganglion barrier exists and blood vessels do not penetrate ganglia[99]. The endogenous independent function of vessels and muscles and exocrine, endocrine and absorptive cells are further tuned by precisely balanced input from the ENS via neurotransmitters and endocrine and paracrine neuroeffectors.

The ENS of the upper gastrointestinal tract is connected to the CNS by two pathways: the parasympathetic via the vagus and the sympathetic via the coeliac ganglion and the splanchnic nerves[116]. Of the two, the vagus is functionally more important to gastric secretion. The myenteric and submucosal plexuses of the stomach and gut wall (Figure 4) are each composed of a network of ganglia densely connected to each other by nervous cell processes, which also connect the two plexuses[117]. In turn, the ganglia are connected to the extraenteric nervous structures by both afferent and efferent axons.

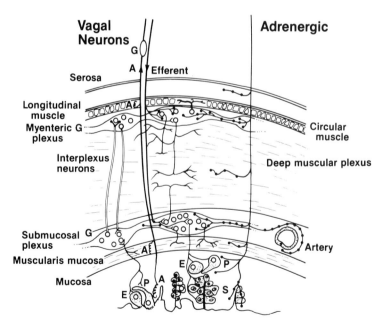

Figure 4 Schematic drawing of autonomic innervation of the stomach by vagal and adrenergic neurons; A = afferent; G = ganglia; P = paracrine; E = endocrine (shown as both 'open' and 'closed' cells); S = secretory cells

The afferent vagal fibres terminate in cell bodies in the nodose ganglion and hence connect to the brainstem.

The efferent fibres of the vagus, representing some 2000 of the 60 000 fibres in the human subdiaphragmatic vagus[2], originate in the DMNV and NA and terminate on the estimated 10^7 ganglia of the gastrointestinal tract via axosomatic, axoaxonal and axodendritic synapses[118]. Given the large numerical disparity, and the sometimes marginal or subtle alteration or loss of gastrointestinal function and only fractional loss of gastric ENS neurons by ultrastructural studies after external denervation, there must be a large amplification of any central signal via the intramural neural networks. There are fewer ganglia in the gastric submucosal than in the intestinal submucosal plexus or either gastric or gut myenteric plexus[118]. Although some adrenergic fibres from the splanchnic nerves apparently bypass the intramural ganglia to innervate directly blood vessels[99,117], as illustrated by fluorescent staining and electron microscopy[118], the vagal efferents apparently all terminate in ganglia.

Although electrical nerve events and muscle contraction can be measured in spatial and temporal relationships[99], the relationships between nerves and exocrine or endocrine secretion or absorption, which are much slower events than contraction, are less amenable to isolation and measurement at the cellular level. This makes it difficult to know which subserve which function or whether any neuron or combination is multifunctional. The coincidence of periodic gastric and pancreatic secretion with periodic motor activity, persisting after vagal interruption and eliminated by atropine or pentolinium, demonstrates at least one area of overlapping motor and secretion activity of the ENS[119]. The vagus appears to serve as the overall regulator of the integration provided by the ENS, since for a time after vagotomy, electrical and motor activity become chaotic[99,117,120]. Thus gastric secretion is eliminated[121] and gastric emptying is markedly impaired. Although gut function apparently recovers or adapts some time after vagotomy, the ENS probably then responds within narrower limits.

Modern histochemical techniques have demonstrated a much more complex chemical picture of the ENS than was generally held until quite recently. Beyond the classification into cholinergic and adrenergic neurons, the same intramural neurons may also contain other transmitters or one or more of the peptides VIP, substance P, gastrin, CCK, somatostatin, bombesin, neurotensin and enkephalin[101,102,107,112], many of uncertain function.[122]

Gastric secretion is controlled at several interacting levels – nervous, hormonal and paracrine (including cell-to-cell communication) – by interstitial tissue environment and by luminal factors[123]. Nervous control of secretion by the vagus is probably entirely mediated by the post-ganglionic and intramural neural networks. Post-ganglionic cholinergic nerve terminals have been shown in proximity to some, but not all, parietal cells[118,124,125]; taken with the pharmacologic evidence of atropine sensitivity[88], both the ganglionic and post-ganglionic stimulation (e.g. with bethanechol) of acid and pepsin secretion are muscarinic. Moreover, parietal cells[53,126] and peptic cells[127,128] can be stimulated directly by cholinergic agents.

Although ACh is clearly the transmitter of the efferent vagal fibres, the peptides gastrin, CCK, GRP, substance P, gastric inhibitory peptide (GIP), VIP, and perhaps others probably occur largely in afferent vagal neurons or in post-ganglionic enteric neurons[102]. The peptides and transmitters in post-ganglionic fibres may act through neurocrine mechanisms directly on effector cells or through stimulating and inhibiting paracrine or endocrine cells, such as gastrin, somatostatin and histamine-secreting cells[126] (Figures 4,5).

Chemical transmitters of neural effects

Acetylcholine
The principal chemicals involved in vagal stimulation of gastric secretion are ACh, gastrin, the bombesin-like GRP, histamine and the inhibitor somatostatin. Vagal stimulation of gastric secretion and motility is mediated at one or more critical steps by ACh. This conclusion follows from the complete suppression of vagally stimulated gastric secretion and motility[46] by atropine at doses of $10-20\,\mu g/kg$[129]. Inhibition by the muscarinic antagonist pirenzepine[28,88], a quaternary compound that does not cross the

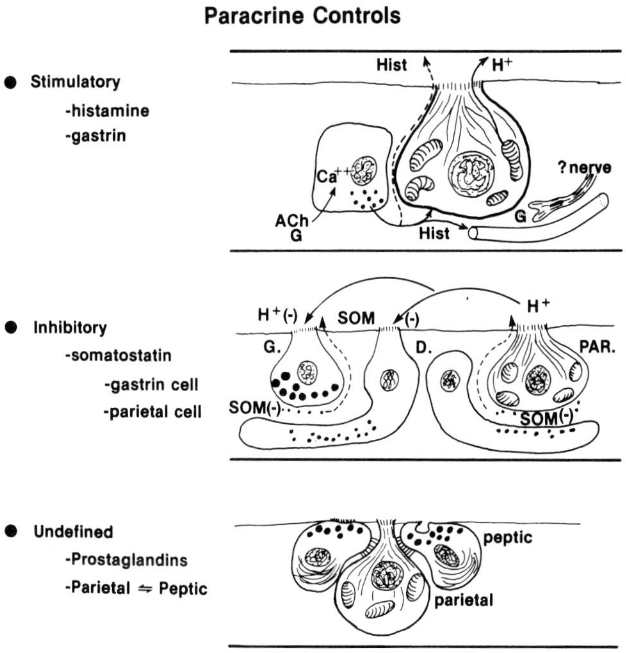

Paracrine Controls

Figure 5 Paracrine controls of gastric secretion include possible stimulatory release of histamine by ACh and perhaps gastrin from a tissue histamine cell. Inhibitory effects of somatostatin may involve both gastrin and parietal cells. Undefined paracrine effects include unknown parietal-peptic cell interactions via gap junctions. In the middle panel, both open (antral) and closed (fundus), G and D cells are shown. ACh = acetylcholine; G = gastrin; HIST = histamine; PAR = parietal; D = D cells; SOM = somatostatin; ($-$) = inhibition

blood–brain barrier (it is not known whether the same applies to the blood–ganglion barrier), indicates that the cholinergic step is peripheral and not central. Inhibition by atropine of vagal stimulation is seen in all species and is independent of the vagal stimulant: 2-DG[88], hypoglycaemia[1,47,130], and sham feeding[73,131] are equally susceptible to atropine inhibition. The sensitivity to atropine, reflected by an ED_{50} of $\sim 1\,nM/kg$[88], clearly defines vagal stimulation of gastric secretion as muscarinic[132]. Bethanechol stimulation of gastric secretion in dogs is equally sensitive to atropine[88].

The susceptibility of basal secretion in humans to atropine with ED_{50} in the range of $\sim 1\,nM/kg$[131,133], shows that basal secretion is sustained by a muscarinic mechanism. That the vagus is in turn largely responsible for basal secretion is shown by the virtual elimination of basal secretion by vagotomy[71,83,85].

The vagus stimulates both acid and pepsin secretion via muscarinic pathways, and both are equally susceptible to atropine. However, histamine H_2 antagonists inhibit only the acid stimulated by the vagus or by cholinomimetics[51]. This suggests that ACh acts either through or with histamine to stimulate parietal cells in intact stomachs, even though there is evidence for direct cholinergic stimulation of isolated parietal cells through specific cholinergic receptors that act on the cell by pathways distinct from those of histamine[126]. Moreover, cholinergic receptors have been localized on parietal cells by electronmicroscopic autoradiography with [^{3}H]-labelled 3-quinuclidinyl benzilate (QNB)[124,134]. Stimulation of peptic cells by ACh apparently occurs without any further intermediation[127] and, during histamine infusion in dogs, where acid is maximally stimulated and pepsin not, superimposition of vagal excitation by 2-DG[34] or insulin[35] results in a strong stimulation of pepsin secretion without change in acid secretion (Figure 6). The added pepsin stimulation is completely inhibited by atropine[34]. Electrical vagal stimulation also increases pepsin secretion under similar circumstances.[135]

Fundic vagotomy in dogs results in a decreased response to stimulation by gastrin or histamine.[121,136] This effect can be reversed by a background infusion of a subthreshold dose ($10\,\mu g\,kg^{-1}\,h^{-1}$) of bethanechol (Figure 7). The exact mechanism whereby fundic vagotomy decreases sensitivity and cholinergic agents reverse the effect is not known. Because atropine also shifts the histamine-[130,137] and pentagastrin-[138] dose-response curves to the right, it must be assumed that the pseudo-competitive inhibitory effects of vagotomy and of atropine are due to a lack of ACh at the cell level.

Contrasting with decreased sensitivity after vagotomy, the administration of bethanechol as background in both dogs and rats potentiates stimulation by histamine and gastrin of gastric acid and pepsin secretion. The effects of bethanechol are twofold: an increase of maximum output of acid and a leftward shift of the dose-response curve of both histamine[136,139] and pentagastrin[121]. Both effects are proportional to the dose of bethanechol and are equally effective before and after vagotomy[136].

Because bethanechol acts at post-ganglionic, rather than ganglionic, sites[140,141], these effects of cholinergics are more likely to be cellular than via the ENS. A cellular site of potentiation by cholinergics can also be

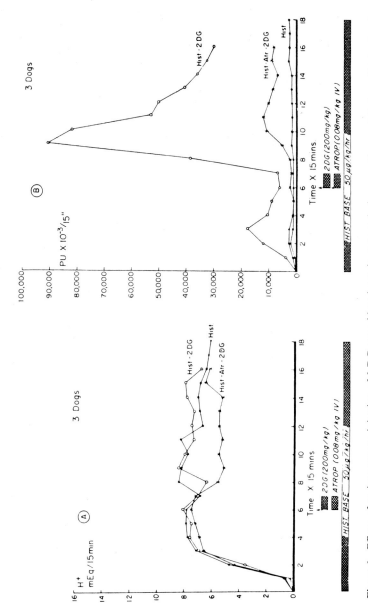

Figure 6 Effects of an intravenous injection of 2-DG on acid and pepsin output during a continuous infusion of histamine. In another experiment, the 2-DG was given with atropine 80 μg/kg (reprinted by permission of the *American Journal of Physiology*[34])

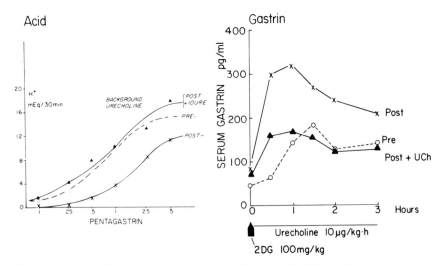

Figure 7 Gastric acid response to graded doses of pentagastrin (left panel) and serum gastrin response to 2-DG (right panel) in 3 dogs before and after fundic vagotomy. After fundic vagotomy, bethanechol (urecholine) 10 μg/kg.h was given as background (Post + UCh) (courtesy of *American Journal of Gastroenterology*[123])

inferred from effects demonstrable in isolated gastric glands[142] and parietal cells[53,126]. It is therefore likely that the pseudo-competitive effects of vagotomy and atropine, the reversal of the vagotomy effect by bethanechol, and potentiation by bethanechol of histamine or pentagastrin effects (in dogs) all occur through actions on the same mechanism. Such a mechanism most likely involves events downstream in the calcium-dependent messenger pathways.

In summary, ACh moderates vagal stimulation of gastric secretion at ganglia as well as by post-ganglionic mechanisms:

(1) by direct receptor-mediated Ca^{2+} dependent action on secretory cells;
(2) as a necessary co-factor and potentiator of histamine or gastrin at a level not yet identified;
(3) by releasing gastrin; and
(4) by paracrine effects on histamine and somatostatin release.

Gastrin

Gastrin plays a major role in both cephalic and gastric phases of gastric secretion. Gastrin stimulates gastric secretion solely by a hormonal mechanism[143] rather than by a paracrine action or by an intragastric portal circulation. Peripheral venous levels, though lower than those in portal venous blood[144], represent the effective concentrations responsible for stimulation of gastric secretion[143,145-147], since gastrin reaches the fundus only through the systemic circulation. ACh and gastrin are synergistic and thus vagal stimulation, using both, produces a vigorous secretory response (Figure 8).

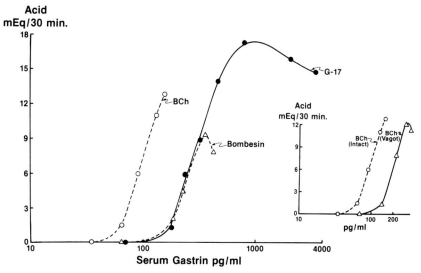

Figure 8 Acid output in fistula dogs related to measured concentrations of serum gastrin. The dogs graded doses (20–160 μg/kg.h) of bethanechol (BCh), bombesin (0.1 to 2 μg/kg.h) and gastrin G-17 (0.05 to 5 μg/kg.h). **Inset**: Bethanechol dose response in 3 dogs before (intact) and after fundic vagotomy (vagot).

Release of gastrin

Gastrin is released into the circulation from G cells, which are almost solely confined to the antrum. Release of gastrin may be stimulated in several ways: nervous, paracrine, and luminal. The principal stimuli are ACh, bombesin-like GRP and protein food products. Gastrin release is modulated or inhibited by somatostatin and by luminal acid. Electrical stimulation of the vagus and excitation of the vagus through cytoglucopenia promote gastrin release[148], proportional to the strength of the vagal signal. Insulin hypolgycaemia[137,149] and 2-DG elevate serum gastrin dose-dependently[129,150]. In dogs sham feeding produces a modest increase in serum gastrin,[151] whereas in humans sham feeding, a weaker stimulus of secretion than hypoglycaemia, causes no significant increase[70,74,152] or, at best, a very small increase (<5–10 pg/ml)[141].

Vagal release of gastrin depends solely on the nerve fibres innervating the antrum and, in dogs, is eliminated by selective antral vagotomy (Figure 9)[88,151,153] thus defining the source of vagally released gastrin as well as the nervous pathway for stimulation. Selective fundic vagotomy, leaving the antrum innervated, results in a greatly augmented vagal release of gastrin (Figure 10)[150]. Bethanechol[129] and bombesin[154] stimulation are also augmented by fundic vagotomy. This effect has been ascribed to the removal by fundic vagotomy of an inhibitor of gastrin release[49,103,155].The augmented vagal- or bombesin-stimulated release of gastrin can be reversed by a background infusion of bethanechol at a dose ($10\,\mu g\,kg^{-1}\,h^{-1}$) that is subthreshold for acid secretion (Figure 7)[121,129]. In an apparent paradox, the anti-cholinergic drug atropine also inhibits the augmented gastrin reponse

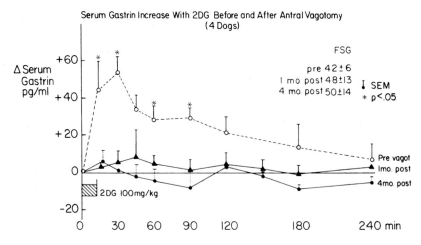

Figure 9 Change in serum gastrin in the 4 h after intravenous injection of 2-DG 100 mg/kg in 4 dogs before and 1 and 4 months after antral vagotomy

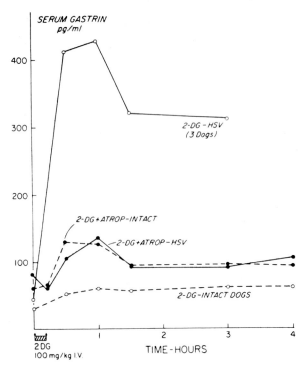

Figure 10 Effect of atropine on serum gastrin after an injection of 2-DG 100 μg/kg given iv over a 10 min period with or without atropine. Studies were performed in conscious fistula dogs before (intact) and after fundic vagotomy (HSV)

to vagal stimulation (Figure 10)[126] but fails to antagonize the increased bombesin response[48]. Thus the disinhibiting effect of fundic denervation on gastrin release is not confined to neural release of gastrin. Because resection of the fundic mucosa also results in augmentation of gastrin release[87,156] inhibition and disinhibition are probably not direct vagal or neural phenomena but apparently involve cholinergic mechanisms and the fundic mucosa.

Acute elevation of serum gastrin 24 h after truncal vagotomy in dogs[157] suggests that gastrin release is under the immediate control of the ENS and that inhibition is under control of the vagus. Vagal excitation during bombesin stimulation of dogs with antral vagotomy and fundic vagus intact did not inhibit gastrin release; thus the vagus does not actively stimulate an inhibitor from the fundus (unpublished observations). The nature of the fundic-cholinergic inhibition of gastrin release thus remains to be discovered.

ENS and paracrine regulation of gastrin release

In further examining the role of the ENS in regulation of gastrin release, major consideration must be given to both bombesin and somatostatin.

Bombesin, a 14-amino acid peptide isolated from the skin of the frog *Bombina bombina*, and the mammalian counterpart GRP, is a potent gastrin releasing peptide with additional effects on other endocrine, exocrine, muscle and neural cells. A family of structurally related peptides of amphibian origin has been isolated and found to have similar actions[158]. Immunohistochemical staining has localized bombesin-like peptides in both myenteric and mucosal plexus neurons in the stomach[159] and in the brain[102], where it has a number of very potent effects[160]. GRP acts as a major intermediate for vagal release of gastrin[125,159,161] and probably represents the atropine-resistant nicotinic component of vagal gastrin release (Figure 10)[159,162]. No role has been defined in gastric secretion for the GRP cells that are found in abundance in the fundus[159,162], since bombesin does not stimulate acid secretion directly and is ineffective after antrectomy[163]. Assays have not been sensitive enough to define a possible hormonal role for circulating GRP. Bombesin directly stimulates smooth muscle contraction, as well as mammalian pancreatic cells[164] and amphibian peptic cells[128].

With the antrum in place, bombesin stimulates gastric acid and pepsin only through release of gastrin, with dose-response curves relating acid output to serum gastrin curves that are superimpasable on those derived from exogenously infused gastrin G-17 (see Figure 8)[143,146,147]. However, bombesin acting via endogenous gastrin does not stimulate either acid or pepsin output to more than 60–80% of gastrin maximum, because at higher doses bombesin produces a concomitant inhibition of acid and pepsin secretion[15,146,147,165]. The failure to reach full response (e.g. see Figure 8) may be due to the co-release at high bombesin doses of somatostatin in the fundus from D cells, which are liberally distributed in proximity to parietal and chief cells[159,166,167].

Somatostatin-secreting D cells are widely distributed in both brain and gut. Somatostatin exhibits remarkably wide effects: inhibiting transport, exocrine, endocrine, neural, immune system, and contractile cells and antagonizing a broad range of stimuli. Nevertheless, somatostatin is not a universal inhibitor; it is at times quite stimulus specific, being relatively ineffective against histamine-stimulated gastric secretion but very potent against cholinergic stimulation. By its strategic location and extensions of the D cell body, the stomatostatin-secreting D cell maintains paracrine contract with both antral G cells and the secretory cells of the fundus[159,166,167]. Somatostatin is therefore well placed to modulate both gastrin release and gastric secretion (see Figure 5). In addition, somatostatin can inhibit the release of ACh at synapses and is thus capable of acting at yet another site concerned with neurohormonal control of secretion.

Antral and fundic D cells differ in one important respect: Antral D cells, like G cells, are of the open type[168], with one surface exposed to the lumen, whereas D cells of the fundus do not open on the lumen[166]. This difference has two possible implications: (1) the D cell of the antrum, but not the fundus, could sense signals from the lumen, e.g. acid[162]; and (2) somatostatin may have a function in the antral lumen. No such function has thus far been defined. A model (Figure 11) represents the apparent interactions resulting from vagal stimulation.

Gastric phase

Stimulation of secretion during the gastric phase of gastric secretion is almost exclusively due to gastrin released by food. Distension and afferent vagal impulses involved in normal eating by themselves probably contribute little in the intact stomach, though some gastrin is released by non-nutrient liquids in the dog[168] and humans[170]. Graded secretory responses to intragastric peptone are mediated by proportional elevations of circulating gastrin[145,171,172].

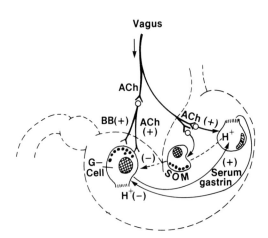

Figure 11 Major factors controlling the release of gastrin by the vagus. Negative feedback inhibiting gastrin release may act directly via acid in the lumen on the open end of the G cell; both H^+ and ACh may act by releasing somatostatin. ACh = acetylcholine; BB = bombesin; SOM = somatostatin; G cell = gastrin cell; (+) and (−) indicate stimulation and inhibition, respectively. Interpretation from results of studies in intact animals

Like the antral D cell, the G cell has one surface, covered by microvilli, that is exposed to the gastrin lumen (e.g. Figure 5)—the so-called open-end endocrine cell of Fujita and Kobayashi[168]. Food products within the lumen acting directly on the open end of the G cell stimulate the cell to secrete gastrin. It is likely that the components of digested food that stimulate the G cell[173] are protein products or amines, though whether they act on cell surface recognition sites or intracellularly is not known. Calcium[173] and ACh[76,151,175] in the lumen also stimulate gastrin release, probably through direct effects on the G cell via the luminally exposed open end. Their effects on antral D cells are unknown.

Vagal denervation prolongs the gastrin response to food[48] due to a combination of delayed gastric emptying and delayed acidification resulting from reduced acid secretion. In the long run, gastric stasis and removal of the acid feedback would produce G cell hyperplasia, leading to a permanently elevated serum gastrin. In the dog, atropine dose responsively inhibits food-stimulated gastrin release irrespective of vagal innervation and independently of pH of the contents[48] .Similar findings have been reported in humans.[176]

The release of gastrin by food (F) and by bombesin (B) is affected oppositely ($\downarrow$, inhibited; 0, no effect) by each of the following: atropine (B0, F$\downarrow$), bethanechol (B$\downarrow$, F0), somatostatin (B$\downarrow$, F0), prostaglandin E_2 (B$\downarrow$, F0), and antral acidification (B0, F$\downarrow$), indicating different pathways for food and bombesin stimulation of the G cell[164,177].

Inhibition by acid of gastrin release

Acidification of the luminal open-end surface[167] of the G cell below pH 3.0 partly and below 2.0 absolutely inhibits gastrin release stimulated by food, ACh, calcium in the lumen or vagal excitation (Figure 12) but does not inhibit gastrin release stimulated by bombesin[48,164,177]. Feedback through acidification of gastric contents thus terminates the gastric phase of gastrin-dependent gastric secretion. Acid inhibition is unaffected by vagal denervation[155,161,175]. Atropine alone may increase fasting serum gastrin[131,133,156,178]; combining acidification and atropine nullifies the effect of both[141] but does not explain either. The concept that somatostatin mediates the effects of acid through a neural cholinergic ENS reflex blocked by atropine[141] is inconsistent with the inhibition of somatostatin release by cholinergics[178-180]. It has also been suggested that acid in the lumen might release somatostatin by acting on the open end of the antral D cell exposed to the gastric lumen[159,162]. Because somatostatin at a dose ($0.5 \mu g \, kg^{-1} \, h^{-1}$) sufficient to inhibit bombesin stimulation did not inhibit food-stimulated gastrin release and acidification inhibited food (but not bombesin[164,177]) stimulation (Figure 12), it is unlikely that somatostatin mediates the inhibitory effect of luminal acid on gastrin release. On balance, it is most probable that acid inhibits the G cell by a direct effect exerted through its surface exposed to the antral lumen.

Histamine

Despite intense research on gastric secretion in general and on histamine in particular, in the dozen years since the development of H_2 receptor

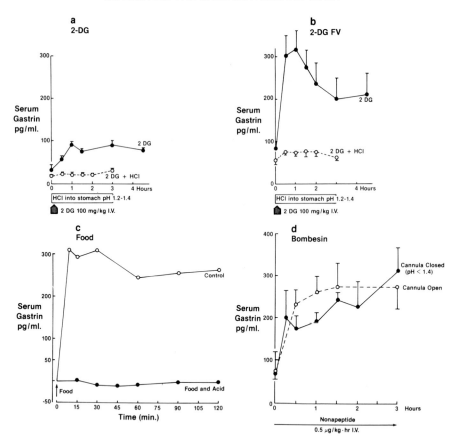

Figure 12 Acidification of antrum to pH < 1.4 in fistula dogs inhibited gastrin release by (a) 2-DG with intact vagi, (b) 2-DG after fundic vagotomy, (c) a meal of 350 g meat, but not (d) bombesin nonapeptide

antagonists, the connection between the vagus and histamine in the stimulation of the stomach remains circumstantial[126,181].

To interpret the evidence implicating histamine in the mediation of vagal stimulation of gastric secretion, acid and pepsin secretion have to be separately considered[36], as well as significant species differences in the metabolism and effects of histamine[126] and different effects in the intact compared to isolated stomachs, mucosa, glands and gastric cells. Another line of evidence derives from the inhibition by H_2 antagonists of the action of histamine and non-histamine stimuli (vagal, cholinergic, gastrin) on acid and pepsin secretion in various models. The synergism between histamine and other agonsits must also be considered. Further evidence is circumstantial: for example, the location of histamine-containing cells[53,126] and neurons[182] in the gastric mucosa and the synthesis and release of histamine from the stomach under various conditions[126]. Nervous control of histamine release is deduced from proximity of post-ganglionic fibres to mast cells in gastric mucosa of rat, guinea pig and rabbit.[17]

Briefly, histamine stimulates acid secretion in all species and in all experimental preparations, including isolated stomachs, mucosae, glands, and cells[183,184]. This effect is competitively and specifically inhibited by histamine H_2-receptor antagonists, the action of which reproduces agonist withdrawal[185]. Moreover, H_2 antagonists inhibit stimulation of acid secretion in intact animals by all stimuli including vagal, cholinergic[51], gastrin, food, and even caffeine in humans[36]. This effect implies that all stimuli of acid secretion in intact animals act through or depend on histamine. From such evidence in intact animals one might conclude that histamine is a critical intermediary in acid stimulation by the vagus and all agonists, that is, all release histamine to stimulate the parietal cell. Alternatively histamine could be an essential co-stimulus and the occupation of the H_2 receptor by an agonist would be obligatory for stimulation via any other receptor. Neither is likely to be generally true and the facts still beg a rational explanation.

Experiments *in vitro* present a somewhat different view of histamine as the 'final common pathway'. Although H_2 antagonists block ganglionic (electrical field or carbachol) stimulation of acid, in isolated mouse stomachs[186] they do not block post-ganglionic (bethanechol) cholinergic stimulation. Moreover, in isolated parietal cells neither cholinergic[53,183] nor gastrin stimulation[126,183,187] is blocked by H_2 antagonists which are also bypassed by cellular cAMP elevation. Histamine intermediation thus occurs in intact stomachs but not at the cellular level, where non-histamine stimuli do bypass H_2 antagonists.

The peptic cell presents a different picture. There are major species differences in the action of histamine on pepsinogen secretion, and H_2-receptor antagonists antagonize only the action of histamine on such cells[68] .Histamine via H_2 receptors stimulates pepsinogen secretion in humans[68] ,monkeys and pigs, among others, but has a biphasic effect on pepsinogen secretion in dogs and cats[36] .In dogs, histamine at low doses stimulates and at high doses inhibits pepsinogen secretion, both apparently via H_2 receptors but presumably of different affinity[188]. Histamine does not stimulate isolated peptic cells[127]. Moreover, histamine H_2 antagonists do not block the stimulation of peptic cells in dogs by cholinergic[51] or vagal stimulation[184]. Because the vagus stimulates acid and pepsin equally well, it is unlikely that histamine mediates vagal stimulation, at least of the peptic cell. Gastrin also stimulates the peptic cell in the dog much more effectively than does histamine, making it unlikely that gastrin acts via the intermediation of histamine. Thus histamine does not appear to be necessary for peptic cell secretion by either the vagus or gastrin.

Circumstantial evidence for a role for histamine in the gastric mucosa that is derived from the presence of histamine-containing cells[53,118,126] or the increase in histamine or histamine-forming capacity, as in the rat[182], does not extend to all species. Vagal stimulation in dogs does not increase venous histamine nor does it alter histidine decarboxylase or N-methyltransferase[189]. Likewise pentagastrin does not release histamine from the canine stomach *in vivo* or *in vitro*.[190]

No single model, therefore, clearly defines a specific role for histamine in vagal stimulation of gastric secretion. Species differences and the apparent discrepancies between *in vivo* and *in vitro* effects of histamine and H_2 antagonists need to be reconciled before a definitive picture can be drawn of the place of histamine in the regulation of gastric secretion.

ANTROFUNDAL INTERACTIONS

The extensive autonomic nervous network in the gastric wall provides a mechanism for the functional integration between anatomic regions of the stomach. Further integration is provided by circulating hormones. Communication between antrum and fundus by a portal intramural circulation has not been established.

Antrofundal reflexes

Distension of separated, vagally innervated antral pouches stimulates acid secretion from the innervated fundus via two mechanisms: gastrin release into the circulation and vagovagal reflexes[102,175,191]. Each can be separately eliminated, the former by luminal acidification and the latter by vagotomy; both together eliminate the antrofundal reflex. Antral distension is much less effective if the antrum is kept in continuity with the rest of the stomach[172]. indicating that the balance between the antrum and fundus is modulated largely via the ENS.

Fundoantral reflexes

In the other direction, distension of an innervated fundic (Pavlov) pouch stimulates the release into the circulation of gastrin[69] from an innervated antral pouch, resulting in turn in acid secretion from the Pavlov pouch. The antral response is eliminated by antral acidification as well as by vagotomy[175]. The pathway is presumed to be via long vagovagal reflexes. Distension of the innervated fundus after antral resection also causes acid and pepsin secretion[80,175,192] presumably via local ENS reflexes. However, distension of the fundus in an intact stomach produces little release of gastrin[80], suggesting a modulating effect of the ENS on vagovagal reflexes.

Antrectomy

A functional antrum is critical to the full response to electrical or central vagal stimulation[76,80,175,192]. Either antral acidification or topical anaesthesia, e.g. cocainization of the antrum, eliminates the gastrin response to most stimuli[175]. Antrectomy sharply reduces the response of the innervated remaining fundus to vagal stimulation, by either sham feeding or insulin hypoglycaemia[135,193], and the fundic responses to the non-vagal stimuli, histamine and gastrin, are also markedly depressed (see Figure 13). The mechanism of

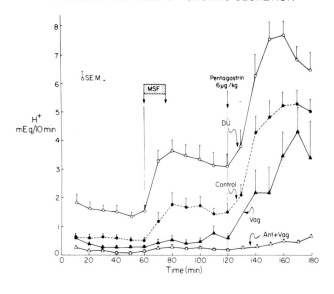

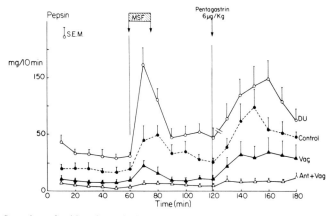

Figure 13 Secretion of acid and pepsin in the basal state (60 min), during and after 15 min modified sham feeding (MSF) (60–120 min), and after pentagastrin 6 μg/kg subcutaneously in 4 groups of subjects. Duodenal ulcer (n = 60), normal controls (n = 40), duodenal ulcer after fundic vagotomy (n = 20) and duodenal ulcer after truncal vagotomy and antrectomy (n = 16)

this effect is unknown, though Sjodin[135] reported that infusions of gastrin or pentagastrin restored the response to sham feeding in antrectomized dogs. This finding has not been reported by others. Even simple separation of the antrum from the body of the stomach reduces the fundic secretory response to stimuli[192]. The effect may be due to disruption of the neural network integrating the two regions of the stomach.

VAGOTOMY

Because vagotomy is used for treating duodenal ulcer[172,195], the role of the vagus in disease and function of the stomach is a matter of considerable interest in medicine.

Truncal vagotomy

If the vagal trunks are interrupted during central vagal stimulation in dogs, gastric secretion ceases almost immediately, indicating that the ENS requires continuous input from the vagus and is not entrained by the vagus for prolonged action. Moreover, if the vagi are cut in rats during stimulation by the combined infusion of histamine, gastrin, and carbachol[196], gastric secretion falls immediately by 90%, an effect that cannot be explained as due to an immediate transmitter deficiency. Acute vagal denervation may induce a transient chaotic state in the ENS by removal of modulatory or oscillatory control and result in dominance of inhibitory effects.

After bilateral truncal vagotomy in dogs, there is neither gastrin released nor acid or pepsin secreted in response to 2-DG central vagal excitation (Figures 14 and 15). Moreover, in such animals, superimposed 2-DG injection does not inhibit secretion stimulated by histamine or pentagastrin infusion (unpublished observations). Thus there is no evidence for a 'vagogastrone'[192] and there are no extravagal pathways for central stimulation or inhibition, for example, by the strong adrenergic stimulation that would be unaffected by gastric vagotomy or the other actions of 2-DG-induced cytoglucopenia, such as growth hormone, vasopressin[197], or renin release[37] and hyperglycaemia and hypokalaemia[34]. In similar experiments with insulin instead of 2-DG, acid secretion is inhibited by a direct K^+ dependent action of insulin[35,36] and not through central vagal excitation.

In humans, bilateral truncal vagotomy produces a decrease in both sensitivity and maximum response to non-vagal stimuli[198]. Basal secretion and vagal responses tend to remain depressed after complete vagotomy[83] ,but partial recovery of the response to histamine or pentagastrin is seen in many vagotomized subjects. Bethanechol has been reported by some[139,193], but not others[199], to restore histamine or gastrin secretory responses to prevagotomy levels. Recovery of secretory[195] and, in many instances, motor function after partial or complete gastric vagotomy has remained unexplained. In rats, recovery of acid secretion within 4–6 weeks has been shown to coincide with regeneration of fundic vagus nerves cut close to the serosa[200] and remaining in proximity to the target organ. In the absence of regeneration, partial functional recovery may represent adaptation of the ENS to assume some of the controlling functions of the full hierarchical system: brain, vagus nerves and ganglia, and peripheral autonomic system. Restoration by bethanechol of sensitivity of the fundus to gastrin and histamine and reversal of hypersensitivity of the antral G cells indicate that the vagus normally exerts its modulation of the ENS via ACh.

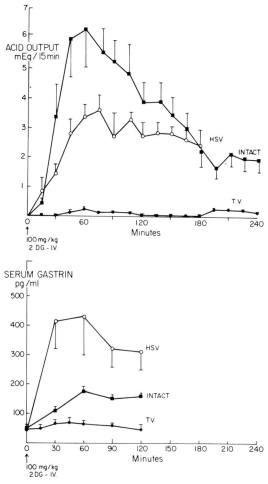

Figure 14   Acid output and gastrin release with 2-DG in dogs before (intact) and after fundic vagotomy (HSV). In the same dogs, subsequent truncal vagotomy (TV) eliminated both acid and gastrin responses (Courtesy of *American Journal of Gastroenterology*[123])

Regional vagotomy

Fundus

Selective vagal denervation of the fundus, leaving the antrum innervated, immediately eliminates the gastric acid and pepsin response to vagal excitation (Figure 7)[136,201]. The sensitivity, but not the maximum response, of the fundus to histamine and gastris is depressed; that is, curves shift to the right (pseudo-competitive inhibition; see Figure 7). This effect is reversed by subthreshold doses of bethanechol[49,121,154], which also reversed the increased gastrin release by 2-DG (see Figure 7). There was also an increased

153

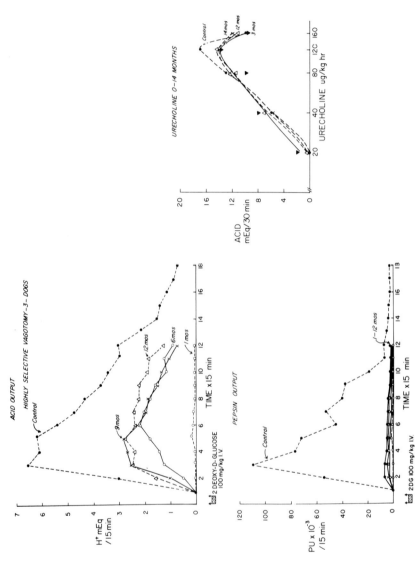

Figure 15 Effect of fundic (highly selective) vagotomy on acid and pepsin responses to 2-DG 100 μg/kg before and 1, 6, 9 and 12 months later. In the right panel, the acid responses to graded doses of bethanechol (urecholine) before and up to 14 months after vagotomy are shown (courtesy of *American Journal of Digestive Diseases*[96])

gastrin response to bombesin[123]; the effect was not purely neural, but this effect too was reversed by bethanechol[129,154].

After a variable period, usually 2–4 months, the vagal responses to 2-DG begin to recover but reach a plateau well below prevagotomy levels[121,136]. Acid secretion recovers to $\sim 60\%$, whereas pepsin secretion recovers to $< 15\%$. However, both acid and peptic cells remain fully responsive to direct stimulation by bethanechol (Figure 15).

Selective antral vagotomy

An experimental operation performed only in animals, antral vagotomy provides an excellent model for studying vagal effects on the fundus[88,151,156]. After selective antral vagotomy, the vagally stimulated release of gastrin by 2-DG (see Figure 9) or insulin hypoglycaemia[151,156] is eliminated. However, the fundic acid and pepsin secretory responses to vagal stimulation by 2-DG or insulin hypoglycaemia[151] remain unimpaired, perhaps because of increased sensitivity of the fundus to cholinergic stimulation. By contrast, the fundic response to pentagastrin was lower (Figure 16).

With the loss of gastrin release after antral vagotomy, it is possible to analyse direct vagal stimulation of the fundus. After antral vagotomy, the secretory response to 2-DG was highly sensitive to atropine[88] with ED_{50} $\sim 1\,nM/kg$. This showed that the direct vagal stimulation of the fundus is muscarinic at pre- and post-ganglionic sites or both.

Neural control of gastric secretion thus involves a complex central network where signals may be generated, and where extensive afferent signals are received, sorted and integrated. From this network through the DMNV complex messages to the periphery are carried via some 2000 nerve fibres in the vagus nerves to modulate the ENS through synapses with the estimated 10^7 ganglia of the ENS. The ENS in turn is a semi-autonomous 'little brain' that exerts detailed control over gastrointestinal function via multiple chemical messengers in post-ganglionic fibres. The interactions between conventional messengers–ACh, histamine and gastrin–and the number of peptides in afferent and efferent nerve fibres, and the endocrine and paracrine are now gradually being brought to light.

Acknowledgements

The author would like to thank Ms Mary Stringer, Ms Nancy Clemons and Mr Jack Smith of the Lister Hill Library at the University of Alabama at Birmingham and Ms Deborah Beam of the Division of Gastroenterology for their assistance in manuscript preparation.

This paper has been adapted from 'Neural and Hormonal Control of

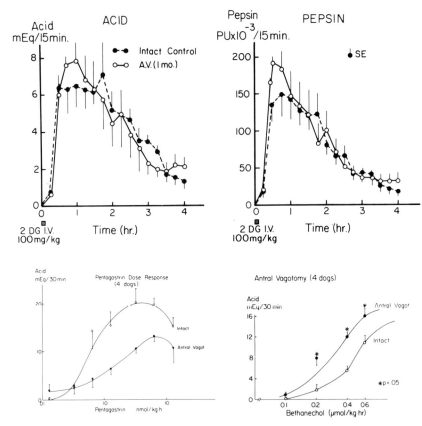

Figure 16 Acid and pepsin output in response to 100 mg/kg 2-DG (top) remained substantially unaltered by antral vagotomy (AV) in 4 dogs. The response to pentagastrin (bottom left) was reduced, while the response to bethanechol (lower right) was increased by antral vagotomy

Gastric Secretion' in *Handbook of Physiology—The Gastrointestinal System III*, John Forte (ed.). American Physiological Society, 1989.

References

1. Brooks, F. P. (1967). Central neural control of gastric secretion. In Code, C. F. and Heidel, W. (ed.) *Handbook of Physiology. Alimentary Canal*, Section 6, Vol. 2, pp. 805–26. Washington, D.C.: Am. Physiol. Soc.
2. Hoffman, H. H. and Schnitzlein, H. N. (1961). The number of nerve fibers in the vagus nerve of man. *Anat. Rec.*, **139**, 429–36
3. Fox, E. A. and Powley, T. L. (1985). Longitudinal columnar organization within the dorsal motor nucleus represents separate branches of the abdominal vagus. *Brain. Res.*, **341**, 269–82
4. Gwyn, D. G., Leslie, R. A. and Hopkins, D. A. (1985). Observations on the afferent and efferent organization of the vagus nerve and the innervation of the stomach in the squirrel

monkey. *J. Comp. Neurol.*, **239**, 163–75

5. Yamamoto, T., Satomi, H., Ise, H. and Takahashi, K. (1977). Evidence of the dual innervation of the cat stomach by the vagal dorsal motor and medial solitary nuclei as demonstrated by the horseradish peroxidase method. *Brain Res.*, **122**, 125–31

6. Ter Horst, G. J., Luiten, P. G. and Kuipers, F. (1984). Descending pathways from hypothalamus to dorsal motor vagus and ambiguus nuclei in the rat. *J. Autonom. Nerv. Syst.* 11:59–75

7. Konturek, S. J., Kwiecien, N., Obtulowicz, W., Mikos, E., Sito, E., Olesky, J. and Popiela, T. (1979). Cephalic phase of gastric secretion in healthy subjects and duodenal ulcer patients role of vagal innervation. *Gut*, **20**, 875–81

8. Swanson, L. W. and Kuypers, H. G. (1980). The paraventricular nucleus of the hypothalamus. *J. Comp. Neurol.*, **194**, 555–70

9. Shiraishi, T. (1980). Effects of lateral hypothalamic stimulation on medulla oblongta and gastric vagal neural responses. *Brain Res. Bull.*, **5**, 245–50

10. Wyrwicka, W. and Garcia, R. (1979). Effect of electrical stimulation of the dorsal nucleus of the vagus nerve on gastric acid secretion in cats. *Exp. Neurol.*, **65**, 315–25

11. Kerr, F. W. and Preshaw, R. M. (1969). Secretomotor function of the dorsal motor nucleus of the vagus. *J. Physiol. (Lond.)* **205**, 405–15

12. Kadekaro, M., Timo-Iaria, C. and de L. Vincentini, M. (1980). Gastric secretion provoked by functional cytoglucopoenia in the nuclei of the solitary tract in the cat. *J. Physiol. (Lond.)*, **299**, 397–407

13. Colin-Jones, D. G. and Himsworth, R. L. (1970). The location of chemoreceptor controlling gastric acid secretion during hypoglycemia. *J. Physiol. (Lond.)*, **206**, 307–409

14. Kadekaro, M., Timo-Iaria, C., Valle, L. E. and Velha, L. P. (1972). Site of action of 2-deoxy-D-glucose mediating gastric secretion in the cat. *J. Physiol. (Lond.)*, **221**, 1–13

15. Kadekaro, M., Timo-Iaria, C. and Valle, L. E. (1975). Neural systems responsible for the gastric secretion provoked by 2-deoxy-D-glucose cytoglucopoenia. *J. Physiol. (Lond.)*, **252**, 565–84

16. Tepperman, B. L. and Evered, M. S. (1980). Gastrin injected into the lateral hypothalamus stimulates secretion of gastric acid in rats. *Science*, **209**, 1142–3

17. Richardson, C. T., Barnett, C. C. and Feldman, M. (1984). Gastric acid secretory responsiveness to food in duodenal ulcer (DU). *Gastroenterology*, **86** (Abstract), 1219

18. Sawchenko, P. E. and Swanson, L. R. (1981). Central noradrenergic pathways for the integration of hypothalamic neuroendocrine and autonomic responses. *Science*, **214**, 685–7

19. Carpenter, M. B. (1985) *Core Text of Neuroanatomy*, 3rd Edn. (Baltimore, MD: Williams & Wilkins)

20. Ridley, P. T. and Brooks, F. P. (1965). Alterations in gastric secretion following hypothalamic lesions producing hyperphagia. *Am. J. Physiol.* **209**, 319–23

21. Brooks, F. P. and Evers, P. W. (eds.) (1977). In *Nerves and the Gut*, p.541.(Thorofare, N. J.: Charles Slack)

22. Ishikawa, T., Nagata, M. and Osumi, Y. (1983). Dual effects of electrical stimulation of ventromedian hypothalamic neurons on gastric acid secretion in rats. *Am. J. Physiol.*, **245**: G265–69

23. Kadekaro, M., Timo-Iaria, C. and Vicentini, M. M. (1977). Control of gastric secretion by the central nervous system. In Brooks, F. P. and Evers, R. W. (eds.) *Nerves and the Gut*, (Thorofare, N.J.: Charles Slack)

24. Shiraishi, T. and Takahashi, T. (1970). Glucose sensing cells and gastric acid secretion. *J. Physiol. Soc. Jpn.*, **32**, 422

25. Kadekaro, M., Savaki, H. and Sokoloff, L. (1980). Metabolic mapping of neural pathways involved in gastrosecretory response to insulin hypoglycaemia in the rat. *J. Physiol. (Lond.)*, **300**, 393–407

26. Simici, D., Popesco, M. and Diculesco, G. (1927). L'action de l'insuline sur la sécrétion de l'estomac a l'état normal et pathologique. *Arch. Maladies App. Digest.*, **17**, 28–43

27. La Barre, J. and de Cespedes, C. (1931). Role du systèmes nerveux central dans l'hypersécrétion gastrique consecutive a l'administration d'insuline. *Comp. Rend. Soc. Biol.*, **106**, 1249–51

28. Gleysteen, J. J., Esser, M. J. and Myrvik, A. L. (1983). Reversible truncal vagotomy in conscious dogs. *Gastroenterology*, **85**, 578–83

29. Chiba, T., Kadowaki, S., Taminato, T., Chihara, K., Seino, Y., Matsukura, S. and Fujita, T. (1981). Effect of antisomatostatin-globulin on gastrin release in rats. *Gastroenterology* **81**, 321–6

30. Colin-Jones, D.G. and Himsworth, R.L. (1969). The secretion of gastric acid in response to a lack of metaboizable glucose. *J. Physiol. (Lond.)*, **202**, 97–109

31. Duke, W. W., Hirschowitz, B. I. and Sachs, G. (1965). Vagal stimulation of gastric secretion in man by 2-deoxy-D-glucose. *Lancet*, **2**, 871–6

32. Himsworth, R. L. (1968). Compensatory reactions to a lack of metabolizable glucose. *J. Physiol. (Lond.)*, **198**, 451–65

33. Himsworth, R. L. (1968). Interference with the metabolism of glucose by a non-metabolizable hexose (3-methylglucose). *J. Physiol. (Lond.)*, **198**, 467–77

34. Hirschowitz, B. I. and Sachs, G. (1965). Vagal gastric secretory stimulation by 2-Deoxy-D-glucose. *Am. J. Physiol.*, **209**, 452–60

35. Hirschowitz, B. I. (1966). Quantitation of inhibition of gastric electrolyte secretion by insulin in the dog. *Am. J. Dig. Dis.*, **11**, 173–82

36. Hirschowitz, B. I. (1967). Continuing gastric secretion after insulin hypoglycemia despite glucose injection. *Am. J. Dig. Dis.*, **12**, 19–25

37. Thompson, D. A., Campbell, R. G., Lilavivat, U., Welle, S. L. and Robertson, G. L. (1981). Increased thirst and plasma arginine vasopressin levels during 2-deoxy-D-glucose-induced glucoprivation in humans. *J. Clin. Invest.*, **67**, 1083–93

38. Himsworth, R. L. and Colin-Jones, D. G. (1969). Factors which determine the gastric secretory response to 2-deoxy-D-glucose. *Gut*, **10**, 1015–18

39. Eisenberg, M. M., Chawla, R. C. and Sugawara, K. (1970). Sustained gastric secretion in response to 2-deoxy-D-glucose. *Gastroenterology*, **59**, 174–9

40. Meyer, J. H. (1981). Control of pancreatic exocrine secretion. In Johnson, L. R. (ed.) *Physiology of the Gastrointestinal Tract*, pp. 821–29. Johnson, L. R. (New York: Raven Press)

41. Burhol, P. G. (1971). Intravenous injection of 2-deoxy-D-glucose in gastric fistula chickens. *Scand. J. Gastroenterol.*, **6** (Suppl. 11), 35–40

42. Hitchcock, M. W. S., Karvonen, M. J. and Phillipson, A. T. (1948). The effect of insulin on the acidity of the abomasal contents of lamb. *Acta Physiol. Scand.* **16**, (Suppl. 53), 33–4

43. Hill, K. J. (1952). The effect of insulin on the secretion of gastric juice in the goat. *Q. J. Exp. Physiol.*, **37**, 143–7

44. Raggi, F. and Kronfeld, D. S. (1966). Higher glucose affinity of hexokinase in sheep brain than in rat brain. *Nature*, **209**, 1353–4

45. Houpt, T. R. (1974). Stimulation of food intake in ruminants by 2-deoxy-D-glucose and insulin. *Am. J. Physiol.*, **227**, 161–7

46. Grahame, G. R., Garrett, J. M. and Hirschowitz, B. I. (1968). 2-Deoxyglucose and histamine effects on gastric motility and secretion in the dog. *Am. J. Physiol.*, **215**, 243–8

47. Bremer, A. (1959). Contribution a l'étude des mecanismes de stimulation de la sécrétion acid de l'estomac. *Acta Gastroenterol. Belg.*, **22**, 467–526

48. Hirschowitz, B. I., Gibson, R. G. and Molina, E. (1981). Atropine suppresses gastrin release by food in intact and vagotomized dogs. *Gastroenterology*, **81**, 838–43

49. Hirschowitz, B. I. and Molina, E. (1980). Gastrin release after truncal vagotomy in fistula dogs: hypersensitivity to bombesin but not bethanechol. *Peptides* **1**, 217–22

50. Himsworth, R. L. (1970). Hypothalamic control of adrenaline secretion in response to insufficient glucose. *J. Physiol. (Lond.)*, **206**, 411–17

51. Hirschowitz, B. I. and Molina, E. (1983). Effects of four H_2 histamine antagonists on bethanechol-stimulated acid and pepsin secretion in the dog. *J. Pharmacol. Exp. Ther.*, **224**, 341–5

52. Gibson, R. G., Colvin, H. W. Jr. and Hirschowitz, B. I. (1974). Kinetics of gastric response in chickens to graded electrical vagal stimulation. *Proc. Soc. Exp. Biol. & Med.*, **145**, 1058–60

53. Soll, A. H. (1983). Receptors modulating acid secretion. In Hirschowitz, B. I. and Spenney, J. G. (eds.) *Receptors and the Upper GI Tract*, pp. 101–15 (New York: Advanced Therapeutics Communications)

54. Debons, A. F., Silver, L., Cronkite, E. P., Johnson, H. A., Brecher, G., Tenzer, D. and Schwartz, I. L. (1962). Localization of gold in mouse brain in relation to gold thioglucose

obesity. *Am. J. Physiol.*, **202**, 743–50
55. Hirschowitz, B. I., Pollard, H. M., Hartwell, S. W. Jr. and London, J. (1956). The action of ethyl alcohol on gastric secretion. *Gastroenterology*, **30**, 244–53
56. Goto, Y. and Debas, H. (1983). GABA-mimetic effect on gastric acid secretion: possible significance in central mechanisms. *Dig. Dis. Sci.*, **28**, 56–9
57. Goto, Y., Tache, Y., Debas, H. and Novin, D. (1985). Gastric acid and vagus nerve response to GABA agonist baclofen. *Life Sci.*, **36**, 2471–5
58. Levine, A. S., Morley, J. E., Kneip, J., Grace, M. and Silvis, S. E. (1981). Muscimol induces gastric acid secretion after central administration. *Brain Res.*, **229**, 270–4
59. Williford, D. J., Ormsbee, H. S. III, Norman, W., Harmon, J. W., Garvey, T. Q. III, Dimicco, J. A. and Gillis, R. A. (1981). Hindbrain GABA receptors influence parasympathetic outflow to the stomach. *Science*, **214**, 193–4
60. Brown, D. A. (1984). Muscarinic excitation of sympathetic and central neurons. *Trends Pharmacol. Sci.*, **1**, (Suppl.), 32–4
61. Brown, D. A. (1986). Neuropharmacology. Acetylcholine and brain cells. *Nature*, **319**, 358–9
62. Hirschowitz, B. I. (1967). The secretion of pepsinogen. In Code, C. F. (ed.) *Handbook of Physiology. Alimentary Canal*, Vol. 2, pp. 889–918. (Washington, D.C.: Am. Physiol. Soc.)
63. Emson, P. C. (ed.) (1983). *Chemical Neuroanatomy*. (New York: Raven Press)
64. Roberts, G. W., Crow, T. J. and Polak, J. M. (1981). Neuropeptides in the brain. In Bloom, S. R. and Polak, J. M. (eds.) *Gut Hormones*, pp. 457–63
65. Kubek, M. J., Rea, M. A., Hodes, Z. I. and Aprison, M. H. (1983). Quantitation and characterization of thyrotropin-releasing hormone in vagal nuclei and other regions of the medulla oblongata of the rat. *J. Neurochem.*, **40**, 1307–13
66. Tache, Y., Vale, W., Rivier, J. and Brown, M. (1980). Brain regulation of gastric secretion: influence of neuropeptides. *Proc. Natl. Acad. Sci. USA*, **77**, 5515–19
67. Feldman, M. and Richardson, C. T. (1986). Role of thought, sight, smell and taste of food in the cephalic phase of gastric acid secretion in humans. *Gastroenterology*, **90**, 428–33
68. Haggstrom, G. D. and Hirschowitz, B. I. (1984). Histamine H_1 and H_2 effects on gastric acid and pepsin, heart rate and blood pressure in humans. *J. Pharmacol. Exp. Ther.*, **221**(1), 120–3
69. Eichhorn, R. and Tracktir, J. (1955). The effect of hypnosis upon gastric secretion. *Gastroenterology*, **29**, 417–21
70. Bonfils, S., Mignon, M. and Roze, C. (1979). Vagal control of gastric secretion. *Int. Rev. Physiol.*, **19**, 61–106
71. Feldman, M., Richardson, C. T. and Fordtran, J. S. (1980). Experience with sham feeding as a test for vagotomy. *Gastroenterology*, **79** (5, Pt. 1), 792–5
72. Feldman, M., Richardson, C. T. and Fordtran, J. S. (1980). Effect of sham feeding on gastric acid secretion in healthy subjects and duodenal ulcer patients: evidence for increased basal tone in some ulcer patients. *Gastroenterology*, **79** (5, Pt. 2), 796–800
73. Helman, C. A. and Hirschowitz, B. I. (1986). Pirenzepine and atropine inhibition of modified sham feeding stimulated gastric acid and pepsin secretion. *Gastroenterology*, **90** (Abstract), 1456
74. Richardson, C. T., Walsh, J. H., Cooper, K. A., Feldman, M. and Fordtran, J. S. (1977). Studies on the role of cephalic-vagal stimulation in the acid secretory response to eating in normal human subjects. *J. Clin. Invest.*, **60**, 435–41
75. Hirschowitz, B. I., Schenker, S. and Boyett, J. D. (1963). A highly active gastric secretagogue extracted from a metastasis of a Zollinger-Ellisom tumor. *Am. J. Dig. Dis.*, **8**, 499–508
76. Uvnas, B. (1942). The part played by the pyloric region in the cephalic phase of gastric secretion. *Acta Physiol. Scand.* **4** (Suppl. XIII)
77. Feldman, M., Richardson, C. T., Taylor, I. L. and Walsh, J. H. (1979). Effect of atropine on vagal release of gastrin and pancreatic polypeptide. *J. Clin. Invest.*, **63**, 294–8
78. Fokina, A., Konturek, S. J., Kwiecien, N. and Radecki, T. (1979). Role of gastric antrum in gastric and intestinal phases of gastric secretion in dogs. *J. Physiol. (Lond.)*, **295**, 229–39
79. Moore, J. G. and Crespin, F. (1980). Influence of glucose on cephalic-vagal-simulated gastric acid secretion in man. *Dig. Dis. Sci.*, **25**, 117–22
80. Grossman, M. I. (1981). Regulation of gastric acid secretion. In Johnson, L. R. (ed.) *Physiology of the Gastrointestinal Tract*, pp. 659–71. (New York: Raven Press)

81. Blair, A. J., Richardson, C. T., Walsh, J. H., Chew, P. and Feldman, M. (1986). Effect of parietal cell vagotomy on acid secretory responsiveness to circulating gastrin in humans. Relationship to postprandial serum gastrin concentration. *Gastroenterology*, **90**: 1001–7

82. Knutson, U. and Olbe, L. (1973). Gastric acid response to sham feeding in the duodenal ulcer subject. *Scand. J. Gastroenterol.*, **8**, 513–22

83. Kronborg, O. (1981). Completeness of vagotomy: anatomy, pathophysiology and consequences. *Scand. J. Gastroenterol.*, **16**, 577–80

84. Maeda-Hagiwara, M. and Watanabe, K. (1983). Bromocriptine inhibits 2-deoxy-D-glucose-stimulated gastric acid secretion in the rat. *Eur. J. Pharmacol.*, **90**, 11–17

85. Powell, D. W. and Hirschowitz, B. I. (1967). Sodium pentobarbital depression of histamine- or insulin-stimulated gastric secretion. *Am. J. Physiol.*, **212**, 1001–6

86. Pappas, T., Hamel, D., Debas, H., Walsh, J. H. and Tache, Y. (1985). Cerebroventricular bombesin inhibits gastric acid secretion in dogs. *Gastroenterology*, **89**, 43–8

87. Soon-Shiong, P. and Debas, H. T. (1980). Fundic inhibition of acid secretion and gastrin release in the dog. *Gastroenterology*, **79**(5, Pt. 1), 867–72

88. Hirschowitz, B. I., Fong, J. and Molina, E. (1983). Effects of pirenzepine and atropine on vagal and cholinergic gastric secretion and gastrin release and on heart rate in the dog. *J. Pharmacol. Exp. Ther.*, **225**, 263–8

89. Brauer, R. F. (1977). Electrically-induced vagal stimulation of gastric acid secretion. In: Brooks, F. P. and Evers, P. W. (eds.) *Nerves and the Gut*, pp. 86–95 (Thorofare, N.J.: Charles Slack)

90. Gamse, R., Lembeck, F. and Cuello, A. C. (1979). Substance P in the vagus nerve: immunochemical and immunohistochemical evidence for axoplasmic transport. *Naunyn-Schmiedeberg Arch. Phramacol.*, **306**, 37–44

91. Olbe, L. and Knutson, U. (1976). Gastric acid response to sham feeding in the dog and the duodenal ulcer patient. *Acta Hepatogastroenterol. (Stuttg.)*, **23**, 455–8

92. Grundy, D. and Scratcherd, T. (1982). Effect of stimulation of the vagus nerve in bursts on gastric acid secretion and motility in the anesthetized ferret. *J. Physiol. (Lond.)*, **333**, 451–61

93. Morrison, T. F. B. (1977). Afferent innervation of the GI tract, In Brooks, F. P. and Evers, P. W. (eds.) *Nerves and the Gut*, pp. 297–326. (Thorofare, N.J.: Charles Slack)

94. Paintal, A. S. (1973). Vagal sensory receptors and their reflex effects. *Physiol. Rev.*, **53**, 159–227

95. Iggo, A. (1957). Gastro-intestinal tension receptors with unmyelinated afferent fibres in the vagus of the cat. *Q. J. Exp. Physiol.*, **42**, 130–43

96. Iggo, A. (1957). Gastric mucosal chemoreceptors with vagal afferent fibres in the cat. *Q. J. Exp. Physiol.*, **42**, 398–409

97. Appia, F., Ewart, W. R., Pittam, B. S. and Wingate, D. L. (1986). Convergence of sensory information from abdominal viscera in the rat brain stem. *Am. J. Physiol.*, **251**, G169–75

98. Harding, R. and Leek, B. F. (1973). Central projections of gastric afferent vagal impulses. *J. Physiol. (Lond.)*, **228**, 73–90

99. Wood, J. D. (1981). Physiology of the enteric nervous system. In Johnson, R. L. (ed.) *Physiology of the Gastrointestinal Tract*, pp. 1–37. (New York: Raven Press)

100. Davison, J. S. (1972). Response of single vagal afferent fibres to mechanical and chemical stimulation of the gastric and duodenal mucosa in cats. *Q. J. Exp. Physiol.*, **57**, 405–16

101. Dockray, G. J. and Sharkey, K. A. (1986). Neurochemistry of visceral afferent neurones. *Prog. Brain Research*. (In press)

102. Ekblad, E., Ekelund, M., Graffner, H., Hakanson, R. and Sundler, F. (1985). Peptide containing nerve fibers in stomach wall of rat and mouse. *Gastroenterology*, **89**, 73–85

103. Dockray, G. J. (1979). Comparative biochemistry and physiology of gut hormones. *Annu. Rev. Physiol.*, **41**, 83–95

104. Dockray, G. J., Gregory, R. A., Tracy, H. J. and Zhu, W. Y. (1981). Transport of cholecystokinin-octapeptide-like immunoreactivity toward the gut in afferent vagal fibers in cat and dog. *J. Physiol. (Lond.)*, **314**, 501–11

105. Altman, J. (1985) Tuning in to neurotransmitters. *Nature*, **315**, 537

106. Maclean, D. B. and Lewis, S. F. (1984). De novo synthesis and axoplasmic transport of (^{35}S) methionine-substance P in explants of nodose ganglion/vagus nerve. *Brain Res.*, **310**, 325–35

107. Rehfeld, J. F. (1983). Gastrin and cholecystokinin in the vagus. *J. Autonom. Nerv. Syst.*, **9**,

113–18

108. Sharkey, K. A., Williams, R. G. and Dockray, G. J. (1984). Sensory substance P innervation of the stomach and pancreas: demonstration of capsaicin-sensitive sensory neurons in the rat by combined immunohistochemistry and retrograde tracing. *Gastroenterology*, **87**, 914–21

109. Zarbin, M. A., Wamsley, J. K. and Kuhar, M. J. (1982). Axonal transport of muscarinic cholinergic receptors in rat vagus nerve: high and low affinity agonist receptors move in opposite directions and differ in nucleotide sensitivity. *J. Neurosci.*, **2**, 934–41

110. Young, W. S., Wamsley, J. K., Zarbin, M. A. and Kuhar, M. J. (1980). Opioid receptors undergo axonal flow. *Science*, **210**, 76–8

111. Zarbin, M. A., Wamsley, J. K., Innis, R. B. and Kuhar, M. J. (1981). Cholecystokinin receptors: presence and axonal flow in rat vagus nerve. *Life Sci.*, **29**, 697–705

112. White, J. D., Stewart, K. D., Krause, J. E. and McKelvy, J. F. (1985). Biochemistry of peptide-secreting neurons. *Physiol. Rev.*, **65**, 553–606

113. Davison, J. S. and Grundy, D. (1978). Modulation of single vagal efferent fibre discharge by gastrointestinal afferents in the rat. *J. Physiol. (Lond.)*, **284**, 69–82

114. Rogers, R. C. and Hermann, G. E. (1985). Vagal afferent stimulation-evoked gastric secretion suppressed by paraventricular nucleus lesion. *J. Autonom. Nerv. Syst.*, **13**, 191–9

115. Harper, A. A., Kidd, C. and Scratcherd, T. (1959). Vago-vagal reflex effects on gastric and pancreatic secretion and gastrointestinal motility. *J. Physiol. (Lond.)*, **148**, 417–36

116. Goyal, R. K. (1983). Neurology of the gut. In Sleisenger, M. H. and Fordtran, J. S. (eds.) *Gastrointestinal Disease*, 3rd Edn., pp. 97–115. (Philadelphia: W. B. Saunders)

117. Gabella, G. (1981). Structure of muscles and nerves in the gastrointestinal tract. In Johnson, L. R. (ed.) *Physiology of the Gastrointestinal Tract*, pp. 197–241 (New York: Raven Press)

118. Radke, R., Stach, W. and Weiss, R. (1980). Innervation of the gastric wall related to acid secretion: a light and electron microscopy study on rats, rabbits and guinea pigs. *Acta Biol. Med. Ger.*, **39**, 687–96

119. Magee, D. F. and Naruse, S. (1983). Neural control of periodic secretion of the pancreas and the stomach in fasting dogs. *J. Physiol. (Lond.)*, **344**, 153–60

120. Roman, C. and Gonella, J. (1981). Extrinsic control of digestive tract motility. In Johnson. L. R. (ed.) *Physiology of the Gastrointestinal Tract* pp. 289–334. (New York: Raven Press)

121. Hirschowitz, B. I. and Hutchison, G. A. (1977). Long term effects of highly selective vagotomy (HSV) in dogs on acid and pepsin secretion. *Am. J. Dig. Dis.*, **22**, 81–95

122. Schultzberg, M. (1983). The peripheral nervous system. In Emson, P. C. (ed.) *Chemical Neuroanatomy*, pp. 1–52 (New York: Raven Press)

123. Hirschowitz, B. I. (1989). Neural and hormonal controls of gastric secretion. In Forte, J. (ed.) *Handbook of Physiology*, (Washington D.C.: Am. Physiol. Soc.)

124. Nakamura, M., Oda, M., Yonei, Y., Tsukada, N., Watanabe, H., Komatsu, H. and Tsuchiya, M. (1984). Demonstration of the localization of muscarinic acetylcholine receptors in the gastric mucosa. *Acta Histochem. Cytochem.*, **17**, 297–309

125. Nishi, S., Seino, Y., Takemura, J., Ishida, H., Seno, M., Chiba, T., Yanaihara, C., Yanaihara, N. and Imura, H. (1985). Vagal regulation of GRP, gastric somatostatin, and gastrin secretion in vitro. *Am. J. Physiol.*, **248**, E425–31

126. Sanders, M. J. and Soll, A. H. (1986). Characterization of receptors regulating secretory function in the fundic mucosa. *Annu. Rev. Physiol.*, **48**, 89–101

127. Hersey, S. J., Norris, S. H. and Gibert, A. J. (1984). Cellular control of pepsinogen secretion. *Annu. Rev. Physiol.*, **46**, 393–402

128. Shirakawa, T. and Hirschowitz, B. I. (1985). Interaction between stimuli and their antagonists on frog esophageal peptic glands. *Am. J. Physiol.*, **249** (6, Pt. 1), G668–73

129. Hirschowitz, B. I. and Gibson, R. G. (1978). Cholinergic stimulation and suppression of gastrin release in gastric fistula dogs. *Am. J. Physiol.*, **235**, E720

130. Hirschowitz, B. I. and Sachs, G. (1969). Atropine inhibition of insulin-, histamine-, and pentagastrin-stimulated gastric electrolyte and pepsin secretion in the dog. *Gastroenterology* **56**, 693–702

131. Hirschowitz, B. I., Molina, E., Ou Tim, L. and Helman, C. A. (1984). Effects of very low doses of atropine on basal and pepsin secretion, gastrin and heart rate in normals and DU. *Dig. Dis. Sci.*, **29** (9), 790–6

132. Arunlakshana, O. and Schild, H. O. (1959). Some quantitative uses of drug antagonists.

Bri. J. Pharmacol., **14**, 48–58

133. Hirschowitz, B. I., Danilewitz, M. and Molina, E. (1982). Inhibition of basal acid, chloride and pepsin secretion in duodenal ulcer by graded doses of ranitidine and atropine with studies of pharmacokinetics of ranitidine. *Gastroenterology*, **82**, 1314–26

134. Nakamura, M., Oda, M., Watanabe, N., Tsukada, N., Yonei, Y. and Tsuchiya, M. (1982). Evidence for direct parasympathetic innervation of parietal cells in the rat glandular stomach. Histochemical and electron microscopic cytochemical study. *Okajimas Folia Anat. Jpn.*, **59**, 167–80

135. Sjodin, L. (1977). Electrical stimulation of nerves and secretion from digestive glands. In Brooks, F. P. (ed.) *Nerves and the Gut*, pp. 1–13

136. Hirschowitz, B. I. and Hutchison, G. A. (1975). Effects of vagotomy on urecholine-modified histamine dose responses in dogs. *Am. J. Physiol.*, **228**, 1313–18

137. Hirschowitz, B. I. (1977). The vagus and gastric secretion. In Brooks, F. P. and Evers, P. W. (eds.) *Nerves and the Gut*, pp. 96–118. (Thorofare, N.J.: Charles Slack)

138. Hirschowitz, B. I. and Hutchison, G. A. (1977). Kinetics of atropine inhibition of pentagastrin-stimulated H^+, electrolytes and pepsin secretion in the dog. *Am. J. Dig. Dis.*, **22**, 99–107

139. Hirschowitz, B. I. and Hutchison, G. A. (1973). A working hypothesis for urecholine effects on histamine stimulation of gastric secretion. *Scand. J. Gastroenterol.*, **8**, 569–76

140. Burleigh, D. E. (1978). Selectivity of bethanechol on muscarinic receptors. *J. Pharm. Pharmacol.*, **30**, 398–9

141. Feldman, M. and Walsh, J. H. (1980). Acid inhibition of sham feeding-stimulated gastrin release and gastric acid secretion: effect of atropine. *Gastroenterology*, **78**, 772–6

142. Baile, C. A., McLaughlin, C. L. and Della-Fera, M. A. (1986). Role of cholecystokinin and opioid peptides in control of food intake. *Physiol. Rev.*, **66**, 172–234

143. Walsh, J. H. (1979). Evidence for the hormonal role of gastrin in regulation of gastric acid secretion. In Miyoshi, A. (ed.) *Gut Peptides: Secretion, Function and Clinical Aspects*, pp. 137–44. (Amsterdam: Elsevier)

144. Becker, H. D., Reeder, D. D. and Thompson, J. C. (1974). Direct measurement of vagal release of gastrin. *Surgery*, **75**, 101–6

145. Feldman, M., Walsh, J. H., Wong, H. C. and Richardson, C. T. (1978). Role of gastrin heptadecapeptide in the acid secretory response to amino acids in man. *J. Clin. Invest.*, **61**, 308–13

146. Hirschowitz, B. I. and Molina, E. (1983). Relation of gastric acid and pepsin secretion to serum gastrin levels in dogs given bombesin and gastrin G17. *Am. J. Physiol.*, **244** (6, Pt. 5), G546–51

147. Hirschowitz, B. I., Ou Tim, L., Helman, C. A. and Molina, E. (1985). Bombesin and G-17 dose responses in duodenal ulcer and controls. *Dig. Dis. Sci.* **30**, 1092–103

148. Rehfeld, J. F. and Amdrup, E. (eds.) (1979). *Gastrins and the Vagus*, p. 315 (London: Academic Press)

149. Stadil, F. and Stage, J. G. (1979). Gastrinomas as model for duodenal ulcer disease. In Rehfeld, J. F. and Amdrup, E. (eds.) *Gastrins and the Vagus*, pp. 199–210 (New York: Academic Press)

150. Hirschowitz, B. I. and Gibson, R. G. (1979). Augmented vagal release of antral gastrin by 2-deoxyglucose after fundic vagotomy in dogs. *Am. J. Physiol.*, **236**, E173–9

151. Tepperman, B. L., Walsh, J. H. and Preshaw, R. M. (1972). Effect of antral denervation on gastrin release by sham feeding and insulin hypoglycemia in dog. *Gastroenterology*, **63**, 973–80

152. Anagnostides, A., Chadwick, V. S., Selden, A. C. and Maton, P. N. (1984). Sham feeding and pancreatic secretion. *Gastroenterology*, **87**, 109–14

153. Debas, H. T., Konturek, S. J., Walsh, J. H. and Grossman, M. I. (1974). Proof of a pyloro-oxyntic reflex for stimulation of acid secretion. *Gastroenterol.*, **66**, 526–32

154. Hirschowitz, B. I. and Gibson, R. G. (1978). Stimulation of gastrin release and gastric secretion: effect of bombesin and a nonapeptide in fistula dogs with and without fundic vagotomy. *Digestion*, **18**, 227–39

155. Debas, H. T., Walsh, J. H. and Grossman, M. I. (1975). Evidence for oxyntopyloric reflex for release of antral gastrin. *Gastroenterology*, **68**, 687–90

156. Debas, H. T., Hollinshead, J., Seal, A., Soon-Shiong, P. and Walsh, J. H. (1984). Vagal control of gastrin release in dog–pathways for stimulation and inhibition. *Surgery*, **95**,

157. Hollinshead, J. W., Debas, H. T., Yamada, T., Elashoff, J., Osadchey, B. and Walsh, J. H. (1985). Hypergastrinemia develops within 24 hours of truncal vagotomy in dogs. *Gastroenterology*, **88** (1, Pt. 1), 35–40

158. Ersparmer, V. and Melchiorri, P. (1973). Active polypeptides of the amphibian skin and their synthetic analogues. *Pure Appl. Chem.*, **35**, 463–94

159. Holst, J. J., Knuhtsen, S., Jensen, S. L., Fahrenkrug, J., Larsson, L.-I. and Nielsen, O. V. (1983). Interrelation of nerves and hormones in stomach and pancreas. *Scand. J. Gastroenterol.*, **82** (Supp.), 85–99

160. Tache, Y., Lesiege, D., Vale, W. and Collu, R. (1985). Gastric hypersecretion by intracisternal TRH: dissociation from hypophysiotropic activity and role of central catecholamine. *Eur. J. Pharmacol.*, **107**, 149–55

161. Duval, J. W., Saffouri, B., Weir, G. C., Walsh, J. H., Arimura, A. and Makhlouf, G. M. (1981). Stimulation of gastrin and somatostatin secretion from the isolated rat stomach by bombesin. *Am. J. Physiol.*, **241**, G242–7

162. Holst, J. J., Jensen, S. L., Knuhtsen, S., Nielsen, O. V. and Rehfeld, J. F. (1983). Effect of vagus gastric inhibitory polypeptide and HCl on gastrin and somatostatin release from perfused pig antrum. *Am. J. Physiol.*, **244**, G515–22

163. Basso, N., Improta, G., Melchiorri, P. and Sopranzi, N. (1974). Gastrin release by bombesin in the antral pouch dog. *Rend. Gastroenterol.*, **6**, 95–8

164. Jensen, R. T., Jones, S. W., Folkers, K. and Gardner, J. D. (1984). A synthetic peptide that is a bombesin receptor antagonist. *Nature*, **309**, 61–3

165. Hirschowitz, B. I. and Molina, E. (1984). Somatostatin, prostaglandin E_2 and atropine inhibition of the gastric actions of bombesin in the dog. *Peptides*, **5** (1), 29–34

166. Larsson, L.-I., Goltermann, N., de Magistris, L., Rehfeld, J. F. and Schwartz, T. W. (1979). Somatostatin cell processes as pathways for paracrine secretion. *Science*, **205**, 1393–5

167. Larsson, L.-I. (1980). Peptide secretory pathways in GI tract: cytochemical contributions to regulatory physiology of the gut. *Am. J. Physiol.*, **239**, G237–46

168. Fujita, T., Kanno, T. and Yanaihara, N. (1983). *Brain-gut Axis*, p. 333. (Tokyo: Biomedical Research Foundation)

169. Hirschowitz, B. I. (1983). Gastrin release in fistula dogs with solid compared to nutrient and non-nutrient liquid meals. *Dig. Dis. Sci.*, **28**, 705–11

170. Schiller, L. R., Walsh, J. H. and Feldman, M. (1980). Distension-induced gastrin release: effects of luminal acidification and intravenous atropine. *Gastroenterology*, **78** (5, Pt. 1), 912–17

171. Lam, S. K., Isenberg, J. I., Grossman, M. I., Lane, W. H. and Walsh, J. H. (1980). Gastric acid secretion is abnormally sensitive to endogenous gastrin released after peptone test meals in duodenal ulcer patients. *J. Clin. Invest.*, **65**, 555–62

172. Richardson, C. T., Peters, M. N., Feldman, M., McClelland, R. N., Walsh, J. H., Cooper, K. A., Willeford, G., Dickerman, R. M. and Fordtran, J. S. (1985). Treatment of Zollinger-Ellison syndrome with exploratory laparotomy, proximal gastric vagotomy, and H_2-receptor antagonists. A prospective study. *Gastroenterology*, **89**, 357–67

173. Lichtenberger, L. M. (1982). Importance of food in the regulation of gastrin release and formation. *Am. J. Physiol.*, **243**, G429–41

174. Levant, J. A., Walsh, J. H. and Isenberg, J. I. (1973). Stimulation of gastric secretion and gastrin release by single oral doses of calcium carbonate in man. *N. Engl. J. Med.*, **289**, 555–8

175. Grossman, M. I. (1967). Neural and hormonal stimulation of gastric secretion of acid. In Code, C. F. (ed.) *Handbook of Physiology. Alimentary Canal*, Section 6, Vol. 2, pp. 835–78 (Washington, D.C.: Am. Physiol. Soc.)

176. Schiller, L. R., Walsh, J. H. and Feldman, M. (1982). Effect of atropine on gastrin release stimulated by an amino acid meal in humans. *Gastroenterology*, **83** (1, Pt. 2), 267–72

177. Hirschowitz, B. I. and Molina, E. (1984). Analysis of food stimulation of gastrin release in dogs by a panel of inhibitors. *Peptides*, **5** (2), 35–40

178. Saffouri, B., Duval, J. W. and Makhlouf, G. M. (1984). Stimulation of gastrin secretion in vitro by intralumenal chemicals: regulation by intramural cholinergic and non-cholinergic neurons. *Gastroenterology*, **87**, 557–61

179. Schubert, M. L., Bitar, K. N. and Makhlouf, G. M. (1982). Regulation of gastrin and somatostatin secretion by cholinergic and noncholinergic intramural neurons. *Am. J.*

Physiol., **243**, G442–7

180. Schubert, M. L. and Makhlouf, G. M. (1982). Regulation of gastrin and somatostatin secretion by intramural neurons: effect of nicotinic receptor stimulation by dimethyl-phenylpiperazinium. *Gastroenterology*, **83**, 626–32

181. Code, C. F. (1977). Reflections on histamine, gastric secretion and the H_2 receptor. *N. Engl. J. Med.*, **296**, 1459–62

182. Hakanson, R., Wahlestedt, C., Westlin, L., Vallgren, S. and Sundler, F. (1983). Neuronal histamine in the gut wall releasable by gastrin and cholecystokinin. *Neurosci. Lett.*, **42**, 305–10

183. Berglindh, T. (1984). The mammalian gastric parietal cell in vitro. *Annu. Rev. Physiol.*, **46**, 377–92

184. Hirschowitz, B. I. (1979). H-2 histamine receptors. *Annu. Rev. Pharmacol. Toxicol.*, **19**, 203–44

185. Hirschowitz, B. I. and Molina, E. (1983). Effect of cimetidine on histamine-stimulated gastric acid and electrolytes in dogs. *Am. J. Physiol.*, **244** (*Gastrointest. Liver Physiol. 7*), G416–20

186. Angus, J. A. and Black, J. W. (1982). The interaction of choline esters, vagal stimulation and H_2-receptor blockade on acid secretion in vitro. *Eur. J. Pharmacol.*, **80**, 217–24

187. Sakaguchi, T. (1982). Alterations in gastric acid secretion following hepatic portal injections of D-glucose and its anomers. *J. Autonom. Nerv. Syst.*, **5**, 337–44

188. Hirschowitz, B. I., Rentz, J. and Molina, E. (1981). Histamine H-2 receptor stimulation and inhibition of pepsin secretion in the dog. *J. Pharmacol. Exp. Ther.*, **218**, 676–80

189. Lorenz, W., Thon, K., Barth, H., Neugebauer, E., Reimann, H.-J. and Kusche, J. (1983). Metabolism and function of gastric histamine in health and disease. In Hirschowitz, B. I. and Spenney, J. G. (eds.) *Receptors of the Upper GI Tract*, pp. 148–73. (New York: Advanced Therapeutics Communications)

190. Redfern, J. S., Thirlby, R., Feldman, M. and Richardson, C. T. (1985). Effect of pentagastrin on gastric mucosal histamine in dogs. *Am. J. Physiol.*, **248**, G369–75

191. Anderson, W., Molina, E., Rentz, J. and Hirschowitz, B. I. (1982). Analysis of the 2-deoxy-D-glucose-induced vagal stimulation of gastric secretion and gastrin release in dogs using methionine-enkephalin, morphine and naloxone. *J. Phramacol. Exp. Ther.*, **222**, 617–22

192. Grossman, M. I. (1979). Vagal stimulation and inhibition of acid secretion and gastrin release: which aspects are cholinergic. In Rehfeld, J. F. and Amdrup, E. (eds.) *Gastrins and the Vagus*, pp. 103–113. (New York: Academic Press)

193. Cabocio, J. L. F., Wolfe, M. M., Hocking, M. P., McGuigan, J. E. and Woodward, E. R. (1981). Effect of antrectomy on the nervous phase of gastric secretion in the dog. *Am. J. Surg.*, **142**, 324–7

194. Preshaw, R. M. (1970). Influence of the antrum on the acid response to distension of the body of the stomach in dogs. *Can. J. Physiol. Pharmacol.*, **48**, 661–9

195. Lyndon, P. J., Greenall, M. J., Smith, R. B., Goligher, J. C. and Johnston, D. (1975). Serial insulin tests over a five-year period after highly selective vagotomy for duodenal ulcer. *Gastroenterology*, **69**, 1188–95

196. Vallgren, S., Ekelund, M. and Hakanson, R. (1983). Mechanism of inhibition of gastric acid secretion by vagal denervation in the rat. *Acta Physiol. Scand.*, **119**, 77–80

197. Puurunen, J. and Leppaluoto, J. (1984). Centrally administered pGE_2 inhibits gastric secretion in the rat by releasing vasopressin. *Eur. J. Pharmacol.*, **104**, 145–50

198. Payne, R. A. and Kay, A. W. (1972). The effect of vagotomy on the maximal acid secretory response to histamine in man. *Clin. Sci.*, **22**, 373–82

199. Feldman, M. and Walsh, J. H. (1982). Effect of bethanechol on gastric acid secretion and serum gastrin concentration after proximal gastric vagotomy. *Ann. Surg.*, **196**, 14–17

200. Joffe, S. N., Crocket, A., Chen, M. and Brackett, K. (1983). *In vitro* and *in vivo* technique for assessing vagus nerve regeneration after parietal cell vagotomy in the rat. *J. Autonom. Nerv. Syst.*, **9**, 27–51

201. Guldvog, I., Gedde-Dahl, D. and Berstad, A. (1980). 'Non-active' pepsin secretion compared with stimulated secretion by bethanechol, histamine, pentagastrin, and 2-deoxy-D-glucose. *Scand. J. Gastroenterol.*, **15**, 939–48

12
Neural control of salivary glandular function

J. R. GARRETT

INTRODUCTION

The secretion of saliva is almost entirely dependent on nerve-mediated mechanisms. Salivary glands are therefore excellent models for studying the effects of nerves on exocrine secretory processes.

A few salivary glands produce a small continuous background flow of saliva independently of nerve impulses, designated spontaneous secretion[1] ;even so the main flow from these glands also depends upon nerve impulses. In contrast with exocrine secretion in most other parts of the gastrointestinal tract, hormones do not normally initiate the flow of fluid from salivary glands, though of course hormones influence the metabolism of the parenchymal cells and so may affect their ability to handle the constituents that normally pass into saliva.

The nerves to the glands are still best considered on the anatomical basis of parasympathetic and sympathetic. Experimentally their effects in isolation are usually very different but when acting together under natural conditions they do so in complementary rather than antagonistic ways[2]. Despite the simple gross anatomical division of the autonomic nerves supplying salivary glands, their final anatomical pathways are not always as well defined as is generally believed[see 4], including the route taken by some sympathetic nerves for parotid glands. It has recently been found in rats that some of the post-ganglionic sympathetic nerves for the parotid arise from the contralateral superior cervical ganglion[5] and presumably these nerves reach the gland by an intracranial course.

Salivary glands, having ducts that can be readily cannulated and nerves that are often freely accessible, are very convenient for making correlative studies, in ways that can be precisely controlled, on the influences of nerves on the glandular cells, the fluid they produce and its constituents. Furthermore, as the glands are paired they provide a built-in control in the same animal for a variety of investigations whether functional, structural or both and for comparing one preceding experimental procedure with another.

A great deal is known about the cholinergic and adrenergic activities of the autonomic nerves on salivary parenchyma *in vivo*[2,6]. Detailed understanding of the cellular and intracellular events has been greatly extended during the last 10 years by *in vitro* studies using pharmacological agents for stimulation[see 7,8]. However, complex interactions occur *in vivo* in response to the different nerves and their different transmitters, which under suboptimal conditions tend to be synergistic and so produce augmentation of the flow and often of the constituents[see 2]. More precise information about neuroeffector secretory responses is obtained from stimulating the nerves *in vivo* than from the use of pharmacological agents which at best give only crude approximations of the nerve-driven events. Stimulation of the nerves in turn has certain limitations, for all nerves in the bundle being stimulated are activated indiscriminately and all at the same rate. Under normal reflex conditions the different modalities come under integrated central control to induce differentiated activities within the glands. Furthermore, within each modality, the impulse traffic in the terminal axons will normally occur asynchronously. Despite these experimental defects the prudent use of nerve stimulation still has an immense value for helping understanding of nerve-mediated events, especially when the functional events can be correlated with the structural changes that occur. The work to be reported in this chapter will largely relate to such an approach.

In the last 10 years there has been an explosion of information about possible non-cholinergic non-adrenergic transmitters, especially peptides. As studied up to 12 years ago, there was little indication that acetylcholine and noradrenaline were not responsible for all of the nerve-mediated events in the glands, other than the century-old problem of an atropine-resistant parasympathetic vasodilatation[9]. In most species the use of appropriate muscarinic or adrenergic antagonists blocked all of the secretory responses to parasympathetic or sympathetic stimulation. Salivary secretion evoked by physalaemin or other exotic peptides in certain species remained a pharmacological oddity[10]. Then, in 1976, Thulin[11,12] made the surprising observation in the rat that parasympathetic salivary secretion was not entirely blocked by large doses of muscarinic plus adrenergic blockers. The importance of this fundamental finding is gradually being unravelled and forms the basis for some recent work to be discussed here.

It is impossible to be comprehensive in a discussion of this nature. It will therefore concentrate on some recent experiments concerning the influence of nerves on the structure and function of salivary glands using some newly developed stimulation protocols, as well as more conventional ones, and the effects of selective denervations.

USE OF PROLONGED PARASYMPATHETIC STIMULATION AT HIGHER FREQUENCY

To study non-adrenergic, non-cholinergic influences

Hitherto most studies using nerve stimulation have been confined to frequencies of 10 Hz or less, because stimulations at higher frequencies were considered unphysiological. However, higher-frequency stimulation is now being used to advantage for answering certain questions about neuro-glandular function.

The auriculotemporal nerve contains most of the post-ganglionic para-sympathetic nerves to the parotid gland of the rat[13]. The ability to stimulate it on the medial side of the mandible avoids any damage to the parotid gland during preparation and confers a unique opportunity for testing a truly post-ganglionic parasympathetic nerve.

Following up the observation by Thulin[11] that an atropine resistant parotid secretion occurs on stimulating the auriculotemporal nerve in the rat, we analysed the phenomenon in greater detail with Ekström and co-workers[14]. This showed that, although the flow of saliva was greatly reduced by atropine, a flow was detectable from 5 Hz onwards and reached a maximum at 40 Hz. Interestingly this frequency was also found to be optimal for secretion in the absence of atropine. Hexamethonium before or after atropine had no influence on the salivary flows obtained, confirming that there was no involvement of ganglia between the point of stimulation and the gland, i.e. the nerve is truly post-ganglionic. The atropine-resistant secretion gradually declined with time but a small flow would persist for a very long time. The results suggested that substance P and VIP may be involved in the non-adrenergic, non-cholinergic response since both these putative transmitters had been detected immunocytochemically in nerves within the parotid gland of the rat[15,16].

Subsequently Ekström and his co-workers showed that section of the auriculotemporal nerve caused more than a 90% reduction of substance P and VIP in the glands[17]. Furthermore, they[18] went on to show that stimulation of the auriculotemporal nerve continuously at 40 Hz for 40 min caused a 75% depletion of substance P and VIP in the gland with little or no further change with more prolonged stimulation. Thus, although these results do not necessarily imply that substance P and VIP are solely responsible for the atropine-resistant parasympathetic secretion of saliva, they indicate that both probably play an important part in the process.

In the course of the above work it was found that the concentration of amylase in parotid saliva from atropinized rats was considerably higher than in saliva from non-atropinized rats. Previously it had been shown that auriculotemporal nerve stimulation at 10 Hz or less in rats produces a copious flow of parotid saliva with a low amylase content and that there is little or no change in the secretory granules in the parotid acini[19,20]. On the other hand sympathetic stimulation was found to cause only a small flow of parotid saliva but it contained a very high content of amylase and there was an extensive degranulation of the acini.

It was decided to test if higher-frequency parasympathetic stimulation would have any effect on the glandular morphology that could be attributed to the release of non-adrenergic, non-cholinergic transmitters[21]. Female Sprague-Dawley rats were used under chloralose anaesthesia. The auriculo-temporal nerve was stimulated at 40 Hz for 80 min and the parotid saliva was collected every 10 min for analyses. All animals received α- and β-adrenergic blockade with dihydroergotamine (1 mg/kg) and propranolol

(1 mg/kg) respectively and half the animals received atropine (1 mg/kg) before stimulation. The physiological results are shown in Figure 1: in the absence of muscarinic blockade, there was a high output of saliva with a moderate output of amylase. In the presence of atropine, the flow of fluid was substantially reduced but in the initial 10 minute period it was about 40% of that in non-atropinized animals. Thereafter the flow rapidly declined so that the total output of saliva was only about 15% of that in the non-atropinized animals. Nevertheless, the total amount of amylase secreted was similar in both sets of animals and a similar degree of parotid acinar degranulation had occurred in both groups (Figure 2). The loss of acinar granules was always rather patchy and never as extensive as after sympathetic nerve stimulation but it was much more evident than after parasympathetic stimulation at 10 Hz or less. On the basis of these results, it was concluded that 'some of the fluid and most of the amylase and acinar granules secreted in the absence of atropine is attributable to release of non-adrenergic, non-cholinergic transmitters from the parasympathetic nerve terminals, when the nerve is stimulated continuously at 40 Hz[21].

It has recently been shown that similar atropine-resistant secretory responses still occur after pretreatment with capsaicin[22]. It is therefore unlikely that the secretory effects were attributable to release of transmitters from afferent fibres in the auriculotemporal nerve.

The extent of the release of non-adrenergic, non-cholinergic transmitters from efferent parasympathetic nerve terminals in the gland under conditions of reflex secretion is unknown. Nevertheless, it seems highly likely that

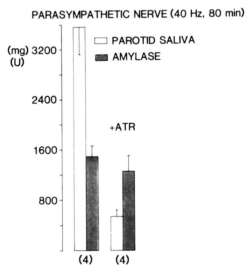

Figure 1 Total secretion of saliva (mg) and amylase (in U) secreted by normal rat parotid glands during auriculotemporal nerve stimulation at 40 Hz for 80 minutes after pretreatment with α- and β-blocking agents. One group ($n = 4$) in the absence of atropine (left-hand columns) and a separate group ($n = 4$) after atropine (1 mg.kg i.v.) (right-hand columns). (Unpublished figure from Ekström et al.[21])

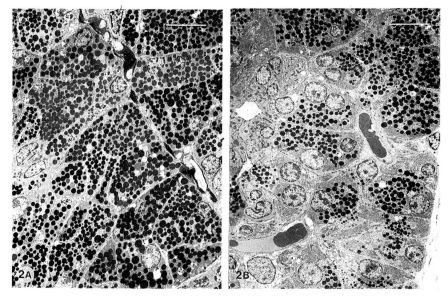

Figure 2 Electron micrographs of acini in parotid glands from a normal rat. Bar = 10 μm. **A**: Left control unstimulated gland showing that the acinar cells are packed with secretory granules. **B**: Right gland after auriculotemporal nerve stimulation at 40 Hz for 80 min, showing a moderately extensive patchy degranulation of the acinar cells. (Unpublished figure from Ekström et al.[21])

variable amounts of peptidergic transmitters are released during normal conditions, especially if bursts of high frequency impulses occur. Their presence will influence the responses of cells that are already receiving cholinergic stimulation. In the sheep it has been found that impulses in individual axons to the parotid gland can reach high frequencies periodically during reflex activity[23]. It has recently been shown in the same species that non-adrenergic, non-cholinergic transmitter release can occur reflexly and induce a detectable effect on parotid secretion[24]. Thus, although our experiments[21] with prolonged high-frequency stimulation produced artificially extreme results, evidence is slowly accruing that less extensive changes may occur, as a part of normal secretory activity, from the release of non-adrenergic, non-cholinergic transmitters from parasympathetic nerve terminals.

In the study of changes in post-ganglionic parasympathetic nerve terminals

Neuropeptides are generally considered to be stored in the large dense-cored vesicles found in axons[25]. There is little information about the influence of nerve impulse formation on these vesicles in peripheral parasympathetic axons. Exocytosis from large dense-cored vesicles has recently been identified in cholinergic autonomic efferent nerves in the adrenal medulla as a result of K^+ treatment[26].

The rat parotid seemed a very convenient model system for testing if prolonged impulse formation has any effects on the numbers of large dense-cored vesicles at neuroeffector sites in post-ganglionic parasympathetic axons. This tissue has the advantage that the neuroeffector sites occur where axons are in intimate association with parenchymal cells in a hypolemmal arrangement (beneath the parenchymal basal lamina). Thus neuroeffector sites in rat parotid glands can be identified with greater confidence than in many other autonomic innervation sites, where the relationship is often less intimate and epilemmal (outside the basal lamina), which makes it problematic whether or not a nerve cell relationship is an actual innervation site. Furthermore, bilateral excision of the superior cervical sympathetic ganglia causes almost total removal of the adrenergic nerves from the glands[27]. Any axons still found in a hypolemmal association with acinar cells after bilateral post-ganglionic sympathectomy can therefore be identified by electron microscopy as parasympathetic, without the need for special staining.

In a recent series of experiments[28], bilateral sympathectomy was undertaken on female Sprague-Dawley rats and 4–6 weeks later the auriculotemporal nerve on one side was stimulated continuously at 40 Hz for 80 min. All animals received propranolol (1 mg/kg) and dihydroergotamine (1 mg/kg) and half the animals also received atropine (1 mg/kg) before starting the nerve stimulation. The flow of saliva was monitored over each 10 minute interval and analysed; the results were similar to those described above. Immediately after cessation of the nerve stimulation parotid tissue was rapidly excised and fixed for electron microscopy. Electron micrographs of 18 unselected hypolemmal axons found sequentially in sections from three different blocks of each gland were examined for their content of large dense-cored vesicles, with diameters of between about 60–100 μm. It was found that whereas only 11% of the axon profiles in the control glands contained no large dense-cored vesicles, the number had increased to 66% on the stimulated side. There was also an 80% reduction in the number of large dense-cored vesicles in the stimulated compared to the unstimulated axons (examples are shown in Figure 3). These results indicate that prolonged impulse formation at the relatively high frequency of 40 Hz causes a depletion of large dense-cored vesicles from the post-ganglionic neuroeffector sites of these parasympathetic axons. This is consistent with the findings by Ekström and co-workers[18] of a 75% depletion of substance P and VIP from the glands under similar conditions of stimulation. Interestingly, the same degree of peptide depletion was found by them to occur within 40 minutes, which is the time during which the non-adrenergic non-cholinergic secretion is most in evidence. Although not established so far, it is possible that the depletion of vesicles in the axons occurs during a similar time span. Presumably the numbers of large dense-cored vesicles present in the axons when the nadir is reached, and thereafter, represent a mixture of those not yet secreted and those having arrived more recently by axon transport.

Although not specifically counted, no obvious differences occurred in the axonal contents of small agranular vesicles, commonly associated with acetylcholine release.

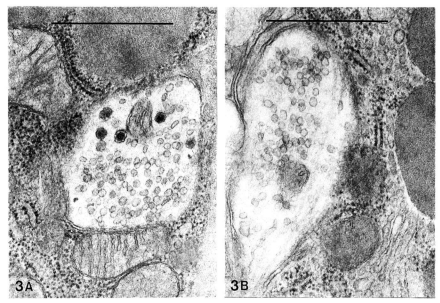

Figure 3 Electron micrographs of hypolemmal axons in rat parotid glands from the same animal, 4 weeks after bilateral sympathetic ganglionectomy. Bar = 1 μm. **A**: Left control unstimulated gland showing five large dense-cored granular vesicles in a terminal axon. **B**: Right gland after auriculotemporal nerve stimulation at 40 Hz for 80 min, showing no large dense-cored granular vesicles in a terminal axon. (Unpublished figure from Ekström et al.[28])

This study shows that stimulation at 40 Hz causes the release of the contents of many of the large dense-cored vesicles from neuroeffector sites in a post-ganglionic parasympathetic nerve without reformation. Presumably this disappearance occurs as a result of an exocytotic process similar to that described by Golding and Pow[26]. It is also reasonable to presume that such release of the contents from large dense-cored vesicles is responsible for much, if not all, of the non-adrenergic non-cholinergic activation of the acinar cells that occurs when this type of stimulation is used.

NERVE STIMULATION IN BURSTS

Edwards and his co-workers[29] have introduced a new procedure for the electrical stimulation of nerves to glands. Instead of continuous stimulation at a set frequency they stimulated the nerves at 10 times the frequency in bursts of 1 s in every 10 s, thereby stimulating the end organ with the same total number of impulses. Results from both types of stimulation were compared. They found that stimulation of the chorda tympani in bursts, at relatively high frequencies, was far more effective in producing vasodilatation in cat submandibular glands of atropinized animals than continuous stimulation at a corresponding lower frequency. Furthermore, the output of VIP from the gland was potentiated by stimulating in bursts and so provided additional evidence to the earlier contention[30,31] that it is the release of this peptide which is largely responsible for the parasympathetic vasodilatation that persists after atropine pretreatment.

Recently we[32] have compared the effects of stimulating the cervical sympathetic nerve in bursts on the secretory and blood flow responses in cat submandibular glands with those occurring on continuous stimulation. At all frequencies from 20–100 Hz in bursts, the flow of saliva was greater than at the corresponding continuous rate over two-minute periods. Continuous stimulation caused an increase in the vascular resistance during the stimulation period followed by an intense transient fall in vascular resistance. In contrast, stimulation in bursts failed to cause an increase in the net vascular resistance during the stimulation period and often caused an overall reduction in the resistance. Immediately after the stimulation period there was a similar transient fall in the vascular resistance, as with continuous stimulation. By spacing the bursts at wider intervals and speeding up the chart speed it was clearly evident that each burst caused an intense short lived vasoconstriction followed by an after-dilatation. β-blockade with propranolol (1 mg/kg) led to a small increase in the vascular resistance during the stimulation period with either type of stimulation but did not affect the after-dilatation. α-blockade with dihydroergotamine (1 mg/kg) revealed a small vasodilator response during stimulation, that could be blocked by propanolol, but the after-dilatation was totally inhibited. Thus, in addition to a small β-adrenoceptor vasodilator component, it was concluded that an active vasodilator component, dependent on α-adrenoceptor activation, is responsible for the after-dilatation which can no longer be attributed to some form of reactive hyperaemia. It seems likely that release of endothelium-derived relaxing factor (EDRF) is involved in this α-adrenergic vasodilatatory activity, but this awaits confirmation.

We have recently tested the effects of stimulating the sympathetic nerve in bursts on rats and found that it also induces a greater, more consistent flow of saliva than continuous stimulation, especially in the submandibular gland in which continuous sympathetic stimulation causes a very erratic secretion[33]. Sympathetic stimulation in bursts therefore has great potential as a method for eliciting a more reliable flow of sympathetic saliva. Some of this beneficial secretory response may relate to the better blood flow during burst stimulation than the inevitable vasoconstriction with continuous stimulation, a problem caused by the unavoidable involvement of vascular nerves during electrical stimulation of the sympathetic trunk.

THE VALUE OF STIMULATING BOTH AUTONOMIC NERVES AT THE SAME TIME

A continuous background of reflex parasympathetic impulses to salivary glands probably occurs in life. Under normal conditions, therefore, any sympathetic impulses reaching the glands are likely to act on cells already receiving a greater or lesser amount of parasympathetic activation. Emmelin and his co-workers have made many experimental studies of superimposing sympathetic stimulation on glands already receiving a background of parasympathetic impulses[2], because this is considered more likely to reflect natural events than stimulating sympathetic nerves in isolation. At suboptimal levels of stimulation this procedure often causes an augmentation of the fluid that is secreted, whereas sympathetic stimulation *per se* at such rates may not even evoke an overt secretion. Furthermore, an augmentation of the protein secreted into the saliva may occur. Such experiments exemplify that the autonomic nerves and the glands work in concert and not in conflict.

Use of single pharmacological agonists and antagonists often leads to the creation of simple arithmetical concepts about the role of the different neurotransmitters in the secretion of different proteins, especially when the studies are done *in vitro*. Thus the secretion of submandibular kallikrein is usually considered as being mediated exclusively by α-adrenergic stimulation. However, the use of double nerve stimulation has caused us to challenge this view[34]. When the sympathetic nerve is stimulated in isolation in the cat there is an erratic flow of saliva, but analysis of individual drops shows that extensive mobilization of glandular kallikrein occurs very rapidly and is followed by a gradual decline. This in itself suggests that a separate population of sympathetic nerves may exist for this express purpose. β-adrenergic blockade appears to slow the flow of fluid but the pattern of mobilization of kallikrein is similar to that in the unblocked situation. α-adrenergic blockade inhibits the flow of saliva on sympathetic nerve stimulation. Using double nerve stimulation with the sympathetic at a low frequency to minimize vasoconstriction, which would impair the flow of saliva, α-adrenergic blockade is then found to inhibit the sympathetic contribution to the secretion of glandular kallikrein. Thus far, all the results obtained appeared to support the idea that secretion of kallikrein is exclusively an α-adrenergic response. However, when a β-blocker was used as the initial blocker during double nerve stimulation it also caused a considerable reduction in the secretion of glandular kallikrein (see Figure 4). Subsequent use of an α-blocker then reduced the output of kallikrein further, to that in parasympathetic saliva *per se*. These results indicate that there is, after all, a β-adrenoceptor component in the secretion of glandular kallikrein from submandibular glands of cats during sympathetic nerve stimulation despite its inability to mobilize kallikrein when stimulated in isolation. This β-response can be considered as having a maximizing influence on the kallikrein secretory effects of α-adrenoceptor stimulation during mixed nerve stimulation. There thus appears to be a synergism between the α- and β-receptor responses from the same sympathetic impulses, as is also likely to occur in life.

RECENT FINDINGS FROM SELECTIVE DENERVATIONS

Studying selective denervations of salivary glands has a long history, starting with Bernard in 1864[35] who showed that an atrophy occurs in submandibular glands after sectioning the chorda tympani. Sympathetic denervations, in contrast, are usually considered not to have much effect on adult glands.

Surgical denervations have helped to identify nerve pathways to the glands.

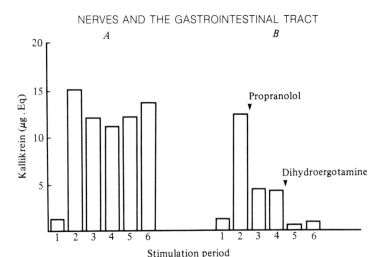

Figure 4 Histograms of the kallikrein output in submandibular saliva from the same cat during consecutive 2 min periods of nerve stimulation, with rest pauses in between. Chorda stimulation at 6 Hz was given during all periods 1–6 and there was super-added sympathetic stimulation at 2 Hz during the periods 2–6. **A**: Control left gland – no blocking drugs were used. **B**: Test right gland – β-blockade (propanolol 1 mg/kg i.v.) was given between periods 2 and 3. α-blockade (dihydroergotamine 1 mg/kg i.v.) was given between periods 4 and 5. (Reproduced from Garrett *et al.*[34] by kind permission of the *Q.J. Exp. Physiol.*)

Study of short-term changes in terminal axons and acini have been informative and a great deal of knowledge about normal influences of the nerves on the glands has been gained from long-term studies[see 4]. In the early stages after post-ganglionic denervation the axons lose their transmitter(s) and a phase is reached whereby this causes activation of glandular cells that can be monitored[36]. Thereafter, sensitivities to conventional transmitters develop by mechanisms that are not yet understood[2]. Sensitivities to putative peptide transmitters[37] have also been found, which supports the likelihood that they have a normal role on the secretory activities of the cells when the innervation is intact.

Some recent experiments that add to existing information will be mentioned.

Parasympathetic denervations

In the cat it has recently been shown that excision of the chorda nerve three weeks previously, leads to an increased secretory response by the submandibular gland to continuous sympathetic stimulation at low frequency (2 Hz)[38]. Use of blocking drugs indicated that muscarinic and β-adrenergic responses are involved in this potentiation. The former may relate to the continuous small release of acetylcholine that occurs from remaining post-ganglionic parasympathetic neurones[39], especially as it may then produce synergistic effects when acting with the sympathetic transmitter on super-sensitive parenchyma[2]. Despite this increased sympathetic secretory response at low-frequency stimulation, there was no change in the secretory capacity during maximal stimulation in bursts[38]. The preceding parasympathetic denervations also enhanced the α-adrenoceptor mediated dilator component in the vascular responses to sympathetic stimulation, whether delivered continuously or in bursts. The dilatation was attributed, as above, to an indirect effect on the endothelium causing release of EDRF or some such agonist. Whether the enhanced vasodilator effect was due to an increased release of the indirect agonist, an increased responsiveness of the vascular smooth muscle, or both, is not known.

Chorda excision in cats has been found to lead to a great decrease in the glandular content of kallikrein despite the continuing ability of the sympathetic nerves to cause its secretion[34]. It can therefore be deduced that, although the secretion of kallikrein is mainly dependent on sympathetic impulses, the glandular parenchyma requires stimulation by transmitters released from parasympathetic nerve impulses for proper resynthesis of kallikrein to occur.

Denervation of glands was found by Bernard[35] to cause 'paralytic secretion', which was eventually shown by Emmelin[40] to be attributable to catecholamines released from the adrenal medulla into the blood, thereby causing an activation of salivary cells made supersensitive by the denervation. Thus it came as a great surprise when we found that the profuse 'paralytic secretion' in rabbit submandibular glands, after preganglionic parasympathectomy, was only partially blocked by adrenergic blockade yet was totally blocked by atropine[41]. We consider, therefore, that under the conditions of our experiments the paralytic secretion was caused by a mixture of the effects of circulating catecholamine and the leakage of acetylcholine from the parasympathetic neurons; the catecholamines on their own, however, were unable to cause secretion and required the additional presence of a muscarinic response. In this way a synergism must have been created for the muscarinic response *per se* was comparatively small.

Sympathetic denervations

In contrast to the generally held view that sympathetic denervation has little or no effect on adult glands, we have now made some interesting observations on rat parotid glands, indicating that metabolic changes do occur in the parenchyma as a result of sympathectomy.

One week after post-ganglionic sympathectomy, parotid saliva produced by auriculotemporal nerve stimulation at 5 Hz showed some distinctive changes in protein composition from the sympathectomised glands[42]. Chromatographic analysis of the saliva revealed a big decrease in the proline-rich protein content and a disproportionately large increase in the amylase concentration. This suggested that normal resynthesis of proline-rich proteins depends on acinar cells receiving stimulation by sympathetic transmitters whereas, in the absence of sympathetic impulses, the parasympathetic transmitters appear to influence the cells to increase their synthesis of amylase.

Prolonged stimulation of the auriculotemporal nerve at 40 Hz after chronic bilateral sympathectomy revealed that other changes also occur[21]. The secretory capacity of the parotid glands was unexpectedly found to be greatly reduced after chronic sympathectomy and the acinar cells showed a marked tendency to vacuolation. However, the non-adrenergic non-cholinergic responses, in the presence of atropine, remained the same as in normal animals.

These experiments indicate that an absence of sympathetic impulses to these glands causes more extensive metabolic effects on the parenchymal cells than had been appreciated.

RECENT FINDINGS FROM THE USE OF CONVENTIONAL NERVE STIMULATION

Parallel or non-parallel secretion

Whether or not the secretion from the same cells always contains the protein constituents in parallel proportions at any one time has been argued for a long time[3]. Recent work with Asking[43,44], using continuous nerve stimulation at 10 Hz or less has shown that differences do exist in the composition of proteins in sympathetic and parasympathetic parotid saliva from rats. The chromatographic patterns show differences in the peaks. There are also differences in the ratios of the amylase iso-enzymes. Sympathetic stimulation is known to cause a degranulation of the parotid acini but little or no degranulation occurs on parasympathetic stimulation at this frequency[19]. It therefore seems possible that some of the protein components reaching the saliva on parasympathetic stimulation may do so from a non-granule pool[45] and this may account for the differences observed.

Synthesis of amylase during parasympathetic stimulation

Although the concentration of amylase is low during prolonged low-frequency parasympathetic stimulation of the rat parotid gland[46,47] the gross amount secreted may become quite large. Nevertheless, no obvious depletion in the glandular content of amylase or of the acinar granules appears to occur. However, when a similar amount of amylase is secreted as a result of sympathetic nerve stimulation, a decrease in glandular amylase and acinar granules does occur. It seems that there must be an increased synthesis of amylase during parasympathetic stimulation and some, at least, seems likely to enter the saliva from a non-granular pool.

Species differences in secretory responses

Species differences in salivary glandular structure and function are enormous, so there are many pitfalls in extrapolating findings from one species to another. In recent years, because so much work has been done on the parotid gland of the rat, it has tended to become the archetypal serous gland. In this way there is a general impression that parasympathetic impulses always cause secretion of fluid without inducing degranulation and that sympathetic impulses always cause degranulation without much movement of fluid. Appreciating that there is a marked difference in the innervation of the parotid gland of the cat compared with that of the rat[48], Emmelin and this author[49] have examined the nerve mediated responses in the parotid gland of the cat. In complete contrast to the rat there was no detectable depletion of acinar granules on prolonged sympathetic stimulation whereas on parasympathetic stimulation there was a rapid and extensive secretion of acinar granules.

The rabbit submandibular gland has a poor reputation for secretion when stimulated sympathetically, because very little extra fluid is expelled from the cannula. However, using histological techniques we have recently shown that an extensive secretion of mucosubstance does in fact occur from the submandibular acinar cells as a result of sympathetic stimulation[50] but, as there is little mobilization of water at the same time, the secreted mucin accumulates in the ducts and distends them. This particular investigation has provided a good example of the value of combining structural assessments with functional studies.

RECENT FINDINGS FROM REFLEX STIMULATION

The ultimate aim for investigating the peripheral role of nerves in the glands is to enable understanding about their actions as they occur in life and this means the events during normal reflex stimulation. Certain glands lend themselves for assessment of the structural changes within the parenchyma when they are stimulated reflexly, during the eating of a meal. In this way we found some time ago that, when rats were starved for 24 h and then fed hard chow for 1–2 h, a considerable amount of parotid acinar degranulation occurred but this was inhibited by sectioning the cervical sympathetic trunk in the neck[51]. Thus, the results from sympathetic nerve stimulation in rats[19] do in fact provide good insight into its role in causing exocytosis of parotid acini under natural conditions. A similar feeding technique has now been used to study secretory events in rabbit submandibular glands after sectioning the cervical sympathetic trunk on one side[52]. This showed that an extensive depletion of acinar mucin occurred on the side with an intact innervation but preganglionic sympathectomy greatly inhibited any such secretion. Thus, again the evidence gained from nerve-stimulation experiments, showing that sympathetic impulses can cause secretion of acinar mucin[50], gave a good indication of events as they occur in life. However, in the rabbit, parasympathetic nerve stimulation will also cause a secretion of mucin from submandibular acinar cells[53]. It would therefore appear that, despite this ability, sympathetic impulses provide the main impetus for the secretion of acinar mucin during chewing, but this may be enhanced under normal conditions by the accompanying parasympathetic stimulation.

During various studies on reflex secretion in rats, a scattered irregular formation of intracellular watery vacuoles was always apparent in the parotid glands. Therefore it seemed worthwhile observing their incidence during natural reflex stimulation in greater detail. The ability of certain serous cells to form watery vacuoles during strong stimulation is well documented[see 54].

We had previously found that this tendency was accentuated in rat parotid glands when parasympathetic stimulation was administered after acinar degranulation[55]. Throughout most work in which vacuolation has been documented it could be considered to have been caused by pathophysiological excess rather than as a result of physiological change. We have now studied a series of rats that were encouraged to chew hard chow for 2 h, after a 24 h fast[56]. The experiments were carried out either at room temperature or in the cold room (0–4°C), since such chilling has been found to induce more vigorous eating. The amount eaten was roughly estimated and this was corroborated by the weight of the stomachs. All glands showed some scattered vacuolation and this became more conspicuous after eating, especially in those animals that had eaten in the cold. Vacuole formation was often associated with, but not dependent on, a degree of acinar degranulation. Cellular debris, including secretory granules, were frequently seen in the vacuoles. As vacuoles could be found in continuity with lumina, it is likely that their contents ultimately reach the saliva. This work has shown that, although vacuole formation may not be an idealistic event, it forms a part of the normal secretory cycle within rat parotid acini. Thus, under physiological conditions the secretion of proteins from parotid acinar cells in rats is not necessarily confined to the orthodox mechanisms of exocytosis as classically witnessed during β-agonist stimulation. Vacuolation, whenever it occurs, may afford a pathway whereby some components enter saliva. If vacuoles rupture this may provide a route by which some of the salivary amylase, normally present in the plasma, reaches the blood. It seems likely that some of the more grossly vacuolated cells will die but the less severely affected may recover[57].

CONCLUDING REMARKS

Use of the well-established, old-fashioned procedure of electrical stimulation of autonomic nerves to salivary glands *in vivo* can still provide useful new information about the roles they play in salivary secretion. This has been enhanced recently by the application of some different stimulation protocols. These include continuous stimulation at a higher frequency, such as 40 Hz, for assessing the effects of non-adrenergic non-cholinergic transmitters thereby released from parasympathetic nerves in rat parotid glands. Such transmitters were found to be mainly responsible for the secretion of amylase and the accompanying exocytosis of acinar granules under these conditions of stimulation. An extensive depletion of the large dense-cored vesicles in terminal parasympathetic axons within the glands has now been found to occur at the same time. Another different protocol – stimulating the nerves in bursts – has produced different results from more conventional continuous stimulation. This has revealed an α-adrenergic vasodilatory component in the vascular response to sympathetic nerve stimulation. Such vasodilatation is now thought to be mediated indirectly via an action on the endothelial cells causing release of EDRF.

Stimulations of both sympathetic and parasympathetic nerves to a gland at the same time have shown that augmentation of fluid formation often occurs when using suboptimal stimulations; augmentation of protein secretion may also occur. Double nerve stimulation has also enabled the detection of a β-adrenergic component in the sympathetic secretion of glandular kallikrein in cats, demonstrating that its secretion is not exclusively an α-adrenergic response, as has usually been considered.

Low-frequency stimulation of the rat parotid gland shows that not all of the protein components secreted in parasympathetic saliva occur in parallel with those present in sympathetic saliva. Much of the amylase in rat parotid saliva during low-frequency parasympathetic stimulation appears to be the result of concurrent synthesis and passage from a non-granule pool.

Besides the better known changes that follow parasympathectomy, selective denervation has now shown that an absence of sympathetic impulses to a gland may also affect its metabolism and secretory capacity. Sympathetic impulses also appear to be an essential stimulus in the parotid gland of the rat for the normal resynthesis of proline-rich proteins whereas, in their absence, parasympathetic impulses then appear to have an increased stimulatory effect on the synthesis of amylase. Denervation experiments in cats indicate that parasympathetic impulses are essential for the resynthesis of kallikrein in submandibular glands.

Both nerve stimulation and reflex stimulation show that sympathetic impulses are mainly responsible for the secretion of parotid acinar granules in rats. In cats, however, parasympathetic impulses are mainly responsible for the degranulation of parotid acini. Histology on submandibular glands of rabbits has provided information, not obtainable in other ways, that acinar mucin is secreted in response to sympathetic impulses. Similar studies after reflex stimulation, from chewing hay, have established the importance of sympathetic impulses in the natural secretion of acinar mucin by rabbit submandibular glands. Reflex studies on rats have further revealed that watery vacuolation can occur in certain secretory cells as a part of normal life, especially when the animals have eaten vigorously. This indicates that not all movement of organic molecules into the saliva necessarily occurs exclusively by means of the neat and tidy process of exocytosis. Vacuolation appears to be an example where even natural secretory drive, when taken beyond certain limits, can produce effects that are not idealistic.

The work presented indicates that, in general, the actions of the different nerves on glandular cells produce harmonious complex interrelated effects, the responses being collaborative rather than conflicting and often synergistic. In life it is likely that there is a well developed central integration of reflex impulse formation in the sympathetic and parasympathetic secretory nerves so that the glandular responses are constantly being modulated to meet the needs of the animal.

Acknowledgements

Collaborative work with colleagues in the Institute of Physiology, Lund has made much of this presentation possible. Their help and travel grants from the Royal Society and the British Council are gratefully acknowledged. The blood flow studies with Dr Edwards in Cambridge were made possible by a visiting Fellowship at Fitzwilliam College. The indispensible help of my colleagues in the Department of Oral Pathology, at King's is also gratefully acknowledged.

References

1. Babkin, B. P. (1950). *Secretory Mechanism of the Digestive Glands*, 2nd Edn. (New York: P. B. Hoeber)
2. Emmelin, N. (1987). Nerve interactions in salivary glands. *J. Dent. Res.*, **66**, 509–17
3. Garrett, J. R. (1987). The proper role of nerves in salivary secretion: A review. *J. Dent. Res.*, **66**, 387–97
4. Garrett, J. R. (1987). Innervation of salivary glands: neurohistological and functional aspects. In Sreebny, L. M. (ed.) *The Salivary System*, pp. 69–93. (Florida: CRC Press)
5. Alm, P., Asking, B., Emmelin, N. and Gjörstrup, P. (1984). Adrenergic nerves to the rat parotid gland originating in the contralateral sympathetic chain. *J. Autonom. Nerv. System.*, **11**, 309–16
6. Burgen, A. S. V. and Emmelin, N. G. (1961). *Physiology of the Salivary Glands.* (London: Edward Arnold)
7. Baum (1987). Regulation of salivary secretion. In Sreebny, L. M. (ed.) *The Salivary System*, pp. 123–34. (Florida: CRC Press)
8. Hand, A. (ed.) (1987). Saliva and Salivary Glands. *J. Dent. Res.*, **66** (2): 385–618
9. Heidenhain, R. (1872). Ueber die Wirkung einiger Gifte auf die Nerven der Glandula submaxillaris. *Pflügers Arch. Ges. Physiol.*, **5**, 309–18
10. Emmelin, N. and Lenninger, S. (1967). The 'direct' effect of physalaemin on salivary gland cells. *Br. J. Pharmac. Chemother.*, **30**, 676–80
11. Thulin, A. (1976). Motor and secretory effects of nerves on the parotid gland of the rat. *Acta Physiol. Scand.*, **96**, 506–11
12. Thulin, A. (1976). Blood flow changes in the submaxillary gland of the rat on parasympathetic and sympathetic nerve stimulation. *Acta Physiol. Scand.*, **97**, 104–9
13. Ekström, J. (1974). Choline acetyltransferase activity in rat salivary glands after cellulose rich diet or treatment with an atropine-like drug. *Q. J. Exp. Physiol.*, **59**, 191–9
14. Ekström, J., Månsson, B., Tobin, G., Garrett, J. R. and Thulin, A. (1983). Atropine-resistant secretion of parotid saliva on stimulation of the auriculo-temporal nerve. *Acta Physiol. Scand.*, **119**, 445–9
15. Hökfelt, T., Johansson, O., Kjellerth, J. O., Ljungdahl, A., Nilsson, G., Nygårds, A. and Pernow, B. (1977). Immunohistochemical distribution of Substance P. In Von Euler, U.S. and Pernow, B. (eds.) *Substance P*, pp. 117–45. (New York: Raven Press)
16. Uddman, R., Fahrenkrug, J. Malm, L., Alumets, J., Håkanson, R. and Sundler, F. (1980). Neoronal VIP in salivary glands: Distribution and release. *Acta Physiol. Scand.*, **110**, 31–8
17. Ekström, J., Brodin, E., Ekman, R., Håkanson, R. and Sundler, F. (1984). Vasoactive intestinal peptide and substance P in salivary glands of the rat following denervation or duct ligation. *Reg. Peptides.*, **10**, 1–10
18. Ekström, J., Brodin, E., Ekman, R., Håkanson, R., Månsson, B. and Tobin, G. (1985). Depletion of neuropeptides in rat parotid glands and declining atropine-resistant salivary secretion upon continuous parasympathetic nerve stimulation. *Reg. Peptides.*, **11**, 353–9
19. Garrett, J. R. and Thulin, A. (1975). Changes in parotid acinar cells accompaning salivary secretion in rats on sympathetic or parasympathetic nerve stimulation. *Cell Tissue Res.*, **159**, 179–93

20. Anderson, L. C., Garrett, J. R., Johnson, D. A., Kauffman, D. L., Keller, P. J. and Thulin, A. (1984). Influence of circulating catecholamines on protein secretion into rat parotid saliva during parasympathetic stimulation. *J. Physiol.*, **352**, 163–71
21. Ekström, J., Garrett, J. R., Månsson, B. and Tobin, G. (1988). The effects of atropine and chronic sympathectomy on maximal parasympathetic stimulation of parotid saliva in rats. *J. Physiol.*, **403**, 105–116
22. Ekman, R., Ekström, J., Håkanson, R., Tobin, G. and Sundler, F. (1988). Effects of capsaicin on neuropeptides and secretory responses of parotid glands. *J. Physiol.*, **401**, 33P.
23. Carr, D. H. (1977). Reflex-induced electrical activity in single units of secretory nerves to the parotid gland. In Brooks, F. P. and Evers, P. W. (eds.) *Nerves and the Gut*, pp. 79–84. (Thorofare, N.J.: Charles Slack)
24. Reid, A. M. and Titchen, D. A. (1986). Reflex stimulation of parotid secretion in sheep after atropine and cervical sympathetic ganglionectomy. *J. Physiol.*, **371**, 129P
25. Fried, G. (1982). Neuropeptide storage in vesicles. In Klein, R. K., Lagercrantz, H. and Zimmerman, H. (eds.) *Neurotransmitter Vesicles*, pp. 361–74. (London: Academic Press)
26. Golding, D. W. and Pow, D. V. (1987). 'Neurosecretion' by a classic cholinergic innervation apparatus. A comparative study of adrenal chromaffin glands in four vertebrate species (teleosts, anurans, mammals). *Cell and Tissue Res.*, **249**, 421–5
27. Garrett, J. R., Harrop, T. J. and Thulin, A. (1985). Secretion of parotid acinar granules in rats during reflex stimulation after chronic sympathectomy. *Q. J. Exp. Physiol.*, **70**, 461–7
28. Ekström, J., Garrett, J. Månsson, B., Rowley, P. S. A., and Tobin, G. (1988). Depletion of large dense-cored vesicles from parasympathetic nerve terminals in rat parotid glands after prolonged stimulation of the auriculo-temporal nerve. *Reg P-eptides*, (In press)
29. Anderson, P.-O., Bloom, S. R., Edwards, A. V. and Järhult, J. (1982). Effects of stimulation of the chorda tympani in bursts on submaxillary responses in the cat. *J. Physiol.*, **322**, 469–83
30. Bloom, S. R. and Edwards, A. V. (1980). Vasoactive intestinal peptide in relation to atropine resistant vasodilatation in the submaxillary gland of the cat. *J. Physiol.*, **300**, 41–53
31. Lundberg, J. M., Änggard, A., Fahrenkrug, J., Hökfelt, T. and Mutt, V. (1980). Vasoactive intestinal polypeptide in cholinergic neurons of exocrine glands: functional significance of coexisting transmitters for vasodilation and secretion. *Proc. Natl. Acad. Aci. USA*, **77**, 1651–5
32. Bloom, S. R., Edwards, A. V. and Garrett, J. R. (1987). Effects of stimulating the sympathetic innervation in bursts on submandibular vascular and secretory function in cats. *J. Physiol.*, **393**, 91–106
33. Anderson, L. C., Garrett, J. R. and Proctor, G. B. (1988). Advantages of burst stimulation for inducing sympathetic salivary secretion in rats. *Q. J. Exp. Physiol.* **73**, 1025–1028
34. Garrett, J. R., Smith, R. E., Kyriacou, K., Kidd, A. and Liao, J. (1987). Factors affecting the secretion of submandibular salivary kallikrein in cats. *Q. J. Exp. Physiol.*, **72**, 357–68
35. Bernard, C. (1864). Du rôle des actions réflexes paralysantes dans le phénomène des sécrétions. *J. Anat. (Paris)*, **1**, 507–13
36. Emmelin, N. (1981). Denervation as a method to produce prolonged stimulation of salivary glands. In Zelles, T. (ed.) *Saliva and Salivation*, pp. 1–9 (Budapest: Akademia Kiade)
37. Ekström, J. (1987). Neuropeptides and secretion. *J. Dent Res.*, **66**, 524–30
38. Edwards, A. V. and Garrett, J. R. (1988). Submandibular responses to stimulation of the sympathetic innervation following parasympathetic denervation in cats. *J. Physiol.*, **397**, 421–31
39. Emmelin, N. (1965). Action of transmitters on the responsiveness of effector cells. *Experientia*, **21**, 57–65
40. Emmelin, N. (1952). 'Paralytic secretion' of saliva. An example of supersensitivity after denervation. *Physiol. Rev.*, **32**, 21–46
41. Garrett, J. R. and Kyriacou, K. (1988). 'Paralytic' secretion after parasympathectomy of rabbit submandibular glands includes a cholinergic component. *Q. J. Exp. Physiol.* **73**, 737–746
42. Proctor, G. B., Asking, B. and Garrett, J. R. (1988). Influences of short-term sympathectomy on the composition of proteins in rat parotid saliva. *Q. J. Exp. Physiol.*, **73**, 139–42
43. Asking, A., Garrett, J. R. and Proctor, G. B. (1986). Non-parallel features in parasympathetic and sympathetic parotid saliva from rats. *J. Physiol.*, **381**, 33P.

44. Asking, B., Masson, P. and Proctor, G. B. (1988). Variations in the isoenzymes of rat parotid amylase depending on the type of autonomic nerve activated. *J. Physiol.* **403**, 52P.
45. Kelly, R. B. (1985). Pathways of protein secretion in eukaryotes. *Science*, **230**, 25–32
46. Asking, B., Clarke, G. and Proctor, G. B. (1987). Amylase in rat parotid saliva on prolonged parasympathetic stimulation. *J. Physiol.* **390**, 172P.
47. Asking, P., and Gjörstrup, P. (1987). Synthesis and secretion of amylase in the rat parotid gland following autonomic nerve stimulation *in vivo. Acta Physiol Scand.*, **130**, 439–45
48. Garrett, J. R. (1972). Neuro-effector sites in salivary glands. In Emmelin, N. and Zotterman, Y. (eds.) *Oral Physiology*, pp. 83–97. (Oxford: Pergamon)
49. Emmelin, N. and Garrett, J. R. (1986). Secretory changes in parotid acini of cats on nerve stimulation. *J. Physiol.*, **376**, 29P.
50. Kyriacou, K., Garrett, J. R. and Gjörstrup, P. (1988). Structural and functional studies of the effects of sympathetic stimulation on rabbit submandibular salivary glands. *Archs. Oral Biol.*, **33**, 271–80
51. Harrop, T. J. and Garrett, J. R. (1974). Effects of preganglionic sympathectomy on secretory changes in parotid acinar cells of rats on eating. *Cell and Tissue Res.*, **154**, 135–50
52. Kryiacou, K. and Garrett, J. R. (1988). Morphological changes in the rabbit submandibular gland after parasympathetic or sympathetic denervation. *Arch. Oral Biol.*, **33**, 281–90
53. Kyriacou, K., Garrett, J. R. and Gjörstrup, P. (1986). Structural and functional studies of the effects of parasympathetic nerve stimulation on rabbit submandibular glands. *Arch. Oral Biol.*, **31**, 235–44
54. Mills, J. W. and Quinton, P. M. (1981). Formation of stimulus-induced vacuoles in serous cells of tracheal submucosal glands. *Am. J. Physiol.*, **241**, C18–24
55. Garrett, J. R., Thulin, A. and Kidd, A. (1978). Variations in parasympathetic secretory and structural responses resulting from differences in the pre-stimulation state of parotid acini in rats. Some factors affecting watery vacuolation. *Cell and Tissue Res.*, **188**, 235–50
56. Garrett, J. R., Harrop, T. J. and Thulin, A. (1987). Electron microscopy of watery vacuole formation in rat parotid acinar cells during reflex stimulation. *Arch. Oral Biol.*, **32**, 611–17
57. Leslie, B. A. and Putney, J. W. (1983). Ionic mechanisms in secretagogue-induced morphological changes in rat parotid gland. *J. Cell Biol.*, **97**, 1119–30

13
How does the brain modify gastric contractions independently of gastric acid secretion?

H.-S. FENG, R. B. LYNN and F. P. BROOKS

The stomach has many functions which, in general, can be divided into the processes of exocrine and endocrine secretion and motility. Studies of isolated cells have established the role of parietal (oxyntic) cells in the secretion of hydrochloric acid and chief cells in the secretion of pepsinogens. Receptors for neuroregulatory peptides and neurotransmitters have been identified on the surface of secretory cells and smooth muscle cells. Endocrine cells responsible for secretion of the hormones gastrin and somatostatin have been identified. The role of the myenteric plexus in the control of gastric function is less known, although electrical field stimulation of isolated stomach preparations has established that nerve-mediated stimulation of acid secretion occurs. The submucosal plexus is poorly developed in the stomach of human, cat and opossum[1] (and personal communication, Michael D. Schuffler). Schemann and Wood (this volume, Chapter 9) report that recordings of electrical activity in ganglion cells of the myenteric plexus of the corpus of the guinea pig stomach differed strikingly from those in the small intestine in three respects: (1) there were no negative after-potentials producing hyperpolarization, (2) there were no slow EPSPs, and (3) there was no evidence for presynaptic inhibition[2].

.Under normal conditions the stomach is called upon to perform strikingly different functions during the interdigestive period compared with those after a meal. During the interdigestive period, gastric acid secretion occurs at a low rate while periodically series of phasic gastric contractions pass from the oesophagus to the ileum, possibly to empty the upper digestive tract of cellular debris and microorganisms. The plasma levels of gastric hormones such as gastrin and somatostatin are usually maintained at low levels.

On the other hand, after a meal, gastric acid secretion reaches its peak rate, gastric phasic contractions are reduced in amplitude, particularly in the body of the stomach, and the migrating motor complexes from the oesophagus to the ileum are replaced by irregular contractions propagated over short distances. Acid secretion increases 10–20-fold and gastric motility shifts from a propulsive to a mixing mode. Gastric acid secretion is classically divided into cephalic, gastric and intestinal phases depending upon the origin of the stimulus. Only more recently has the concept of a cephalic phase of gastric motility been advanced. The changes in gastric motor activity involving circular and longitudinal smooth muscle in response to a meal are now beginning to be defined.

For the last 30 years, my colleagues and I have studied the role of extrinsic nerves (the vagi) and the brain in the control of gastric function. We have been impressed with the divergence in secretory and motor responses during stimulation of different portions of the brain stem and hypothalamus. In contrast, stimulation of efferent vagal trunks seems to stimulate both the amplitude of phasic contractions, especially in the antrum, and to increase gastric acid secretion. In this communication we consider the divergent patterns in some detail.

The most striking divergence between acid secretion and gastric phasic contractions occurs during the response of the stomach to sham feeding in conscious dogs. Figure 1, taken from a 1950 paper by Lorber, Komarov and Shay, shows the decrease in amplitude of phasic contractions of the body and antrum of the stomach during 3 min of sham feeding of a dog with a gastric fistula and an oesophagostomy, despite an increase in acid output. The latency of the secretory response was 5–10 min, while the effect on motility was seen within a few seconds. On the basis of similar results in four dogs the authors suggested that 'different vagal centers exist to control these gastric functions'[3].

Thirteen years later Olbe and Jacobson used pressure-sensitive endosondes to follow phasic gastric contractions in nine conscious dogs with vagally innervated (Pavlov) pouches and oesophagostomies[4]. There was a reduction in the amplitude of phasic contractions during sham feeding despite an increase in acid secretion. In contrast, insulin-induced hypoglycaemia was followed by an increase in the force and frequency of phasic contractions as well as an increase in acid output. These results also suggest different vagally mediated mechanisms for the control of acid secretion and phasic gastric contractions. Poster presentations at the meeting on modified phase feeding in human subjects were thought to show excitatory effects on pressures[5] and myoelectrical activity[6].

.Observations on patients with functional upper gastrointestinal disorders also suggest that disturbances in gastric motor function can occur independently of abnormalities in acid secretion[7]. This evidence suggests also that brain–gut relationships may result in divergent effects in gastric motor and secretory functions.

ELECTRICAL STIMULATION OF EFFERENT VAGAL TRUNKS

We and others have carried out extensive investigations of the effect of electrical stimulation of vagal efferents in the neck of anesthetized cats. The studies of Martinson[8] are sometimes cited as an example of divergent effects

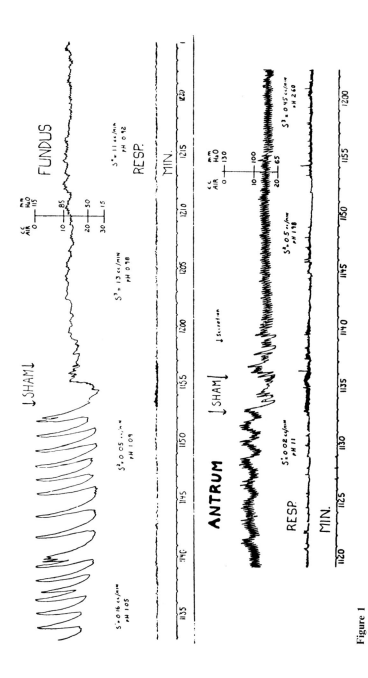

Figure 1

of vagal stimulation on secretion and motility. He reported that gastric motility as measured with a large balloon in the corpus was controlled by 'low threshold' and 'high threshold' fibres in the vagus. The low threshold fibres when stimulated by impulses with a pulse duration of less than 1 ms increased gastric tone but had no effect on acid output, while the high threshold fibres when stimulated with pulse durations of 2–4 ms increased gastric acid output but lowered gastric tone. Experiments in our laboratory using a similar balloon, but using extraluminal force transducers on the antrum to record phasic contractions, showed that stimulation of high threshold fibres increased the force of antral contractions (Figure 2) while lowering basal pressure in the balloon[9]. We subsequently showed that intra-aortic eserine shifted the response of phasic antral contractions to vagal stimulation so that pulse durations of 0.2 ms increased their amplitude[10] compared to 1–4 ms without eserine. Figure 3 shows the shift in dose response. These results suggest that the amount of acetylcholine released by nerve stimulation determines the increase in amplitude of phasic congractions.

Subsequently we compared acid output during efferent vagal stimulation with that obtained during a maximal stimulating infusion of pentagastrin as shown in Figure 4. Vagal stimulation could produce near maximal acid output using 1 mA, 5 Hz, and 4 ms[11]. Similarly, stimulation with the same parameters produced phasic antral contractions of the same amplitude and force as a maximal stimulating infusion of bethanechol[12] as shown in Figure 5. Martinson found that the same parameters of electrical stimulation increased gastric mucosal blood flow[13]. These results indicate that in vagal efferent trunks the parameters of electrical stimulation for producing maximal gastric output, maximal force of phasic antral contractions, and increase in gastric mucosal blood flow are the same. The same parameters also doubled the arterial plasma concentration of immunoreactive gastrin[14].

BRAIN STIMULATION

With this background we began to explore control of gastric function by stimulation of discrete areas of the medulla. Our initial results of electrical stimulation within the dorsal motor nucleus of the vagus in anaesthetized cats gave equivocal results[15]. Pagani and his associates reported that electrical stimulation of the dorsal motor nucleus of the vagus in cats using parameters of 100 μA, 50 Hz and 0.2 ms increased the force of antral contractions but had no effect on acid secretion. Using parameters of 1 mA, 5 Hz and 4 ms, we obtained significant increases in gastric acid output as well as increased force of antral contractions[16]. When we used the same parameters as Pagani et al., we also obtained no increase in acid secretion[17] .These experiments have been criticized for the large currents used. However, more recently we have obtained similar results with microinjections of thyrotropic releasing hormone (TRH) and the GABA-ergic antagonist bicuculline[18,19]. With both agents, doses required to stimulate acid secretion were greater than those needed to increase the force of antral contractions.

Pagani et al[20] .also reported that electrical stimulation of the nucleus

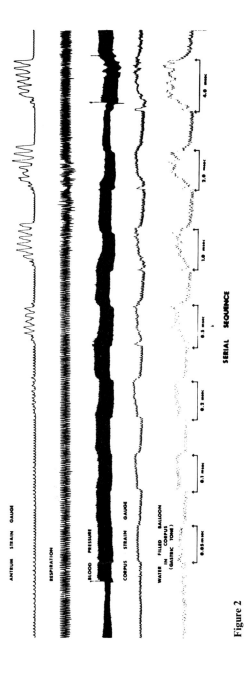

Figure 2

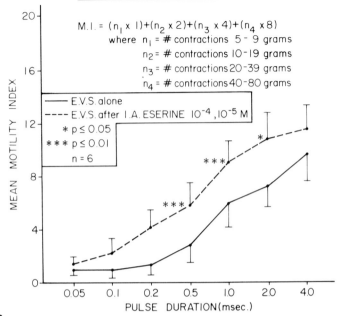

Figure 3

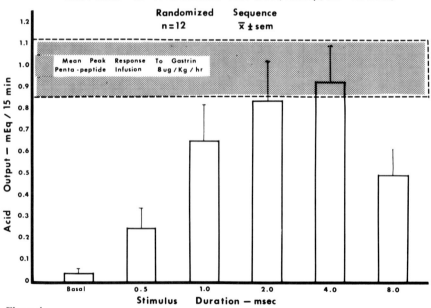

Figure 4

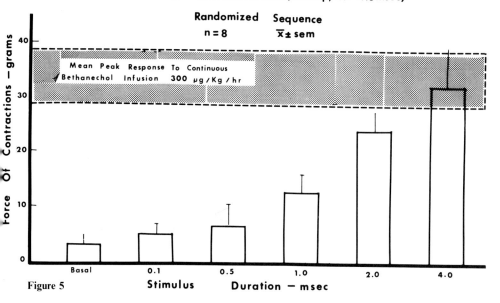

Figure 5

ambiguus with low-current, high-frequency electrical stimulation increased the force of antral contractions. We found that stimulation of the nucleus ambiguus with other these parameters or those we had found effective in stimulating acid secretion in the dorsal motor nucleus of the vagus were ineffective in increasing acid output[17]. Ishikawa et al. have recently reported that TRH injected into the nucleus ambiguus increased acid output in the rat[21]. The lack of response to electrical stimulation of acid secretion in the cat has yet to be tested with chemical stimulation.

Finally, we have demonstrated that electrical stimulation of an area of the lateral hypothalamus in cats with 1 mA, 10 Hz and 8 ms increased the force of antral contractions without increasing acid output[22] (Figure 6). This pathway is mediated through the vagi and blocked by atropine. Bicuculline microinjections also failed to stimulate acid output, but since the volume of gastric content increased while the pH rose to above 8, bicarbonate secretion may have occurred[23].

Greenwood and Davison have recently published a review of the relationship between gastrointestinal motility and secretion, and concluded that increased motor activity in the stomach is frequently associated with increased acid and pepsin secretion[24]. Although pepsin is considered a marker of cholinergic stimulation in the dog[23], it should be noted that in the spider monkey histamine is equally effective as insulin hypoglycaemia in stimulating pepsin secretion[25]. They suggested that acid secretion might have been masked by cardiovascular effects in Pagani et al.'s experiments. In our experiments cardiovascular effects were most consistent during stimulation

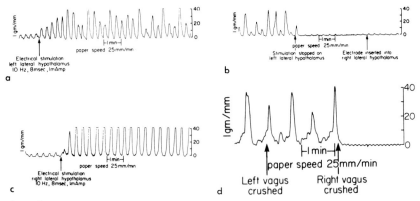

Figure 6

of the nucleus ambiguus at high frequencies.

It appears to us that divergence of effects on gastric motor function and acid output are seen with stimulation within the brain but not at the level of vagal trunks. This is consistent with specificity of control mechanisms at levels within the brain and with clinical observations in patients with functional gastrointestinal disorders. The difference in sensitivity between motor and secretory responses to electrical and chemical stimulation in the brainstem also may be important in accounting for divergence in physiological gastric responses.

References

1. Christensen, J., and Rick, G. D. (1985). The cell density in submucous plexus throughout the gut of cat and opossum. *Gastroenterology*, **89**, 1064–9
2. Schemann, M. and Wood, J. D. (1988). Neurophysiology of the enteric nervous system the stomach. Presented at the *Symposium on Nerves and the Gastrointestinal Tract*. Titisee, West Germany, 2–4 June
3. Lorber, S. H., Komarov, S. A. and Shay, H. (1950). Effect of sham feeding on gastric motor activity of the dog. *Am. J. Physiol.*, **162**, 447–51
4. Olbe, L. and Jacobson, B. (1963). Intraluminal pressure waves of the stomach in dogs studied by endoradiosondes. *Gastroenterology*, **44**, 787–96
5. Sielaff, F., Berndt, H. and Bytel, Th. (1988). Effect of sham feeding on interdigestive gastroduodenal motility. Presented as a poster at *Symposium on Nerves and the Gastrointestinal Tract*. Titisee, West Germany, 2–4 June
6. Stern, D. M., Koch, K. L., Crawford, H. E., Vasey, M. W., and Stewart, W. R. (1988). Sham feeding: cephalic-vagal influences on gastric myoelectric activity in man. Presented as a poster at *Symposium on Nerves and the Gastrointestinal Tract*. Titisee, West Germany, 2–4 June
7. Brooks, F. P. (1983). Central nervous system and the digestive tract in Chey, W. Y. (ed.) *Functional Disorders of the Digestive Tract*, pp. 21–27 (New York: Raven Press)
8. Martinson, J. (1965). Studies on the efferent control of the stomach. *Acta Physiologica Scand.*, **65**, (Suppl. 225), 1–24
9. Lombardi, D. M. and Brooks, F. P. (1980). Low and high threshold fibers in the vagi revisited. *Physiologist*, **23**, 38
10. Lombardi, D. M., Feng, H.-S. and Brooks, F. P. (1981). Phasic vs. tonic contractions of the cat stomach in response to electrical vagal stimulation. *Fed. Proc.*, **40**, 576

11. Bauer, R. F. (1977). Electrically-induced vagal stimulation of gastric acid secretion. In Brooks, F. P. and Evers, P. W. (eds.) *Nerves and the Gut*, pp. 86–95 (Thorofare, N.J.: Charles Slack)

12. Lombardi, D. M., Gindea, A. and Brooks, F. P. (1978). Stimulation of gastric antral contractions and acid secretion by bethanechol in anesthetized cats. *Physiologist*, **21**, 73

13. Martinson, J. (1965). The effect of graded vagal stimulation on gastric motility, secretion and blood flow in the cat. *Acta Physiol. Scand.* **65**, 300–9

14. Bauer, R. F., McGuigan, J. E. and Brooks, F. P. (1977). The serum gastrin after electrical vagal stimulation in cats. *Gastroenterology*, **72**, 1028

15. Lombardi, D. M., Feng, H.-S. and Brooks, F. P. (1982). Dissociation of secretory and motor responses to stimulation of the dorsal motor nucleus of the vagus in anesthetized cats. *Gastroenterology*, **82**, 1120

16. Pagani, F. D., Norman, W. P., Kasbekar, D. K. and Gillis, R. A. (1985). Localization of sites within the dorsal motor nucleus of vagus that affect gastric motility. *Am. J. Physiol.* **249**, (*Gastrointest. Liver Physiol.*, **12**), 673–84

17. Feng, H.-S., Han, J. and Brooks, F. P. (1987). Stimulation of the dorsal motor nuclei (DMV) but not the nucleus ambiguus increases gastric acid output. *Fed. Proc.*, **46**, 1065

18. Lynn, R. B., Han, J., Feng, H.-S. and Brooks, F. P. (1988). TRH injections into the dorsal motor nucleus of the vagus (DMV) increases gastric acid output and the force of gastric contractions in anesthetized cats. *Gastroenterology*, **94**, A274

14
Control of bile secretion by sympathetic liver nerves

K. BECKH, G. SCHUSTER and R. ARNOLD

INTRODUCTION

The liver parenchyma is innervated by autonomic nerves of the sympathetic and the parasympathetic nervous system[1-4]. In several studies using *in vivo* and *in vitro* models, regulation of hepatic metabolic pathways by liver nerves were reported (see reviews[5-7]). In the *in situ* perfused rat liver electrical stimulation of the perivascular nerves around the hepatic artery and portal vein was shown to cause an increase of glucose and lactate output[8], a decrease of ketone body production[9], of urea formation and ammonia uptake[10] as well as of oxygen uptake[11,12] and an overflow of noradrenaline into the hepatic vein[13].

Although it was histochemically demonstrated that the biliary system receives sympathetic and parasympathetic nerves[5] little is known about the nervous regulation of bile secretion[6]. In *in vivo* models and in the perfused liver circulating hormones regulate the bile flow[14-17]. For example, glucagon and insulin increase the bile flow[17].

It was the aim of the investigation to demonstrate the regulation of the bile secretion by hepatic nerves. To exclude hormonal signals we used the *in situ* perfused rat liver as model.

MATERIALS AND METHODS

Livers of male Wistar rats weighing 190–240 g were perfused with a medium containing Krebs–Henseleit bicarbonate buffer equilibrated with 95% O_2 and 5% CO_2 as previously described[8]. The flow rate was $4 \, \mathrm{ml \, min^{-1} \, g^{-1}}$ liver. In a series of experiments by lowering the portal pressure the flow rate was adjusted to the values indicated in the text and Table 1, respectively. A plastic tube was placed in the bile duct. The bile was collected over periods of five minutes. The hepatic nerves were electrically stimulated by a platinum electrode placed around hepatic artery and portal vein (20 Hz, 20 V, 2 ms).

Table 1 Bile flow and glucose output during artificially lowered portal flow mimicking the flow reduction during nerve stimulation. Values are means $\pm$ SEM of five experiments, each

	Change of flow rate (ml min^{-1} g^{-1})	Change of glucose output (μmol min^{-1} g^{-1})	Change of bile flow (μl min^{-1} g^{-1})
Stimulation			
	-1.90 ± 0.37	$+1.23 \pm 0.14$	-0.32 ± 0.04
Artificial			
	-1.29 ± 0.06	$+0.08 \pm 0.02$	-0.06 ± 0.02
	-2.09 ± 0.08	$+0.37 \pm 0.08$	-0.21 ± 0.03

In a series of experiments, the electrode was placed around the bile duct insulated from the hepatic artery and portal vein. Cholic acid was infused in two different concentrations (1μmol l^{-1}, 10μmol l^{-1}). The bile flow was quantitated gravimetrically. In effluent samples glucose and lactate, in bile probes bile acids were determined by standard enzymatic methods.

RESULTS AND DISCUSSION

Electrical stimulation of the perivascular hepatic nerves around the hepatic artery and portal vein resulted in an increase of glucose production and in a decrease of portal flow (Figure 1). The enhancement of glucose release is due to an activation of glycogenolysis via glycogen-phosphorylase[8]. The nerve stimulation led also to a reduction of the bile flow (-34%, Figure 1). The bile acid secretion was diminished simultaneously (-40%, Figure 1). These experiments were done in the absence of bile acids in the portal vein.

In order to exclude an unspecific reaction of the biliary system, i.e. an effect on the smooth muscle of the bile duct, the electrode was placed around the bile duct in a segment where anatomically the bile duct is not joined with hepatic nerves[6]. The portal vein and the hepatic artery were insulated. This electrical stimulation had no effect on the glucose and lactate output. The portal flow, the bile flow as well as the bile acid secretion were unaltered (data not shown). These experiments showed that the nerve effects on the biliary system were dependent on the ramification of the sympathetic and parasympathetic nerves around the hepatic artery and portal vein. A locally induced contraction of the bile duct was excluded as a major mode of action on the biliary system.

The bile flow reduction after nerve stimulation was caused either by a direct or an indirect mechanism. The former could be mediated by a direct mode of action of the neurotransmitter, released at the synapses in close contact to the parenchymal cells regulating the intracellular bile formation and secretion into the bile canaliculi. The direct contact of the nerve endings to the hepatocytes was shown to be the major mechanism for the described metabolic effects as the increase of glucose and lactate output[19]. The indirectly mediated reduction could be caused by the diminution of the hemodynamic parameters since it is known that the activation of the sympathetic nervous system results in a decrease of blood supply[20]. This effect was shown to be

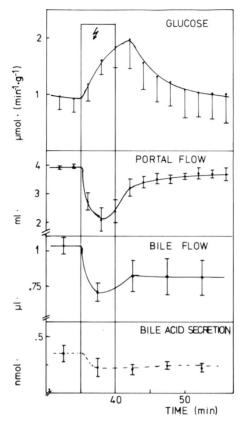

Figure 1 Glucose output, portal flow and bile flow as well as bile acid secretion during nerve stimulation over 5 min (column) after an equilibration period of 30 min. Values are means ± SEM of five experiments

accomplished with a heterogeneous perfusion of the hepatic regions[8,21]. However, the driving force of bile formation is not supposed to be the hydrostatic pressure[22]. The bile salts are the major choleretic agents of the bile secretion[20]. The transport of these substances is active. During the nerve stimulation the heterogenous perfusion could lead to a reduced energetic state of the hepatocytes reducing the energy-consuming export of the bile salts. This situation was mimicked by an artificially lowered portal pressure resulting in a reduction of portal flow. Table 1 shows that the reduction of portal flow in a range of the nerve-mediated decrease of perfusion flow led to a comparable decline of the bile flow. These results suggest that the hemodynamic changes possibly mediate indirectly the nerve effect on bile flow. Further studies should elucidate the dependence of bile formation on hemodynamic changes. As mentioned above, the main driving force for bile flow are the bile acids. We therefore examined whether the nerve-mediated bile flow reduction is modulated by different concentrations of bile acids in

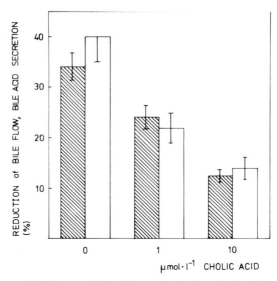

Figure 2 Change of bile flow and bile acid secretion during electrical stimulation of hepatic nerves in the absence and presence of cholic acid ($1\,\mu$mol$\,$l^{-1}, $10\,\mu$mol$\,$l^{-1}). Values are means $\pm$ SEM of 5, 4 and 4 experiments, respectively

the portal vein. As shown in Figure 2, increasing concentrations of cholic acid in the portal vein decreased the relative reduction of bile flow. Under these conditions, bile acids in the portal vein and nerve stimulation had antagonistic effects on bile flow and bile acid secretion.

CONCLUSION

In the perfused rat liver it was shown that the sympathetic hepatic nerves regulate the carbohydrate metabolism and the bile secretion. In contrast with the carbohydrate metabolism the bile flow and the bile acid secretion seemed to be mediated via the nerve-induced alteration of the hemodynamics.

Acknowledgements

We thank Ms Susanne Kneip for her excellent technical assistance.

References

1. Forssmann, W. G. and Ito, S. (1977). Hepatocyte innervation of primates. *J. Cell. Biol.*, **74**, 299–313
2. Metz, W. and Forssmann, W. G. (1980). Innervation of the liver in guinea pig and rat. *Anat. Embryol.*, **160**, 239–52
3. Forssmann, W. G. (1986). Innervation der Leber. *Z. Gastroenterol. Suppl.*, **21**, 190–1
4. Reilley, F. D., McCuskey, A. P. and McCuskey, R. S. (1978). Intrahepatic distribution of

nerves in the rat. *Anat. Rec.*, **191**, 55–671
5. Lautt, W. W. (1980). Hepatic nerves: A review of their functions and effects. *Can. J. Physiol. Pharmacol.*, **56**, 679–82
6. Lautt, W. W. (1983). Afferent and efferent neural roles in liver function. *Progr. Neurobiol.*, **21**, 323–48
7. Jungermann, K., Gardemann, A., Beuers, U., Ballé, C., Sannemann, J., Beckh, K. and Hartmann, H. (1987). Regulation of the liver metabolism by the hepatic nerves. *Adv. Enz. Reg.*, **26**, 63–88
8. Hartmann, H., Beckh, K. and Jungermann, K. (1982). Direct control of glycogen metabolism in the perfused rat liver by the sympathetic innervation. *Eur. J. Biochem.*, **123**, 521–6
9. Beuers, U., Beckh, K. and Jungermann, K. (1986). Control of ketogenesis in the perfused rat liver by the sympathetic innervation. *Eur. J. Biochem.*, **158**, 19–24
10. Ballé, C. and Jungermann, K. (1986). Control of urea production, glutamine release and ammonia uptake in the perfused rat liver by the sympathetic innervation. *Eur. J. Biochem.*, **158**, 13–18
11. Beckh, K., Hartmann, H., Jungermann, K. and Scholz, R. (1984). Regulation of oxygen consumption in perfused rat liver: decrease by α-sympathetic nerve stimulation and increase by the α-agonist phenylephrine. *Pflügers Arch. Eur. J. Physiol.*, **401**, 104–6
12. Ji, S., Beckh, K. and Jungermann, K. (1984). Regulation of oxygen consumption and microcirculation by α-sympathetic nerves in isolated perfused rat liver. *FEBS Lett.*, **167**, 117–22
13. Beckh, K., Balks, H. J. and Jungermann, K. (1982) Activation of glycogenolysis and norepinephrine overflow in the perfused rat liver during repetitive perivascular nerve stimulation. *FEBS Lett.*, **149**, 261–5
14. Okolicsanyi, L., Lirussi, F., Trazzabosco, M., Jemmolo, R. M., Orlando, R., Nassuato, G., Muraca, M. and Crepaldi, G. (1986). The effect of drugs on bile flow and composition. *Drugs*, **13**, 430–48
15. Yamatani, K., Sato, N., Takahashi, K., Hara, M. and Sasaki, H. (1985). Effect of gastrointestinal hormones on choleresis from the isolated perfused rat liver. *Regul. Pept.*, **10**, 237–42
16. Calhoun, P. and Hanks, J. B. (1984). Hormonal contributions to biliary secretion. *Surg. Gastroenterol.*, **3**, 8–16
17. Thomsen, O. O. and Larsen, J. A. (1982). Interaction of insulin, glucagon, and DBcAMP on bile acid-independent bile production in the rat. *Scand. J. Gastroenterol.*, **17**, 687–93
18. Brauer, R. W., Leong, G. F. and Holloway, R. J. (1954). Mechanics of bile secretion: effect of perfusion pressure and temperature on bile flow and secretion pressure. *Am. J. Physiol.*, **177**, 103–12
19. Beckh, K., Beuers, U., Engelhardt, R. and Jungermann, K. (1987). Mechanism of action of sympathetic hepatic nerves on carbohydrate metabolism in perfused rat liver. *Biol. Chem. Hoppe-Seyler*, **368**, 379–86
20. Richardson, P. D. I. and Withrington, P. G. (1982). Physiological regulation of the hepatic circulation. *Annu. Rev. Physiol.*, **44**, 57–69
21. Reilly, F. D., McCuskey, R. S. and Cilento, E. V. (1981). Hepatic microvascular regulation mechanisms: I. Adrenergic mechanisms. *Microvasc. Res.*, **21**, 487–501
22. Strange, R. C. (1984). Hepatic bile flow. *Physiol. Rev.*, **64**, 1055–102

15
Importance of cholinergic and adrenergic tone in the regulation of human interdigestive pancreatic secretion

P. LAYER and E. P. DIMAGNO

INTRODUCTION

Interdigestive exocrine pancreatic secretion cycles in concert with the phases of periodic proximal gastrointestinal motility. During phase I motor quiescence coincides with low pancreatic enzyme outputs, motility activity during phase II is variable and during phase III contractions occur at a maximum rate for a brief period. Pancreatic enzyme outputs are moderate during phase II and peak during early phase III[1,2]. The regulation of interdigestive motor and secretory activity is undetermined, but likely includes neural and humoral factors. Since motility and secretion of gastric juice, pancreatic juice and bile are parallel[3], a common mechanism may regulate interdigestive motility and secretion.

Our aim was to determine if, in normal human subjects, during interdigestive phase II motility pancreatic secretion parallels spontaneously irregular motor activity and if plasma concentrations of motilin, a hormone that may regulate interdigestive motility and pancreatic secretion, or human pancreatic polypeptide (hPP) are associated with motility or pancreatic secretion. In a second step, we wanted to study the effects of exogenous changes in cholinergic and adrenergic tone on motor and pancreatic secretory activities and plasma concentrations of motilin and hPP.

COUPLING OF SPONTANEOUS MOTILITY AND PANCREATIC SECRETION DURING PHASE II

Fifteen fasting volunteers were intubated with a gastroduodenal multilumen catheter assembly that allowed gastric and duodenal marker perfusion, sampling (for determination of trypsin output) at 10 min intervals and motility recordings.

After identification of interdigestive phase II motility, motor activity in the antrum was graded according to frequency of contractions as low, intermediate, or high, as described earlier[4]. Plasma samples were analysed for concentrations of motilin and hPP.

Antral motility during phase II showed the expected spontaneous irregular variations in pressure activity. Changes in motility were closely associated with parallel changes in pancreatic enzyme output throughout phase II. Mean trypsin output was 58 ± 14 U/min during low, 144 ± 23 U/min during intermediate and 362 ± 52 U/min during high grade II (Figure 1). Moreover, phases of interdigestive motility during the overall cycle were also tightly coupled with pancreatic secretion with minimal rates during phase I and peak rates during phase III, as expected.

Plasma motilin varied throughout phase II. There was no correlation between motilin and the grades of phase II motility (Figure 2) or pancreatic secretion ($p > 0.1$).

Plasma hPP fluctuated irregularly during phase II. In contrast to motilin, however, there was a significant correlation among hPP, motility and trypsin output ($p < 0.001$; Figure 3).

COUPLING OF MOTILITY AND PANCREATIC SECRETION DURING EXOGENOUS CHANGES IN CHOLINERGIC TONE

In a second study, 17 fasting subjects underwent gastroduodenal intubation as described above. Each subject was randomized to receive two hours intravenous infusion of saline (control studies), a cholinergic agonist (bethanechol at 5 or $40 \mu g/kg/h$) or a cholinergic antagonist (atropine at 4 or $16 \mu g/kg/h$) alone or in combination according to a 3×3 factorial design.

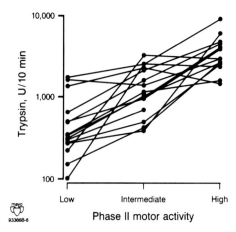

Figure 1 Duodenal trypsin output during low-, intermediate-, and high-grade phase II motor activity. Mean values within each subject ($n = 15$) for each motility grade. Level of significance was $p < 0.001$. (Reprinted with permission from reference 4)

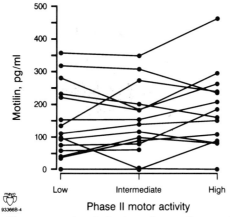

Figure 2 Plasma motilin concentration during low-, intermediate-, and high-grade phase II motor activity. Mean values within each subject ($n = 15$) for each motility grade. Values were not significant. (Reprinted with permission from reference 4)

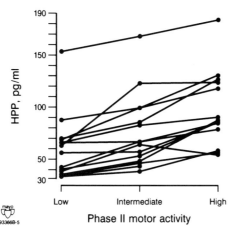

Figure 3 Plasma human pancreatic polypeptide (HPP) concentrations during low-, intermediate-, and high-grade phase II motor activity. Mean values within each subject ($n = 15$) for each motility grade. Level of significance was $p < 0.001$. (Reprinted with permission from reference 4)

Motility and pancreatic enzyme outputs were analysed for the test period and coupled within each subject with a preceding control period with intravenous NaCl for a complete interdigestive motility cycle.

Coupled with saline, bethanechol at the higher dose doubled trypsin output ($p < 0.05$), increased motor activity, but did not abolish the cyclical interdigestive pattern of motility. Atropine caused a dose-dependent decrease in pancreatic secretion ($p < 0.05$) and abolished motor activity. Neither bethanechol nor atropine altered plasma motilin concentrations. By contrast, hPP was significantly increased during intravenous bethanechol ($p < 0.005$), and decreased during intravenous atropine ($p < 0.05$).

INTERDIGESTIVE MOTILITY AND PANCREATIC SECRETION DURING EXOGENOUS CHANGES IN ADRENERGIC TONE

In a third study of 16 subjects we investigated the effect of exogenously modulating α and β adrenergic tone on interdigestive pancreatic secretion. Each subject underwent gastrointestinal intubation as described above and were randomized to receive intravenous infusions of phentolamine (0.5 mg/min), propranolol (80 µg/min), epinephrine (50 kg/min), or saline as control alone or in combinations according to a 2^3 factorial design. Phentolamine doubled (72 vs. 36 U/min; $p < 0.05$), whereas propranolol had no effect on interdigestive secretion. However, there was a significant interaction between the effects of propranolol and epinephrine and when only test periods were compared, epinephrine decreased trypsin secretion ($p < 0.05$).

CONCLUSION

Human interdigestive gastrointestinal motility and pancreatic secretion are tightly coupled during the overall interdigestive cycle, within irregular phase II motor activity and during exogenous changes of cholinergic or adrenergic tone. During cholinergic modulation, motor and secretory changes are always associated with parallel changes in plasma hPP, but not motilin. These findings suggest a common control mechanism for interdigestive proximal gastrointestinal function and the participation of cholinergic pathways in its regulation.

The preliminary results from the adrenergic study suggest that a balance between α- and β-adrenergic input is necessary for the regulation of normal interdigestive trypsin secretion. α input is definitely inhibitory as α blockade in the presence of normal (no epinephrine) or increased α- + β-input (epinephrine infusion) increases pancreatic secretion. On the other hand, β input does not appear to have a significant effect on interdigestive secretion. These data are in agreement with our previous data in patients with traumatic cervical cord lesions above the level of the sympathetic outflow to the gastrointestinal tract, in whom we found loss of normal cyclical interdigestive motility[5] and exocrine pancreatic secretion[6]. Together these data suggest that resting adrenergic α-input to the pancreas is required for normal interdigestive pancreatic secretion.

References

1. DiMagno, E. P., Hendricks, J. C., Go, V. L. W. and Dozois, R. R. (1979). Relationships among canine fasting pancreatic and biliary secretions, pancreatic duct pressure and duodenal phase III motor activity—Boldyreff revisited. *Dig. Dis. Sci.*, **24**, 689–93
2. Keane, F. B., DiMagno, E. P., Dozois,R. R. and Go, V. L. W. (1980). Relationships among canine interdigestive exocrine pancreatic and biliary flow, duodenal motor activity, plasma pancreatic polypeptide, and motilin. *Gastroenterology*, **78**, 310–16
3. Vantrappen, G. R., Peeters, T. L., Janssens, J. (1979). The secretory component of the interdigestive migrating motor complex in man. *Scand. J. Gastroenterol.*, **14**, 633–67

4. Layer, P., Chan, A. T. H., Go, V. L. W. and DiMagno, E. P. (1988). Human pancreatic secretion during phase II antral motility of the interdigestive cycle. *Am. J. Physiol.*, **154,** G249–53
5. Fealey, R. D., Szurszewski, J. H., Merritt, J. L. and DiMagno, E. P. (1984). Effect of traumatic spinal cord transection on human upper gastrointestinal motility and gastric emptying. *Gastroenterology*, **87,** 69–75
6. Fealey, R. D., Szurszewski, J. H., Marritt, J. L. and DiMagno, E. P. (1982). Supraspinal sympathetic nervous control of human interdigestive and postprandial exocrine pancreatic secretion: The effect of traumatic spinal cord transection. *Pamphlet of Abstracts from the Joint Meeting of the American Pancreatic Association and the National Pancreatic Cancer Project, NCI*, p. 20.

16
Action of cutting the extrinsic nerves of the pancreas on the pancreatic enzyme response to intestinal stimulants: a short review

M. V. SINGER, W. NIEBEL and H. GOEBELL

The relative contributions of the vagus and splanchnic nerves on the one hand and gastrointestinal hormones (e.g. cholecystokinin, CCK) on the other as mediators of the pancreatic enzyme response to intestinal stimulants are still incompletely determined. Although there is plenty of evidence that CCK or CCK-like hormones, when given intravenously, do stimulate pancreatic enzyme secretion in humans and animals, the *physiological role* of *CCK* as a classical hormonal regulator is still not definitely established. This is mainly due to the lack of sensitive and specific radioimmunoassays for this peptide. In addition, with a few exceptions[1] the blood samples were not sufficiently treated to prevent degradation of CCK. Thus, large molecular forms of CCK were only detected recently[1,2]. On the basis of data from CCK-assays published during the last years, it is apparent that a meal increases plasma CCK concentration five- to tenfold above basal in humans and animals[3-5]. The range of the basal values, however, is still very large and was found to be $0.2 \, pmol/l$[5] or even $8 \, pmol/l$[26]. As long as it has not been shown that exogenous CCK infused in doses that produce post-prandial plasma concentrations of CCK does stimulate the pancreatic enzyme response, the physiological role of CCK will be unsettled.

During the last ten years, considerable experimental evidence has been accumulated demonstrating the existence of *enteropancreatic, cholinergic, vago-vagal reflexes* as quantitatively important mediators of the pancreatic enzyme response to intestinal stimuli such as amino acids, fatty acids and HCl[6-11]. Enteropancreatic reflexes are also critical for obtaining rapid pancreatic response as chyme begins flowing into the duodenum.[12] This evidence has mainly come from three different kinds of studies.

1. Studies in which the effect of truncal vagotomy and the anticholinergic

205

drug, atropine, on the pancreatic secretory response to exogenous and endogenous stimulants in dogs with an autotransplanted uncinate processus of the pancreas has been compared with the responses in dogs with an intact innervated pancreas[8-11].

2. Studies in which the latency of the pancreatic secretory response to intestinal stimulants has been compared with that to intraportal CCK or secretin[7,12].

3. Studies in which the pancreatic secretory response to intestinal and intravenous (exogenous) stimulants has been recorded before and after cutting the extrinsic nerves of the pancreas[6,9,13-16].

The transplanted pancreas which is extrinsically denervated, was used to monitor plasma hormone levels because it can respond only to humoral (= hormonal) stimulants. The transplanted pancreas was as sensitive as the intact pancreas to exogenous stimulation by caerulein, a CCK analogue. Neither truncal vagotomy[11] nor atropine[8] altered protein secretion from either the intact or transplanted pancreas in response to exogenous caerulein. Truncal vagotomy and atropine, however, depressed by about 50% the protein response to intestinal tryptophan and oleate in the intact pancreas but had no effect on the response of the transplanted pancreas. The secretory response of the transplanted pancreas to intestinal perfusion with tryptophan or oleate was only 40–50% of the enzyme response of the innervated intact pancreas when expressed as a percentage of capacity to respond to exogenous hormonal stimulation (Figure 1). These findings are consistent with the idea that approximately 50% of the enzyme response of the innervated, intact pancreas to intestinal amino acids and fatty acids is mediated by neural pathways, which are vagovagal and cholinergic since they are blocked by truncal vagotomy and atropine. These studies also suggest that vagotomy

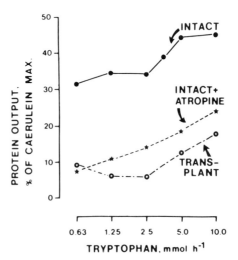

Figure 1 Protein output, percentage of caerulein maximum, from pancreatic transplant and intact innervated pancreas in response to intestinal perfusion with graded amounts of tryptophan with and without atropine (data were calculated from Ref. 8)

and atropine do not interfere with the release of hormones such as CCK in response to intestinal stimulants, as has been postulated for many years.

An indirect proof for the involvement of an enteropancreatic reflex in the pancreatic enzyme response to intestinal stimulants came from studies on the *latency of pancreatic enzyme response* to intestinal stimulants[7]. In conscious dogs, the latencies of pancreatic amylase response to intraduodenal bolus injection of either tryptophan (0.30 min) or oleate (0.33 min) were significantly shorter than that following an intraportal bolus of CCK (0.53 min) (Figure 2). Atropine and truncal vagotomy increased the latency to tryptophan and oleate tenfold but did not affect the latency to intraportal CCK. These observations stronly suggest that the early phase of pancreatic enzyme response to intestinal amino acids and fatty acids is unlikely to be humoral (blood-borne) and therefore is probably nervous. The actions of vagotomy and atropine support the concept that an enteropancreatic reflex is involved and that it is cholinergic and vago-vagal[7,9,14].

Large amounts of intraduodenal HCl have also been shown to stimulate pancreatic enzyme secretion and release of CCK[17-21]. Truncal vagotomy or atropine diminished the pancreatic enzyme response to low, but not high, loads of HCl[10,21]. These findings suggest that cholinergic nerves are also involved in the pancreatic enzyme response to low loads of HCl.

In humans, enteropancreatic vagal reflexes probably are also important mediators of the pancreatic response to intestinal stimulants[22,23].

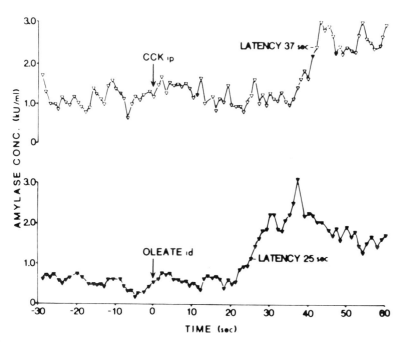

Figure 2 Latency of pancreatic amylase response, in seconds, to intraduodenal injection of 1 mmol of sodium oleate or intraportal injection of 0.66 Ukg^{-1} of CCK in representative experiments in the same dog. Each point represents a drop of pancreatic juice (from ref. 7)

Although these studies in dogs and humans indicated that enteropancreatic, cholinergic, vagovagal reflexes existed, it was not clear until recently whether these enteropancreatic reflexes are only vagovagal. Possible extravagal pathways are indicated in Table 1. As can be seen, the splanchnic nerves especially may contain afferent and efferent arcs of the enteropancreatic reflexes. However the action of splanchnectomy on the response to intestinal amino acids has been studied only recently. During the last five years, our research group has studied the action of stepwise extrinsic pancreatic denervation of the pancreatic secretory response to intestinal (endogenous) and intravenous (exogenous) stimulants in dogs. In dogs equipped with chronic gastric and pancreatic fistulas, according to Thomas[24], pancreatic secretory studies were performed before and after truncal vagotomy (thus cutting the main secretory nerves of the pancreas) and after cutting all the extrinsic nerves of the pancreas, i.e. truncal vagotomy plus coeliac and superior mesenteric ganglionectomy. In another set of dogs only coeliac and superior mesenteric ganglionectomy was performed, thus removing all sympathetic innervation of the pancreas. At each stage of innervation, the pancreatic secretory studies were repeated in the presence of atropine, an anticholinergic drug. The basic assumption of these studies was that atropine is not only capable of counteracting the muscarinic activity produced by the cholinergic fibres of the vagus and the splanchnic nerves, but can suppress the remaining intrinsic post-ganglionic nerves of the pancreas which still release sufficient acetylcholine after removal of the extrinsic pancreatic nerves. Thus we hoped to be capable of discerning between the muscarinic activity produced by the cholinergic fibres of the vagus and the splanchnic nerves on the one hand and the intrapancreatic nerves on the other. Plasma levels of different hormones such as CCK were also monitored in these studies.

The main results of the effects of stepwise extrinsic pancreatic denervation on the pancreatic enzyme response to endogenous and exogenous stimulants in dogs are given in Table 2.

The pancreatic protein response to intravenous caerulein, a CCK-analogue, was not altered by truncal vagotomy alone, coeliac and superior mesenteric ganglionectomy alone or a combination of both surgical procedures. Atropine did not significantly alter the protein response to caerulein at any stage of innervation[9,14].

Coeliac and superior mesenteric ganglionectomy did not alter the pan-

Table 1 Possible extravagal pathways for enteropancreatic reflexes

Afferent	Site of afferent–efferent connection	Efferent
Splanchnic	Spinal cord	Preganglionic splanchnic
Splanchnic	Prevertebral ganglia	Post-ganglionic splanchnics
Cell bodies in submucous plexus of duodenum or jejunum	Prevertebral ganglia	Post-ganglionic splanchnics
Cell bodies in submucous plexus of duodenum	Ganglia in pancreas	Post-ganglionic pancreatic nerves

Table 2 Pancreatic protein response to intravenous caerulein and intraduodenal tryptophan with and without intravenous atropine in conscious dogs with intact pancreatic nerves, after truncal vagotomy alone or coeliac and superior mesenteric ganglionectomy alone or a combination of both surgical procedures (for detailed information see refs. 9, 15)

	Caerulein (intravenous)	Tryptophan (intraduodenal)
Intact nerves		
+ atropine	No effect	Depressed (low loads)
Truncal vagotomy		
− atropine	No effect	Depressed (low loads)
+ atropine	No effect	No further depression
Truncal vagotomy plus coeliac and superior mesenteric ganglionectomy		
− atropine	No effect	Depressed (low loads)
+ atropine	No effect	No further depression
Coeliac and superior mesenteric ganglionectomy		
− atropine	No effect	No effect
+ atropine	No effect	Depressed (low loads)

ENZYMES

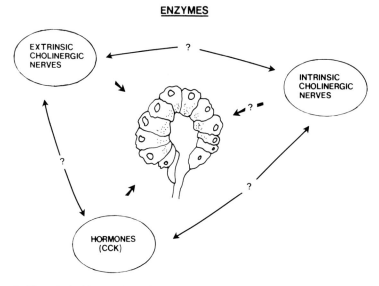

Figure 3 Hypothetical interactions of extrinsic and intrinsic cholinergic nerves and hormones, such as CCK, on pancreatic enzyme secretion

creatic protein response to intestinal tryptophan. Truncal vagotomy significantly reduced the protein response to low, but not high loads of tryptophan. Additional ganglionectomy after vagotomy did not cause a further reduction of the already reduced pancreatic protein response to low loads of tryptophan. Before, but not after, truncal vagotomy atropine significantly reduced the pancreatic protein response to low loads of tryptophan[9,15].

Intraduodenal perfusion with tryptophan caused a dose-dependent increase in plasma CCK concentrations. Neither any of the different surgical procedures nor atropine given in intact animals or after stepwise cutting the extrinsic nerves of the pancreas, had any significant effect on the plasma CCK levels basally and in response to intestinal tryptophan[9].

CONCLUSIONS AND HYPOTHESES

These recent studies allow the following conclusions. Neither the extrinsic (vagal and splanchnic) nor the intrinsic (cholinergic) pancreatic nerves significantly alter the pancreatic protein response to exogenous caerulein (or CCK). The sympathetic nerves of the pancreas most likely do not mediate the pancreatic secretory response to intestinal aminao acids, since coeliac and superior mesenteric ganglionectomy alone did not alter the pancreatic protein response to intraduodenal tryptophan. In conjunction with the studies on the transplanted pancreas and the latency of enzyme response to intestinal amino acids, intraduodenal tryptophan most likely stimulates pancreatic enzyme response via activation of long, vagovagal, enteropancreatic, cholinergic reflexes with both, afferent and efferent fibres running within the vagus nerves; extravagal pancreatic nerves not being involved. The release of CCK by intestinal tryptophan is not under cholinergic and splanchnic control.

Altogether, these recent findings suggest that under physiological conditions it is probably the interplay of neural and hormonal mechanisms which regulates the pancreatic enzyme response to intestinal stimulants such as amino acids, fatty acids and HCl. Neurohormonal interaction occurs probably in each instance whether low or high loads of intestinal stimulants are given[25]. Enteropancreatic, cholinergic, vagovagal reflexes are the main mediators of the pancreatic enzyme response to low loads of amino acids, fatty acids and HCl. Both, afferent and efferent limbs of these reflexes run in the vagus nerve. CCK is probably the main mediator of the pancreatic enzyme response to high loads of amino acids, fatty acids and HCl. The neurohormonal interaction at each dose level might explain why only small amounts of CCK are needed to stimulate the pancreatic enzyme response during the digestion of a meal.

Whether, as far as pancreatic enzyme secretion is concerned, an additive or potentiating interaction between the extrinsic cholinergic vagal nerves and the intrinsic cholinergic nerves of the pancreas does exist has not been experimentally substantiated. Whether the intrinsic cholinergic nerves potentiate the enzyme response to hormones such as CCK is completely unknown. A potentiating interaction between extrinsic cholinergic vagal nerves and CCK is likely, but has not been studied systematically (Figure 3).

Thus, a main goal of pancreatic research for the next years will be to determine the relative contribution of the extrinsic and intrinsic pancreatic nerves and of hormones as mediators of the pancreatic secretory response to a meal.

Acknowledgement

All the authors' scientific work cited has been supported by a grant (Si 228) from the German Society for Research (Deutsche Forschungsgemeinschaft).

References

1. Eysselein, V. E., Eberlein, G. A., Hesse, W. H., Singer, M. V., Goebell, H. and Reeve, Jr., J. R. (1987). Cholecystokinin-58 is the major circulating form of cholecystokinin in canine blood. *J. Biol. Chem.*, **262**, 214–17
2. Eysselein, V. E., Reeve, Jr., J. R. and Eberlein, G. (1986). Cholecystokinin — gene structure and molecular forms in tissue and blood. *Z. Gastroenterol.*, **24**, 645–59
3. Jansen, J. B. M. J. and Lamers, C. B. H. W. (1983). Radioimmunoassay of cholecystokinin in human tissue and plasma. *Clin. Chim. Acta*, **131**, 305–16
4. Schafmayer, A., Becker, H. D., Werner, M., Fölsch, U. R. and Creutzfeldt, W. (1985). Plasma cholecystokinin levels in patients with chronic pancreatitis. *Digestion*, **32**, 136–9
5. Walsh, J. H., Lamers, C. B. and Valenzuela, J. E. (1982). Cholecystokinin — octapeptidelike immune reactivity in human plasma. *Gastroenterology*, **82**, 438–44
6. Singer, M. V., Niebel, W., Hoffmeister, D. and Goebell, H. (1985). Effect of atropine on pancreatic bicarbonate response to HCl after cutting the extrinsic nerves of the pancreas. *Gastroenterology*, **88**, 1588
7. Singer, M. V., Solomon, T. E., Wood, J. and Grossman, M. I. (1980). Latency of pancreatic enzyme response to intraduodenal stimulants. *Am. J. Physiol.*, **238**, G23–9
8. Singer, M. V., Solomon, T. E. and Grossman, M. I. (1980). Effect of atropine on secretion from intact and transplanted pancreas in the dog. *Am. J. Physiol.*, **238**, G18–22
9. Singer, M. V., Niebel, W., Jansen, J. B. M. J., Hoffmeister, D., Gotthold, S., Goebell, H. and Lamers, C. B. H. W. (1988). Pancreatic secretory response to intravenous caerulein and intraduodenal tryptophan before and after stepwise removal of the extrinsic nerves of the pancreas in dogs. *Am. J. Physiol.* (In press)
10. Solomon, T. E. and Grossman, M. I. (1977). Cholecystokinin and secretin release are not affected by vagotomy or atropine (Abstract). *Gastroenterology*, **72**, 1134
11. Solomon, T. E. and Grossman, M. I. (1979). Effect of atropine and vagotomy on response of transplanted pancreas. *Am. J. Physiol.*, **236**, E186–90
12. Singer, M. V. (1983). Latency of pancreatic fluid secretory response to intestinal stimulants in the dog. *J. Physiol. (Lond.)*, **339**, 75–85
13. Niebel, W., Beglinger, C. and Singer, M. V. (1988). Pancreatic bicarbonate response to HCl before and after cutting the extrinsic nerves of the pancreas in dogs. *Am. J. Physiol.*, **254**, 436–43
14. Singer, M. V., Niebel, W., Gotthold, S., Hoffmeister, D. and Goebell, H. (1987). Extrinsic nerves as mediators of the pancreatic secretory response to intravenous caerulein and intraduodenal tryptophan (Abstract). *Gastroenterology*, **92**, 1642
15. Singer, M. V., Niebel, W., Kniesburges, S., Hoffmeister, D. and Goebell, H. (1986). Action of atropine on the pancreatic secretory response to secretin before and after cutting the extrinsic nerves of the pancreas in dogs. *Gastroenterology*, **90**, 355–61
16. Singer, M. V., Niebel, W., Uhde, K. H., Hoffmeister, H. and Goebell, H. (1985). Dose response effects of atropine on pancreatic response to secretin before and after truncal vagotomy. *Am. J. Physiol.*, **248**, G532–8
17. Barbezat, G. O. and Grossman, M. I. (1975). Release of cholecystokinin by acid. *Proc. Soc. Exp. Biol. Med.*, **148**, 463–7
18. Chen, Y. F., Chey, W. Y., Chang, T. M., Lee, K. S. (1985). Duodenal acidification releases cholecystokin. *Am. J. Physiol.*, **249**, 629–33
19. Fried, G. M., Ogden, W. D., Greeley, G. and Thompson, J. C. (1983). Correlation of release and actions of cholecystokinin in dogs before and after vagotomy. *Surgery*, **93**, 786–91
20. Meyer, J. H., Way, L. W. and Grossman, M. I. (1970). Pancreatic bicarbonate response to various acids in duodenum of the dog. *Am. J. Physiol.*, **219**, 964–70
21. Singer, M. V., Solomon, T. E., Rammert, H., Caspary, F., Niebel, W., Goebell, H. and

Grossman, M. I. (1981). Effect of atropine on pancreatic response to HCl and secretin. *Am. J. Physiol.*, **240**, G376–80

22. Dooley, C. P. and Valenzuela, J. E. (1984). Duodenal volume and osmoreceptors in the stimulation of human pancreatic secretion. *Gastroenterology*, **86**, 23–7
23. Valenzuela, J. E., Lamers, C. B., Modlin, I. M. and Walsh, J. H. (1983). Cholinergic component in the human pancreatic secretory response to intraintestinal oleate. *Gut*, **24**, 807–11
24. Thomas, J. E. (1941). An improved cannula for gastric and intestinal fistulas. *Proc. Soc. Exp. Biol.*, **46**, 260–1
25. Beglinger, Ch., Grossmann, M. I. and Solomon, T. E. (1984). Interaction between stimulants of exocrine pancreatic secretion in dogs. *Am. J. Physiol.*, **246**, G173–9
26. Byrnes, D. J., Henderson, L., Borody, T., Rehfeld, F. F. (1981). Radioimmunoassay of cholecystokinin in human plasma *Clin. Chim. Acta*, **111**, 81–9

17
Cholinergic and hormonal regulation of post-prandial gallbladder contraction in humans

C. B. H. W. LAMERS and J. B. M. J. JANSEN

Several neural and hormonal mechanisms exert excitatory or inhibitory actions on the gallbladder *in vivo* or *in vitro*[1]. The excitatory stimuli comprise acetylcholine, α-adrenergic agents, cholecystokinin, gastrin, histamine (H_1), motilin, neurotensin, prostaglandins, substance K and substance P; whereas adenosine, ATP, β-adrenergic agents, histamine (H_2), pancreatic polypeptide, secretin, VIP and somatostatin exert inhibitory effects on the gallbladder. However, it is questionable whether, apart from acetylcholine and cholecystokinin, these substances play a major role in the post-prandial gallbladder contraction in humans.

Although it has been known for decades that cholecystokinin and the cholinergic system are involved in post-prandial gallbladder contraction and the presence of receptors for CCK and acetylcholine on the gallbladder muscle has been well established *in vitro*[1], the exact role of both stimulants is only delineated in more recent years. The progress in our understanding of the regulation of gallbladder contraction is mainly due to the development of sensitive and specific radioimmunoassays for CCK[2], real-time ultra-sonographic determination of gallbladder volumes[3] and the availability of synthetic, specific antagonists of the binding of CCK to its receptors[4,5]. At present only few specific radioimmunoassays sufficiently sensitive to measure the low CCK concentrations in human plasma are available[2,6-9]. Real-time ultrasonography is now widely used to quantitate gallbladder dynamics[3,10], whereas some investigators employ cholescintigraphy to determine gallbladder emptying[11,12]. Two types of CCK-receptor antagonists have been used in *in vivo* studies of the gall-bladder: non-peptide CCK-receptor antagonists, of which L-364 718 is most widely used[4]; and glutaramic acid derivatives of which CR-1409 and CR-1505 are most frequently employed[5]. Furthermore, the significance of the cholinergic system for gallbladder stimulation can be studied by the application of drugs activating the cholinergic receptors on the gallbladder muscle, such as bethanechol[11], and specific inhibitors of the cholinergic system, such as atropine[11]. Finally, disorders with abnormalities of CCK secretion or cholinergic activation of the gallbladder have contributed to our understanding of gallbladder regulation.

PHYSIOLOGICAL ROLE OF CHOLECYSTOKININ AND THE CHOLINERGIC SYSTEM IN POST-PRANDIAL GALLBLADDER CONTRACTION

The availability of specific and sensitive radioimmunoassays for CCK and the development of specific CCK-receptor antagonists have enabled investigators to determine whether CCK is involved in the physiological regulation of gallbladder contraction. Measurements of increases in plasma CCK concentrations after feeding followed by studies of infusion of exogenous CCK in doses leading to plasma CCK increments in the physiological, i.e. post-prandial, range have unequivocally demonstrated that physiological CCK increments do stimulate gallbladder contraction[13]. Hopman et al.[14] found that ingestion of a mixed meal consisting of a hamburger, an omelette, two slices of bread and 150 ml of milk increased plasma CCK from a basal level of 2.3 ± 0.1 pM to a peak value of 5.9 ± 0.4 pM and reduced gallbladder volume by about 70%. This rise in plasma CCK was clearly above the threshold CCK-increment of 1.3 pM for gallbladder contraction when CCK was administered exogenously[15]. Although the effect of CCK-receptor antagonists on post-prandial gallbladder contraction has not been reported in humans, a study in dogs showed that the CCK-receptor antagonist L-364 718 inhibited post-prandial gallbladder contraction by about 70%[16]. Furthermore, an unpublished study employing the CCK-receptor antagonist CR-1505 (Beglinger et al.) showed that this compound halved bile secretion into the duodenum in response to an intraduodenal nutrient load in healthy human subjects.

The physiological role of the cholinergic system for gallbladder contraction can be determined by studying the effect of sham feeding on the gallbladder. Studies on the effect of sham feeding by the chew and spit technique on the gallbladder have shown that activation of the cholinergic system does induce gallbladder emptying, as assessed by cholescintigraphy[17], and gallbladder contraction, as quantitated by real-time ultrasonography[9,14]. It can therefore be concluded that both CCK and the cholinergic system are physiological stimulants of gallbladder contraction in humans.

CONTRIBUTION OF CCK AND THE CHOLINERGIC SYSTEM TO THE VARIOUS PHASES OF GALLBLADDER CONTRACTION

Post-prandial stimulation of gallbladder contraction comprises a cephalic, a gastric and an intestinal phase.

Cephalic phase

The cephalic phase of gallbladder contraction can be studied by sham feeding or insulin hypoglycaemia. Insulin hypoglycaemia has been shown to be a more potent, although less physiological, stimulant of gallbladder contraction than sham feeding by the chew and spit technique[18]. These stimuli induce gallbladder contraction without affecting plasma CCK levels[9,14]. The finding that the gallbladder response to sham feeding is abolished by treatment with atropine indicates that cephalic stimulation of gallbladder contraction is mediated by the cholinergic system[9,14]. The degree of gallbladder contraction to sham feeding varies considerably in the various studies. Using cholescintigraphy, Fisher et al.[17] found that gallbladder emptying during sham feeding was similar to post-prandial emptying during the first hour after meal ingestion. Hopmen et al.[14] using real-time ultrasonography, reported that sham feeding induced a gallbladder contraction of 30%, which amounted to about half of that seen after ingestion of the same meal. In contrast, Yamamura et al.[9] also employing real-time ultrasonography, found a gallbladder contraction of only 12% after sham feeding compared to 44% after ingestion of a fat meal.

Gastric phase

The gastric phase of gallbladder contraction can be studied by studying the effect of gastric distension on gallbladder volumes. Yamamuri et al.[9] found that ingestion of 400 ml of water within a 1–2 min period induced a gallbladder contraction of maximally 25% lasting for less than 1 h, compared to a contraction of maximally 44% lasting for more than 3 h after ingestion of a fatty meal. The gallbladder contraction in response to the water load was not accompanied by increases in plasma CCK and was fully abolished by atropine treatment, indicating that the gastric phase of gallbladder contraction is mediated by the cholinergic system. This finding is in agreement with the existence of a cholinergic, vagovagal, pylorocholecystic reflex as demonstrated in the dog[19]. It is, however, questionable whether a large oral water load is a selective stimulant of the gastric phase of gallbladder contraction.

Intestinal phase

Several studies have shown that intraduodenal instillation of nutrients stimulate secretion of CCK and gallbladder contraction[8,20–22], suggesting that CCK is involved in the intestinal phase of gallbladder emptying. However, it has also been shown that blockade of the cholinergic receptors with atropine affects gallbladder contraction induced by feeding and administration of exogenous CCK[11,22–24]. In a well-designed study, Hopman et al.[22] have delineated the relative contributions of CCK and the cholinergic system to the intestinal phase of gallbladder contraction. These workers compared the effect of atropine on gallbladder contraction induced by intraduodenal fat and infusion of exogenous CCK, giving rise to plasma CCK concentrations similar to those seen after the fat meal. Atropine was found to inhibit fat-induced gallbladder contraction by about 45%. This inhibition was not due to reduction of fat-induced CCK release, but resulted from a diminished sensitivity of the gallbladder to CCK. In fact, a similar reduction in the sensitivity of the gallbladder to endogenous and exogenous CCK was found.

The conclusion of the above-mentioned study, that both CCK and the cholinergic system are involved in the intestinal phase of stimulation of gallbladder contraction, was supported by an as-yet unpublished investigation by Beglinger *et al.* showing that the CCK-receptor antagonist CR-1505 inhibits the gallbladder response to an intraduodenal nutrient load in healthy human subjects by about 50%. At present it is unknown whether a cholinergic, vagovagal, enterocholecystic reflex mechanism, as found in the dog, is also present in humans.

GALLBLADDER CONTRACTION IN DISORDERS WITH IMPAIRED CCK SECRETION OR CHOLINERGIC ACTIVATION

Impaired CCK secretion

It has been demonstrated that patients with mucosal atrophy of the upper small intestine due to coeliac disease have a greatly impaired CCK secretion in response to feeding, whereas coeliac patients on a gluten-free diet with normal mucosal architecture show normal CCK secretion[10,25]. It has further been found that in coeliac patients with small intestinal mucosal atrophy the impaired CCK response to feeding is accompanied by a greatly reduced gallbladder contraction, pointing to an important role of CCK in post-prandial gallbladder contraction[10,25].

Impaired cholinergic activation

Numerous studies on the effect of truncal vagotomy on gallbladder contraction have been published[1]. Most studies on vagotomized patients showed that fasting gallbladder volume was increased, while gallbladder emptying after feeding or exogenous CCK was either unchanged or reduced. A more recent study found that in vagotomized patients gallbladder emptying as assessed by cholescintigraphy was reduced, whereas the gallbladder response to exogenous CCK was increased[11]. However, all these studies have to be interpreted with great caution, since vagotomy has been shown to influence gastric emptying[11] and post-prandial CCK secretion[26]. Studies on the regulation of gallbladder contraction in autonomic neuropathy are surprisingly scarce. In a preliminary study we found that post-prandial gallbladder contraction in patients with autonomic neuropathy due to diabetes mellitus was only marginally affected[27].

CONCLUSION

Both CCK and the cholinergic system are involved in the post-prandial stimulation of gallbladder contraction. The cholinergic system is of utmost importance in the cephalic and gastric phases of post-prandial gallbladder contraction, whereas both CCK and the cholinergic system interact in the intestinal phase of stimulation of gallbladder contraction.

References

1. Ryan, J. P. (1987). Motility of the gallbladder and the biliary tree. In Johnson, L. R. (ed). *Physiology of the Gastrointestinal Tract*, 2nd Edn., pp. 695–721. (New York: Raven Press)
2. Jansen, J. B. M. J. and Lamers, C. B. H. W. (1983). Radioimmunoassay of cholecystokinin in human tissue and plasma. *Clin. Chim. Acta*, **131**, 305–16
3. Everson, G. T., Bravermann, D. Z., Johnson, M. L. and Kern, F. (1980). A critical evaluation of real-time ultrasonography for the study of gallbladder volume and contraction. *Gastroenterology*, **79**, 40–6
4. Lotti, V. J., Pendleton, R. G., Gould, R. J., Hanson, H. M., Chang, R. S. L. and Clineschmidt, B. V. (1987). In vivo pharmacology of L364,718, a new potent nonpeptic peripheral cholecystokinin antagonist. *J. Pharmacol. Exp. Ther.*, **241**, 103–9
5. Makovec, F., Chiste, R., Bani, M., Revel, L., Setnikar, I. and Rovati, L. A. (1986). New glutaramic and aspartic derivatives with potent CCK-antagonist activity. *Eur. J. Med. Chem.*, **21**, 9–20
6. Byrnes, D. J., Henderson, L., Borody, T. and Rehfeld, J. F. (1981). Radioimmunoassay of cholecystokinin in human plasma. *Clin. Chim. Acta*, **111**, 81–9
7. Schafmayer, A., Werner, M. and Becker, H. D. (1982). Radioimmunological determination of cholecystokinin in tissue extracts. *Digestion*, **24**, 146–54
8. Wiener, I., Inoue, K., Fagan, C. J., Lilja, P., Watson, L. C. and Thompson (1981). Release of cholecystokinin in man. Correlation of blood levels with gallbladder contraction. *Ann. Surg.*, **194**, 321–7
9. Yamamura, T., Takahashi, T., Kusunoki, M., Kantoh, M., Seino, Y. and Utsunomiya, J. (1988). Gallbladder dynamics and plasma cholecystokinin responses after meals, oral water, or sham feeding in healthy subjects. *Am. J. Med. Sci.*, **295**, 102–7
10. Hopman, W. P. M., Brouwer, W. F. M., Rosenbusch, G., Jansen, J. B. M. J. and Lamers, C. B. H. W. (1985). A computerized method for rapid quantification of gallbladder volume from real-time sonographs. *Radiology*, **154**, 236–7
11. Fisher, R. S., Rock, E. and Malmud, L. S. (1985). Cholinergic effects on gallbladder emptying in humans. *Gastroenterology*, **88**, 391–6
12. Maton, P. N., Selden, A. C., Fitzpatrick, M. L. and Chadwick, V. S. (1985). Defective gallbladder emptying and cholecystokinin release in celiac disease. *Gastroenterology*, **88**, 391–6
13. Kerstens, P. J. S. M., Lamers, C. B. H. W., Jansen, J. B. M. J., de Jong, A. J. L., Hessels, M. and Hafkenscheid, J. C. M. (1985). Physiological plasma concentrations of cholecystokinin stimulate pancreatic enzyme secretion and gallbladder contraction in man. *Life Sci.*, **36**, 565–9
14. Hopman, W. P. M., Jansen, J. B. M. J., Rosenbusch, G. and Lamers, C. B. H. W. (1987). Cephalic stimulation of gallbladder contraction in humans: Role of cholecystokinin and the cholinergic system. *Digestion*, **38**, 197–203
15. Hopman, W. P. M., Kerstens, P. J. S. M., Jansen, J. B. M. J., Rosenbusch, G. and Lamers, C. B. H. W. (1985). Effect of graded physiological doses of cholecystokinin on gallbladder contraction measured by ultrasonography; determination of threshold, dose-response relationships and comparison with intraduodenal bilirubin output. *Gastroenterology*, **89**, 1242–7
16. Pendleton, R. G., Bendesky, R. J., Schaffer, L., Nolan, Th. E., Gould, R. J. and Clineschmidt, B. V. (1987). Roles of endogenous cholecystokinin in biliary, pancreatic and gastric function: studies with L-364,718, a specific cholecystokinin receptor antagonist. *J. Pharmacol. Exp.*

Ther., **241**, 110–6

17. Fisher, R. S., Rock, E. and Malmud, L. S. (1986). Gallbladder emptying response to sham feeding in humans. *Gastroenterology*, **90**, 1854–7
18. Vermeulen, M., Hopman, W. P. M., de Jong, A. J. L., Yap, S. H. and Lamers, C. B. H. W. (1985). Vagale stimulatie van pancreas en galblaas bij patienten met achalasie. *Ned. Tijdschr. Geneesk.*, **129**, 1657
19. Debas, H. T. and Yamagishi, T. (1979). Evidence for a pylorocystic reflex for gallbladder contraction. *Ann. Surg.*, **190**, 170–6
20. Hopman, W. P. M., Jansen, J. B. M. J. and Lamers, C. B. H. W. (1984). Effect of equimolar amounts of long chain triglycerides and medium chain triglycerides on plasma cholecystokinin and gallbladder contraction. *Am. J. Nutr.*, **39**, 356–9
21. Hopman, W. P. M., Jansen, J. B. M. J. and Lamers, C. B. H. W. (1984). Effect of atropine on plasma cholecystokinin response to intraduodenal fat in man. *Digestion*, **29**, 19–25
22. Hopman, W. P. M., Jansen, J. B. M. J., Rosenbusch, G. and Lamers, C. B. H. W. (1986). Role of cholecystokinin and the cholinergic system in the intestinal phase of gallbladder contraction in man. *Gut*, **27**, A603
23. Gullo, L., Bolondi, L., Priori, P., Casanova, P. and Labo, G. (1984). Inhibitory effect of atropine on cholecystokinin-induced gallbladder contraction in man. *Digestion*, **29**, 209–13
24. Marzio, L., Digimmarco, A. M., Neri, M., Cuccurollo, F. and Malfertheiner, P. (1985). Atropine antagonizes cholecystokinin and caerulein induced gallbladder evacuation in man: a real-time ultrasonographic study. *Am. J. Gastroenterol.*, **80**, 1–4
25. Jansen, J. B. M. J., Hopman, W. P. M. and Lamers, C. B. H. W. (1984). Impaired cholecystokinin secretion and gallbladder contraction in response to intraduodenal fat in patients with coeliac disease. *Digestion*, **30**, 95
26. Hopman, W. P. M., Jansen, J. B. M. J. and Lamers, C. B. H. W. (1984). Plasma cholecystokinin response to a liquid fat meal in vagotomized patients. *Ann. Surg.*, **200**, 693–7
27. Jansen, E. H., Tjon a Tham, R. T., Jansen, J. B. M. J., Lemkes, H. H. P. J. and Lamers, C. B. H. W. (1988). Gallbladder function in diabetes mellitus. *Neth. J. Med.* (In press)

18
Neural control of duodenal mucosal bicarbonate secretion: effects of some brain peptides

G. FLEMSTRÖM, G. JEDSTEDT and L. KNUTSON

INTRODUCTION

Gastric and duodenal mucosa secretes bicarbonate to the lumen by processes that depend on tissue metabolism[1]. The secretion increases pH in the mucous gel adherent to the epithelial surface and it is important in the protection against luminal acid. Electrical stimulation of the vagal nerves in cats[2,3] and rats[4,5] increases the secretion, whereas electrical stimulation of the splanchnic nerves, intravenous administration of α_2-adrenergic agonists or eliciting sympathetic reflexes act inhibitory. Evidence for autonomic nervous control of the secretion has been obtained also in humans. Sham feeding is a stimulant of gastric[6,7] as well as duodenal[8] mucosal bicarbonate secretion in healthy volunteers, which strongly suggests vagal influence. Sympathetic influence is indicated by the recent demonstration[9] that intravenous injection of the α_2-agonist clonidine in humans inhibits the duodenal secretion.

A relationship between hypothalamic lesions and occurrence of acute peptic ulceration in humans is well established. More recently, it has been shown that administration of some brain peptides in rats[10,11] and dogs[12] markedly alters gastric secretion of acid and induces or prevents formation of gastric ulcers. The ability of the gastric and duodenal mucosa to maintain its integrity reflects the balance between aggressive factors such as luminal acid and pepsin and protective mechanisms such as mucosal secretion of mucus and bicarbonate. It seemed possible, therefore that some peptides might act also on central nervous control of mucosal defence. The aim of the present study was to test for the presence of central nervous influence on duodenal mucosal bicarbonate secretion in the rat by intracerebroventricular infusion of some peptides known to occur in brain tissue.

METHODS OF STUDY

Male rats (Sprague–Dawley 300 g) were kept in cages with mesh bottoms and deprived of food for 20–24 h before experiments but had free access to drinking water. They were anaesthetized with 5-ethyl-5(1' methyl-propyl)-2-thiobarbiturate (Inactin, Byk-Gulden, Konstantz, FRG) 120 mg/kg intraperitoneally. They were tracheostomized and body temperature was maintained at 37°C by a heated pad controlled by a rectal thermistor. The abdomen was opened by a midline incision and the pylorus was ligated. A 12 mm segment of proximal duodenum starting 15–18 mm distal to the pylorus, and thus devoid of Brunner's glands, was cannulated *in situ* between two glass tubes connected to a reservoir. Fluid (5 ml of isotonic NaCl) maintained at 37°C was rapidly circulated by a gas lift. Bicarbonate secretion into the luminal perfusate was titrated continuously at pH 7.4 with 50 mM HCl (NaCl to isotonicity) under automatic control by a pH-stat system (Radiometer, Copenhagen, Denmark)[13]. The transepithelial electrical potential difference (PD) across the duodenal lumen and the inferior Vena cava and the mean arterial blood pressure were continuously recorded.

A metal cannula was inserted into the right lateral cerebral ventricle by a stereotaxic instrument. A skin incision was made over the right parietal bone and the 1 mm hole was drilled through the bone, 0.5 mm posterior to the bregma and 1.5 mm lateral to the midsagittal suture. A stainless steel cannula was inserted stereotaxically and cemented to the skull. Artificial cerebrospinal fluid was infused through this cannula at the rate of 1 μl/min and effects of the following peptides were tested: β-endorphin, bombesin, cholecystokinin (CCK) octapeptide, corticotropin-releasing factor (CRF), and thyrotropin-releasing hormone (TRH). All peptides, except TRH, were purchased from Peninsula Lab. Europe Inc., Merseyside, UK; TRH was obtained from Sigma Chemical Co., St. Louis, USA. They were dissolved in artificial cerebrospinal fluid also containing 0.5 mg/ml of bovine serum albumin. The amount of peptide infused was always 1 μg/h.

RESULTS

Intracerebroventricular infusion of TRH increased the bicarbonate secretion by the duodenal mucosa, as illustrated in Figure 1. The stimulation was associated with a small increase in the transepithelial electrical potential difference. Adding prostaglandin E_2 (PGE_2, 10 μM) to the perfusate further increased the secretion. This was always used as a test of the viability of the duodenum. Stimulation of the duodenal secretion also occurred with CRF while bombesin (Figure 2) caused transient stimulation followed by some inhibition of the secretion. Intracerebroventricular infusion of CCK octapeptide or β-endorphin was without effects on the bicarbonate secretion. Cervical vagotomy abolished the stimulatory effect of TRH and bombesin.

COMMENTS

The present study provides evidence there is a central nervous control of the duodenal mucosal bicarbonate secretion influenced by some specific peptides and, at least in part, mediated by the vagal nerves. The presence of a central

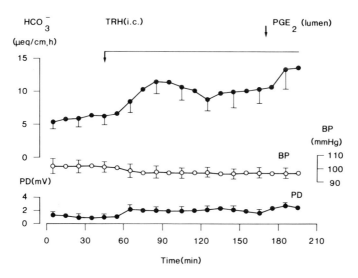

Figure 1 Intracerebroventricular infusion of thyrotropin releasing hormone (TRH) increased duodenal mucosal alkaline secretion in the anaesthetized rat. Adding prostaglandin E_2 (10 μM) at the end of the experiment further increased the secretion; means $\pm$ S.E. of bicarbonate secretion to the lumen, mean arterial blood pressure (BP) and transepithelial electrical potential difference (PD) are given ($n = 8$)

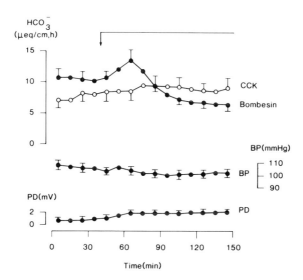

Figure 2 Intracerebroventricular infusion of bombesin has a biphasic effect on duodenal mucosal alkaline secretion, whereas CCK-octapeptide was without effect; means $\pm$ S.E. are shown ($n = 8$ with both peptides)

221

MUCOSAL PROTECTION — CNS CONTROL

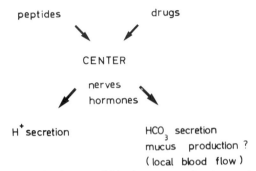

Figure 3 Gastric and duodenal mucosal bicarbonate secretion (as previously known from gastric acid secretion) are under central nervous influence, there may therefore be a balance at the central nervous level between the control of protective bicarbonate secretion and that of acid secretion

nervous control is in line with previous observations in dogs[14] and humans[6-8] that duodenal, as well as gastric mucosal alkaline secretion, are stimulated by sham-feeding. It has also been reported that intrahypothalamic injection of CRF causes an increase in the gastric bicarbonate content in the rat[15]. The experiments in the present study cannot exclude, however, that centrally elicited effects on the secretion in part are mediated by sympathetic nerves. Intravenous infusion of α_2-agonists[4] or electrical stimulation of the splanchnic nerves[5] thus inhibits the duodenal mucosal bicarbonate secretion in rats and cats while the α_1-agonist phenylephrine[4] has a small stimulatory action. Adrenergic β-blockade by propanol is without effect.

It is well known that intracerebroventricular or intrahypothalamic injection of a variety of peptides affects the gastric secretion of acid and induces or prevents gastric ulceration[10-12]. TRH induces ulceration while bombesin, CRF and β-endorphin prevent stress-induced ulceration. Some, but not all, of these effects of centrally administered peptides are inhibited by vagotomy or ganglionic blockade. Ulcer formation or prevention of ulcer formation may reflect effects on gastroduodenal mucosal defence mechanisms as well as on the gastric secretion of acid. The ability of the mucosa to maintain its integrity is considered to reflect the balance on the mucosal level between mucosal defence mechanisms and luminal acid (and pepsin). As Figure 3 illustrates, there may be a similar balance on the central nervous level between controls of mucosal defence and secretion of acid. This could relate to the long-established relationship between hypothalamic lesions and acute peptic ulcer formation and in humans and experimental animals.

Acknowledgements

This work was supported by the Swedish Medical Research Council (04X-3515).

References

1. Flemström, G. (1987). Gastric secretion of bicarbonate. In Johnson, L. R. (ed.) *Physiology of the Gastrointestinal Tract, 2nd Edn.*, pp. 1011–29. (New York: Raven Press)
2. Nylander, O., Flemström, G., Delbro, D. and Fändriks, L. (1987). Vagal influence on gastroduodenal HCO_3^- secretion in the cat in vivo. *Am. J. Physiol.*, **252**, (*Gastrointest. Liver Physiol.*, **15**), G522–8
3. Fändriks, L., Jönson, C. and Nylander, O. (1987). Effects of splanchnic nerve stimulation and of clonidine on gastric and duodenal HCO_3^- secretion in the anesthetized cat. *Acta Physiol. Scand.*, **130**, 251–8
4. Nylander, O. and Flemström, G. (1986). Effects of alpha-receptor agonists and antagonists on duodenal surface epithelial HCO_3^- secretion in the rat in vivo. *Acta Physiol. Scand.*, **126**, 433–41
5. Jönson, C. and Fändriks, L. (1987). Bleeding inhibits vagally-induced duodenal HCO_3^- secretion via activation of the splanchnic nerves in anaesthetized rats. *Acta Physiol. Scand.*, **130**, 259–64
6. Forssell, H., Stenquist, B. and Olbe, L. (1985). Vagal stimulation of human gastric bicarbonate secretion. *Gastroenterology*, **89**, 581–6
7. Feldman, M. (1985). Gastric H^+ and HCO_3^- secretion in response to sham feeding in humans. *Am. J. Physiol.*, **248**, (*Gastrointest. Liver Physiol.*, **11**), G188–91
8. Ballesteros, M. A., Hogan, D. L., Koss, M. A., Chen, H. S. and Isenberg, J. I. (1988). Vagal stimulation of human duodenal bicarbonate secretion (DBS) acts by non-cholinergic mechanisms. *Gastroenterology*. **94**, 420
9. Knutson, L., Flemström, G. and Thorén, L. (1988). Duodenal mucosal bicarbonate secretion: Mechanisms of control in animals and humans. *J. R. Coll. Surg.* (In press)
10. Tache, Y., Simard, P. and Collu, R. (1979). Prevention by bombesin of cold-restraint stress-induced hemorrhagic lesions in rats. *Life Sci.*, **24**, 1719–26
11. Tache, Y. (1987). The peptidergic brain–gut axis: influence on gastric ulcer formation. *Chronobiol. Internat.*, **4**, 11–17
12. Lenz, H. J., Klapdor, R., Hester, S. E., Webb, J. V., Galyean, R. F., Rivier, J. E. and Brown, M. R. (1986). Inhibition of gastric acid secretion by brain peptides in the dog. Role of the autonomic nervous system and gastrin. *Gastroenterology*, **91**, 905–12
13. Flemström, G., Garner, A., Nylander, O., Hurst, B. C. and Heylings, J. R. (1982). Surface epithelial HCO_3^- transport by mammalian duodenum in vivo. *Am. J. Physiol.*, **243**, (*Gastrointest. Liver Physiol.*, **6**), G348–58
14. Konturek, S. J. and Thor, P. (1986). Relation between duodenal alkaline secretion and motility in fasted and sham-fed dogs. *Am. J. Physiol.*, **251**, (*Gastrointest. Liver Physiol.* **14**), G591–6
15. Gunion, M. W., Tache, Y. and Kauffman, G. L. (1985). Intrahypothalamic corticotropin-releasing factor (CRF) increases gastric bicarbonate content. *Gastroenterology*, **88**, 1407

Section III
Enteric neuroeffector control

19
Neural basis of enteric motor function

J. D. WOOD

INTRODUCTION

The intestine of humans and virtually all vertebrates is adapted for organized propulsion of intraluminal contents. Propulsion is achieved by the co-ordinated application of myogenic forces that results in appropriate movement of chyme or faeces through the intestinal tube. Neural circuitry resident in the gut wall controls the musculature for generation of propulsive motility. Total failure of the mechanisms responsible for peristaltic propulsion results in stasis, which presents a life-threatening situation for the individual. Subnormal functional deficits in the neural circuitry are the probable explanation for a variety of poorly understood motor disorders now classified as 'functional'. This chapter reviews concepts of enteric neurophysiology basic to understanding of the functional disorders.

PERISTALSIS IS A STEREOTYPED BEHAVIOUR

Peristalsis is a synonym for propulsive motility. The peristaltic reflex has long been recognized, although progress in clarifying the details of the underlying neuronal and muscular mechanisms has been slow. A continuum of reviews of the literature provide a chronology of the development of understanding of peristaltic behaviour[1-9]. The classic peristaltic reflex occurs in response to radial distension of the intestinal wall. Inflation of a balloon in the intestinal lumen results in circular muscle contraction on the oral side of the balloon, while aboral to the distension, the circular muscle relaxes and the longitudinal muscle contracts. Kosterlitz and Robinson[10] referred to the longitudinal contraction as the preparatory phase of the reflex.

A bolus placed in the lumen of the large bowel *in vitro* to simulate faeces will be propelled in the anal direction[11,12]. During propulsion, contraction of the circular muscle occurs above the bolus, while the circular muscle relaxes and the longitudinal shortens below the bolus.

Peristaltic propulsion can be viewed as a stereotyped behavioural complex that propagates along the intestine (Figure 1). The longitudinal and circular muscle layers behave in a stereotypical pattern during propulsion of the luminal contents. This pattern is established by 'hardwired' synaptic connections within the circuitry of the enteric nervous system.

The longitudinal muscle of the muscularis externa and perhaps the longitudinal component of the muscularis mucosae contract in the segment below the advancing intraluminal contents. The circular muscle in this segment relaxes simultaneously with longitudinal shortening. Under these conditions, the intestinal tube behaves geometrically like a cylinder with constant surface area[13]. Shortening of the longitudinal axis leads to expansion of the cross-sectional diameter of the tube. Shortening of the longitudinal muscle coincident with relaxation of the circular muscle expands the lumen and functions to establish a 'receiving segment' that accommodates the oncoming material. Neuronal inhibition of the circular muscle in the receiving segment ensures that contraction of this much stronger muscle does not antagonize the lumen expanding function of longitudinal contraction in the receiving segment.

The circular muscle layer in the segment above the advancing intraluminal content contracts as part of the stereotyped behaviour of peristalsis. The longitudinal muscle layer in this segment relaxes simultaneously with contraction of the circular muscle. The outcome is conversion of this intestinal region to a 'propulsive segment' that functions to propel the intraluminal material into the 'receiving segment below'. Intestinal segments below the advancing bolus of material become receiving segments and then propulsive segments in succession, as the peristaltic behavioural complex propagates along the intestine.

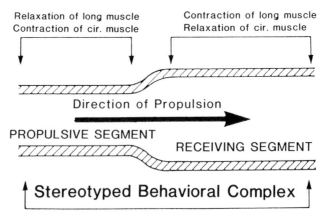

Figure 1   Peristaltic propulsion is a stereotyped pattern of motor behaviour that propagates along the intestine. This behavioural complex is determined by an enteric neural circuit that co-ordinates contraction and relaxation of the musculature for transient formation of propulsive and receiving segments. Relaxation of the longitudinal muscle in concert with contraction of the circular muscle occurs in the propulsive segment, while the longitudinal muscle is contracted coincident with circular muscle relaxation in the receiving segment

The stereotypic behavioural complex (Figure 1) propagates over variable distances in either the oral or aboral direction at various times in the life of the animal. Direction and distance of propagation are determined by conditions in the bowel that may be physiologically normal or result from pathological situations. In all cases, the prevailing peristaltic behaviour in the intestine is undoubtedly adaptive for homeostasis at the level of the whole body.

Long-distance propulsion is an adaptive response to the presence of noxious or potentially damaging substances or organisms within the intestinal lumen. The migrating myogenic spike bursts that appear in response to introduction of enterotoxins or intestinal parasites are the electrical correlates of long-distance propulsion. When strain gauges are attached experimentally next to the electrodes on the serosa, the migrating spike bursts are seen as the electrical correlate of giant migrating contractions or power contractions depending on the terminology of the authors[14-16].

The peristaltic behavioural complex can travel in either the ortho- or retrograde direction. Long-distance propulsion occurs in the retrograde (oral) direction in the intestine during emesis[17]. Retrograde propulsion also occurs as an adaptive response to an intestinal obstruction. In the piebald mouse model for Hirschsprung's disease, the direction of peristaltic propulsion reverses as the forward moving faecal material encounters the transition zone of the aganglionic terminal segment[12].

The occurrence of retrograde propulsion in the intestine suggests that the same basic neural circuit is 'wired' directionally to produce either forward or reverse propulsion. Neural mechanisms, and perhaps also hormonal actions, are expected to activate one or the other sets of circuits while suppressing the counter circuit.

The distance of travel of the stereotyped propulsive behavioural complex is intermediate when it occurs within the activity front of the migrating motor complex during the interdigestive state of small intestinal motility[18]. In this case, it starts each time at the oral boundary of the activity front and propagates to the aboral boundary of the advancing front. The propulsive complexes are limited to the confines of the activity front as it inches down the intestine.

Short-distance travel of the peristaltic behavioural complex occurs during the segmentation pattern of motility characteristic of the digestive state. In the digestive state, contractions of the circular muscle are often described as segmental or mixing contractions. These produce a pattern of movement of chyme that would be observed at the starting point of a peristaltic behavioural complex. In this case, the chyme is propelled into the aboral receiving segment and also into the relaxed segment oral to the propulsive segment. This interpretation pictures segmentation as a situation in which the distance of propagation of the peristaltic behavioural complex is ultrashort.

THE BRAIN IN THE GUT

The 'brain-in-the-gut' concept refers to the capability of the intrinsic nervous system of the gut for performance of integrative functions independent of any input from the central nervous system. This concept, which is central to gastrointestinal neurobiology, implies that local circuits within the ENS automatically control and co-ordinate the contractile activity of the various muscle layers, as well as other gastrointestinal effector systems. These circuits are designed to respond appropriately both to sensory information from gastrointestinal receptors and to command signals from the central nervous system. Some are programmed (hardwired') for generation of the stereotyped behavioural complex of peristalsis.

The fundamental principles of neurophyisology are the same for the ENS and the CNS. Sensory receptors generate information on the minute-to-minute state of the intestinal wall and lumen and code the information in the form of action potentials. Interneurons are synaptically connected into networks that process the sensory information and intelligently control the activity of motor neurons. Motor neurons are the final common pathways to the effector systems and may initiate, sustain or inhibit the behaviour of the effector. The effector system of concern in this chapter is the intestinal musculature.

NEURONAL CONSTITUENTS

Alexander S. Dogiel described three morphological types of enteric ganglion cells which have come to be known as Dogiel type I, II and III neurons in the brain in the gut (Figure 2). Neurons with Dogiel type I morphology have cell bodies with many short, stubby dendrites and a single long process (axon) that projects through interganglionic fibre tracts and many rows of

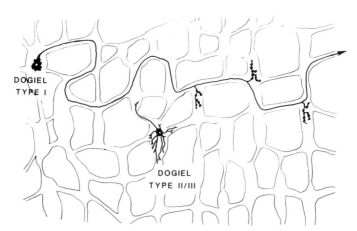

Figure 2 Morphological types of enteric neurons have specific projections within the myenteric plexus. Dogiel type I neurons have cell bodies with many short club-shaped dendrites and a single long axon that projects through interganglionic connectives and many ganglia for distances of 2–3 cm along the intestine. Cell somas of Dogiel type II and III neurons have long and short processes that project for varying distances. Type III cells have intermediate length processes relative to type II. Subpopulations of Dogiel type I neurons contain 5-HT, VIP and enkephalin. Substance P is found in multipolar neurons with Dogiel type II or III morphology

ganglia for several centimetres along the longitudinal axis of the intestine. The somas of neurons with Dogiel type II morphology have long and short processes positioned in a variety of configurations. Type III ganglion cells are also multipolar but with intermediate length processes which terminate in the same or adjacent ganglia. There is great variation in size and detailed morphology within the Dogiel classification which limits its usefulness to that of facilitating general discussion.

Functional significance of the neuronal morphology relative to a network theory of propulsive motility will be elaborated later on in the chapter. The reader will be made aware in several other chapters of this volume that enteric neurons can be divided into many more than three types on the basis of the kinds of neurotransmitters they contain (see Chapter 1 by Furness *et al.* and Chapter 20 by Szurszewski).

ELECTRICAL AND SYNAPTIC BEHAVIOUR

The cellular neurophysiology of enteric neurons is basically the same as for neurons elsewhere in the nervous system. An intracellular microelectrode placed in an enteric neuronal cell body may record three different electrical events (Figure 3). These are action potentials generated by the somal membrane, electrotonic invasion of the somal membrane by action potentials in the neurites and synaptic potentials.

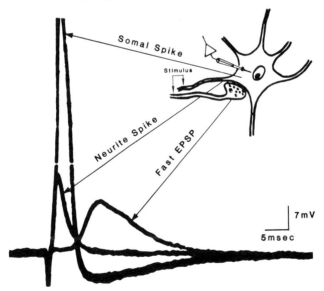

Figure 3   Three kinds of electrical events are recorded in the cell bodies of enteric neurons with intracellular microelectrodes. Electrical stimulation of the interganglionic connective evoked action potentials in both a neurite projecting from the cell body and an axon that synapsed with the cell body. Activation of the synapse evoked a fast EPSP in the cell soma. Electrotonic spread of current from the inbound spike in the process fired an action potential in the somal membrane

Action potentials of the somal membrane are spike-like, are less than 5 ms in duration and they overshoot zero membrane potential (Figure 3). The functional significance of somal action potentials is the relay of coded information arriving in one neurite to neurites at opposite poles of the cell body. The somal membrane may also be the site of initiation of action potentials. These spike codes propagate away from the cell body in processes that eventually synapse with other neurons or form neuroeffector junctions. At the synapse or neuroeffector junction, the spike code is transformed to a chemical message carried by action potential evoked release of neurotransmitter.

Electronic invasion by neurite action potentials results from propagation of action potentials toward the cell body in one of the processes of the multipolar neuron. The processes of multipolar neurons in the ENS, unlike many neurons in the CNS, are electrically excitable and conduct action potentials. The action potentials may be triggered experimentally by focal electrical stimulation of the neurite or may occur spontaneously under physiological conditions (see refs. 8 and 9 for a comprehensive review). The electrotonic potentials (Figure 3) are produced by the passive spread of electrical current into the cell body as the action potential in the neurite approaches the cell body, but fails to reach threshold to fire the somal membrane.

Synaptic potentials are produced by the release of neurotransmitter substances at synapses on the cell body (Figure 3). These may be produced experimentally by focal electrical stimulation of the presynaptic axon or may occur spontaneously. Synaptic potentials may depolarize the membrane and therefore fit the criteria for excitatory post-synaptic potentials or they may hyperpolarize and fit the definition of inhibitory post-synaptic potentials (see refs. 8,9 for a comprehensive review of synaptic potentials in enteric neurons).

BASIC PERISTALTIC CIRCUIT

The term 'basic peristaltic circuit' refers to a hardwired circuit that automatically reproduces the stereotyped behavioural complex described above for peristaltic propulsion each time the circuit is activated. The detailed organization of the synaptic connections in the basic network is not yet entirely unravelled. Nevertheless, information obtained in the past decade on morphological types of neurons, localization and identification of neurotransmitters and on cellular neurophysiology provide clues to the organization of the circuits that programs the behaviour. The basic circuit will probably turn out to be relatively simple when it is more thoroughly understood. The basic circuit in Figure 4, together with Figure 6, illustrates the minimal requirements the circuitry should meet and suggests that it need not be complex.

The main requirement is for interneuronal connections that generate longlasting trains of spikes in excitatory motor neurons to the longitudinal muscle and in inhibitory motor neurons to the circular muscle of the receiving segment. This must occur ahead of the advancing intraluminal material and

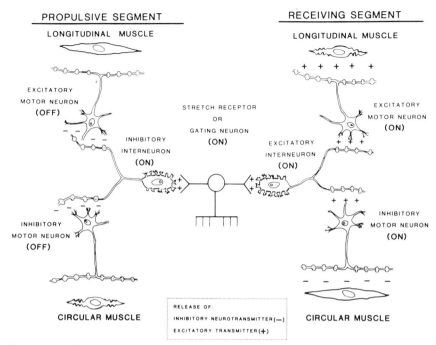

PROPULSIVE SEGMENT

LONGITUDINAL MUSCLE

EXCITATORY
MOTOR NEURON
(OFF)

INHIBITORY
INTERNEURON
(ON)

STRETCH RECEPTOR
OR
GATING NEURON
(ON)

EXCITATORY
INTERNEURON
(ON)

INHIBITORY
MOTOR NEURON
(OFF)

CIRCULAR MUSCLE

RECEIVING SEGMENT

LONGITUDINAL MUSCLE

+ + + + +

EXCITATORY
MOTOR NEURON
(ON)

INHIBITORY
MOTOR NEURON
(ON)

CIRCULAR MUSCLE

RELEASE OF:
INHIBITORY NEUROTRANSMITTER (—)
EXCITATORY TRANSMITTER (+)

Figure 4 A fundamental synaptic circuit consisting of sensory neurons, interneurons and motor neurons generates the stereotyped behavioural pattern of perstalsis

be timed to occur synchronously around the circumference of the receiving segment. As the bolus moves into the receiving segment, the same motor neurons must be abruptly shut off in order for the receiving segment to be converted to a propulsive segment.

The basic peristaltic circuit does not require many different kinds of neuronal units to function effectively. It demands that the same units and basic connections be repeated continuously along the length and in parallel around the circumference of the bowel. The apparent histoanatomical complexity of the enteric nervous system that has baffled investigators for nearly 100 years may be a reflection of repetition rather than complexity of the basic circuit diagram.

SYNAPTIC EVENTS

Results of neurophysiological studies suggest that chemical transfer and transformation of information within the basic circuits takes place at axosomatic, axodendritic and axo-axonal synapses. The events at these synapses consist of fast synaptic potentials with durations less than 50 ms and slow synaptic potentials lasting several seconds or minutes. They may be excitatory post-synaptic potentials (EPSPs) or inhibitory post-synaptic potentials (IPSPs).

233

Presynaptic inhibitory events are mediated by receptors located on the enteric axons at or near the release site for neurotransmitters. They may involve axo-axonal transmission or be involved in negative feedback mechanisms of autoinhibition of transmitter release (for reviews, see refs. 8,9).

Fast EPSPs

Fast EPSPs are depolarizing potentials that have durations in the millisecond time domain and occur in the ganglion cells of the stomach and small and large intestine. They can be recorded in both the myenteric and submucosal plexuses. They are most prevalent in S type 1 neurons, but are often seen in AH type 2 neurons. All of the fast EPSPs are mediated by the nicotinic cholinergic actions of acetylcholine.

Fast EPSPs are the equivalents of 'bytes' of information in the rapid processing of data within the enteric circuits. They may or may not reach threshold for the discharge of action potentials. Fast EPSPs do not reach threshold when the neural membranes are hyperpolarized during slow inhibitory post-synaptic potentials. They are more apt to reach spike threshold when the membranes are depolarized during slow excitatory post-synaptic potentials.

Slow EPSPs

Slow EPSPs are evoked by electrical stimulation of axons in experimental studies of enteric synaptic events. This releases neurotransmitters which produce a slowly rising membrane depolarization that is sustained for several seconds to minutes after termination of the stimulation. The membrane depolarization is associated with increased input resistance and markedly augmented excitability. Prolonged trains of action potentials that continue for several seconds after offset of stimulation are characteristic of the slow EPSPs (Figure 5).

The prolonged discharge of spikes during the slow EPSP actuates the release of neurotransmitter from the neuron's axon for the duration of the spike discharge. This is expected to produce longlasting excitation or inhibition at neuronal synapses and neuromuscular junctions. The peristaltic

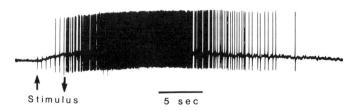

Stimulus   5 sec

Figure 5 Slow EPSPs are characterized by trains of action potentials that persist for several seconds after termination of stimulation of the slow synaptic input

behavioural complex consists of sluggish components that span time courses of several seconds from start to completion. The train-like discharge during slow EPSPs is the neural correlate of the longlasting events in the propulsive and receiving segments of the peristaltic complex.

Chemical messengers that may be peptidergic, aminergic or cholinergic mimic the slow EPSPs when applied experimentally to the neurons. Amines which produce slow EPSP-like behaviour are 5-hydroxytryptamine (5-HT) and histamine. The peptides so far identified are substance P, vasoactive intestinal peptide, bombesin, cholecystokinin and calcitonin gene-related peptide. The strongest evidence for a neurotransmitter function exists for acetylcholine, 5-HT and substance P. Acetylcholine produces its slow EPSP-like effects through action at M_1 muscarinic receptors[19].

Histamine mimics the slow EPSP[20] but is probably not a neurotransmitter as such. It is found in mast cells in close proximity to enteric neurons and may function as a messenger in communication between the immune system and nervous system of the gut (see Chapter 24 by Castro).

INFORMATION TRANSFER RELATIVE TO HISTOANATOMY

Slow EPSPs often occur in multipolar neurons of the Dogiel type II and III classification. Subpopulations of these neurons in the myenteric plexus have been shown by immunocytochemical methods to contain substance P[21]. Dogiel type I neurons differ in receiving much more fast excitatory synaptic input at the cell soma and in forming subpopulations that contain 5-HT.

Immunocytochemical studies show that the 5-HT containing axons of Dogiel type I neurons project in the aboral direction for great distances through many ganglia and their connectives[22]. The regions of axon in the interganglionic connectives are smooth whereas those in the ganglia where the neurotransmitter is likely to be released are varicose. The projections of the Dogiel type I neurons suggest that these neurons are specialized for transmission of information for long distances up and down the intestine. Projections of the substance-P-containing Dogiel II or III neurons suggests a local function for these neurons that does not extend much beyond the ganglion of residence of the cell body.

NETWORK THEORY

Simultaneous excitation or inhibition of the musculature around the circumference of the receiving and propulsive segments of the peristaltic behavioural complex is a functional necessity for achieving the balanced forces required for effective propulsion. Enteric network theory suggests that build-up of slow EPSPs in a synaptically coupled network of multipolar neurons drives excitation of the longitudinal muscle and inhibition of the circular muscle around the circumference of the receiving segment of the peristaltic complex. Figure 6 is an hypothetical model of a synaptically coupled network of neurons that provide prolonged drive to excitatory or inhibitory motor

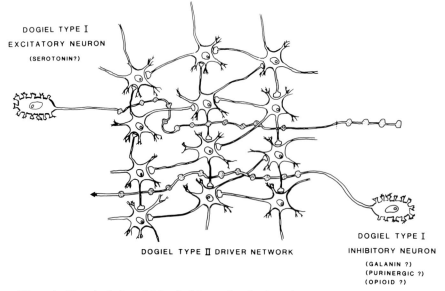

DOGIEL TYPE I
EXCITATORY NEURON
(SEROTONIN?)

DOGIEL TYPE II DRIVER NETWORK

DOGIEL TYPE I
INHIBITORY NEURON
(GALANIN ?)
(PURINERGIC ?)
(OPIOID ?)

Figure 6 Hypothetical model for feed-forward activation of a synaptic network of neurons with Dogiel type II or III morphology around the intestinal circumference. This is a driver network for activation of excitatory and inhibitory motor neurons around the circumference. Serotonin released from axons with Dogiel type I morphology evokes slow EPSPs in neurons of the driver network. These Dogiel II/III neurons then release substance P, which leads to rapid build-up of excitation (slow EPSPs) in the entire network. Activity within the network is terminated with appropriate timing by slow inhibitory synaptic input from neurons pictured with Dogiel type I morphology. Putative inhibitory transmitters are galanin, opioid peptides and purinergic substances

neurons around the circumference of a length of bowel. These neurons fit the description of the substance P containing Dogiel type II and III neurons that generate slow EPSPs. They are shown connected in a positive feed forward array organized such that development of slow synaptic excitation in a few neurons would release substance P and lead to rapid build-up of excitation in the entire network.

The driver networks are proposed to be multipolar neurons like Dogiel type II or III; nevertheless, the exact association of morphological type with function is unknown. In spite of this, it is obvious that the driver network must be activated initially by synaptic inputs that are appropriately timed for the appropriate spatial organization of the behaviour within the receiving or propulsive segment. Subpopulations of neurons with Dogiel type I morphology are pictured as neurons that transmit the timing signals to the driver networks along the intestine as the peristaltic complex advances. These neurons evoke slow EPSPs in a few neurons of the driver network and this leads to rapid build-up of slow EPSPs and spike discharge in the entire network. The probable neurotransmitter released by the Dogiel type I signal neurons is 5-HT. This is based on the localization of 5-HT in this morphological type and on the slow EPSP-like action of 5-HT.

Spike discharge in neurons of the driver network must be terminated swiftly to enable the receiving segment to convert to a propulsive segment. This is presumably achieved by appropriately timed turn-on of inhibitory Dogiel type I neurons that are diagrammed as projecting in the oral direction in Figure 6. Action potential discharge in these neurons release neurotransmitters for slow inhibitory synaptic potentials (slow IPSPs) that terminate spike activity in neurons of the driver network and return them to the resting state.

Slow IPSPs

Slow IPSPs in the enteric circuits are the inverse of slow EPSPs. Like slow EPSPs, they are evoked experimentally by electrical stimulation of the axons of the inhibitory neurons and release of the inhibitory neurotransmitter. They are characterized by a slowly developing membrane hyperpolarization that persists after termination of the stimulation. The membrane hyperpolarization is associated with a decrease input resistance that reflects an increase in K^+ conductance. Hyperpolarization moves the membrane away from action potential threshold and the lowered resistance of the membrane requires that relatively larger ionic currents be generated to depolarize the membrane back to spike threshold.

Several different chemical messenger substances which may be peptidergic or purinergic mimic the slow IPSPs in intestinal myenteric neurons. Enkephalins, dynorphin and morphine all mimic the slow IPSPs when applied to enteric neurons[23]. Galanin is a 29 amino acid polypeptide that simulates slow synaptic inhibition in virtually all of the neurons of the myenteric plexus[24].

Application of adenosine, ATP and other purinergic analogues also mimic the slow IPSPs when applied to myenteric neurons. This occurs in virtually all AH type 2 neurons and appears to result from suppression of the enzyme adenylate cyclase and reduction in intraneuronal levels of cyclic adenosine $3',5'$-monophosphate[25].

GATING MECHANISMS DETERMINE PROPULSIVE DISTANCE

The discussion above pointed out that the propulsive behavioural complex propagates over a variable distance dependent upon the digestive state and influenced by pathogenic factors. Gating mechanisms, for which there are enteric neurophysiological correlates, have been postulated as the controlling factors that determine the distance of spread of the propulsive behavioural complex along the intestine[9]. According to this theory, gates control transmission of 'start' signals between blocks of peristaltic circuits that are repeated along the bowel. As described above, a block of peristaltic circuitry in an intestinal segment is envisioned as being hardwired for conversion of a length of intestine first to a receiving segment and then, with appropriate timing, to a contractile segment as the propagating complex passes. If the gate were opened, peristalsis would continue; if the gate to the circuitry in the next segment remained closed, then peristalsis would stop at that segment.

PRESYNAPTIC INHIBITION

The neurophysiological correlate of gating is presynaptic inhibition. Presynaptic inhibition refers to suppression of neurotransmitter release from axonal terminals or varicosities by the action of chemical messengers at receptors on the axon. Presynaptic inhibition may involve axo-axonal transmission, occur in the form of autoinhibition or involve endocrine or paracrine release of substances that act at presynaptic receptors. Presynaptic inhibition has the effect of blocking the forward transfer of information at chemical synapses in the continuum of circuits along the intestine.

Chemical messengers that may be peptidergic, aminergic or cholinergic produce presynaptic inhibition at synaptic connections within the enteric circuitry. Norepinephrine acts at alpha$_2$ presynaptic adrenoceptors to suppress both fast and slow EPSP[26,27]. Presynaptic α_2-receptors represent the synaptic interface between the post-ganglionic sympathetic fibres and the enteric nervous system[28]. Adrenergic suppression of enteric synaptic transmission is responsible for inactivation of the neural circuits that programme the stereotyped behavioural complex and for blockade of propagation by closure of synaptic gates. Activation of the sympathetic input by the central nervous system or by intestinointestinal reflex loops through the prevertebral ganglia (see Chapter 20) thereby shuts down propulsive behaviour. This occurs in association with continuous discharge of intrinsic inhibitory motor neurons to the musculature, with the overall effect of producing a state of intestinal motor paralysis in conjunction with reduced splanchnic blood flow.

Serotonin suppresses both fast and slow EPSPs in the myenteric plexus[29]. The prokinetic drug Cisapride also suppresses fast EPSPs and behaves like a serotonergic agonist in this respect[30]. It is unclear if this property of Cisapride is related to its therapeutic value as a promotility agent.

Opiates or opioid peptides suppress some fast EPSPs in the guinea-pig small intestine myenteric plexus, but not in the cat[31,32].

Acetylcholine acts at muscarinic presynaptic receptors to suppress fast EPSPs in the myenteric plexus[33]. This may occur in a form of autoinhibition where acetylcholine released at synapses with nicotinic post-synaptic receptors feeds back on to presynaptic muscarinic receptors to suppress release of acetylcholine in negative feedback manner. The presynaptic muscarinic receptors behave like the M$_2$ subtype[19].

Histamine acts at histaminergic presynaptic receptors of the H$_3$ subtype to suppress fast EPSPs[34]. This may reflect another mechanism by which chemical communication occurs between cellular components of the immune system and the ENS. (See Chapter 24.)

CONCLUSION

The old classical concept of neural control of gastrointestinal motility emphasizes the CNS. This concept, which still persists at the textbook level, views gut ganglia as relay distribution centres for preprocessed information emanating from the brain and spinal cord. Parasympathetic preganglionic fibres are represented as synapsing directly with 'post-ganglionic' neurons that innervate the musculature. This view which places the 'computer' entirely in the central nervous system, is no longer defensible and should be discarded.

Most of the microprocessor-like circuits that determine the motor behaviour of the intestine are intramural within the enteric nervous system. These are synaptic circuits that utilize mechanisms of chemical transfer and transformation of information that are essentially the same as found in the brain and spinal cord. This is the essence of the 'brain-in-the-gut' concept.

Neural connections for organized propulsion of intraluminal contents are 'wired' into the circuits of the 'little brain'. The peristaltic reflex is a 'hardwired' circuit that is basic to propulsive motor function. It occurs as a stereotyped sequence of muscular behaviours in response to stimulation of intestinal mechanoreceptors and, undoubtedly, other inputs as well. Radial distention is an adequate stimulus for generating the pattern of behaviour which consists of contraction of the circular muscle oral to the stimulus while shortening of the longitudinal muscle and inhibition of the circular muscle occur aboral to the stimulus. This behaviour is produced by a fundamental circuit that is expressed repeatedly along the intestine to accomplish unidirectional propulsion of intraluminal contents. Long-distance propulsion is achieved by linking basic peristaltic reflex circuits that are redundant along the bowel. Operation of synaptic gates between the linked circuits determines the distance of propulsion.

Acknowledgements

My thanks to Dr H. Falk for sponsoring the meeting on Nerves and the Gastrointestinal Tract and to Prof. Dr M. Singer and Dr Goebell for a fine job of organizing the meeting. Gratitude is expressed also to the Digestive Diseases Institute of the National Institutes of Health for support of my work on enteric neurobiology since 1973.

Figures 1,2,4 & 6 are adapted from *Unit* 20, *Gastrointestinal Neurophysiology* of the Undergraduate Teaching Project under sponsorship of The American Gastrointestinal Association. Distribution of Unit 20, authored by J. D. Wood and D. L. Wingate, began in 1988. Distributor is Millner-Fenwick, Inc., 2125 Greenspring Drive, Timonium, Maryland 21093 USA.

References

1. Bayliss, W.M. and Starling, E.H. (1900). The movements and the innervation of the large intestine. *J. Physiol. (Lond.)*, **26**, 107–18
2. Bayliss, W.M. and Starling, E.H. (1900). The movements and the innervation of the small intestine. *J. Physiol. (Lond.)*, **26**, 125–38
3. Alverez, W.C. (1948). *An Introduction to Gastroenterology*, 4th Edn. (London: Heinemann)
4. Hukuhara, T., Yamagami, M. and Nakayama, S. (1958). On the intestinal intrinsic reflex. *J. Physiol. (Japan)*, **8**, 9–20
5. Kosterlitz, H.W. and Lees, G.M. (1964). Pharmacological analysis of intrinsic intestinal

reflexes. *Pharmacol. Rev.*, **16**, 301–39
6. Hirst, G.D.S. (1979). Mechanisms of peristalsis. *Br. Med. Bul.*, **35**, 263–68
7. Costa, M. and Furness, J.B. (1982). Nervous control of intestinal motility. In Bertaccini, G. (ed.) *Mediators and Drugs in Gastrointestinal Motility I, Handbook of Experimental Pharmacology*, Vol. 59, pp. 279–382. (Berlin: Springer-Verlag)
8. Wood, J.D. (1987). Physiology of the enteric nervous system. In Johnson, L.R. (ed.) *Physiology of the Gastrointestinal Tract*, 2nd Edn., pp. 67–109. (New York: Raven Press)
9. Wood, J.D. (1987). Neurophysiological theory of intestinal motility. *Jpn. J. Smooth Muscle Res.*, **23**, 143–86
10. Kosterlitz, H.W. and Robinson, J.A. (1959). Reflex contractions of the longitudinal muscle coat of the isolated guinea-pig ileum. *J. Physiol. (Lond.)*, **146**, 369–79
11. Friggo, G.M. and Lecchini, S. (1970). An improved method for studying the peristaltic reflex in the isolated colon. *Br. J. Pharmacol.*, **39**, 346–56
12. Brann, L.R. and Wood, J.D. (1976). Motility of the large intestine of piebald lethal mice. *Am. J. Dig. Dis.*, **23**, 633–40
13. Wood, J.D. and Perkins, W.E. (1970). Mechanical interactions between longitudinal and circular axes of the small intestine. *Am. J. Physiol.*, **235**, E345–53
14. Palmer, J.M. and Castro, G.A. (1986). Anamnestic stimulus-specific myoelectric responses associated with intestinal immunity in the rat. *Am. J. Physiol.*, **250**, G266–73
15. Mathias, J.R. and Sninsky, C.A. (1985). Motility of the small intestine: a look ahead. *Am. J. Physiol.*, **248**, G495–500
16. Sarna, S.K. (1987). Giant migrating contractions and their myoelectric correlates in the small intestine. *Am. J. Physiol. (Gastrointest. Liver Physiol)*, **16**, G697–705
17. Lang, I.M., Sarna, S.K. and Condon, R.E. (1986). Gastrointestinal motor correlates of vomiting in the dog: Quantification and characterization as an independent phenomenon. *Gastroenterology*, **90**, 40–7
18. Schemann, M. and Ehrlein, H.J. (1986). Mechanical characteristics of Phase II and Phase III of the interdigestive migrating motor complex in dogs. *Gastroenterology*, **91**, 117–23
19. North, R.A., Slack, B.E. and Surprenant, A. (1985). Muscarini M–V1–V and M–V2–V receptors mediate depolarization and presynaptic inhibition in guinea-pig enteric nervous system. *J. Physiol. (Lond.)*, **368**, 435–52
20. Nemeth, P.R., Ort, C.A. and Wood, J.D. (1984). Intracellular study of effects of histamine on electrical behaviour of myenteric neurons in guinea-pig small intestine. *J. Physiol. (Lond.)*, **355**, 411–25
21. Llewellyn-Smith, I., Furness, J.B., Murphy, R., O'Brien, P.E. and Costa, M. (1984). Substance P-containing nerves in the human small intestine. *Gastroenterology*, **86**, 421–35
22. Furness, J.B. and Costa, M. (1982). Neurons with 5-hydroxytryptamine-like immunoreactivity in the enteric nervous system; their projections in the guinea-pig small intestine. *Neuroscience*, **7**, 341–49
23. Mihara, S. and North, R.A. (1986). Opioids increase potassium conductance in submucous neurons of guinea-pig caecum by activating delta-receptors. *Br. J. Pharmacol.*, **88**, 315–22
24. Palmer, J.M., Schemann, M., Tamura, K. and Wood, J.D. (1986). Galanin mimics slow synaptic inhibition in myenteric neurons. *Eur. J. Pharmacol.*, **124**, 379–80
25. Palmer, J.M., Wood, J.D. and Zafirov, D.H. (1987). Purinergic inhibition in the small intestinal myenteric plexus of the guinea-pig. *J. Physiol. (Lond.)*, **387**, 357–69
26. Hirst, G.D.S. and McKirdy, H.C. (1974). Presynaptic inhibition at a mammalian peripheral synapse. *Nature (Lond.)*, **250**, 430–31
27. Wood, J.D. and Mayer, C.J. (1979). Adrenergic inhibition of serotonin release from neurons in guinea-pig Auerbach's plexus. *J. Neurophysiol.*, **42**, 594–693
28. Wood, J.D. (1983). The synaptic interface between the sympathetic and enteric divisions of the autonomic nervous system. In Chey, W.Y. (eds.) *Functional Disorders of the Digestive Tract*, pp. 87–91. (New York: Raven Press)
29. North, R.A., Henderson, G., Katayama, Y. and Johnson, S.M. (1980). Electrophysiological evidence for presynaptic inhibition of acetylcholine release by 5-hydroxytryptamine in the enteric nervous system. *Neuroscience*, **5**, 581–86
30. Nemeth, P.R., Ort, C.A., Zafirov, D.H. and Wood, J.D. (1985). Interactions between serotonin and cisapride on myenteric neurons. *Eur. J. Pharmacol.*, **108**, 77–83
31. Cherubini, E., Morita, K. and North, R.A. (1985). Opioid inhibition of synaptic transmission in the guinea-pig myenteric plexus. *Br. J. Pharmacol.*, **85**, 805–17

32. Wood, J.D. (1979). Intracellular study of effects of morphine on electrical activity of myenteric neurons in cat small intestine. *Gastroenterology*, **79**, 1222–30

33. Morita, K., North, R.A. and Tokimasa, T. (1982). Muscarini presynaptic inhibition of synaptic transmission in myenteric plexus of guinea-pig ileum. *J. Physiol. (Lond.)*, **333**, 141–9

34. Tamura, K., Palmer, J.M. and Wood, J.D. (1988). Presynaptic inhibition produced by histamine at nicotinic synapses in enteric ganglia. *Neuroscience*, **25**, 171–9

20
Colonic mechanosensory afferent fibres to prevertebral ganglion cells

J. H. SZURSZEWSKI

INTRODUCTION

This chapter provides a brief review of peripheral reflex activity between the inferior mesenteric ganglion and colon of the guinea-pig. Following a brief historical review of the notion that local reflexes occur between gut structures and abdominal prevertebral ganglia, data are reviewed which raise the possibility that colonic mechanosensory afferents fall into two subpopulations based on transmitter identification. One population is cholinergic, the other is non-cholinergic and non-adrenergic (NANC). Both substance P (SP) and vasoactive intestinal peptide (VIP) are probable transmitter candidates of the NANC pathway. A more extensive review of the literature on peripheral reflexes through abdominal prevertebral ganglia and a thorough exposition of the data substantiating the physiological function of cholinergic and non-adrenergic, non-cholinergic mechanosensory afferents has been published[1].

There is very strong support for the concept that prevertebral ganglia mediate local reflexes with the gastrointestinal tract. Between 1857 and 1971, there arose suggestive evidence that abdominal prevertebral ganglia participated in peripheral reflex activity with gastrointestinal structures. Although the gastrointestinal tract was not the organ system studied, the Russian physiologist, Sokownin, found that even after decentralization of the inferior mesenteric ganglion, stimulation of the central end of a transected hypogastric nerve caused the urinary bladder to contract by an action of motor nerves in the uncut contralateral hypogastric nerve[2,3]. Sokownin's observations represent the first physiological evidence for peripheral reflex activity through prevertebral ganglia without involvement of the central nervous system. Although Langley and Anderson repeated the same experiments and obtained similar results, they suggested the reflex was pseudo-reflex involving collateral branches of bifurcating central efferent nerves[4]. Job and Lundberg, using electrophysiological techniques, established unequivocally the existence of a 'Sokownin' reflex. Using extracellular recording techniques, their results showed the existence of two populations of fibres. One population consisted of small high-threshold C-fibres. It is these fibres that form the basis of the 'Sokownin' reflex[5]. These small C-fibres escaped the attention of Lloyd who also supported Langley and Anderson's notion of a pseudo-reflex[6]. The second population of fibres consisted of lower-threshold B-fibres that bifurcate in the inferior mesenteric ganglion. These fibres are the basis of pseudo-reflex. The bifurcating fibres were of central origin, whereas the small C-fibres making up the peripheral reflex arc were of peripheral origin. Thus was born the concept that abdominal peripheral ganglia mediate local visceral reflexes. Kuntz[7] and his colleagues[8,9] provided evidence for peripheral reflexes between different regions of the gastrointestinal tract and prevertebral ganglia. In cats whose prevertebral ganglia were completely decentralized, Kuntz and his co-workers showed that distension of the distal half of a transected colon caused inhibition of the proximal half of the colon. A similar inhibitory reflex was found to occur in cats between the coeliac ganglion and segments of small intestine[9].

Peripheral reflexes between prevertebral ganglia and the motor apparatus of the gastrointestinal tract has also been demonstrated in other species including dog[10-13], guinea-pig[14-16] and mouse[17]. There are inhibitory reflexes through prevertebral ganglia between segments of large intestine of the dog and guinea-pig; between the duodenum and gastric antrum; and between segments of the small intestine. Also, distension of the rectum leads to relaxation of the ileum by way of the inferior mesenteric ganglion. The prevertebral ganglia also appear to mediate reflex activity between the gastrointestinal tract and its accessory organs[9,18] and the ganglia may also mediate mesenteric vascular reflexes[19].

Extrinsic electrophysiological recordings from all nerve trunks attached to the prevertebral ganglia reveal a complex arrangement of ascending and descending nerve pathways between the prevertebral ganglia and various regions of the gastrointestinal tract[20,21]. This extensive network provides lines of communication that form the basis for a number of gastrointestinal reflexes including the gastroileal, gastrocaecal, gastrocolonic, duodenal-jejunal, ileocaecal, colocolonic and colorectal reflexes. It must be emphasized that, although decentralized prevertebral ganglia are capable of mediating local peripheral reflexes, the ability to demonstrate such reflexes and the physiological importance of such reflexes depends upon spatiotemporal summation of central and peripheral inputs. Thus, the peripheral reflexes should not be viewed as a series of separate, physiologically distinct reflexes. Rather, they should be viewed as peripheral pathways linking near and distant regions of the gastrointestinal tract in consort with central synaptic input. The functional effect of spatial summation of central and peripheral input is to prime the prevertebral ganglion cells, thereby allowing them to adjust their firing frequency and hence modulate gastrointestinal motility (function).

CHOLINERGIC MECHANOSENSORY AFFERENT NERVES TO THE INFERIOR MESENTERIC GANGLION

The existence of local peripheral reflex activity mediated through the prevertebral ganglia received considerable support when it was shown that individual sympathetic ganglion cells receive ongoing nicotinic fast EPSPs from cholinergic mechanosensory afferents arising from the wall of the colon (Figures 1 and 2)[22,23]. Since these recordings were made from an inferior mesenteric ganglion attached to a segment of distal colon *in vitro*, the observed synaptic input could only have arisen from colonic afferents because all connections between the ganglion and other visceral structures and the CNS were severed. The colonic afferents responsible for the synaptic input are slowly adapting mechanoreceptors. Experimentally induced (Figure 2) increases in colonic intraluminal pressure[14,15,22,24,25] and spontaneous increases in colonic intraluminal pressure[26] increase the frequency of fast synaptic events. The schematic diagram in Figure 3 summarizes the proposed neural connections among colonic cholinergic mechanoreceptors, prevertebral sympathetic neurons and enteric cholinergic neurons. Since nicotinic antagonists applied to the colon markedly depress afferent synaptic input to the prevertebral ganglion (Figure 2), a cholinergic synapse is present in the enteric plexus. However, there are also direct cholinergic projections because low-level mechanosensory afferent activity remains even during nicotinic blockade (Figure 2)[22].

The anatomical basis of the peripheral reflex loop has been established. When the fluorescent marker True Blue is injected into the inferior mesenteric ganglion, ganglion cells in the myenteric plexus are labelled[27]. Occasionally, a fluorescent-labelled ganglion cell can be found in the submucous ganglia.

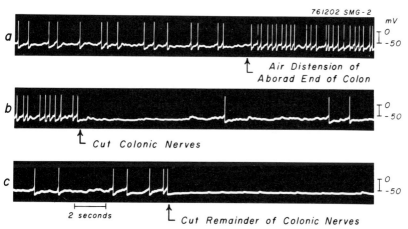

Figure 1 Excitatory synaptic input from an attached segment of distal colon to a sympathetic neuron in a guinea-pig inferior mesenteric ganglion.
(a) Distension increased frequency of firing.
(b) Most of the fibres running in the colonic nerve were cut during maintained distension.
(c) All but a single fibre was cut (from Kreulen and Szurszewski[38])

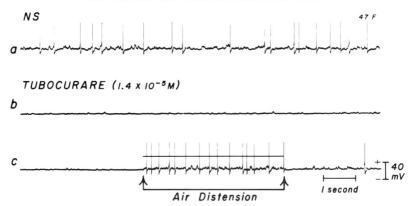

Figure 2 Effect of adding tubocurarine to the perfusate passing over a segment of colon on excitatory synaptic input to a sympathetic neuron in a guinea-pig inferior mesenteric ganglion. A two-compartment organ chamber allowed for addition of the antagonist to the solution bathing only the colon.
(a) Synaptic input when the colonic segment was bathed in normal Krebs solution.
(b) 5 min after adding tubocurarine to the colon side of the two-compartment chamber.
(c) Effect of air distension of the segment of distal colon during nicotinic blockade.
Note that tubocurarine significantly suppressed synaptic input to the ganglion indicating the existence of a cholinergic, nicotinic synapse along the mechanosensory pathway. Note also that during nicotinic blockade, distension caused an immediate increase in excitatory synaptic input suggesting that the fibres projecting out of the colonic segment to the inferior mesenteric ganglion were mechanosensory. All recordings from the same cell. Recording in panel C continuous with recording in panel B (from Szurszewski and Weems[37])

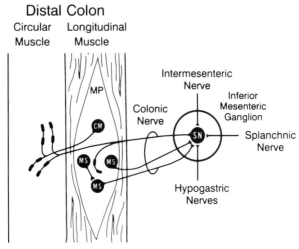

Figure 3 Schematic diagram of neural connections between the inferior mesenteric ganglion and colon of guinea pigs. CM, enteric cholinergic motor neuron; MS, enteric cholinergic mechanosensory pathway; SN, sympathetic neuron; MP, myenteric plexus. Synaptic contact between the enteric MS neurons is cholinergic nicotinic

NANC MECHANOSENSORY AFFERENT NERVES TO THE INFERIOR MESENTERIC GANGLION

In addition to cholinergic mechanosensory afferents from the colon, many sympathetic neurons in the inferior mesenteric ganglion also receive colonic afferents which are NANC. The evidence at present suggests that these afferents may utilize SP, VIP, cholecystokinins (CCK), bombesin and dynorphin as transmitters. An extensive review of the literature supporting the existence of these neuropeptides or similar substances in colonic afferent nerves making synaptic contact with sympathetic neurons in the inferior mesenteric ganglion appears elsewhere[1]. Unlike the synaptic action of acetylcholine, the time course of action of SP, VIP and CCK extends over tens of seconds (20 s to 4 min). It appears that under normal physiological conditions, the slow, longlasting depolarization which these neuropeptides produce does not by itself generate action potentials. Rather, the slow depolarization facilitates conversion of subthreshold nicotinic fast EPSPs to action potentials. Thus, the function of the slow EPSPs caused by NANC colonic afferent nerves is to modulate the amount of information transferred through the ganglion over extended periods. The slow NANC EPSP increases the synaptic efficacy of the cholinergic pathways.

Evidence is accumulating supporting the hypothesis that separate populations of colonic afferent nerves function as mechanosensory afferents, one population containing VIP and the other containing SP. The evidence supporting this hypothesis has been reviewed in detail elsewhere[1] so only a brief synopsis is provided here. With regard to VIP, a population of sympathetic neurons in the guinea-pig inferior mesenteric ganglion responds with a slow EPSP following repetitive electrical stimulation of the lumbar colonic nerve[25]. The slow EPSP is unaffected by nicotinic and muscarinic antagonists[25]. Since both desensitization to exogenously applied VIP and application of rabbit VIP antiserum (Figure 4) significantly depress the electrically induced noncholinergic slow EPSP, it appears that VIP may be a transmitter contributing to the slow NANC EPSP. The physiological significance of these results lies in the observation that radial distension of a segment of distal colon induces a slow NANC depolarization that is suppressed by VIP antiserum[25] (Figure 5). Thus, VIP or a related peptide should be considered a candidate neurotransmitter mediating colonic reflexes in the guinea-pig inferior mesenteric ganglion.

Another candidate neurotransmitter mediating colonic reflexes appears to be SP or a related peptide[28]. Increases in colonic intraluminal pressure between 2 and 20 cmH$_2$O causes a progressive increase in amplitude of the slow NANC EPSP. Capsaicin treatment *in vivo* and desensitization by high concentrations of SP decrease the number of neurons in the inferior mesenteric ganglion that exhibits NANC mechanosensory responses[28] (Figure 6) and also attenuates the amplitude of the slow EPSP.

Direct evidence for release of SP or a closely related peptide in the inferior mesenteric ganglion in response to colonic distension has recently been reported in abstract form[29]. Using electrophysiological and radioimmunological techniques, it was reported that NANC slow EPSPs induced by colonic

247

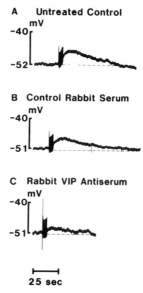

A Untreated Control

B Control Rabbit Serum

C Rabbit VIP Antiserum

├────┤
25 sec

Figure 4 Effect of VIP antiserum on a noncholinergic slow EPSP recorded from a sympathetic ganglion cell in a guinea pig inferior mesenteric ganglion. Hexamethonium (2×10^{-4} M) and atropine (2×10^{-6} M) were present throughout to block nicotinic and muscarinic receptors, respectively. **A**: Repetitive electrical stimulation of the lumbar colonic nerve (20 Hz, 4 s) evoked a noncholinergic slow EPSP which was 4 mV in amplitude. **B**: During application of rabbit antiserum by pressure ejections for 2 min, the slow EPSP was 4.5 mV in amplitude. **C**: The amplitude of the slow EPSP was reduced to 2 mV during pressure ejection of rabbit VIP antiserum. All recordings made from the same cell (from Love and Szurszewski[25])

distension were associated with an increase in SP-like immunoreactivity in the superfusate which passed over the inferior mesenteric ganglion. Colonic distension significantly increased the SP-like immunoreactivity from a basal level of 268 ± 175 pg/ml to 593 ± 324 pg/ml. The SP-like material released by colonic distension co-eluted with synthetic porcine SP on HPLC.

Lack of complete abolition by capsaicin of distension-induced depolarizing responses and lack of complete suppression by desensitization to SP indicate that SP is but one of a number of putative peptide neurotransmitters for the NANC mechanosensory depolarization. As mentioned above, VIP should also be considered a strong candidate.

The SP-containing terminals in the prevertebral ganglia represent axon collaterals of primary afferent visceral sensory neurons that traverse the ganglia on their way from visceral structures to the spinal ganglia[30,31]. Retrograde transport of True Blue dye, combined with immunocytochemical localization of SP indicate that the majority of SP-containing fibres are unmyelinated primary afferents with their cell bodies located in thoracic (T_6 to T_{12}) and lumbar (L_2 and L_3) dorsal root ganglia[32-34]. Since capsaicin treatment depletes the inferior mesenteric ganglion of immunoreactive SP material[35,36] and since it significantly attenuates colonic induced slow depolarization, the intriguing possibility arises that the SP pathway mediates

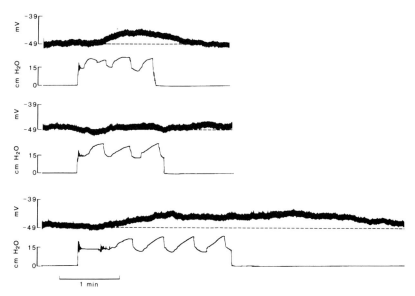

Figure 5 Effect of VIP antiserum on a slow depolarization evoked by distension of an attached segment of distal colon. Throughout the experiment hexamethonium (2×10^{-4} M) and atropine (2×10^{-6} M) were present in the Krebs solution bathing only the inferior mesenteric ganglion. The upper trace in all three panels represents intracellular recording from a sympathetic ganglion cell. The bottom trace in all three panels represents colonic intraluminal pressure. **A**: Colonic distension evoked a 4 mV slow depolarization. **B**: Pressure ejection of rabbit VIP antiserum onto the neuron greatly attenuated the distension-induced depolarization. **C**: Two minutes after wash-out of the antiserum, colonic distension evoked a slow depolarization that was 5 mV in amplitude. All recordings taken from the same neuron (from Love and Szurszewski[25].)

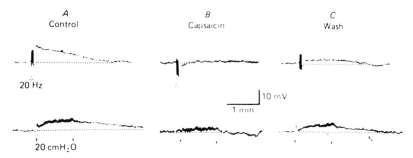

Figure 6 Effect of capsaicin on noncholinergic slow EPSPs in a sympathetic neuron in a guinea pig inferior mesenteric ganglion. In the upper trace in panels A, B and C, supramaximal stimulation of both hypogastric nerves caused a slow EPSP. The lower trace in all three panels is the response to distension of a segment of attached distal colon. Note, in panel B, that 10 min after adding capsaicin both the electrically evoked slow EPSP (upper trace) and the distension-induced slow depolarization (lower trace) were abolished and significantly attenuated, respectively (from Kreulen and Peters[28])

249

both mechanosensory and nociceptive information. It is reasonable to hypothesize that mechanosensory information can be modulated separately in the inferior mesenteric ganglion from information referred to the CNS.

SUMMARY AND CONCLUSIONS

Prevertebral ganglia should no longer be considered relay and distributing stations. Experimental evidence supports the hypothesis that prevertebral ganglionic neurons participate in peripheral reflexes, integrate synaptic messages arriving from a variety of sources and utilize several neurotransmitters. Colonic mechanosensory neurons projecting to the inferior mesenteric ganglion are cholinergic and peptidergic (Figure 7). The prevertebral ganglia are far more complex than hitherto believed and future experimentations are likely to uncover even greater complexity.

Acknowledgements

I wish to thank the many colleagues who worked in my laboratory making the observations reported on in this chapter. In particular, David Kreulen, Jacob Krier, Jeffrey Love, Wolf Stapelfeldt and William Weems. I am grateful to Jan Applequist for her highly skilled assistance in the preparation of this manuscript and to Philip Schmalz for collaboration in some of the experiments. I am especially grateful to the National Institutes of Health

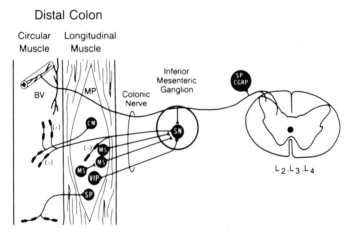

Figure 7 Schematic diagram of cholinergic mechanosensory, SP and VIP mechanosensory afferent pathways projecting to sympathetic neurons in the guinea pig inferior mesenteric ganglion. Note that of the two SP pathways shown, only the central pathway consisting of axon collaterals to cells in the inferior mesenteric ganglion is proposed as being mechanosensory to the prevertebral ganglion. SP, substance P; CGRP, calcitonin gene-related peptide; L_2, L_3, L_4, second to fourth regions of the lumbar spinal cord; SN, sympathetic neuron; MS, cholinergic enteric mechanosensory neurons; CM, enteric cholinergic motor neuron; MP, myenteric plexus; BV, blood vessel

and National Institute of Digestive Diseases and Kidney for support through Public Health Service Grant DK 17632.

References

1. King, B.F. and Szurszewski, J.H. (1988). Physiology of prevertebral ganglia in mammals with special reference to inferior mesenteric ganglion. In Wood, J. (ed.) *Handbook of Gastrointestinal Physiology*. Vol. 4, pp. – . (Baltimore: American Physiological Society) (In press)
2. Sokownin, N. Cited by Kowalesky, N. and Arnstein, C. (1874). *Pfluegers Arch.*, **8**, 600
3. Sokownin, N.M. (1877). Materials for the physiology of micturition and ischuria. *Izu. Nauch. Zap. Imper. Kazan Univ.*, **44**, 1243–83
4. Langley, J.N. and Anderson, H.K. (1894). On reflex action from sympathetic ganglia. *J. Physiol. (Lond.)*, **16**, 410–40
5. Job, C. and Lundberg, A. (1952). Reflex excitation of cells in the inferior mesenteric ganglion on stimulation of the hypogastric nerve. *Acta Physiol. Scand.*, **26**, 366–82
6. Lloyd, D.P.C. (1937). The transmission of impulses through the inferior mesenteric ganglia. *J. Physiol. (Lond.)*, **91**, 296–313
7. Kuntz, A. (1940). The structural organization of the inferior mesenteric ganglia. *J. Comp. Neurol.*, **72**, 371–82
8. Kuntz, A. and Saccamanno, G. (1944). Reflex inhibition of intestinal motility mediated through decentralized prevertebral ganglia. *J. Neurophysiol.*, **7**, 163–70
9. Kuntz, A. and Van Buskirk, C. (1941). Reflex inhibition of bile flow and intestinal motility mediated through decentralized coeliac plexus. *Proc. Soc. Exp. Biol. Med.*, **46**, 519–23
10. Semba, T. (1954). Intestino-intestinal inhibitory reflexes. *Jpn. J. Physiol.*, **4**, 241–5
11. Semba, T. (1954). Studies on the entero-gastric reflexes. *Hiroshima J. Med. Sci.*, **2**, 323–7
12. Shapiro, H. and Woodward, E.R. (1955). Inhibition of gastric motility by acid in the duodenum. *J. Appl. Physiol.*, **8**, 121–7
13. Schapiro, H. and Woodward, E.R. (1959). Pathway of enterogastric reflex. *Proc. Soc. Exp. Biol. Med.*, **101**, 407–9
14. Kreulen, D.L. and Szurszewski, J.H. (1979). Nerve pathways in celiac plexus of the guinea pig. *Am. J. Physiol.*, **237**, E90–7
15. Kreulen, D.L. and Szurszewski, J.H. (1979). Reflex pathways in the abdominal prevertebral ganglia: evidence for a colo-colonic inhibitory reflex. *J. Physiol. Lond.*, **295**, 21–32
16. Kreulen, D.L., Muir, T.C. and Szurszewski, J.H. (1983). Peripheral sympathetic pathways to gastroduodenal region of the guinea pig. *Am. J. Physiol.*, **245**, (*Gastrointest. Liver Physiol.*, **8**), G369–75
17. Miller, S.M. and Szurszewski, J.H. (1987). Colonic mechanosensory input to the superior mesenteric ganglion in the mouse. *Physiologist*, **30**, 214
18. Warkentin, J., Huston, J.H., Preston, F.W. and Ivy, A.C. (1943). The mechanism of bile flow inhibition upon distension of the colon or stimulation of its nerve supply. *Am. J. Physiol.*, **138**, 462–4
19. Keef, K.D. and Kreulen, D.L. (1986). Venous mechanoreceptor input to neurones in the inferior mesenteric ganglion of the guinea-pig. *J. Physiol. (Lond.)*, **377**, 49–59
20. Davison, J.S. and Hersteinsson, P. (1975). Functional organization of the guinea-pig inferior mesenteric ganglion. *J. Physiol. Lond.*, **250**, 27P–28P
21. King, B.F. and Szurszewski, J.H. (1988). Peripheral reflex pathways involving abdominal viscera. The transmission of impulses through prevertebral ganglia in guinea pig. *Am. J. Physiol.* (Submitted)
22. Crowcroft, P.J., Holman, M.E. and Szurszewski, J.H. (1971). Excitatory input from the distal colon to the inferior mesenteric ganglion in the guinea-pig. *J. Physiol. (Lond.)*, **219**, 443–61
23. Dick, E. and Miller, R.F. (1981). Peptides influence retinal ganglion cells. *Neurosci. Lett.*, **26**, 131–5
24. Kreulen, D.L. and Szurszewski, J.H. (1979). Electrophysiological and morphological basis for organization of neurons in prevertebral ganglia. In Janowitz, H.D. and Sachar, D.B.

(eds.) *Frontiers of Knowledge in the Diarrheal Diseases: International Colloquium in Gastroenterology*, pp. 211–26. (Upper Montclair, NJ: Projects in Health)

25. Love, J.A. and Szurszewski, J.H. (1987). The electrophysiological effects of vasoactive intestinal polypeptide in the guinea-pig inferior mesenteric ganglion. *J. Physiol. (Lond.)*, **394**, 67–84

26. Weems, W.A. and Szurszewski, J.H. (1977). Modulation of colonic motility by peripheral neural inputs to neurons of the inferior mesenteric ganglion. *Gastroenterology*, **73**, 273–8

27. Dalsgaard, C.-J. and Elfvin, L.-G. (1982). Structural studies on the connectivity of the inferior mesenteric ganglion of the guinea pig. *J. Autonom. Nerv. Syst.*, **5**, 265–78

28. Kreulen, D.L. and Peters, S. (1986). Non-cholinergic transmission in a sympathetic ganglion of the guinea-pig elicited by colon distension. *J. Physiol. (Lond.)*, **374**, 315–34

29. Stapelfeldt, W.H., Go, V.L.W. and Szurszewski, J.H. (1988). Colonic distension releases substance P in the guinea pig inferior mesenteric ganglion. *Gastroenterology*, **94**, A441

30. Matthews, M.R. and Cuello, A.C. (1982). Substance-P immunoreactive peripheral branches of sensory neurons innervate guinea-pig sympathetic neurons. *Proc. Natl. Acad. Sci. USA*, **79**, 1668–72

31. Tsunoo, A., Konishi, S. and Otsuka, M. (1982). Substance P as an excitatory transmitter of primary afferent neurons in guinea-pig sympathetic ganglia. *Neuroscience*, **7**, 2025–37

32. Dalsgaard, C.-J., Hökfelt, T., Elfvin, L.-G., Skirboll, L. and Emson, P. (1982). Substance-P containing primary sensory neurons projecting to the inferior mesenteric ganglion: evidence from combined retrograde tracing and immunohistochemistry. *Neuroscience*, **7**, 647–54

33. Hökfeldt, T., Elde, R.P., Johansson, O., Luft, R., Nilsson, G. and Arimura, A. (1976). Immunohistochemical evidence for separate populations of somatostatin-containing and substance P-containing primary afferent neurons in the rat. *Neuroscience*, **1**, 131–6

34. Léránth, C. and Féher, ? (1983). Synaptology and sources of vasoactive intestinal polypeptide and substance P containing axons of the cat coeliac ganglion. An experimental electron microscopic immunohistochemical study. *Neuroscience*, **10**, 947–58

35. Gamse, R.A., Wax, A., Zigmond, R.E. and Leeman, S.E. (1981). Immunoreactive substance P in sympathetic ganglia: distribution and sensitivity toward capsaicin. *Neuroscience*, **6**, 437–41

36. Holzer, P., Bucsics, A. and Lembeck, F. (1982). Distribution of capsaicin-sensitive nerve fibres containing immunoreactive substance P in cutaneous and visceral tissues of the rat. *Neurosci. Lett.*, **31**, 253–7

37. Szurszewski, J.H. and Weems, W.A. (1976). A study of peripheral input to and its control by post-ganglionic neurones of the inferior mesenteric ganglion. *J. Physiol. (Lond.)*, **256**, 541–56

38. Kreulen, D.L. and Szurszewski, J.H. (1979). Nerve pathways in celiac plexus of the guinea pig. *Am. J. Physiol.*, **237**, E90–7

21
Synaptic transmission in neurons of the submucous plexus

A. SURPRENANT

INTRODUCTION

The submucous plexus of the guinea-pig ileum has been favoured by electrophysiologists as an ideal preparation in which to study transmitter actions on submucosal neurons. A glance down the dissecting microscope immediately reveals some of the main reasons for this choice. The underlying mucosa and overlying circular smooth muscle and myenteric plexus layer easily pull away, leaving a muscle-free sheath of connective tissue which contains the submucous neurons with their interconnecting nerve fibres and the submucosal vasculature. Such a preparation is free of mechanical barriers such as muscle movements, thereby allowing long-term, stable intracellular recordings to be made from the submucous neurons. There are virtually no diffusion barriers in this very thin preparation (the total thickness of this connective tissue sheath with blood vessels and neurons is less than 15 μm); thus, drugs and transmitter substances can be applied precisely and interpretations of pharmacological results are much simplified. In addition, a detailed knowledge of the anatomical and immunohistochemical projections to and from these neurons is available[1] as well as a considerable body of information regarding the actions of these nerves on intestinal mucosa, which is one of their primary effector tissues[2,3].

There are four main synaptic functions associated with submucosal neurons; three of these are post-synaptic and one is presynaptic. Post-synaptic functions are fast excitatory transmissions, inhibitory synaptic transmission and slow excitatory transmission. On the other side of the synapse, a fourth major function of these neurons appears to be inhibition of transmitter release via activation of presynaptic receptors. The aim of this chapter is to describe briefly what is known about the mechanisms of these forms of transmission, the sources of the transmitters and the types of receptors present on the post-synaptic membranes of nerve fibres in the submucous plexus of the guinea-pig ileum.

253

FAST EXCITATORY TRANSMISSION

The classical nicotinic response is recorded by an intracellular microelectrode from over 90% of all submucous neurons when acetylcholine is applied by ionophoresis or pressure-ejection (Figure 1A), or when it is released from nerve fibres in response to stimulation of the interconnecting nerve fibres (Figure 1C). The synaptically mediated nicotinic response, the first synaptic potential (fEPSP), is a brief depolarization lasting about 30–60 ms caused by a transient increase in the membrane conductance for cations, mainly sodium, as well as potassium and calcium. It is blocked by the traditional nicotinic blockers such as hexamethonium and curare. Additionally, an identical depolarization is produced in all the same cells by ionophoresis of 5-HT[4,5,6]; this fast depolarization is reversibly blocked by ICS 205-930, the 5-HT$_3$ receptor antagonist (Figure 1B). Hexamethonium does not block this 5-HT$_3$ depolarization nor does ICS 205-930 alter the nicotinic depolarization, although curare blocks both responses[6]. While both of these responses can be recorded in all of the same cells, the fEPSP seems only to be nicotinic in that no ICS 205-930 sensitive fEPSP has been described. However, because cholinergic projections outnumber 5-HT ones by many thousand-fold, it remains a distinct possibility that, if a means for selectively stimulating 5-HT fibres were to be found, a 5-HT$_3$-mediated fEPSP might be discovered.

How many cholinergic fibres innervate a single submucous neuron? The experiment illustrated in Figure 2A indicates how it is possible to determine the minimum number of functional cholinergic fibres projecting onto a single

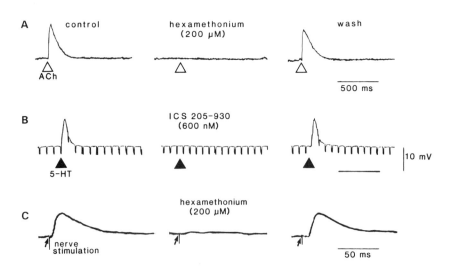

Figure 1 Nicotinic depolarizations (upper row), 5-HT$_3$ depolarizations (middle row) and fEPSPs (lower row) recorded from a submucous plexus neuron. Arrowheads in upper and middle represent pressure-ejection pulses (single 5 ms duration pulse) of acetylcholine and 5-HT respectively. Curare can abolish all of these responses; hexamethonium but not ICS 205-930 blocks both the nicotinic depolarization and the fEPSP

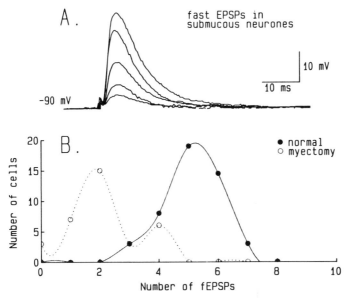

Figure 2 A: fast EPSPs recorded from one submucous plexus neuron in response to increasing stimulus intensity pulses applied to one interconnecting fibre tract. Each trace is the average of 10 identical stimuli delivered at a frequency of 0.1 Hz and so individual fluctuations in EPSP amplitude are obviated. In this particular experiment, five distinct cholinergic fibres can be distinguished as impinging onto this submucous neuron. Note that the membrane potential is artificially held at a very hyperpolarized level (-90 mV) so as to prevent initiation of action potentials from the larger EPSPs. **B**: Data taken from Bornstein, Furness and Costa[8]; these experiments show that approximately half of the cholinergic input impinging onto submucous neurons is derived from myenteric neurons (see text fur further description)

neuron. When single stimuli of increasing intensity are applied onto the interconnecting nerve strands, stepwise increases in fEPSP amplitude are recorded. These steps have been shown to correspond to recruitment of individual cholinergic fibres[7]. From experiments of this type we have estimated that a minimum average number of cholinergic fibres impinging onto one submucous neuron is about 7 (7.28 $\pm$ 0.9; $n = 14$).

What is or are the sources of this (nicotinic) cholinergic input? The Flinders group (Adelaide, South Australia) have investigated this question by carrying out similar experiments to those illustrated in Figure 2A in normal guinea-pigs and in guinea-pigs in which the overlying myenteric plexus had been removed[8]. The rationale behind this type of surgical denervation is that cholinergic cell bodies (i.e. ChAT-immunoreactive soma) are present in both the myenteric and the submucous plexus[1]; however it has not been possible to demonstrate ChAT-immunoreactive nerve terminals. Thus, immunohisto-chemical studies have not been able directly to determine the source of the nicotic input onto submucous neurons. On the other hand, electrophysiolog-ical characterization of the number of distinct fEPSPs combined with removal of the only source of cholinergic fibres other than submucous neurons could provide this information. Figure 2B illustrates some of the pertinent results of that study. In control animals, most of the submucous neurons showed about five to six cholinergic fibres, while in the myectomized animals generally only two to three fibres could be discerned. This means that about half the cholinergic fibres projecting onto submucous neurons originate from myenteric neurons; the other half almost certainly being the cholinergic interneurons in the submucous plexus itself. It should be noted in this regard that no vagal fibres have been observed in the submucous plexus of the guinea-pig ileum, although they can be seen to project onto a small proportion of ileal myenteric neurons (A. Kirchgessner and M.D. Gershon, unpublished).

INHIBITORY SYNAPTIC TRANSMISSION

Inhibitory synaptic potentials (IPSPs) are recorded from all VIP-containing submucous neurons[17]. The IPSPs can be considered one of the strongest forms of synaptic input onto submucous neurons; the marked decrease in membrane resistance which accompanies the IPSP and the very large (hyperpolarizing) amplitude of this synaptic response almost guarantees blockade of action potential initiation or transmission during its time course of action. It has recently become clear that there are two distinct IPSPs present in submucous neurons: in one case the source of and transmitter responsible for the IPSP has been directly determined; in the other the source has been directly demonstrated and the responsible transmitter indirectly implicated.

The adrenergic IPSP

Three decades after von Euler received the Nobel Prize for his work in establishing noradrenaline as a neurotransmitter, the only synaptic potential which has been unequivocally established as being due to noradrenaline released from sympathetic nerves is the adrenergic inhibitory synaptic potential (aIPSP) in submucous plexus neurons. In addition to the biochemical and histochemical evidence for the presence, synthesis and release of sympathetically derived noradrenaline onto submucous neurons[1], the solid physiological evidence is as follows.

Mimicry
The aIPSP is a membrane hyperpolarization lasting approximately 1 s following a latency of 45–100 ms after application of a single nerve stimulus and it results from an increased membrane conductance to potassium ions[4,9]. The specific potassium conductance which underlies the aIPSP is one which shows all the properties of the classical, voltage-dependent, 'inwardly rectifying' potassium conductance; activation of this potassium conductance (and appearance of the aIPSP) requires the presence of a pertussis-toxin sensitive GTP-binding protein[9]. Finally, the catecholamine uptake inhibitor,

neurons which produce membrane hyperpolarizations: noradrenaline, soma-tostatin and opiates[1,4,9,11,12]. Each of these substances hyperpolarizes the neuronal membrane by increasing the same G-protein dependent, inwardly rectifying, potassium conductance that underlies the aIPSP[9,11]. However, only noradrenaline can precisely mimic the time course of the aIPSP and cocaine enhances the (exogenously applied) noradrenaline response but neither the somatostatin nor the opiate, response[9,10,13].

Selective antagonism

The aIPSP is selectively abolished by the α_2-adrenoceptor antagonists yohimbine, phentolamine and idazoxan, as is the noradrenaline-evoked hyperpolarization[8,13,14]. These α_2-adrenoceptor antagonists do not alter the hyperpolarizations produced by somatostatin or opiates and the aIPSP and noradrenaline potentials are not altered by a variety of other receptor antagonists, such as α_1- and β-adrenoceptor, cholinergic, dopaminergic, serotonergic and opiate receptor antagonists[9,11,13,14]. Moreover, all catecho-lamine-containing nerve fibres in the submucous plexus disappear after selective sympathetic denervation[1,15] and no aIPSPs can be observed[8,13].

Selective stimulation

Figure 3 illustrates the arrangement of the preparation and stimulating electrodes that allows selective stimulation of the sympathetic nerves to the submucous plexus. This method of selective sympathetic stimulation elicits aIPSPs in the submucous neuron (Figure 3, upper recording) but not the EPSPs which are always associated with focal stimulation of the interganglionic connectives (Figure 3, lower recording). The IPSP recorded from submucous neurons using this method of stimulation is blocked by α_2-

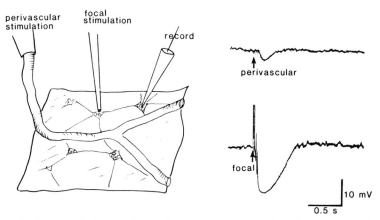

Figure 3 Experiment showing the results of selective stimulation of the sympathetic nerve supply to submucous neurons. Perivascular stimulation selectively activates sympathetic fibres; this type of stimulation evokes an adrenergic IPSP without evidence of fast or slow EPSPs. Focal stimulation activates myriad nerve fibres in the submucous plexus; this type of stimulation evokes the typical sequence of synaptic potentials: fEPSP followed by aIPSP followed by sEPSP

adrenoceptor antagonists. No IPSP has been recorded when using this method of stimulation on a submucous plexus preparation which has been sympathectomized (Surprenant, unpublished observations).

The ability to stimulate a chemically distinct set of nerve fibres in the intestine is currently a feature uniquely of the sympathetic nerves.

The non-adrenergic, non-cholinergic IPSP

Hirst originally described an IPSP which could be recorded in submucous plexus neurons after sympathectomy[16]. More recently it has been shown that this IPSP is not altered by adrenergic or cholinergic blocking agents[8,11] and, therefore, in keeping with the most often used nomenclature, it seems reasonable to refer to it as the nancIPSP until the transmitter responsible for it has been directly determined.

Unlike the adrenergic IPSP, the nancIPSP is only occasionally observed when a single nerve stimulus is applied (e.g. Figure 4). The time course of the nancIPSP evoked by multiple stimuli is generally some 10–100 times slower than the aIPSP, most often showing a biphasic time course (Figure 4)[8,18]. The underlying ionic mechanism is identical to that of the aIPSP, i.e. an increased membrane conductance to potassium ions, the potassium conductance being a G-protein dependent, inwardly rectifying, type.

Of the many receptor blocking agents examined, none has been found capable of inhibiting the nancIPSP[8,18,19]. Importantly, the opiate receptor antagonist, naloxone, does not alter the nancIPSP, thus providing rather strong evidence against an opiate peptide as the transmitter underlying this synaptic potential.

Somatostatin would therefore seem to be the most likely candidate as the transmitter of this nancIPSP, if only on the basis of exclusion of noradrenaline and opiates. In fact, there is a stronger basis than simple exclusion for suspecting somatostatin as the transmitter substance. The Flinders group has found that no IPSPs can be recorded from submucous plexus neurons after a myectomy has been performed in addition to extrinsic sympathetic denervation[19]. These surgical denervations result in a complete loss of somatostatin-containing nerve terminals in the submucous plexus[1]. This study also shows that the fibres giving rise to the transmitter which mediates the nancIPSP in submucous neurons must arise from myenteric cell bodies.

SLOW EXCITATORY SYNAPTIC TRANSMISSION

At least 90% of all submucous neurons show a slow depolarization, the sEPSP, when the nerve fibres are stimulated with single or multiple pulses (Figure 5). Many substances, including SP, VIP, CGRP, muscarine, 5-HT, neurotensin, CCK and GRP, are capable of mimicking the sEPSP in time course and ionic mechanism (e.g. Figure 5); the depolarization appears to be due to a decrease in an ill-defined potassium conductance[14,20,21]. However, there is no solid evidence to implicate any one of these substances as a

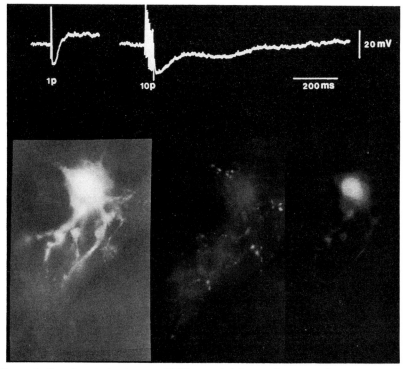

Figure 4 Experiment showing nancIPSP recorded from submucous plexus neuron after extrinsic sympathectomy. Note the biphasic nature of the nancIPSP evoked by multiple stimuli. The neuron from which the recordings of the nancIPSPs was made was also filled with Lucifer Yellow (left photograph) and the preparation was then prepared for tyrosine hydroxylase (TH) immunostaining (right photograph); the absence of TH-immunostaining confirms the success of the sympathetic denervation (reproduced with permission from reference 19 and, with permission, from unpublished results of J. C. Bornstein)

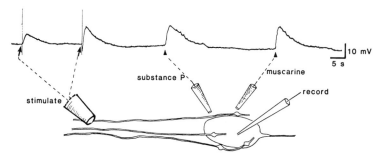

Figure 5 Example of responses to nerve stimulation and local pressure-ejection pulses of substance P or muscarine recorded from a submucous plexus neuron. Synaptic potentials were evoked by single and multiple (3 pulses at 20 s) stimuli; both stimuli evoked sEPSPs (in addition to fEPSPs; idazoxan was present to block the aIPSP). Very similar depolarizations were produced by 'puffs' (single 5 ms duration pulse) of SP or muscarine

transmitter. Indeed, until means for selective stimulation of specific fibres becomes available, it may well be impossible directly to determine a transmitter role for any of these substances, even if selective receptor antagonists were available for all of these substances. There are several reasons for this.

First, unlike fEPSPs, sEPSPs seldom show stepwise increases in their amplitude upon increasing intensity of single stimuli, thus making it impossible to estimate the number of fibres giving rise to the recorded response and, additionally, making it unlikely that the sEPSP is due to release of transmitter from one or a few discrete fibres. Secondly, unlike the aIPSP and nancIPSP, there are few consistent differences in the time courses of sEPSPs recorded from S type submucous neurons, thus making it unlikely that removal of a distinct input, either by selective lesioning or development of a specific receptor antagonist, would reveal a separable component to the sEPSP. Thirdly, all the substances listed above appear to close the same set of potassium channels in the membrane (references 6,14,21 and Shen and Surprenant, unpublished results). What this means is that if, as is likely, the *in vitro* method of nerve stimulation releases many of these peptides, then one could, for example, remove any 9 out of 10 of these peptide inputs and not expect markedly to alter the amplitude or time course of the nerve-evoked sEPSP. It is now clear from electrophysiologic experiments and from immunohistochemical mapping studies that it is naive to assume that the sEPSP in each submucous neuron results from the release of one, or even a few, primary transmitter substances.

Although we know much less about the sEPSP than we do about the fEPSPs or IPSPs, there is one consistently observed feature of the sEPSP and of the responses to SP, VIP, muscarine and 5-HT which may be of considerable physiological significance. Studies of the current–voltage relationships obtained for the inward current recorded in response to applications of SP, muscarine and 5-HT as well as for the sEPSP suggest that the potassium conductance decrease underlying all of these responses occurs at a site distant from the microelectrode recording site, presumably at dendritic locations[6,20,22]. The experiment illustrated in Figure 6 also suggests this.

An ionophoretic electrode was filled with 5-HT; ionophoresis releases small amounts of 5-HT over an extremely localized area. A blunter microelectrode (labelled 'puff) was also filled with 5-HT; pressure-ejection releases small amounts of 5-HT over a relatively diffuse area. In situation 1, the ionophoretic electrode was placed within 2–5 μm of the cell surface; an ionophoretic pulse evoked a brief depolarization which was abolished by the 5-HT$_3$ receptor antagonist, ICS 205-930. No other 5-HT response could then be evoked even with very much larger ionophoretic pulses. The ionophoretic pipette was then moved several microns away from the cell soma; the ionophoretic pulse now produced a very slow depolarization which was not altered by ICS 205-930. Finally, pressure-ejection of 5-HT (labelled 3) evoked a brief depolarization followed by a much longer-lasting depolarization. In this case the fast depolarization, but not the slow depolarization, was blocked by ICS 205-930. The functional consequences of receptors mediating the sEPSP

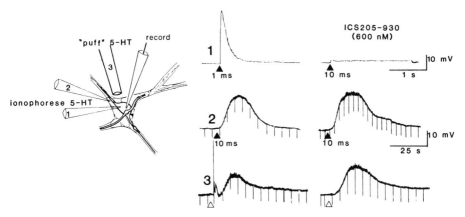

Figure 6 Experiment showing differential responses to application of 5-HT at various sites in the vicinity of the impaled neuron. Schematic illustrates the experiment, voltage recordings show the results. **1**: Brief depolarization produced by ionophoresis of 5-HT close to the cell soma; only the 5-HT$_3$ mediated depolarization could be evoked (even when the duration of the ionophoretic pulse was increased to 200 ms; data not shown). **2**: The ionophoretic pipette was moved some distance away from the soma and a 10 ms duration pulse of 5-HT produced a slow depolarization which was unaltered by the 5-HT$_3$ blocker. **3**: Pressure-ejection (single 10 ms duration pulse) of 5-HT produced both components of the 5-HT depolarization, the initial component being blocked by 5-HT$_3$ receptor blockade. Left row of responses in 1–3 were obtained in the absence of, while right row of responses were obtained in the presence of, ICS 205-930

being localized to the dendritic regions would be to enhance transmission through the dendrites, thus ensuring spread of otherwise subthreshold excitatory events into the cell soma.

SUMMARY

The main function of intestinal mucosa is to maintain water and electrolyte homeostasis, by absorbing sodium, chloride and other ions from the luminal surface or by secreting chloride and other ions into the intestinal lumen. Activation of submucous neurons can alter secretory and absorptive processes of the intestinal mucosa[2,3]. The nicotinic input is most likely the primary form of final excitation onto its efferent projection, the mucosa, both through direct nicotinic excitation of the secretomotor neurons and through nicotinic excitation of the interneurons. Here, cholinergic neurons of the myenteric plexus also play a major role, as much of the cholinergic input onto submucous neurons derives from myenteric neurons. In the body, in most species, there is normally a net absorptive state; much of this net absorption is due to the dominating sympathetic tone. It is likely that a significant proportion of this tonic inhibitory transmission is the result of α_2-adrenocept-or-mediated IPSPs keeping the submucous plexus neurons hyperpolarized below threshold for action potential initiation. It also seems probable that, under some circumstances, perhaps as a result of sympathetic neuropathy, another type of inhibitory transmission in the form of the nancIPSP may take over the role of maintaining submucous neurons under tonic inhibition. This nancIPSP derives from the myenteric plexus and it is highly possible that the transmitter may be somatostatin.

The physiological relevance of the sEPSP is less clear but is most likely operative under conditions of extended or excessive secretory activity where it would function to enhance cholinergic transmission throughout the ganglia and its efferent projections, as well as to release secretomotor transmitters on to mucosal receptors.

Acknowledgements

Unpublished work reported in this chapter supported by US Department of Health and Human Services grant NS25996.

References

1. Furness, J.B. and Costa, M. (1987). *The Enteric Nervous System.* (New York: Churchill Livingstone)
2. Keast, J. (1987). Mucosal innervation and control of water and ion transport in the intestine. *Rev. Physiol. Biochem. Pharmacol.,* **109**, 1–59
3. Cooke, H. (1986). Neurobiology of the intestinal mucosa. *Gastroenterology,* **90**, 1057–81
4. Hirst, G.D.S. and McKirdy, H.C. (1975). Synaptic potentials recorded from neurones of the submucous plexus of guinea pig small intestine. *J. Physiol.,* **249**, 369–85
5. Neild, T.O. (1978). The action of 5-hydroxytryptamine and possible 5-hydroxytryptamine antagonists on neurones of the guinea-pig submucous plexus. *Gen. Pharmacol.,* **12**, 281–4
6. Surprenant, A. and Crist, J. (1988). Electrophysiological characterization of functionally distinct 5-hydroxytryptamine receptors on guinea-pig submucous plexus. *Neuroscience,* **24**, 283–95
7. Shok, V.I. (1973). *Physiology of Autonomic Ganglia.* (Tokyo: Igaku Shoin)
8. Bornstein, J.C., Furness, J.B. and Costa, M. (1987). Sources of excitatory synaptic inputs to neurochemically identified submucous neurons of guinea-pig small intestine. *J. Autonom. Nerv. Sys.,* **18**, 83–91
9. Surprenant, A. and North, R.A. (1988). Mechanism of synaptic inhibition by noradrenaline acting at α_2-adrenoceptors. *Proc. R. Soc. Lond. B.* (In press)
10. Surprenant, A. and Williams, J.T. (1987). Inhibitory synaptic potentials recorded from mammalian neurones prolonged by blockade of noradrenaline uptake. *J. Physiol.,* **382**, 87–103
11. Mihara, S., North, R.A. and Surprenant, A. (1987). Somatostatin increases an inwardly rectifying potassium conductance in guinea-pig submucous plexus neurones. *J. Physiol.,* **390**, 335–55
12. Mihara, S. and North, R.A. (1986). Opioids increase potassium conductance in guinea-pig caecum submucous neurones by activating δ-receptors. *Br. J. Pharmacol.,* **88**, 315–22
13. North, R.A. and Surprenant, A. (1985). Inhibitory synaptic potentials resulting from α_2-adrenoceptor activation in guinea-pig submucous plexus neurones. *J. Physiol.,* **358**, 17–33
14. Mihara, S., Katayama, Y. and Nishi, S. (1986). Slow postsynaptic potentials in neurones of the submucous plexus of guinea-pig caecum and their mimickry by noradrenaline and various peptides. *Neuroscience,* **16**, 1057–66
15. Furness, J.B. and Costa, M. (1978). Distribution of intrinsic nerve cell bodies and axons which take up aromatic amines and their precursors in the small intestine of the guinea-pig. *Cell Tissue Res.,* **188**, 527–43
16. Hirst, G.D.S. and Silinsky, E.M. (1975). Some effects of 5-hydroxytryptamine, dopamine and noradrenaline on neurones in the submucous plexus of guinea-pig small intestine.

J. Physiol., **251**, 817–32

17. Bornstein, J.C., Costa, M. and Furness, J.B. (1986). Synaptic inputs to immunohistochem-ically identified neurones in the submucous plexus of the guinea-pig small intestine. *J. Physiol.*, **381**, 465–82

18. Mihara, S., Nishi, S., North, R.A. and Surprenant, A. (1987). A non-adrenergic, non-cholinergic slow inhibitory postsynaptic potential in neurones of the guinea-pig submucous plexus. *J. Physiol.*, **390**, 357–65

19. Bornstein, J.C., Costa, M. and Furness, J.B. (1988). Intrinsic and extrinsic inhibitory synaptic inputs to submucous neurones of the guinea-pig small intestine. *J. Physiol.*, **398**, 371–90

20. Surprenant, A. (1984). Slow excitatory synaptic potentials recorded from neurones of guinea-pig submucous plexus. *J. Physiol.*, **351**, 343–61

21. Surprenant, A., North, R.A. and Katayama, Y. (1987). Observations on the actions of substance P and [D-Arg^1,D-Pro^2,D- Trp^{7,9},Leu^{11}] substance P on single neurons of the guinea pig submucous plexus. *Neuroscience*, **20**, 189–99

22. Shen, K-Z. and Surprenant, A. (1988). Properties of the potassium conductance decreased by real and putative neurotransmitters in submucous plexus neurones. *Soc. Neurosci. Abstr.* **14**, 111–16

22
Neuroeffector relations in the intestinal mucosa *in vitro*

H. J. COOKE

Maintenance of body fluid homeostasis is governed by the efficiency of transport of solutes and water by the gastrointestinal epithelium. More than 95% of the fluid and solutes which are ingested in the diet or which reach the intestinal lumen as a result of salivary, gastric, biliary, pancreatic and intestinal secretion is absorbed, and only a small fraction is excreted. The net movement of ions and water across the mucosal lining is dependent on opposing processes in two cell populations distinguished by their inherent transport properties. Thus, absorption occurs in the villous cells of the small intestine and surface cells of the colon, whereas secretion occurs in the crypt cells of both the small and large intestine[1].

The transport function of intestinal epithelial cells is regulated by the enteric nervous system (ENS), which comprises two ganglionated plexuses, the myenteric and submucosal plexuses. These serve to co-ordinate the transport and motility functions of the intestine. In addition, the presence of intrinsic nerves in association with enteroendocrine cells and immune elements within the lamina propria raises the possibility that chemical messengers acting locally can modify epithelial function directly or modulate intrinsic neural activity that influences ion transport[2,3].

This chapter focuses on the current state of knowledge of intrinsic neural pathways that influence ion transport *in vitro*. It will address reflex pathways that regulate basal rates of ion transport as well as examine interactions of putative transmitters at neuropeithelial junctions and within the ganglionic circuitry. Communication between myenteric ganglia and submucosal ganglia that may be important in co-ordinating motility patterns with transport function will also be addressed.

INTRINSIC REFLEX REGULATION OF BASAL ION TRANSPORT

The presence of reflex pathways that regulate ion transport was suggested from the early observations that tactile stimulation or distension of extrinsically denervated canine Thiry–Vella loops stimulated fluid secretion[4]. As fluid secretion could be prevented by hexamethonium, it seemed likely that nicotinic cholinergic synapses within the enteric ganglia were involved in the transmission and integration of information[4]. Since these early observations, other studies have confirmed the regulation of basal ion transport by the ENS. Most of these studies utilized tetrodotoxin, which prevents action-potential dependent release of transmitters, to demonstrate tonic neural influences on mucosal function. Addition of tetrodotoxin to the serosal bathing medium of muscle-stripped preparations of human, rabbit and guinea-pig small intestine or human and rat colon set up in flux chambers, resulted in a decrease in short-circuit current[5–9]. The ionic basis for this change in transport after tetrodotoxin administration was attributed to an increase in sodium and chloride absorption in the guinea-pig and rabbit ileum[6,7]. Removal of the submucosal ganglia from rat colon resulted in an increase in sodium and chloride absorption compared to segments of tissue with intact submucosal ganglia. This observation, along with others in the canine colon, provides additional support for the involvement of enteric neural pathways in regulation of basal ion transport[9,10].

Muscarinic receptor blockade did not alter baseline short-circuit current in either the rabbit or the guinea-pig small intestine; it therefore seems unlikely that these pathways involve release of acetylcholine at neuroepithelial junctions in these two species[6,7]. In contrast to these findings, however, atropine reduced basal transport rates in the human ileum, and the possibility must be considered that cholinergic secretomotor neurons are involved in reflex regulation of transport in this segment in humans[8].

The question of whether cholinergic interneurons that release acetylcholine at nicotinic synapses within the submucosal ganglia are necessary for transfer of information to the epithelium has not been resolved. Although early *in vivo* studies in the dog suggested that information transfer within the ganglia occurred at nicotinic cholinergic synapses, this is less certain in other species, because the appropriate *in vitro* experiments have not always been done to address this point[4]. In the rabbit ileum, hexamethonium had no effect on basal short-circuit current[7]. In guinea-pig ileum, the reduction in short-circuit current evoked by tetrodotoxin was initially greater than after treatment with hexamethonium[11]. Either nicotinic cholinergic transmission plays a minor role in ganglionic processing of information in these species or peptidergic synaptic transmission predominates.

The predominant influence of the ENS is to suppress sodium and chloride absorption and to limit the absorptive capacity of the intestines. Although a number of studies support this conclusion, others have failed to observe an influence of the ENS on basal ion transport in the same region of intestine and in same species[12–14]. Failure to observe tonic neural influences on ion transport may be related either to differences in sensory detection of the chemical composition of the lumen and stretch of the gut wall or to differences in diet and body fluid homeostasis that could alter hormonal status and neuronal influences on ion transport[15,16].

It is likely that intrinsic reflex pathways are suppressed by input from the extrinsic sympathetic nerves *in vivo*[17–19]. The presence of noradrenergic nerve terminals surrounding cell bodies of submucosal neurons, and the ability of norepinephrine to shut down the synaptic circuitry and inhibit neurally controlled intestinal transport function, suggests that the sympathetic nerves act as a brake on the ENS[17-19]. Studies in transplanted Thiry–Vella loops of rats on an immunosuppressive regimen support this conclusion: intestinal allografts or isografts that were extrinsically denervated secreted ions and water, whereas control segments with intact extrinsic nerves did not[20].

RESPONSES TO ELECTRICAL FIELD STIMULATION

In order to study neural pathways involved in regulation of ion transport, electrical field stimulation has been used to depolarize neurons, and pharmacological agonists and antagonists have been administered to assess the role of specific neurotransmitters. Unlike reflex mechanisms that involve a subset of neurons, electrical field stimulation is a non-selective stimulus that depolarizes all neurons, and this can lead to release of excitatory and inhibitory transmitters. The magnitude of the changes in ion transport will be a composite response that reflects the contribution of both excitatory and inhibitory transmitters.

In general, electrical field stimulation results in inhibition of ion absorption or stimulation of ion secretion, depending on the region of intestine examined. In the duodenum of the frog, stimulation of bicarbonate secretion occurred after depolarization of the intrinsic innervation, and this may be an important protective mechanism for neutralizing acid chyme that is emptied from the stomach[21]. Electrogenic chloride secretion was the predominate effect of intrinsic neural stimulation in the remaining small intestine and distal colon of several mammalian species[7,12,22]. This contrasted with the proximal colon of the guinea-pig, where neural stimulation resulted in inhibition of neutral sodium and chloride absorption[23]. In the turtle colon, which lacks crypt glands, submucosal cholinergic neurons were implicated in inhibition of electrogenic sodium absorption[24]. Stimulation of secretion probably is important in lubrication of the luminal contents, maintenance of luminal fluidity, dilution of noxious agents and removal of invading organisms.

NEUROEPITHELIAL JUNCTIONS

There is considerable evidence to date in a variety of species including humans, rabbits, guinea-pigs and ground squirrels that cholinergic motor neurons are involved in regulation of ion transport[8,23,25-29]. Approximately 50% of the neurons projecting to the mucosa contained choline acetyltransferase, the synthetic enzyme for acetylcholine, and released this transmitter in response to depolarizing stimuli[30,31]. Interaction of muscarinic agonists with muscarinic receptors, which are present on epithelial cells, mimicked the responses to neural stimulation and resulted in inhibition of absorption and/or stimulation of secretion[22,26,27,32].

Failure of muscarinic cholinergic blockade to abolish the response to neural stimulation suggested that peptidergic transmitters also contributed to the secretory response. Cholinergic neurons contain a variety of peptides that could be released simultaneously with acetylcholine, and could therefore function as transmitters at neuroepithelial junctions. Of the peptides that co-localize with choline acetyltransferase, it is uncertain whether substance P is a likely candidate at neuroepithelial junctions for the secretory response, because it stimulates anion secretion[19,33,34]. Evidence that substance P is a functional transmitter has been reported for the guinea-pig small intestine, but this does not appear to be the case for the rabbit ileum[33-35].

Other peptides present in intrinsic cholinergic neurons include calcitonin gene-related peptide (CGRP), neuropeptide Y, somatostatin and cholecysto-kinin[19]. Although many of these peptides have not been studied in sufficient detail to define their specific roles in neurally evoked secretion, somatostatin and neuropeptide Y can be eliminated as candidate transmitters, because they enhance absorption or inhibit secretion[36,37]. If somatostatin and neuropeptide Y are released at neuroepithelial junctions from cholinergic motor neurons, they would be expected to attenuate the secretory response. Calcitonin gene-related peptide does not appear to alter basal ion transport in muscle-stripped segments of guinea-pig distal colon with intact submucosal ganglia, but additional studies in other segments of intestine and species are needed to confirm these findings[38].

Another subset of submucosal neurons contains vasoactive intestinal peptide (VIP) which co-localizes with dynorphin or galanin in the guinea pig and with neuropeptide Y in the rat[19,39,40]. With the eception of VIP, none of these peptides appear to evoke electrogenic ion secretion, and are therefore unlikely transmitter candidates for the neurally evoked respon-ses[37,41,42].

Considerable evidence implicates VIP as a transmitter at neuroepithelial junctions. The presence of VIP and its release from enteric neurons has been reported[19,40,43]. Interaction of VIP with its receptors on epithelial cells has been shown to elevate intracellular cyclic AMP and to enhance secretion[44-46]. While these observations suggest that VIP may initiate signal transduction in the epithelium during neural stimulation, lack of potent VIP antagonists have precluded definitive conclusions regarding its role in neurally evoked responses. Although VIP antiserum was ineffective in altering neurally evoked secretion in the guinea-pig ileum, the putative VIP antagonist, VIP (10–28), caused a small reduction in neurally evoked secretion and a small rightward shift of the concentration-response curve for VIP in guinea-pig distal colon[44,47]. These observations in the guinea-pig colon are consistent with a role for VIP at neuroepithelial junctions in mediating secretory responses. Nevertheless, additional studies are needed to confirm these findings in other segments and species before VIP can unequivocally be established as an important peptidergic transmitter involved in stimulation of intestinal secretion.

EPITHELIAL INTERACTIONS OF NEUROTRANSMITTERS

Co-localization of peptides with conventional neurotransmitters in enteric neurons raises the possibility that these messengers are released simultaneously from the same or different subsets of neurons during electrical field stimulation. Interactions of simultaneously released transmitters could lead to potentiation or attenuation of the epithelial responses. Studies in the guinea-pig ileum suggest that VIP or other substances that elevate intracellular cyclic AMP (isobutyl methylxanthine and cholera toxin) enhanced cholinergic transmission[5,44]. This effect was attributed to transmitter interaction at the level of the epithelial cells, because VIP enhanced the response to bethanechol, a muscarinic cholinergic agonist, during neural blockade[44].

Another example of neurotransmitter interactions involves neuropeptide Y. Neuropeptide Y decreased neurally evoked chloride secretion in the guinea-pig colon by approximately 95%[37]. During neural blockade, neuropeptide Y reduced the chloride secretory responses evoked by VIP and bethanechol[37]. These observations suggest that simultaneous release of neuropeptide Y with either VIP or acetylcholine would lead to attenuation of the peptidergic or cholinergic responses. This is an area of research that must be addressed in order to define the interactions of the large array of putative messengers found in enteric neurons.

GANGLIONIC INTERACTIONS

A variety of receptors for classical neurotransmitters or peptides are present on submucosal neurons, but it is not known whether all of these function in regulation of ion transport[11]. Both cholinergic and peptidergic neurons that influence epithelial function are depolarized by serotonin, by acetylcholine interacting at nicotinic and muscarinic receptors, and by substance P[27,34,48,49]. In contrast, inhibition of cholinergic and peptidergic neurons occurs in response to norepinephrine, somatostatin and enkephalins[31,50].

MYENTERIC-SUBMUCOSAL INTERACTIONS

Serotonergic and enkephalinergic neurons originate in the myenteric ganglia and project to submucosal ganglia in most species[41,51]. The well-recognized increase in absorption evoked by opiates can be explained by their action at delta receptors on submucosal neurons without any direct effect on the epithelium[41]. In contrast, stimulation of serotonergic receptors on cholinergic and peptidergic submucosal neurons leads to intestinal secretion[48,49]. These interconnecting pathways between myenteric and submucosal ganglia provide excitatory and inhibitory input to cholinergic and peptidergic neurons involved in regulation of ion transport, and this may be the basis for co-ordinating motility patterns with transport function.

Another pathway which projects from the myenteric ganglia to submucosal ganglia or directly to the mucosa, and which is involved in regulation of ion transport has been identified by the actions of CGRP in whole thickness colonic segments of guinea-pig colon[38]. CGRP evoked an increase in short-circuit current only in whole thickness preparations with intact myenteric and submucosal ganglia, but not in muscle-stripped preparations without

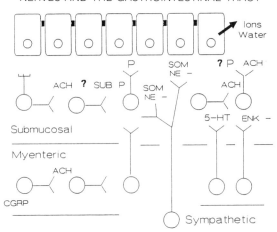

Figure 1 Model of neural control of the intestinal epithelium. See text for discussion of model. P, peptide; ACH, acetylcholine, 5-HT, 5-hydroxytryptamine or serotonin; ENK, enkephalins; CGRP, calcitonin gene-related peptide; SUB P, substance P

myenteric ganglia[38]. This response could be reduced by furosemide suggesting an involvement of chloride secretion, and could be blocked by hexamethonium and tetrodotoxin. The pathway identified by CGRP appears to involve release of acetylcholine at nicotinic synapses from cholinergic interneurons. Additional studies are necessary to identify interconnecting pathways between the two ganglionated plexuses and to define their functional significance in regulation of epithelial transport.

SUMMARY

The enteric nervous system subserves a pivotal role in modulation of intestinal transport, but current understanding of the specific regulatory pathways is still limited. Nevertheless, it is possible to assimilate a model that generalizes current concepts on how the ENS regulates epithelial ion transport. In this model, a subset of motor neurons continuously inhibits sodium and chloride absorption and limits the absorptive capacity of the intestine (Figure 1). The afferent limb of this reflex pathway involves sensory detection of the chemical composition of the lumen or mechanical stresses on the gut wall, and processing and integration of this information by peptidergic and cholinergic interneurons within the ganglia. Activation of the efferent limb or the motor neuron releases a peptidergic transmitter in proximity to epithelial cells and results in a decrease in absorptive capacity.

Activity of the submucosal ganglia can be modulated by input from the myenteric ganglia (Figure 1) via serotonergic excitatory and enkephalinergic inhibitory pathways that modify ion transport. Additional pathways identified by the actions of CGRP suggest communicating interactions between myenteric and submucosal ganglia that are involved in regulation of transport function. Finally, the activity of the ENS can be modulated by input from the extrinsic sympathetic neurons which contain norepinephrine and somatostatin and function as a brake to suppress epithelial transport mediated by the ENS.

Acknowledgements

This research was supported by a grant from the National Institutes of Health, R01-DK37240.

References

1. Frizzell, R.A. and Schultz, S.G. (1979). Models of electrolyte absorption and secretion by gastrointestinal epithelia. In Crane, R.K. (ed.) *International Review of Physiology. Gastrointestinal Physiology III*, Vol. 19, pp.205–25. (Baltimore University Park Press)
2. Wade, P.R. and Westfall, J.A. (1985). Ultrastructure of enterochromaffin cells and associated neural and vascular elements in the mouse duodenum. *Cell Tissue Res.*, **241**, 557–63
3. Bienenstock, J., Tomioka, M., Matsuda, H., Stead, R.H., Quinonez, G., Simon, G.T., Coughlin, M.D. and Denberg, J.A. (1987). The role of mast cells in inflammatory processes: Evidence for nerve/mast cell interactions. *Int. Arch. Allergy Appl. Immun.*, **82**, 238–43
4. Caren, J.F., Meyer, J.H. and Grossman, M.I. (1974). Canine intestinal secretion during and after rapid distension of the small bowel. *Am. J. Physiol.*, **227**, 183–8
5. Carey, H.V. and Cooke, H.J. (1986). Submucosal nerves and cholera toxin-induced secretion in guinea pig ileum in vitro. *Digest. Dis. Sci.*, **31**, 732–6
6. Carey, H.V. and Cooke, H.J. (1986). Enteric neural reflex pathways influence basal ion transport in guinea pig ileum. *XXX Congress Intern. Union Physiol. Sci.*, **16**, 105
7. Hubel, K.A. (1978). The effects of electrical field stimulation and tetrodotoxin on ion transport by the isolated rabbit ileum. *J. Clin. Invest.*, **62**, 1039–47
8. Hubel, K.A. and Shirazi, S. (1982). Human ileal ion transport in vitro: Changes with electrical field stimulation and tetrodotoxin. *Gastroenterology*, **83**, 63–8
9. Andres, H., Bock, R., Bridges, R.J., Rummel, W. and Schreiner, J. (1985). Submucosal plexus and electrolyte transport across rat colonic mucosa. *J. Physiol. (Lond.)*, **364**, 301–12
10. Rangachari, P.K. and McWade, D. (1986). Epithelial and mucosal preparations of canine proximal colon in Ussing chambers: Comparison of responses. *Life Sci.*, **38**, 1641–52
11. Cooke, H.J. (1986). Neurobiology of the intestinal mucosa. *Gastroenterology*, **90**, 1057–81
12. Cooke, H.J., Shonnard, K. and Wood, J.D. (1983). Effects of neuronal stimulation on mucosal transport in guinea-pig ileum. *Am. J. Physiol.*, **245**, G290–6
13. Zimmerman, T.W. and Binder, H.J. (1983). Effect of tetrodotoxin on cholinergic and agonist-mediated colonic electrolyte transport. *Am. J. Physiol.*, **244**, G386–91
14. Perdue, M.H. and Gall, D.G. (1986). Rat jejunal mucosal response to histamine and anti-histamines in vitro. Comparison with antigen-induced changes during intestinal anaphylaxis. *Agents Actions*, **19**, 5–9
15. Mei, N. (1985). Intestinal chemosensitivity. *Physiol. Rev.*, **65**, 211–37
16. Levens, N.R. (1984). Modulation of jejunal ion and water absorption by endogenous angiotension after dehydration. *Am. J. Physiol.*, **246**, G700–9
17. North, R.A. and Surprenant, A. (1985). Inhibitory synaptic potential resulting from alpha$_2$-adrenoceptor activation in guinea-pig submucous plexus neurones. *J. Physiol. (Lond.)*, **358**, 17–34
18. Sjovall, H. (1984). Sympathetic control of jejunal fluid and electrolyte transport. *Acta Physiol. Scand.*, **535** (Suppl.), 1–63
19. Keast, J.R., Furness, J.B. and Costa, M. (1984). Origins of peptide and norepinephrine nerves in the mucosa of the guinea pig small intestine. *Gastroenterology*, **86**, 637–44
20. Watson, A.J.M., Lear, P.A., Montgomery, A., Elliott, E., Dacre, J., Farthing, M.J.G. and Wood, R.F.M. (1988). Water, electrolyte, glucose and glycine absorption in rat small intestinal transplants. *Gastroenterology*, **94**, 863–9

21. Crampton, J.R., Gibbons, L.G. and Rees, W.D.W. (1988). Neural regulation of duodenal alkali secretion: Effects of electrical field stimulation. *Am. J. Physiol.*, **254**, G162–7

22. Kuwahara, A., Bowen, S., Wang, J., Condon, C. and Cooke, H.J. (1987). Epithelial responses evoked by stimulation of submucosal neurons in guinea pig distal colon. *Am. J. Physiol.*, **252**, G667–74

23. Kuwahara, A. and Radowicz-Cooke, H.J. (1988). Epithelial transport in guinea-pig proximal colon: Influence of enteric neurones. *J. Physiol. (Lond.)*, **395**, 271–84

24. Venglarik, C.J. and Dawson, D.C. (1987). Cholinergic regulation of Na absorption by turtle colon: Role of basolateral K conductance. *Am. J. Physiol.*, **251**, C563–70

25. Cooke, H.J. (1984). Influence of enteric cholinergic neurons on mucosal transport in guinea pig ileum. *Am. J. Physiol.*, **246**, G263–7

26. Carey, H.V., Tien, X.-Y., Wallace, L.J. and Cooke, H.J. (1987). Muscarinic receptor subtypes mediating the mucosal response to neural stimulation of guinea pig ileum. *Am. J. Physiol.*, **253**, G323–9

27. Kuwahara, A., Tien, X.-Y., Wallace, L.J. and Cooke, H.J. (1987). Cholinergic receptors mediating secretion in guinea pig colon. *J. Pharmacol. Exp. Ther.*, **242**, 600–6

28. Carey, H.V. and Cooke, H.J. (1987). Neural control of intestinal ion transport in the ground squirrel, a season hibernator. *Z. Gastroenterol.*, **25**, 621

29. Hubel, K.A. (1983). Effects of scorpion venom on electrolyte transport by rabbit ileum. *Am. J. Physiol.*, **244**, G501–6

30. Furness, J.B., Costa, M. and Eckenstein, F. (1983). Neurons localized with antibodies against choline acetyltransferase in the enteric nervous system. *Neurosci. Lett.*, **40**, 105–10

31. Gaginella, T.S. and Wu, Z.-C. (1983). [D-Ala^2,D-Met^5 NH$_2$] Enkephalin inhibits acetylcholine release from the submucous plexus of rat colon. *J. Pharm. Pharmacol.*, **35**, 823–5

32. Rimele, T.J., O'Dorisio, M.S. and Gaginella, T.S. (1981). Evidence for muscarinic receptors on rat colonic epithelial cells: Binding of [^{3}H] quinuclidinyl benzilate. *J. Pharmacol. Exp. Ther.*, **218**, 426–34

33. Keast, J.R., Furness, J.B. and Costa, M. (1985). Different substance P receptors are found on mucosal epithelial cells and submucous neurons of the guinea-pig small intestine. *Naunyn-Schmiedeberg's Arch. Pharmacol.*, **329**, 382–87

34. Perdue, M.H., Galbraith, R. and Davison, J.S. (1987). Evidence for substance P as a functional neurotransmitter in guinea pig small intestinal mucosa. *Regulatory Peptides*, **18**, 63–74

35. Hubel, K.A. (1984). Electrical stimulus-secretion coupling in rabbit ileal mucosa. *J. Pharmacol. Exp. Ther.*, **231**, 577–82

36. Guandalini, S., Kachur, J.F., Smith, P.I., Miller, R.J. and Field, M. (1980). In vitro effects of somatostatin on ion transport in rabbit intestine. *Am. J. Physiol.*, **238**, G67–74

37. McCulloch, C.R., Kuwahara, A., Condon, C.D. and Cooke, H.J. (1987). Neuropeptide modification of chloride secretion in guinea pig distal colon. *Regulatory Peptides*, **19**, 35–43

38. McCulloch, C.R. and Cooke, H.J. (1989). Human-alpha-CGRP influence colonic secretion by acting on myenteric neurons. *Reg. Peptides* (In Press)

39. Melander, T., Hokfelt, T., Rokaeus, A., Fahrenkrug, J., Tatemoto, K. and Mutt, V. (1985). Distribution of galanin-like immunoreactivity in the gastro-intestinal tract of several mammalian species. *Cell Tissue Res.*, **239**, 253–70

40. Ekblad, E., Hakanson, R. and Sundler, F. (1984). VIP and PHI coexist with an NPY-like peptide in intramural neurones of the small intestine. *Regulatory Peptides*, **10**, 47–55

41. Miller, R.J. and Brown, D.R. (1984). Opiates and the gut. *Viewpoints on Digestive Diseases*, **16**, 5–8

42. Carey, H.V., Cooke, H.J. and Rivier, J. (1987). Effects of a VIP-antagonist on non-cholinergically mediated secretion in guinea pig ileal mucosa. *Fed. Proc.*, **46**, 1077

43. Gaginella, T.S., O'Dorisio, T.M. and Hubel, K.A. (1981). Release of vasoactive intestinal polypeptide by electrical field stimulation of rabbit ileum. *Regulatory Peptides*, **2**, 165–74

44. Cooke, H.J., Zafirova, M., Carey, H.V., Walsh, J.H. and Grider, H. (1987). Vasoactive intestinal polypeptide actions on the guinea pig intestinal mucosa during neural stimulation. *Gastroenterology*, **92**, 361–70

45. Beubler, E. (1980). Influence of vasoactive intestinal polypeptide on net water flux and cyclic adenosine 3′,5′-monophosphate formation in the rat jejunum. *Naunyn-Schmiedeberg's Arch. Pharmacol.*, **313**, 243–7

46. Binder, H.J., Lemp, G.F. and Gardner, J.D. (1980). Receptors for vasoactive intestinal peptide and secretin on small intestinal epithelial cells. *Am. J. Physiol.*, **238**, G190–6

47. Cooke, H.J. and Kuwahara, A. (1987). Vasoactive intestinal peptide: A neural mediator of secretion in the guinea pig distal colon. *Z. Gastroenterol.*, **25**, 622

48. Cooke, H.J. and Carey, H.V. (1985). Pharmacological analysis of 5-hydroxytryptamine actions on guinea-pig ileal mucosa. *Eur. J. Pharmacol.*, **111**, 329–37

49. Keast, J.R., Furness, J.B. and Costa, M. (1985). Investigations of nerve populations influencing ion transport that can be stimulated electrically, by serotonin and by a nicotinic agonist. *Naunyn-Schmiedeberg's Arch. Pharmacol.*, **331**, 260–6

50. Keast, J.R., Furness, J.B. and Costa, M. (1986). Effects of noradrenaline and somatostatin on basal and stimulated mucosal ion transport in the guinea-pig small intestine. *Naunyn-Schmeideberg's Arch. Pharmacol.*, **333**, 393–9

51. Gershon, M.D., Dreyfus, C.F., Pickel, V.M., Joh, T.H. and Reis, D. (1977). Serotonergic neurons in the peripheral nervous system: Localization of tryptophan hydroxylase in the gut. *Proc. Natl. Acad. Sci. USA*, **74**, 3086–9

23
Enteric nervous control of mucosal functions of the small intestine *in vivo*

O. LUNDGREN

There is both morphological and functional evidence for the view that the enteric nervous system (ENS) represents a rather independent part of the autonomic nervous system. For example, it can be calculated that the relationship between the number of extrinsic efferent nerve fibres and the number of neurons in the ENS is 1:300 in the cat[1]. Many physiological observations also indicate that ENS can function independently from the central nervous system. An important example of this is the peristaltic reflex which functions also in intestines devoid of any extrinsic innervation.

The peristaltic reflex represents a co-ordinated response of nerves and muscles, which is confined to the gastrointestinal wall. It seems probable that the control of other intestinal functions may also be exerted by reflexes within the ENS. This chapter discusses the ENS control of two intestinal functions mainly localized to the intestinal mucosa: blood flow and fluid and electrolyte transport. At the end the possibility that also epithelial cell migration may be controlled by the ENS is commented upon. The extrinsic nervous control of fluid and electrolyte transport will not be commented upon here since it has been the subject of recent reviews[1,2].

ENS CONTROL OF BLOOD FLOW

Mechanical stimulation of the intestinal mucosa by, for example, a glass rod, induces a vasodilatation in extrinsicly denervated intestinal segments of the cat[3]. The vasodilatation occurs mainly in the intestinal villi (Biber, Lundgren and Svanvik, unpublished observations). Quantitatively, total intestinal blood flow is doubled. This response reflects the activation of an intramural nervous reflex, to judge by experiments using tetrodotoxin (a blocker of sodium gates in nerves) and lidocaine (a local anaesthetic) which abolish the mechanically induced vasodilatation[3]. The vasodilatation is, on the other hand, not influenced by nicotinergic, muscarinic or adrenergic receptor blockers[3], which indicates that the neurotransmitter at the effector cell (vascular smooth muscles) is non-cholinergic and non-adrenergic. A similar nervous vasodilatation can also be evoked by transmural electrical field stimulation *in vivo*[4], an observation which further strengthens the conclusion that enteric vasodilator nerves can control vascular smooth muscles.

The vasodilatation caused by mechanical mucosal stimulation may be mediated by an axon reflex as arranged in the skin. To test if this was the case, Biber[5] performed experiments on intestinal segments which had been denervated periarterially 2–3 weeks prior to acute experiments on anaesthetized cats. The denervation procedure was tested by showing the absence of any vascular effect on stimulating the regional sympathetic vasoconstrictor fibres. Biber[5] demonstrated that it is possible also to evoke a vasodilatation in these segments, which rules out an axon reflex arrangement of the type found in the skin.

Various receptor blocking agents were tested with regard to the intestinal vasodilatation caused by mechanical stimulation of the mucosa. Among those only 5-HT tachyphlyaxis and certain 5-hydroxytryptamine (5-HT) blocking agents (e.g. 2-bromo-lysergic acid diethylamide) blocked the response[3,6]. Two sites of action for 5-HT seem possible. It may be a neurotransmitter in the reflex arc or it may be released from enterochromaffin (EC) cells upon mechanical stimulation. In the latter case Biber and co-workers[6] proposed that the released 5-HT activates dendrites situated just underneath the EC cell. These two possible arrangements of the reflex are illustrated in the left part of Figure 1.

It was pointed out earlier that the neurotransmitter at the effector cells in the studied vasodilator reflex is non-cholinergic and non-adrenergic. Several observations indicate that the neurotransmitter is vasoactive intestinal polypeptide (VIP), a substance known to cause vasodilatation. Mechanical stimulation of the mucosa induces the release of VIP from the small intestine of the cat concomitant to the hyperaemia[7]. Giving apamin, a peptide in bee venom, blocks the flow increase seen on mechanical or electrical field stimulation and also inhibits the release of VIP[8]. Apamin is suggested to act via a presynaptic VIP receptor controlling VIP release ('autoregulation of transmitter release'). Finally, giving 5-HT in doses that evoke an intestinal vasodilatation also causes the release of large amounts of VIP from the intestine[7]. All these findings are compatible with the two models for the vasodilator reflex illustrated in the left part of Figure 1.

The physiological function of the nervous vascular reflex of Biber *et al.*[3-6] is probably to increase blood flow at the site of a food bolus in the intestinal lumen to facilitate the absorption of nutrients. It also seems possible that the vasodilatation accompanying every migrating myoelectric complex in the conscious dog[9] is mediated via the same nervous vasodilator reflex.

It was pointed out above that the vasodilator mechanism described by Biber *et al.*[3-6], is not mediated by an axon reflex. However, indirect evidence for an axon reflex controlling blood flow in the feline small intestine has been reported by Rozsa *et al.*[10-12]. Capsaicin, a drug which causes the release of neurotransmitters from thin afferent fibres (C-fibres), evokes an intestinal

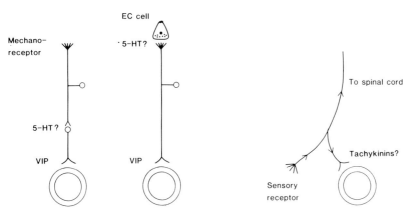

Figure 1 The intrinsic nervous control of intestinal blood vessels schematically illustrated. **Left**: two possible arrangements of the reflex vasodilatation elicited by mechanical stimulation of the intestinal mucosa. 5-hydroxytryptamine (5-HT) is either a neurotransmitter in the reflex arc or is released from the enterochromaffin (EC) cell which functions as a mechanoreceptor. Vasoactive intestinal polypeptide (VIP) is probably the transmitter at the vascular smooth muscle cells. **Right**: an axon reflex which, via the release of tachykinins, probably evokes an intestinal vasodilatation. This reflex can be activated by luminal chemical stimuli; for details, see text

vasodilatation when given into the intestinal lumen. This effect is blocked by intraluminal lidocaine but not by hexamethonium. According to Rozsa et al.[11], capsaicin-induced vasodilatation is caused by the release of substance P, cholecystokinin and VIP, presumably from nerves. The capsaicin sensitive afferents seem also to be stimulated by luminal solutions containing bile and oleic acid, inferring that this reflex is activated by chemicals in the luminal contents (Figure 1).

ENS CONTROL OF EPITHELIAL TRANSPORT *IN VIVO*

There exists a large body of experimental evidence obtained *in vitro* which supports the view that enteric nerves control epithelial transport in the intestine, as reviewed elsewhere in this volume. To what extent these nerves are part of intrinsic and/or extrinsic control systems cannot be judged from *in vitro* experiments. However, observations *in vivo* also suggest that intrinsic nervous reflexes control epithelial transport. The intramural nervous reflexes studied so far have all caused net fluid secretion. One of the first studies which suggested the presence of intramural secretory reflexes in the small intestine was published by Caren et al.[13]. They showed in denervated canine intestines that tactile stimulation of the mucosa increases fluid secretion. This effect was blocked by atropine, hexamethonium or lidocaine (all drugs given i.v.). A mechanically induced fluid secretion in the rat was also oberved by Beubler and Juan[14]. Sjövall et al.[15] showed that atropine administration enhances fluid uptake from the feline gut via nerves that cannot be activated by stimulating the vagal fibres to the gut; suggesting the presence of an ongoing cholinergic influence on epithelial fluid transport during 'resting' control conditions. In other studies on cats, Sjövall et al.[16,17] obtained indirect evidence for the presence of a secretory nervous reflex activated by glucose in the lumen. The evidence suggests that this reflex pathway does not contain any cholinergic synapse[17]. Finally, Eklund and co-workers[18,19] demonstrated that placing lipophilic analogues of cyclic 3'5' adenosine monophosphate (cAMP) or cyclic 3'5'-guanosine monophosphate (cGMP) in the lumen of periarterially denervated intestines evokes an intestinal fluid secretion that is markedly diminished by three 'blockers' of nervous activity: TTX, hexamethonium and lidocaine. These experiments tended to mimic the increase of cyclic nucleotides that may occur in the epithelial cells both during physiological and pathophysiological circumstances.

These observations demonstrate that there exist intramural nervous reflexes elicited by luminal stimuli that cause fluid secretion in the small intestine, but they do not provide any information on the details of how such reflexes are arranged. However, observations made in vitro with electrophysiological techniques (mainly performed on guinea-pigs) and with so-called Ussing chambers (rabbit, rats, guinea-pigs, humans), as well as results obtained in vivo studying mainly fluid transport (rats, cats), are beginning to form a coherent picture.

A model of this is presented in Figure 2 mainly based on studies performed by Bornstein et al.[20,21] and on work performed in our laboratory. It should be stressed that the figure presents the simplest model that can be constructed from the available evidence. For example, the illustrated reflex arcs may contain several interneurons but the experimental approaches available cannot analyse the neuronal circuitry in such detail. These reflexes will now be discussed beginning with the efferent part of the proposed reflexes since we know more about the efferent than the afferent portion of the reflexes.

The efferent part of the secretory intramural reflexes

There are at least two final common nervous pathways, one cholinergic and one non-cholinergic, which influence epithelial fluid and electrolyte transport in the small intestine. The nerve cell bodies of these neurons are mainly located in the submucosal plexus, although one cannot exclude that there are also myenteric neurons that directly influence the intestinal epithelium[22].

In the guinea-pig, the cholinergic and non-cholinergic pathways (Dogiel type III neurons) from submucosal neurons seem to be possible to track by mapping neuropeptide Y (NPY; probably also containing acetylcholine, cholecystokinin, calcitonin gene related peptide, somatostatin) and VIP immunoreactivity (non-cholinergic neuron also containing dynorphin) in submucosal neurons, respectively, although this approach does not map the submucosal neurons containing only substance P and acetylcholine. Furthermore, immunohistochemistry can be made on the neurons that have

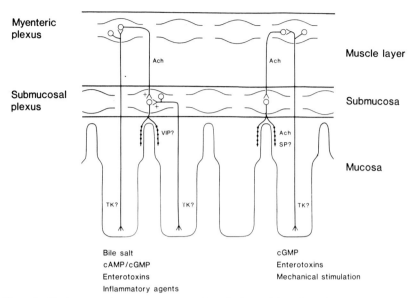

Figure 2 The intramural secretory nervous reflexes in the small intestine schematically depicted. Experimental evidence suggests that there are at least two types of submucosal neurons influencing epithelial function, one cholinergic and one non-cholinergic; they are illustrated in the right and left part of the figure, respectively. The afferent neuron of the two illustrated reflexes is proposed to be a peptidergic one using a tachykinin (TK) as neurotransmitter. Electrophysiological evidence suggests that the cholinergic submucosal neuron is mainly controlled by cholinergic neurons with cell somas located in the myenteric plexus. The non-cholinergic submucosal neuron is influenced by other than cholinergic neurons to judge from electrophysiological observations. A TK neuron is proposed to act directly on the submucosal neuron. (This figure is based mainly on observations made in our laboratory and on electrophysiological studies by Bornstein et al.[21,22])

been characterized with electrophysiological techniques. It can then be shown that inputs evoking fast and slow excitatory post-synaptic potentials (EPSPs; proposed neurotransmitters acetylcholine and substance P/serotonin, respectively) and inhibitory post-synaptic potentials (IPSPs; proposed neurotransmitter norepinephrine) can be recorded from VIP-ergic neurons[20]. Removing the myenteric plexus reduces significantly the number of inputs eliciting fast and slow EPSPs, indicating that the somas of many of the neurons influencing the VIP-ergic submucosal neurons via nicotinergic receptors are located in the myenteric plexus[21]. This nervous arrangement is illustrated in the left panel of Figure 2. The adrenergic influence (IPSPs), which is extrinsic, was not influenced by the removal of the myenteric plexus in the experiments by Bornstein et al.[20,21].

The arrangement of the non-cholinergic control of epithelial transport illustrated in Figure 2 agrees with the *in vivo* studies performed in our laboratory. We have shown that several secretagogues evoke fluid secretion to a large extent via an activation of the ENS[23-28]. This holds true not only for bacterial toxins but also for inflammatory mediators. Most of these effects are not influenced by atropine but all are diminished by hexamethonium, a nicotinergic receptor blocker (Figure 3[29]). Furthermore, one of the most efficient ways of inhibiting fluid secretion induced by, for example, cholera toxin, bile salt or sodium ricinoleate is to place lidocaine, a local anaesthetic, on the serosal surface (Figure 4[30]). The inhibition of secretion occurs within minutes in line with the proposal made in Figure 2 that many of the cholinergic neurons are located in the myenteric plexus close to the serosal surface.

The submucosal neurons, which influence the intestinal epithelium via the release of acetylcholine, are only influenced by nerve cells acting via fast cholinergic EPSPs. The cell somas of many of these 'nicotinergic' neurons are also located in the myenteric nerve plexus[21], as illustrated in the right panel of Figure 2. This arrangement is also supported by the findings in our studies of cholinergic secretory reflexes confined to the intestinal wall[15].

The above description suggests that all secretory nervous reflexes contain a cholinergic synapse. However, this may not be the case. Sjövall and co-workers[16,31] have provided experimental evidence for a secretory nervous reflex elicited by glucose in the intestinal lumen. This is not influenced by hexamethonium which, of course, does not exclude that the reflex has one or several synapses with unknown transmitter. Glucose elicits secretion also in *in vitro* preparations stripped of their muscle coat[32], which suggests that the reflex may be confined to the mucosa–submucosa. The left panel of Figure 2 shows such a non-cholinergic reflex.

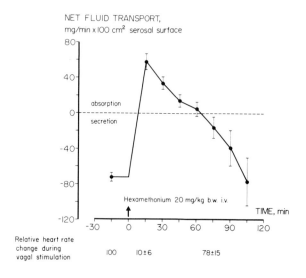

Figure 3 The effect of hexamethonium on cholera toxin induced secretion in rats. The relative decrease in heart rate induced by electrical stimulation of the cervical vagus before and after giving the drug is also indicated. Mean + S.E. $n = 6$[24]

280

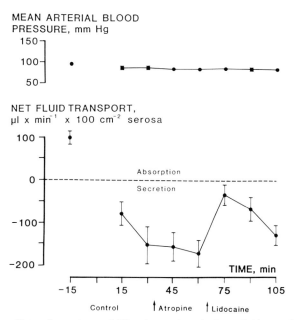

Figure 4 The effects of atropine and lidocaine on intestinal net fluid secretion induced by luminal perfusion with a modified Krebs-Henseleit solution containing 6 mM sodium ricinoleate. The perfusion was started at time 0. The observation at -15 min represents the net fluid transport during the last 15 min of a perfusion period with a modified Krebs-Henseleit solution devoid of sodium ricinoleate. Bars denote $\pm$ SE; $n = 6$

The neurotransmitter at the epithelial effector cell

As discussed elsewhere there are a great number of substances which are potential transmitters at the effector cells, that is, the enterocytes in the intestinal crypts. This discussion can be summarized by stating that the evidence for acetylcholine as a secretory transmitter in the intestines is convincing, fulfilling all the criteria for a transmitter function. Substance P(SP) and vasoactive intestinal polypeptide (VIP) are probably also neurotransmitters but the experimental evidence is still not fully conclusive.

The afferent part of the secretory intramural reflexes

It is apparent from the studies reviewed above that both mechanical and chemical stimuli applied from the lumen side may evoke a secretory response in the intestinal mucosa via an activation of the ENS. The following discussion addresses itself to the questions of how the ENS is activated and which neurotransmitters participate in the afferent part of the secretory reflexes.

The sensor for the secretion evoked by the tactile mucosal stimulation is most probably a mechanoreceptor. In line with this Wood and co-workers reported that several neurons in the myenteric plexus begin firing on mechanical distortion[33]. Furthermore, distension of the gut evokes afferent firing in vagal nerves[34]. The rate of firing is proportional to the degree of distension. Paintal[35] also described mucosal mechanoreceptors not sensitive to distension but to movements of the mucosa itself. Such a receptor could of course be involved in the secretory and vascular responses evoked by tactile stimulation of the mucosa.

Chemical receptors are known to be present in the intestine, to judge from experiments where rate of firing in vagal or sympathetic fibres have been shown to be dependent on the presence of various solutes in the intestinal lumen (for review, see ref. 36). The morphological counterparts of these chemical sensors are not established. Lipophilic solutes may diffuse across the epithelial lining to activate, directly or indirectly, sensory nerve endings in the villus tissue. With regard to water-soluble compounds unable to cross the epithelial lining, we have proposed[37], that the epithelial cells containing peptidergic hormones and/or amines may act as chemical sensors which, upon releasing the contents from their granules across the basolateral cell membrane, activate the nerves (dendrites) located just underneath the epithelial layer[38]. Figure 5 illustrates in a schematic way the proposed arrangement. The cleft between these so-called 'receptor cells' and the subepithelial dendrites may be looked upon as a primitive synapse. The nerves represent the 'afferent' limbs of intramural reflexes influencing intestinal fluid transport and possibly also motility.

The nature of the afferent sensory neuron in the intramural sensory reflexes is not known at present and one can only speculate on the neurotransmitters involved. One possible candidate is SP and/or other tachykinins, which are known to be contained in afferent fibres to the CNS, probably conveying pain. This proposal has received support in cat studies performed in our laboratory. Close i.a. SP infusion evokes a fluid secretion in the cat small intestine that is accompanied by a release of VIP, an observation which

"Receptor cell"

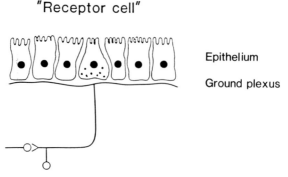

Epithelium

Ground plexus

Figure 5 A highly schematic illustration of the 'receptor cell' concept. Receptor cells are proposed to be the cells which are characterized by a triangular form with granules in the part of the cell facing the tissue. The granules contain amines and/or peptides. Luminal stimuli may release the contents of the granules into the subepithelial space where dendrites are located. The dendrite is part of a plexus situated just underneath the epithelial cells and the synapse of the afferent neuron is located in one of the large nerve plexuses of the intestinal wall

suggests that SP acts via a nervous mechanism. This contention is also supported by the concomitant inhibition by TTX of SP-induced fluid secretion and VIP release. These variables are also diminished by hexamethonium[39], which further suggests that the SP receptors are located on a neuron 'proximal' to the cholinergic one, as proposed in Figure 2.

The physiological significance of the discussed nervous secretory reflexes in the small bowel is not known. We have proposed that the reflexes are part of the defence system of the body; the intestinal mucosal surface representing an 'outer' surface. Potentially noxious agents are diluted by the induced fluid secretion. Furthermore, some of the agents that we have investigated also evoke motility of a propulsive type (see, for example, ref. 27).

ENS CONTROL OF EPITHELIAL CELL MIGRATION

The turnover of epithelial cells in the gastrointestinal tract is fast. The cells are formed by mitosis at the base of the crypts. During a lifespan of 48–72 h the enterocytes migrate from their place of formation to the tips of the villi where they slough and lyse. A large number of factors have been inferred to regulate the rate of enterocyte formation including nerves although the experimental evidence for a nervous control is very scarce.

We have studied cell migration in the rat small intestine using the method of pulse labelling cells in mitosis with [^{3}H]thymidine. The migration of the labelled cells along the crypt–villus axis was studied with two techniques. In one the mucosa of frozen intestinal segments was cut perpendicular to the long axis of the villus and the distribution of radioactivity was determined by scintillation counting; the other technique used was autoradiography.

The experimental design was based on our earlier demonstration, described above, that cholera toxin placed in the intestinal lumen induces a fluid secretion that, to about 70% is mediated via intramural nervous reflexes (cf. Figures 2 and 3). Consequently, one segment was exposed to a cholera toxin concentration that was known to induce fluid secretion and another segment in the same animal served as control. Both autoradiography and tissue sectioning revealed that the migration rate of the cells in the cholera segment was faster than that observed in the control. This effect was abolished by giving hexamethonium in a dose that has been shown to inhibit cholera fluid secretion. We therefore propose that ENS not only controls blood flow, motility and epithelial transport but also influences rate of cell migration probably via an effect on mitosis rate in the intestinal crypts.

Acknowledgements

The research reported in this review and performed in the author's laboratory was supported by a grant from the Swedish Medical Research Council (2855). The author is greatly indebted to a number of collaborators: Mats Jodal, Björn Biber, Sergio Bustamante, Ingemar Brunsson, Jean Cassuto, Stefan

Eklund, John Fara, Jan Fahrenkrug, Madeleine Forshult, Lars Karlström, Staffan Redfors, Henrik Sjövall, Anders Sjöqvist, Joar Svanvik, Mayuree Tantisira and Richard Tuttle.

References

1. Lundgren, O. (1988). Nervous control of intestinal transport. *Bailliére's Clin. Gastroenterol.*, **2**, 85–106
2. Sjövall, H., Jodal, M. and Lundgren, O. (1988). Sympathetic control of intestinal fluid and electrolyte transport. *NIPS*, **2**, 214–7
3. Biber, B., Lundgren, O. and Svanvik, J. (1971). Studies on the intestinal vasodilatation observed after mechanical stimulation of the mucosa of the gut. *Acta Physiol. Scand.*, **82**, 177–90
4. Biber, B., Fara, J. and Lundgren, O. (1973). Intestinal vasodilatation in response to transmural electrical field stimulation. *Acta Physiol. Scand.*, **87**, 277–82
5. Biber, B. (1973). Vasodilatory mechanisms in the small intestine. *Acta Physiol. Scand.*, (Suppl. 401)
6. Biber, B., Fara, J. and Lundgren, O. (1974). A pharmacological study of vasodilator mechanisms in the cat. *Acta Physiol. Scand.*, **90**, 673–83
7. Eklund, S., Fahrenkrug, J., Jodal, M., Lundgren, O., Schaffalitzky de Muckadell, O.B. and Sjöqvist, A. (1980). Vasoactive intestinal polypeptide, 5-hydroxytryptamine and reflex hyperemia in the small intestine of the cat. *J. Physiol.*, **302**, 549–57
8. Sjöqvist, A., Fahrenkrug, J., Jodal, M. and Lundgren, O. (1983). Effect of apamin on release of vasoactive intestinal polypeptide (VIP) from cat intestines. *Acta Physiol. Scand.*, **119**, 69–76
9. Fioramonti, J. and Bueno, L. (1984). Relation between intestinal motility and mesenteric blood flow in the conscious dog. *Am. J. Physiol.*, **246**, G108–13
10. Rozsa, Z., Jancso, G. and Varro, V. (1984). Possible involvement of capsaicin-sensitive sensory nerves in the regulation of intestinal blood flow in the dog. *Naunyn-Schmiedeberg's Arch. Pharmacol.*, **326**, 352–6
11. Rozsa, Z., Varro, A. and Jancso, G. (1985). Use of immunoblockade to study the involvement of peptidergic afferent nerves in the intestinal vasodilatory response to capsaicin in the dog. *Eur. J. Pharmacol.*, **115**, 59–64
12. Rozsa, Z., Sharkey, K.A. and Varro, V. (1986). Evidence for a role of capsaicin-sensitive mucosal afferent nerves in the regulation of mesenteric blood flow in the dog. *Gastroenterology*, **90**, 906–10
13. Caren, J.F., Meyer, J.H. and Grossman, M.I. (1974). Canine intestinal secretion during and after rapid distension of the small bowel. *Am. J. Physiol.*, **227**, 183–8
14. Beubler, E. and Juan, H. (1978). PGE-release, blood flow and transmucosal water movement after mechanical stimulation of the rat jejunal mucosa. *Naunyn-Schmiedeberg's Arch. Pharmacol.*, **305**, 91–5
15. Sjövall, H., Brunsson, I., Jodal, M. and Lundgren, O. (1983). The effect of vagal nerve activation on net fluid transport in the jejunum of the cat. *Acta Physiol. Scand.*, **117**, 351–7
16. Sjövall, H., Redfors, S., Jodal, M. and Lundgren, O. (1983). On the mode of action of the sympathetic fibres on intestinal fluid transport: Evidence for the existence of a glucose stimulated secretory nervous pathway in the intestinal wall. *Acta Physiol. Scand.*, **119**, 39–48
17. Sjövall, H. (1984). Evidence for separate sympathetic regulation of fluid absorption and blood flow in the feline jejunum. *Am. J. Physiol.*, **247**, G510–4
18. Eklund, S., Cassuto, J., Jodal, M. and Lundgren, O. (1984). The involvement of the enteric nervous system in the intestinal secretion evoked by cyclic adenosine 3′,5′-monophosphate. *Acta Physiol. Scand.*, **120**, 311–16
19. Eklund, S., Jodal, M. and Lundgren, O. (1986). The net fluid secretion caused by cyclic 3′5′-guanosine monophosphate in the rat jejunum in vivo is mediated by a local nervous reflex. *Acta Physiol. Scand.*, **128**, 57–63

20. Bornstein, J.C., Costa, M. and Furness, J.B. (1986). Synaptic inputs to immunohistochemically identified neurones in the submucous plexus of the guinea-pig small intestine. *J. Physiol.*, **381**, 465–82

21. Bornstein, J.C., Furness, J.B. and Costa, M. (1987). Sources of excitatory synaptic inputs to neurochemically identified submucous neurons of guinea-pig small intestine. *J. Autonom. Nerv. Syst.*, **18**, 83–91

22. Furness, J.B. and Costa, M. (1987). *The Enteric Nervous System.* (New York: Churchill Livingstone)

23. Cassuto, J., Jodal, M., Tuttle, R. and Lundgren, O. (1981). On the role of intramural nerves in the pathogenesis of cholera toxin-induced intestinal secretion. *Scand. J. Gastroenterol.*, **16**, 377–84

24. Cassuto, J., Jodal, M. and Lundgren, O. (1982). The effect of nicotinic and muscarinic receptor blockade on cholera toxin induced intestinal secretion in rats and cats. *Acta Physiol. Scand.*, **114**, 573–7

25. Cassuto, J., Siewert, A., Jodal, M. and Lundgren, O. (1983). The involvement of intramural nerves in cholera toxin induced intestinal secretion. *Acta Physiol. Scand.*, **117**, 195–202

26. Eklund, S., Jodal, M. and Lundgren, O. (1985). The enteric nervous system participates in the secretory response to the heat stable enterotoxins of *Escherichia Coli* in rats and cats. *Neuroscience*, **14**, 673–81

27. Karlström, L. (1986). Mechanisms of bile salt-induced secretion in the small intestine. *Acta Physiol. Scand.*, **126**, (Suppl. 549), 1–48

28. Brunsson, I., Sjöqvist, A., Jodal, M. and Lundgren, O. (1987). Mechanisms underlying the small intestinal fluid secretion caused by arachidonic acid, prostaglandin E_1 and prostaglandin E_2 in the rat in vivo. *Acta Physiol. Scand.*, **130**, 633–42

29. Cassuto, J., Jodal, M., Tuttle, R. and Lundgren, O. (1982). 5-hydroxytryptamine and cholera secretion. *Scand. J. Gastroenterol.*, **17**, 695–703

30. Karlström, L., Cassuto, J., Jodal, M. and Lundgren, O. (1983). The importance of the enteric nervous system for the bile salt induced secretion in the small intestine of the rat. *Scand. J. Gastroenterol.*, **18**, 117–23

31. Sjövall, H., Jodal, M. and Lundgren, O. (1984). Further evidence for a glucose-activated secretory mechanism in the jejunum of the cat. *Acta Physiol. Scand.*, **120**, 437–43

32. Cooke, H.J. (1986). Neurobiology of the intestinal mucosa. *Gastroenterology*, **90**, 1057–81

33. Wood, J.D. (1987). Physiology of the enteric nervous system. In Johnson, L.R. (ed.) *Physiology of the Gastrointestinal Tract*, Vol. 1, 2nd Edn., pp. 67–109. (New York: Raven Press)

34. Iggo, A. (1975). Gastrointestinal tension receptors with unmyelinated afferent fibers in the vagus of the cat. *Q. J. Exp. Physiol.*, **42**, 130–43

35. Paintal, A.S. (1957). Responses from mucosal mechanoreceptors in the small intestine of the cat. *J. Physiol.*, **139**, 353–68

36. Cooke, H.J. (1987). Neural and humoral regulation of small intestinal electrolyte transport. In Johnson, L.R. (ed.) *Physiology of the Gastrointestinal Tract*, Vol. 2, 2nd Edn., pp. 1307–50 (New York: Raven Press)

37. Cassuto, J., Jodal, M., Sjövall, H. and Lundgren, O. (1981). Nervous control of intestinal secretion. *Clin. Res. Rev.*, **1**, (Suppl. 1), 11–21

38. Lundberg, J.M., Dahlström, A., Bylock, A., Ahlman, H., Pettersson, G., Larsson, I., Hansson, H.-A. and Kewenter, J. (1978). Ultrastructural evidence for an innervation of epithelial enterochromaffin cells in the guinea pig duodenum. *Acta Physiol. Scand.*, **104**, 3–12

39. Brunsson, I., Eklund, S., Fahrenkrug, J., Jodal, M., Lundgren, O. and Sjöqvist, A. (1987). Effects of substance P on intestinal secretion, blood flow, motility and release of vasoactive intestinal polypeptide in vivo in rat and cat. *J. Physiol.*, **390**, P255

24
Intestinal neuroimmune interactions

G. A. CASTRO

CURRENT STATUS

Opening remarks by Jankovic[1] from proceedings of the second international workshop on neuroimmunmoodulation emphasize that the immune system is functionally comprised of: (1) T and B lymphocytes; (2) accessory non-lymphoid cells, such as macrophages and epithelial cells; (3) an array of paracrine factors; (4) hormones; and (5) cholinergic, adrenergic and peptidergic nerves, all working within an atmosphere of electrical and magnetic fields. Such a cosmic view of immunology has led to coinage of the terms immunophysiology[2], neuroimmunoendocrinology[3], and psychoneuroimmunology[4], in addition to neuroimmunomodulation[5]. These combining terms, while representing attempts to integrate information from immunology with that from other disciplines to explain certain biological phenomena, embrace the seminal physiological concept of *co-ordination of systems*. That concept, which is highlighted and amply illustrated by Adolph[6] in his tr eatise on physiological integrations in action, implies that any functional response requires the co-ordination of a complex array of cellular and subcellular events (Figure 1).

Whereas Jankovic's[1] statement about the cosmic nature of the immune system prefaced 100 papers (756 pages) on neuroimmune interactions, it is significant that none of those reports focused specifically on interactions in the gastrointestinal (GI) tract. This emphasizes that the involvement of the enteric nervous system (ENS) in mucosal immune phenomenona is only beginning to be recognized. Stead et al.[7] reviewed the potential for nerve–mucosal immune system communication, based primarily on evidence of common receptors for neuropeptide transmitters and intimate anatomic associations between elements of both systems. The aim of the report described here is to highlight recently acquired physiological information indicating that neural pathways are strategically involved in the transduction of antigenic signals into physiological changes in the GI tract. For the sake of brevity the thrust of this presentation will centre around the rat–*Trichinella*

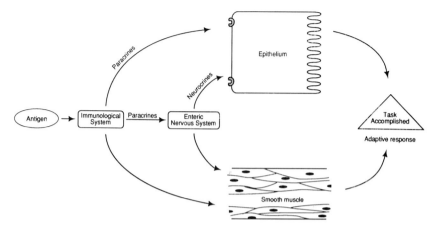

Figure 1 A view of neuroimmune interactions in the gastrointestinal tract, based on the concept of co-ordination of systems. The task accomplished presumably relates to physiological adaptation. Although not shown, the system may be modulated through endocrine or extrinsic neural pathways

spiralis, host–parasite system to illustrate mucosal neuroimmune interactions in the gut.

CHARACTERISTICS OF NEUROEFFECTOR SYSTEM

To understand how neuroeffector control systems are modulated by immune elements and why such modulation is significant, the following questions must be addressed: (1) Where do antigens that sensitize and challenge the mucosal immune system originate? (2) How do antigens affect the immune system? (3) How is the effector tissue altered? (4) How are the immune and nervous systems linked with the effector tissue? (5) What physiological task is accomplished? Also for pragmatic reasons, it is worth asking what variables affect the expression of the antigen-stimulated effector response and how that response might be modified or manipulated by extrinsic factors.

MODEL SYSTEMS

Immunological factors: antigen origin and action

Several reports, using various models, provide insight into neuroimmune interactions in the gut. A few deal with smooth muscle as the target tissue[8-10]. Most, however, involve anaphylactically induced changes in epithelial ion transport[11-26]. Whereas the latter represent the primary focus of this communication, all[8-26] these reports have their roots in the historic Schultz-Dale reaction[27,28]. In the studies of epithelial tissue, the jejunum[17,19-21,23-26], ileum[12,16] and colon[11,12-15,18,22] have been examined. Antigens used to sensitize these tissues are β-lactoglobulin (βLG)[11-16] and *Trichinella spiralis* antigen[17-19] in the guinea-pig, and ovalbumin[23-26], *Trichinella* antigen[20,21] and *Nippostrongylus brasiliensis* antigen[22] in the rat. Various antigen delivery systems have been used to induce sensitization. Feeding guinea-pigs cow's milk causes them to become hypersensitive to βLG. Rats are sensitized to ovalbumin through peritoneal injection of this protein along with an adjuvant and to *Trichinella* and *Nippostrongylus* through infection. Antigens used to challenge tissues from *Trichinella*-infected hosts are derived from somatic tissues of infective, L_1 larvae. Those used to challenge *Nippostrongylus*-infected rats are excretory–secretory products or somatic antigens from adult worms of both sexes. These antigens interact with antibodies bound to receptors on mucosal mast cells of sensitized hosts to trigger an anaphylactic reaction. Where identified[8-26], the specific immunoglobulin isotype triggering anaphylaxis is IgG_1 in the guinea-pig[14,17] and IgE in the rat[20,21,24].

Effector response: epithelial changes

The antigen that triggers anaphylaxis in each of those systems described is quite specific, but the target tissue responses evoked have many similarities. The epithelial response measured in most studies cited[11-26] was a change in ion transport; primarily an increase in net anion secretion. Transport changes induced by antigenic challenge were measured electrophysiologically[11-22,25,26] or by tracing unidirectional fluxes of radioactive ions[22,24]. In the electrical measurements, transport was quantified by determining the change in transmural short-circuit current (I_{sc}) required to offset the voltage, developed from the net transmural movement of ions and/or to a change in tissue electrical resistance, i.e. a change in I_{sc} (ΔI_{sc}) is a measure of net ion transport.

When isolated full-thickness jejunal segments from rats sensitized to *Trichinella* are mounted in Ussing chambers and challenged with *Trichinella*-derived antigen added to the serosal solution, anaphylaxis is expressed as a change in I_{sc}[21]. The ΔI_{sc} is due to net Cl^- secretion inasmuch as the antigen-induced response is blocked by agents which prevent entry of Cl^- into the epithelium via carrier-mediated processes at the basolateral membrane or prevent Cl^- exit through ion-specific channels on the apical membrane.

Neuroimmunological linkage

Mast cell-derived mediators transducing antigenic signals into changes in epithelial ion transport include, histamine[11,19,21,25], 5-hydroxytryptamine (5-HT)[15,21,26] and prostaglandins[19,21,26]. The interaction of these mediators with the ENS in signal transduction was examined in six[12,15,16,21,25,26] of the studies cited[11-26] by observing the effects of the muscarinic cholinergic antagonist, atropine[12,21] and/or the neurotoxin, tetrodotoxin (TTX)[15,16,25,26] on antigen-stimulated ion transport.

Ovalbumin sensitivity

Two studies involving ovalbumin-sensitized rats present different results. In one, the antigen-stimulated transmural ΔI_{sc} was attributed in part to histamine and was weakly sensitive to TTX treatment[25]. In the other, 5-HT and prostaglandin E_2 (PGE_2) were the reported chemical mediators of the ΔI_{sc} response[26] which, in this case, was insensitive to TTX. Based on these results from the ovalbumin-sensitive rat, a role for the ENS in antigen signal transduction remains equivocal.

Studies of intestinal smooth muscle in ovalbumin-sensitized guinea-pigs provide some intriguing results in relation to the regulation of local anaphylactic reactions. Zilletti et al.[8] reported that γ-aminobutyric acid (GABA) inhibited ovalbumin-induced Schultz-Dale reactions and histamine release in longitudinal strips of guinea-pig ileum. This anti-allergic response, in which GABA presumably acts as a neurotransmitter, was ablated by treating the tissue with TTX. GABA anti-allergic effects could be mimicked by GABA-A (isoguvacine) or GABA-B [(-)-baclofen] agonists and inhibited by antagoists[9] (GABA-A, bicuculline; GABA-B, Δ-amino valeric acid) of either receptor type.

β-lactoglobulin sensitivity

βLG challenge of ileum from milk-sensitized guinea-pigs elicited an ion transport change that was blunted by TTX[16]. In separate studies histamine[12] and 5-HT[15], respectively, were reported to mediate the βLG-induced ΔI_{sc} in colonic epithelium. Atropine was ineffective in blocking the effect presumably mediated by histamine, whereas TTX significantly reduced the response mediated by 5-HT. Histamine, but not 5-HT, is present in mast cells from guinea-pigs[27]. 5-HT must therefore be released from other cell types in this species[15].

Baird et al.[15] observed through rigorously designed experiments that both TTX and ICS 205-930 (Sandoz AG, Basle), a $5-HT_3$ (Neural receptor) antagonist, inhibited βLG-induced Cl^- secretion in sensitized guinea-pig colon. Since $5-HT_3$ receptors (M receptors) are localized on substance P-containing nerve terminals in guinea-pig intestine[29] it is possible that part of the anaphylactically released 5-HT acts directly on efferent neurons to release substance P which effects epithelial Cl^- secretion[30]. The sum of the effects of TTX in the three experiments with milk-fed guinea-pigs supports the conclusion that enteric nerves are involved in the response to βLG challenge.

Trichinella sensitivity

Studies of antigen stimulated changes in Cl^- secretion in Trichinella-infected rats[21] have established the presence of neuroimmunological pathways in the gut. An association between the immune system and the ENS to effect Cl^- secretion could be rationalized from evidence that (1) antigenic challenge of sensitized gut tissue leads to rapidly evoked changes in physiological function[27,28]; (2) mast cell-mediated immune responses are prominent in enteric helminth infections in general[31,32] and in trichinosis specifically[33]; (3) 5-HT, histamine and PG are released or generated *de novo* as a result of mast cell degranulation[34,35]; (4) 5-HT, histamine and PG act as Cl^- secretagogues on intestinal epithelium[36-40]; (5) nerves are involved in epithelial secretion of Cl^- [41,42]; and (6) stimulation of epithelial Cl^- secretion by diverse agents such as prostaglandins, cAMP, Ca^{++} and bacterial enterotoxins involves common intraepithelial pathways[43,44].

The Cl^- secretory response evoked by *Trichinella* antigen is biphasic, with peak responses occurring at ~ 1.5 min and ~ 5.0 min after stimulation. The fast phase (I) is completed in about 2–3 min whereas the slow phase (II) is sustained, lasting for at least 15 min.

Experimentally, it was demonstrated that in association with antigen-induced Cl^- secretion in *Trichinella*-sensitized rat jejunum, histamine, 5-HT and PGE_2 accumulate in the bathing solution[21]. When applied exogenously to unsensitized rat jejunum, both 5-HT and histamine mimic the fast phase of Cl^- secretion while PGE_2 simulates the slow phase. Furthermore, antagonists of 5-HT (cinanserin and metergoline) and of histamine (diphenhydramine) specifically reduce the Cl^- secretory response to those respective secretagogues. The 5-HT and histamine antagonists also blunt the fast phase of Cl^- secretion induced by antigen without altering the slow phase. In contrast indomethacin, an inhibitor of prostaglandin synthesis, almost completely eliminates the slow phase response to antigenic challenge.

5-HT- and histamine-evoked Cl^- secretion were partially inhibited by atropine and TTX, whereas these neural blockers had no effect on PGE-mediated secretion. When tested against antigen-induced Cl^- secretion the peak of the fast phase (I) response in the rat–*Trichinella* system was inhibited $\sim 60\%$ by atropine and $\sim 80\%$ by TTX, whereas that of the slow phase (II) response was reduced only 20%. These results indicate that the ENS is involved in antigen-stimulated responses. A functional overview of antigen-evoked Cl^- secretion is presented in Figure 2.

Palmer *et al.*[45], in an exciting and novel approach, examined the influence of antigenic stimulation on myenteric neurons in the small intestine. Micro-electrodes were used to directly record electrical and synaptic activity in myenteric nerves in *Trichinella*-infected guinea-pigs as the sensitized tissue was challenged with *Trichinella* antigen administered by superfusion or by pressure microinjection. Recordings from AH type II neurons revealed specific, antigen-evoked patterns of membrane depolarization and repolarization along with increased input resistance. Antigen also suppressed nicotinic cholinergic fast excitatory post-synaptic potentials evoked by electrical stimulation.

Direct stimulation of intestinal smooth muscle by anaphylactically released chemical mediators in albumin sensitized guinea-pigs[8,9], is in line with observations in murine trichinosis. Schultz–Dale type reactions expressed by longitudinal smooth muscle from trichinized rat intestine and mediated by 5-HT were unaffected by atropine or TTX[10]. In contrast isolated, fluid-filled segments of guinea-pig small intestine, sensitized to and challenged with *Trichinella* antigen, were responsive to the neurotoxin. Changes in fluid-propelling behaviour evoked by antigenic challenge and mimicked by

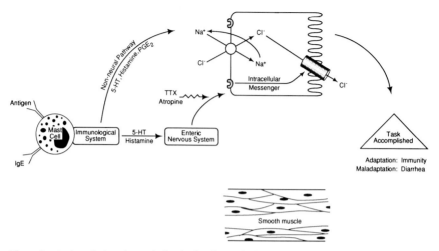

Figure 2 Antigen-induced, anaphylactically triggered Cl⁻ secretion in jejunum of rats sensitized by infection with *Trichinella spiralis* and challenged with *Trichinella* antigen. Cl⁻ secretion is mediated by 5-Hydroxytryptamine (5-HT) and histamine released from mast cells and by prostaglandin (PGE$_2$) synthesized *de novo* following mast cell activation. A major component of 5-HT- and histamine-mediated secretion is inhibited by either atropine or tetrodotoxin (TTX), implying involvement of neural pathways. The antigen-evoked component of secretion attributed to PGE$_2$ is only weakly affected by atropine and TTX, therefore, that component and the TTX insensitive part of 5-HT-and histamine-mediated Cl⁻ secretion are considered to be mediated primarily through non-neural pathways. Pathways similar to those explaining the transduction of antigenic signals into epithelial responses are beginning to be identified for intestinal smooth muscle. Antigen-induced Cl⁻ secretion may be reflective of epithelial changes that bear on immunity to the intraepithelial parasite, but which may also be pathological in scope (summarized from Castro *et al.*[21])

histamine were inhibited in the presence of TTX (unpublished results).

Despite convincing evidence that the ENS participates in transduction of antigenic stimuli into epithelial responses, it is not yet possible to unambiguously identify specific pathways involved. An interpretation of the neuroimmunological data from the rat–*Trichinella* experiments within the context of current models of nerve-modulated Cl⁻ secretion[46,47] must account for 5-HT- and histamine-evoked Cl⁻ secretion in the absence of evidence that gut epithelium possesses receptors for these amines. Thus, one is compelled to consider that the atropine- and TTX-insensitive components of Cl⁻ secretion mediated by 5-HT and histamine also involve an indirect, possibly neural, pathway. A TTX-insensitive pathway might involve neurons with short processes which use graded, non-spiking conductive mechanisms[48].

Histamine appears to effect Cl⁻ secretion through H$_1$ receptors. Although involvement of H$_2$ receptors can be ruled out by experimental results, a possible role for H$_3$ receptors cannot be eliminated. H$_3$ receptors on presynaptic terminals of nicotinic cholinergic neurons in the gut suppress acetylcholine release when activated[49]. Thus, histamine might contribute to Cl⁻ secretion by blocking synaptic transmission in multineuronal pathways which normally inhibit Cl⁻ secretion.

The mode of action of antigen-released 5-HT appears to be more complex than that of histamine. The inhibition of Cl^- secretion by cinanserin suggests that a 5-HT_2 receptor might be involved[29]. Since such receptors have not been identified nor on Cl^--secreting epithelial cells it might be appropriate at this time to consider the presence of 5-HT_2 receptors on other cell types in the gut mucosa or submucosa. It was recently suggested that 5-HT_1 and 5-HT_3 receptors on AH type II neurons of the myenteric plexus be designated 5-HT_{P1} and 5-HT_{P2} receptors[50]. Functionally 5-HT binding to 5-HT_{P1} and 5-HT_{P2} receptors is specifically antagonized by 5-HT dipeptide and ICS 205-930, respectively. Although the fast phase of antigen-induced Cl^- secretion in *Trichinella*-sensitized rat jejunum could be blocked substantially by 5-HT_1 and 5-HT_2 antagonists, a role for ICS 205-930 sensitive Cl^- secretion, as reported by others[15], cannot be ruled out.

It is difficult to explain why either 5-HT_2 or H_1 antagonists alone inhibit, almost completely, fast Cl^- secretion in the rat–*Trichinella* model, since either 5-HT or histamine can mimic the antigen-induced response. It may be that 5-HT and histamine act synergistically through a common pathway that is, in large part, TTX- and atropine-sensitive.

Task accomplished

A question in search of an answer relates to what physiological function is accomplished through neuroimmune interactions. Although the task accomplished in the rat–*Trichinella* model is not yet clear, the rapid onset of epithelial secretion following antigenic challenge coincides with functional immunity to the parasite[51]. Thus, the association between the epithelial response and rapid worm rejection supports the hypothesis that anaphylactically induced epithelial changes create a microenvironment inhospitable to the parasite. In short, the timely elicitation of immune reactions which involve nerve-mediated modulation of epithelial function may represent an adaptive response that interferes with the infectivity of this nematode, which lives within epithelial cells during the intestinal phase of its life-cycle.

In addition to potential involvement in acquired resistance to reinfection, the changes in target tissue function mediated by anaphylactic reactions may contribute to pathological states. Cl^- secretion is a case in point. That secretory process may represent an 'enteric tear' system which during homeostatic states cleanses and protects the mucosal surface, but under uncontrolled conditions converts to a maladaptive, diarrheal state. The latter condition clearly could be viewed as harmful to the host and contributory to pathological signs and symptoms.

Potential for external modulation

Once neuroimmunologically controlled processes are identified, the possibility exists for mimicking, pharmacologically, 'useful' ones and curbing those contributing to pathological states. Such processes appear to be potentially

Table 1 Pharmacological modulation of gut anaphylaxis

Targeted Effect (tissue)[a]	Agent[b]	Action[b]
Inhibition of mediator release (E)	Doxantrazole[25]	Inhibits MMC degranulation
Antagonism of mediators (E)	Pyrilamine[19]	H_1 receptor blocker
	Diphenhydramine[21]	H_1 receptor blocker
	Cinanserin[21]	5-HT$_2$ receptor blocker
	Indomethacin[21]	Inhibits PG synthesis
Inhibition of neural stimulatory pathways (E)	Atropine[21]	Muscarinic blocker
	TTX[15,16,21]	Neural blockade
	ICS 205-930[15]	5-HT$_3$ (5-HT$_{P2}$;[50] neural receptor) blocker
Activation of neural inhibitory pathways (SM)	GABA agonist[9] [isoquvacine; (-)-baclofen]	Inhibits anaphylaxis through unknown mechanism
Modulation of effector tissue (E)	Furosemide[21]	Inhibits Cl$^-$ entry (BLM)
	DPC[21]	Inhibits Cl$^-$ conductance (apical membrane)

[a]E, epithelium; SM, smooth muscle.
[b]MMC, mucosal mast cell; PG, prostaglandin; Ach, acetylcholine; TTX, tetrodotoxin; GABA, γ-aminobutyric acid; DPC, diphenylamine-2-carboxylate; BLM, basolateral membrane

susceptible to pharmacological control at the level of the immune system, neural system and effector tissues (Table 1).

SUMMARY

Paracrine substances released from immunologically reactive cells in the intestine of sensitized animals regulate epithelial and smooth muscle function. Rapid responses of both tissues to antigenic challenge represent functional analogues of the classic Schultz–Dale reaction, which is the prototype of immediate hypersensitivity in the GI tract. Although the rat–*Trichinella spiralis* system was focused on as a model of anaphylaxis, an overriding observation was that responses, which are analogous in effect though different in cause, are evoked by different antigens in different species sensitized through a variety of antigen delivery systems. The sum of results from studies of different host species support a working hypothesis that antigen-induced release of histamine, 5-HT and prostaglandin E_2 stimulate Cl$^-$ secretion by gut epithelium. Histamine and 5-HT exert effects partly through enteric nerves. While most evidence implicates enteric nerves in mediating local anaphylaxis, GABA-ergic neurons in the myenteric plexus purportedly have anti-anaphylactic properties. The immunophysiological responses described are potentially susceptible to pharmacologic control at the level of the immune system, neural system and effector tissue.

Whereas the anatomical components of intestinal neuroimmunological pathways are present in the immune host, their integrative functions are expressed only upon antigenic challenge. Thus, that expression may be viewed as a highly regulated exploitive adaptation, supporting the premise[3] that the immune system is a functional extension of the neural sensory system.

Acknowledgements

Original work from the author's laboratory alluded to in text was supported by the US Public Health Service Research Grant No. AI-11361 from the National Institute of Health.

References

1. Jankovic, B.D. (1987). Opening remarks. In Jankovic, B.D., Markovic, B.M. and Spector, N.H. (eds.) *Neuroimmune Interactions: Proceedings of the Second International Workshop on Neuroimmunomodulation*, pp. 1–2 (New York: The New York Academy of Sciences)
2. Castro, G.A. (1982). Immunological regulation of epithelial function. *Am. J. Physiol.*, **243** (*Gastrointest. Liver Physiol.*, **6**), G321–9
3. Blalock, J.E. (1984). The immune system as a sensory organ. *J. Immunol.*, **132**, 1067–8
4. Ader, R. (ed.) (1981). *Psychoneuroimmunology*. (New York: Academic Press)
5. Spector, N.H. and Korneva, E.A. (1981). Neurophysiology, immunophysiology and neuroimmunomodulation. In Ader, R. (ed.) *Psychoneuroimmunology*, pp. 449–73 (New York: Academic Press)
6. Adolph, E.F. (1982). Physiological integrations in action. In *The Physiologist* (Suppl.), Vol. 25 (Bethesda: The American Physiological Society)
7. Stead, R.H. Bienenstock, J. and Stanisz, A.M. (1987). Neuropeptide regulation of mucosal immunity. *Immunol. Rev.*, **100**, 333–59
8. Zilletti, L., Luzzi, S., Franchi-Micheli, S., Rizzotti, M., Rosi, E. and Spagnesi, S. (1984). Influence of GABA on anaphylactic histamine release in vitro. *Agents Actions*, **14**, 478–80
9. Luzzi, S., Franchi-Micheli, W., Ciuffi, M., Rosi, E. and Zilletti, L. (1987). Effect of various GABA-receptor agonists and antagonists on anaphlyactic histamine release in the guinea-pig ileum. *Agents Actions*, **20**, 181–4
10. Vermillion, D., Sciccitano, R. and Collins, S.M. (1987). Immunological control of motility: 5-HT mediates antigen-specific contraction of smooth muscle in sensitized gut. *Gastroenterology*, **92**, 1682 (Abstract)
11. Cuthbert, A.W., McLaughlan, P. and Coombs, R.R.A. (1983). Immediate hypersensitivity reaction to β-lactoglobulin in the epithelium lining the colon of guinea pigs fed cow's milk. *Int. Arch. Allergy Appl. Immunol.*, **72**, 34–40
12. Baird, A.W., Coombs, R.R.A., McLaughlan, P. and Cuthbert, A.W. (1984). Immediate hypersensitivity reactions to cow milk proteins in isolated epithelium from ileum of milk-drinking guinea pigs: comparisons with colonic epithelia. *Int. Arch. Allergy Appl. Immunol.*, **75**, 255–63
13. Kessel, D. and Cuthbert, A.W. (1984). Sidedness of the reaction to β-lactoglobulin in sensitized colonic epithelia. *Int. Arch. Allergy Appl. Immunol.*, **74**, 113–19
14. Baird, A.W., Barclay, W.S. and Blazer-Yost, B.L. (1987). Affinity purified immunoglobulin G transfers immediate hypersensitivity to guinea pig colonic epithelium in vitro. *Gastroenterology*, **92**, 635–42
15. Baird, A.W. and Cuthbert, A.W. (1987). Neuronal involvement in type 1 hypersensitivity reactions in gut epithelia. *Br. J. Pharmacol.*, **92**, 647–55
16. Baird, A.W., Cuthbert, A.W. and MacVinish, L.J. (1987). Type 1 hypersensitivity reactions in reconstructed tissues using syngeneic cell types. *Br. J. Pharmacol.*, **91**, 857–69
17. Russell, D.A. and Castro, G.A. (1985). Anaphylactic-like reaction of small intestine epithelium in parasitized guinea pigs. *Immunology*, **54**, 573–9
18. Russell, D.A. and Castro, G.A. (1987). Comparison of jejunal and colonic epithelial immediate hypersensitivity responses. *Gastroenterology*, **92**, 1605 (Abstract)
19. Russell, D.A. (1986). Mast cells in the regulation of intestinal electrolyte transport. *Am. J.*

Physiol., **251** (*Gastrointest. Liver Physiol.*, **14**), G253–62

20. Harari, Y., Russell, D.A. and Castro, G.A. (1987). Anaphylaxis mediated epithelial Cl⁻ secretion and parasite rejection in rat intestine. *J. Immunol.*, **138**, 1250–5
21. Castro, G.A., Harari, Y. and Russell, D. (1987). Mediators of anaphylaxis-induced ion transport changes in small intestine. *Am. J. Physiol.*, **253**, (*Gastrointest. Liver Physiol.*, **16**), G540–8
22. Baird, A.W., Cuthbert, A.W. and Pearce, F.L. (1985). Immediate hypersensitivity reactions in epithelia from rats infected with *Nippostrongylus brasiliensis. Br. J. Pharmacol.*, **85**, 787–95
23. Perdue, M.H., Chung, M. and Gall, D.G. (1984). Effect of intestinal anaphylaxis on gut function in the rat. *Gastroenterology*, **86**, 391–7
24. Perdue, M.H. and Gall, G.D. (1986). Intestinal anaphylaxis in the rat: jejunal response to in vitro antigen exposure. *Am. J. Physiol.*, **250**, (*Gastrointest. Liver Physiol.*, **13**), G427–31
25. Perdue, M.H. and Gall, G.D. (1986). Rat jejunal mucosal response to histamine and anti-histamines *in vitro*. Comparisons with antigen-induced changes during intestinal anaphylaxis. *Agents Actions*, **19**, 5–9
26. Catto-Smith, A.G., Patrick, M.K., Hardin, J.A. and Gall, D.G. (1988). Mediators responsible for electrolyte transport abnormalities induced by intestinal anaphylaxis. *Gastroenterology*, **94**, Part 2, A62 (Abstract)
27. Schultz, W.H. (1910). Physiological studies in anaphylaxis. I. The reaction of smooth muscle on the guinea pig sensitized with horse-serum. *J. Pharmacol. Exp. Ther.*, **1**, 549–67
28. Dale, H.H. (1913). The anaphylactic reaction of plain muscle in guinea pig. *J. Pharmacol. Exp. Ther.*, **4**, 167–223
29. Richardson, B.P. and Engel, G. (1986). The pharmacology and function of 5-HT₃ receptors. *Trends Neurosci.*, **9**, 424–8
30. Walling, M.W., Brasitus, T.A. and Kimberg, D.V. (1977). Effects of calcitonin and substance P on the transport of Ca, Na and Cl across rat ileum in vitro. *Gastroenterology*, **73**, 89–94
31. Askanase, P.W. (1980). Immunopathology of parasitic diseases: Involvement of basophils and mast cells. *Springer Seminars Immunopathol.*, **2**, 417–42
32. Befus, D. (1986). Immunity in intestinal helminth infections: present concepts, future directions. *Trans. R. Soc. Trop. Med. Hyg.*, **80**, 735–41
33. Sharp, A.D. and Olson, L.J. (1962). Hypersensitivity response in *Toxocara, Ascaris* and *Trichinella*-infected guinea pigs to homologous challenge. *J. Parasitol.*, **48**, 326–7
34. Lee, T.D.G., Sweeter, M.G. and Befus, D. (1986). Mast cell responses to helminth infection. *Parasitol. Today*, **2**, 186–91
35. Foreman, J.C. (1984). Functional aspects of mast cells, mediator contents and mediator effects. *Acta Otolaryngol. Suppl.*, **414**, 93–101
36. Musch, N.W., Miller, R.J., Field, M. and Siegel, M.I. (1982). Stimulation of colonic secretion by lipoxygenase metabolites of arachidonic acid. *Science*, **217**, 1255–6
37. Donowitz, M., Tai, Y.H. and Asarkof, N.A. (1980). Effect of serotonin on active electrolyte transport in rabbit ileum gallbladder and colon. *Am. J. Physiol.*, **239**, (*Gastrointest. Liver Physiol.*, **2**), G463–72
38. Hardcastle, J., Hardcastle, P.T. and Redfern, J.S. (1981). Action of 5-hydroxytryptamine on intestinal ion transport in the rat. *J. Physiol.* (*Lond.*), **320**, 41–55
39. Cooke, H., Nemeth, P.R. and Wood, J.D. (1984). Histamine action on guinea pig ileal mucosa. *Am. J. Physiol.*, **246** (*Gastrointest. Liver Physiol.*, **9**), G372–7
40. Cuthbert, A.W. and Margolius, H.S. (1982). Kinins stimulate net chloride secretion by the rat colon. *Br. J. Pharmacol.*, **75**, 587–98
41. Hubel, K.A. (1978). The effects of electrical field stimulation and tetrodotoxin on ion transport by the isolated rabbit ileum. *J. Clin. Invest.*, **62**, 1039–47
42. Sjovall, H., Jodal, M. and Lundgren, O. (1987). Sympathetic control of intestinal fluid and electrolyte transport. *News Physiol. Sci.*, **2**, 214–17
43. Field, M. (1980). Regulation of small intestinal ion transport by cyclic nucleotides and calcium. In Field, M., Fordtran, J.S. and Schultz, S.G. (eds.). *Secretory Diarrhea*, pp. 21–30. (Bethesda: American Physiological Society)
44. Frizzell, R.A., Heintze, K. and Stewart, C.P. (1980). Mechanism of intestinal chloride secretion. In Field, M., Fordtran, J.S. and Schultz, S.G. (eds.), *Secretory Diarrhea*, pp. 11–19 (Bethesda: American Physiological Society)
45. Palmer, J.M., Tamura, K. and Wood, J.D. (1988). Electrical and synaptic properties of

myenteric plexus neurons from guinea-pig small intestine during infection with *Trichinella spiralis*. *FASEB J.*, **2**, A325 (Abstract)

46. Cooke, H.J. (1986). Neurobiology of the intestinal mucosa. *Gastroenterology*, **90**, 1057–81
47. Keast, J.R. (1987). Mucosal innervation and control of water and ion transport in the intestine. *Rev. Physiol. Biochem. Pharmacol.*, **109**, 1–59
48. Roberts, A. and Bush, B.M.H. (eds.) (1981). *Neurones Without Impulses: Their Significance for Vertebrate and Invertebrate Nervous Systems.* (Cambridge: Cambridge University Press)
49. Tamura, K., Palmer, J.M. and Wood, J.D. (1988). Presynaptic inhibition produced by histamine at nicotinic synapses in enteric ganglia. *Neuroscience*, **25**, 171–9
50. Mawe, G.M., Branchek, T.A. and Gershon, M.D. (1986). Peripheral neuronal serotonin receptors: Identification and characterization with specific antagonists and agonists. *Proc. Natl. Acad. Sci.*, **83**, 9799–803
51. Russell, D.A. and Castro, G.A. (1979). Physiological characterization of a biphasic immune response to *Trichinella spiralis* in the rat. *J. Inf. Dis.*, **139**, 304–12

Summary of Section III

J. D. WOOD

The purpose of this session was to present an expert overview of current concepts of neural determination of behaviour of the intestinal effector systems. This was planned to include the musculature, mucosal epithelium, blood vasculature and immune system. The session was arranged to provide an overview of cellular neurophysiology and functional organization of synaptic networks in the myenteric and submucosal plexuses and in the prevertebral ganglia. These neurophysiological presentations served as basic background for the lectures on neurally mediated behaviours of the major effector systems.

J.D. Wood of The Ohio State University opened the session with discussion of electrical and synaptic behaviour of neurons in the myenteric plexus and presented this in the context of network theory for control of intestinal motility. He was followed by J. H. Szurszewski from the Mayo Clinic, who developed concepts of interactions between the enteric nervous system and prevertebral ganglia, as well as synaptic integration within the prevertebral ganglia. A. Surprenant, from the Oregon Health Sciences University, then presented her lecture on the electrical and synaptic properties of ganglion cells in the submucosal plexus. While doing so, she introduced an exciting new preparation for investigation of intrinsic neural influence on mucosal blood vessels. H.J. Cooke of The Ohio State University built on the presentation of Dr Surprenant in presenting current concepts of neuroeffector relations that determine mucosal electrolyte secretion and absorption. She focused on results from *in vitro* investigation of reflex pathways to the mucosa and on the neurotransmitters/neuromodulators involved in the synaptic circuits and at neuroepithelial junctions. O. Lundgren, of Göteborg University, complimented Dr Cooke's lecture with an insightful view of neural control of mucosal behaviour and blood flow as interpreted from investigations carried out *in vivo*. J.S. Davison, of the University of Calgary and co-chairman of the session, followed with his lecture on neural mechanisms responsible for co-ordination and integration between motor behaviour of the musculature and functional behaviour of the mucosal epithelium. G.A. Castro, from the University of Texas Medical School, ended the session with a presentation of the highly interesting new frontier of interactions between the intestinal immune system and the enteric nervous system.

NEURAL BASIS OF ENTERIC MOTOR FUNCTION

J.D. Wood used slides from the newly developed Unit # 20[1] of the Undergraduate Teaching Project of the American Gastroenterological

Association for his lecture. This Unit entitled, 'Gastrointestinal Neurophysiology: The Little Brain in the Gut' presents a neurophysiological theory of intestinal motility based on knowledge of electrical and synaptic behaviour of enteric neurons, localization of neurotransmitters and histoanatomy of the neuronal units that make up the networks of circuitry.

This presentation illustrated how the known neurobiological functions at the cellular level can be integrated into a coherent view of circuit operations, when considered in the context of well-established neurophysiological principles. Fast excitatory post-synaptic potentials (EPSPs) were explained as the 'bytes' of information in the rapid processing of information within the logic circuits. Information transfer at these synapses was shown to be modulated extensively by a variety of presynaptic receptors for several different putative neurotransmitters found in the ENS and in external inputs that interface with it. Slow EPSPs were pictured, as producing dramatic augmentation of excitability, which results in action potential discharge for several seconds. These longlasting spike trains in the ganglion cell body release neurotransmitters from the cell's axon/s for commensurate periods and this is a mechanism for prolonged excitatory or inhibitory drive at the junctions with the effector systems. Receptors for several putative neurotransmitters/neuromodulators, that are responsible for the slow EPSPs, are localized to subpopulations of enteric neurons. Slow synaptic inhibition, which is the inverse of slow synaptic excitation, also utilizes a variety of receptors for a different set of putative messengers.

This talk concluded with a discussion of demands of a neural circuit for organization of peristaltic propulsion and of synaptic gating mechanisms that might account for determination of distance of spread of a peristaltic motor complex. One of the important directions for future research should be development of new technology and approaches to tracing the spatial transfer of information within the dimensions of the myenteric plexus. It will be necessary to do this actively, perhaps with imaging technology and voltage-sensitive tracers, as the circuit operates to organize the behaviour of the musculature to achieve propulsion. There is little question that unravelling of the peristaltic circuit will be a major key for future clarification of the physiology and pathophysiology of intestinal motor function.

INTEGRATION OF SYMPATHETIC NEURAL OUTFLOW TO THE GI TRACT

J.H. Szurszewski's lecture stressed the critical concept that prevertebral ganglia are independent integrative centres for processing synaptic information derived from intestinal sensory receptors and the CNS. He emphasized that the traditional concept of prevertebral ganglia, as simple relay distri-

---

[1] UTP Unit # 20 *Gastrointestinal Neurophysiology: The Little Brain in the Gut* was prepared by J.D. Wood and D.L. Wingate in conjunction with the Subcommittee on Undergraduate Education, chaired by D.H. Alpers. It is distributed for the American Gastroenterological Association by Milner-Fenwick, Inc. 2125 Greenspring Drive, Timonium, Maryland 21093, USA.

bution centres for transfer of information from preganglionic to post-ganglionic sympathetic neurons, is no longer tenable in light of present knowledge.

Professor Szurszewski skilfully developed an elegant picture of the significance of the prevertebral ganglia in the schema of intestinal neurobiology. He showed how sympathetic projections from the ganglia release norepinephrine and co-localized neuropeptides to suppress synaptic functions in the enteric circuits as well as directly influence intestinal blood vessels and the mucosal epithelium. Co-localization is specific within the sympathetic neurons. Those that innervate the blood vessels express neuropeptide Y in co-stores with norepinephrine, whereas the neurons innervating submucosal ganglia and the epithelium express somatostatin.

He proceeded to show how the sympathetic ganglion cells not only project information to the intestine, but also receive information derived from sensory neurons in the intestine. This information comes from two kinds of sensory afferent fibres. One kind has its cell body in the ENS and behaves like a mechanoreceptor that fires in response to distention of the intestinal wall. The second kind have cell bodies in dorsal root ganglia (DRG). As these project to the spinal cord, they appear also to send collaterals that synapse in the prevertebral ganglia. Sensory fibres from the intramural mechanoreceptors utilize acetylcholine as a neurotransmitter that evokes classical fast nicotinic cholinergic EPSPs; whereas, the sensory fibres of DRG origin appear to release substance P, which evokes slow EPSPs in the sympathetic ganglion cells. Substance P behaves like a neuromodulator in this respect in that it greatly increases the safety factor for the fast cholinergic EPSPs to evoke spikes in the sympathetic ganglion cell and thereby increase the probability that reflex information will be relayed back to the intestine.

Doctor Szurszewski continued his stimulating story by revealing evidence that peptidergic synaptic input from the CNS also modulates the input–output relations of the sympathetic ganglion cells. These inputs are in addition to the classical nicotinic cholinergic inputs from neurons in the intermediolateral cell columns of the spinal cord. He presented strong evidence from his own laboratory that central inputs modulate transmission in the ganglia through release of neurotensin and opioid peptides. Neurotension potentiates the release of substance P, whereas the enkephalins suppress the release of substance P.

Dr Szurszewski finished with an intriguing hypothesis for dual function of the substance P connections in the ganglia. During hyperactivity of intestinal effectors (e.g. muscular spasm or enhanced H_2O/electrolyte secretion) substance P inputs to the prevertebral ganglia enhance transmission in the ganglion–gut loop to increase the sympathetic 'braking' action on the effector activity. The same substance P fibres also convey afferent information to the CNS, where it may be interpreted as visceral pain. Central processing of this information, as well as other decisions within the 'big brain', may lead to the generation of central outflow to the ganglia that further adjusts transmission through the gut–ganglion reflex path. Future research will, undoubtedly, continue to address the neurobiology of the central and peripheral mechanisms involved in integration and control of the sympathetic outflow from the prevertebral ganglia to the gut. The motivation for this kind of research will be the potential for clearing up some of the puzzles that surround nervous-system-related disorders such as the irritable bowel syndrome, chronic constipation and nervous diarrhoea. Not to mention stress-related exacerbations of inflammatory bowel disease, especially in the colon.

CELLULAR NEUROPHYSIOLOGY/PHARMACOLOGY OF SUBMUCOSAL NEURONS

A. Surprenant's lecture was based on her highly productive studies of intracellularly recorded electrical and synaptic behaviour in ganglion cells in the submucosal plexus. Her talk was an important prelude to the subsequent presentations of Drs Cooke and Lundgren on neural control of mucosal function. She described at the single neuronal level, neurophysiological behaviour which must be integral to the circuit operations that organize secretory and absorptive behaviour as well as co-ordinate local blood flow in support of these processes.

One of Dr Surprenant's main 'take home' lessons was that a spectrum of neurotransmitters/neuromodulators are involved in the chemical transfer of information to submucosal neurons. These included adrenergic, aminergic, cholinergic and peptidergic agents, some of which had preference for particular receptor subtypes. For example: (1) norepinephrine acts at α_2-receptors on submucosal neurons; (2) serotonin binds preferentially to $5HT_3$ receptors to produce fast depolarizing responses and to other unidentified subtypes in producing slow depolarizing responses and presynaptic inhibition; (3) acetylcholine acts at M_1 muscarinic receptors to produce slow EPSP-like responses, whereas presynaptic muscarinic receptors are more like M_2 receptors; (4) enkephalinergic receptors on submucosal neurons are of the delta subtype, in contrast to myenteric neurons which possess the μ subtype.

She emphasized also that most of the 'slow' synaptic potentials are generated by conductance changes in potassium channels in the somal membranes of the submucosal neurons. Opening of potassium channels is responsible for the membrane hyperpolarization of slow inhibitory post-synaptic potentials (IPSPs) and closure of the potassium channels is part of the mechanism involved in the depolarization during slow EPSPs. She called attention to the very important fact that receptors, for more than one neurotransmitter, are coupled to the same potassium channel and this coupling may involve inhibitory guanosine triphosphate-binding proteins. For example, application of norepinephrine, somatostatin or enkephalin produce slow IPSP-like responses by opening the same potassium channels. The inhibitory responses to somatostatin and norepinephrine are interesting in light of Dr Szurszewski's demonstration that these two transmitters are co-localized and presumably released from sympathetic axons in the mucosa. Doctor Suprenant alluded to this in relating that somatostatin is present both in neurons with cell bodies in the intestine and in the sympathetic projections from prevertebral ganglia. Since, enteric neurons do not express norepinephrine, this neurotransmitter disappears from the intestine after experimental ablation of the sympathetic innervation. In this circumstance, both the levels of somatostatin in the intrinsic innervation and the sensitivity of the receptors for somatostatin are enhanced. This is indicative of compensatory changes suggestive of the adaptive significance of paired innervation with dual transmitters and receptors, but the same synaptic action.

Dr Surprenant's lecture revealed several neurobiological differences between the submucosal and myenteric plexuses. No doubt this is a reflection of the specialized functions of each in a primary role of controlling the mucosal epithelium or the muscularis externa respectively. This talk illustrated much progress derived from direct recording from the neurons of the submucosal plexus. It also suggests that continued application of this methodology will continue to produce new findings that will maintain present momentum in advancement of understanding of gastrointestinal physiology.

Dr Surprenant concluded her talk by describing an exciting new submucosal preparation consisting of submucosal ganglia and blood vessels. This is the first preparation for direct observation of the effects of stimulation of intrinsic ganglion cells on the contractile responses of intestinal blood vessels. She described her preliminary observations of changes in the calibre of arterioles during focal electrical stimulation of individual submucosal ganglia. If she microejected norepinephrine, the arterioles constricted. Focal stimulation of a submucosal ganglion relaxed the norepinephrine-induced constriction and the diameter of the arteriole increased. The M_1 muscarinic antagonist pirenzipine blocked the vasodilation. Inhibition of acetylcholinesterase enhanced the dilation to ganglionic stimulation, consistent with Dr Surprenant's interpretation that the relaxation of the vessels is cholinergically mediated. The promise of this preparation will undoubtedly be recognized in future research on the neurophysiology and pharmacology of intrinsic mechanisms of control of intestinal blood flow.

NEUROEFFECTOR RELATIONS IN THE INTESTINAL MUCOSA
IN VITRO

H.J. Cooke, at The Ohio State University, and K.A. Hubel, at the University of Iowa, have been the pioneers in development and application of methods of electrical field stimulation of intramural neurons in conjunction with measurements of ionic currents and fluxes in Ussing chambers. In her symposium lecture, Dr Cooke reviewed the new insights into neural control of the mucosa that have emerged from application of these methods in combination with innovative pharmacological analysis.

She began by presenting evidence that ongoing activity in the ENS is the drive for suppression of neutral NaCl absorption across the mucosa of *in vitro* preparations. It was pointed out that spontaneous spike discharge recorded from enteric neurons in electrophysiological studies of Dr Surprenant and others is probably the neural correlate of the ongoing secretory activity. She suggested that some of the ongoing secretory activity may reflect absence of the sympathetic 'brake' that is normally functional *in vivo*. This was reminiscent of the lecture of Prof. Szurszewski, where he stressed the significance of co-localization of norepinephrine and somatostatin in the sympathetic innervation of the mucosa and submucosal plexus and of Dr Surprenant's description of the inhibitory action of both norepinephrine and somatostatin on excitability of submucosal ganglion cells.

The next major topic was identification of neurotransmitter function both in the synaptic circuitry and at the neuroepithelial junctions. According to Dr Cooke, the Ussing chamber studies, in combination with electrical field stimulation, have unequivocally identified acetylcholine release and activation of muscarinic receptors as a major mode of neuroepithelial transmission in the stimulation of secretion of chloride and water. Circumstantial evidence for vasoactive intestinal peptide as an excitatory neurotransmitter in stimulation of chloride secretion is strong, but remains equivocal due to unavailability of specific VIP antagonists. Inhibitory neuroeffector transmission appears to also be operational in the form of release of neuropeptide Y from intrinsic neurons of the submucosal plexus.

Within the synaptic circuitry, the Ussing chamber studies point to serotonin, acetylcholine and substance P as excitatory neurotransmitters. The actions of acetylcholine involve both nicotinic and muscarinic receptors. Enkephalin and norepinephrine are implicated as inhibitory transmitters at synapses in the control circuits. Results of the Ussing chamber studies show the inhibitory actions of enkephalin to be mediated by delta opioid receptors and the norepinephrine inhibition to be an α_2 effect. These findings are entirely consistent with the results obtained by Dr Surprenant and associates in their electrophysiological studies of submucosal neurons.

Dr Cooke proceeded to describe interactions between neurotransmitters, some of which are proposed to be co-localized in individual neurons of the submucosal nervous system. She used examples of acetylcholine and VIP, where the responses to VIP are greatly potentiated when it is applied after recovery from a cholinergic response. The direct inhibitory effect of neuropeptide Y on VIP and cholinergic induced secretion was also used as an example of messenger interactions.

Dr Cooke concluded by reviewing evidence for intercommunication between the myenteric and submucosal plexuses in control of secretory activity. Her example was calcitonin gene-related peptide (CGRP) which, when added to whole-thickness preparations, stimulates chloride secretion. This action of CGRP is blocked by tetrodotoxin and suppressed by hexamethonium. It does not occur if the myenteric plexus has been removed prior to setting the preparation up in the Ussing chamber. Her interpretation of these results were as follows: (1) Ganglion cells with receptors for CGRP in the myenteric plexus are excited to discharge spikes. Electrophysiological studies have demonstrated slow EPSP-like actions of CGRP on myenteric neurons. (2) The spike information is transmitted in projections to the submucosal plexus. (3) The spike information is transformed at nicotinic cholinergic synapses in route to motor neurons in the submucosal plexus. (4) The termination of the pathway is a motor neuron that releases an unidentified neurotransmitter at receptors on the cells of the intestinal crypts.

Dr Cooke suggested that this might be a reflection of network interactions in the co-ordination of intestinal motor and secretory functions. Applicable to this suggestion was Dr Surprenant's report that about one-half of the synaptic inputs to submucosal ganglion cell come from the myenteric plexus.

Dr Cooke's presentation illustrated the value of investigating responses of the effector system to neural stimulation *in vitro* and Dr Surprenant's talk showed us the merit of direct electrophysiological study of the neurons that make up the control circuits. The two talks, taken together, reveal the value of analysing results of Ussing chamber studies in light of direct electrophysiological recording from the neurons and vice versa. New insights have emerged from unification of the two approaches which are of sufficient significance to justify future expansion of application of the two methodologies in parallel.

NEUROEFFECTOR RELATIONS IN THE INTESTINAL MUCOSA
IN VIVO

O. Lundgren reviewed interpretations of results obtained by the group in Göteborg during several years of investigation of intestinal mucosal secretion and blood flow *in vivo*. He began by reviewing a vasodilatory reflex that can be evoked by gently stroking the mucosal surface of the large intestine of the cat and small bowel of the rat. The mechanoreceptor induced vasodilatation is abolished by nervous blockade with tetrodotoxin and by serotonergic desensitization. Prof. Lundgren presented evidence indicating that the involvement of serotonin was at an interneuron in the pathway and that the final motor neuron released vasoactive intestinal peptide to relax the vascular muscle. He pointed out that the identification of the mechanoreceptor for this response was unknown and suggested the possibility that the receptors might be serotonin-containing enterchromaffin cells. In this model, serotonin released from the enterochromaffin cells would activate the motor neuron to release vasoactive intestinal peptide. These models recalled Dr Surprenant's descriptions of the excitatory actions of serotonin on submucosal ganglion cells and the occurrence of slow EPSPs in neurons that contain vasoactive intestinal peptide.

Besides serotonin and vasoactive intestinal peptide, Prof. Lundgren suggested that substance P may also be involved in neural influences on blood flow. He presented results showing increased blood flow induced by treatment with capsacian. Since capsacian releases substance P from sensory fibres with cell bodies in the dorsal root ganglia but not from intrinsic enteric neurons, it was proposed that an axon reflex involving connections between spinal sensory fibres within the intestinal wall and the blood vessels might be responsible for the vasodilatation. This would be analogous to Dr Szurszewski's story where collaterals of spinal afferents release substance P in the prevertebral ganglia.

The second part of Prof. Lundgren's presentation addressed the well-documented observations that the mucosal stimulatory action of several secretogogues involves the ENS. Secretion of chloride and water in response to cholera toxin, enterotoxigenic *E. coli* and bile acids is suppressed by nervous blockade, by nicotinic synaptic blockade and muscarinic blockade at the neuroepithelial junctions. Consistent with this are observations that cholera toxin induces the release of vasoactive intestinal peptide and that this action of the toxin is blocked by tetrodotoxin.

Professor Lundgren concluded his lecture by presenting provocative evidence that cell migration from the intestinal crypts and along the villi is influenced by the ENS. His results showed that treatment with cholera toxin increase the rate of epithelial cell migration from the crypts and that this effect is abolished by neural blockade with tetrodotoxin.

Due consideration of the trilogy of lectures by Surprenant, Cooke and Lundgren underscores the desirability of integrating discoveries at reduced levels of organization to achieve better understanding of emergent properties of the functional system *in vivo*. There is little question that the present trend for research on nerves and the gastrointestinal tract to be conducted at reduced levels of organization will continue. It is to be hoped that it will be recognized that investigations at the cellular and molecular levels are little more than exercises if physiology and pathophysiology of the whole organ *in situ* is ignored in the process.

INTEGRATION OF MOTOR AND SECRETORY ACTIVITY IN THE GI TRACT

Gastrointestinal motility and secretion have traditionally been treated as different research subdisciplines of gastrointestinal biology. J. Davison's lecture addressed the relation between motility and secretion. He began with the premise that motility and secretion are linked functions and proceeded to present the underlying reasoning.

His first point was that a clear association between gastric motility and secretion is established for both humans and experimental animals. Two mechanisms that could account for the association were then presented. The first of these was activation of parallel pathways and the second was sequential activation of secretion by motor activity. Dr Davison suggested that vagovagal reflexes could utilize either of the two mechanisms. Observations that atropine blocks muscular responses to efferent vagal traffic without complete blockade of secretomotor responses is consistent with parallel paths but is inconclusive.

He described experiments in the ferret intestine where spontaneous patterns of small intestinal contractile activity occurred in association with fluctuations in transmural potential difference indicative of changes in ion secretion. Both of these were abolished simultaneously by transection of both vagal nerves or by administration of atropine or tetrodotoxin. In vagotomized ferrets, Dr Davison and his associates demonstrated that cyclically occurring contractions were followed by fluctuations in transmural potential difference. He concluded that this involved co-ordination within the enteric nervous system which could be interpreted as sequential activation. The sequence of events were considered to be: (1) contraction of the musculature activates 'in series' tension receptors which are known to be present in the intestinal wall; (2) spike information generated by the 'in series' mechanoreceptors is processed by local interneuronal circuits, probably in the myenteric plexus; (3) outflow from the internuncial circuits drives the motor innervation of the intestinal crypts to evoke secretion of chloride and water.

In summary, Dr Davison considered two co-existing neural mechanisms for coupling motility to secretion. The first was parallel but separate pathways to the muscle and epithelium, that could be activated simultaneously by integrated outflow in the vagal nerves. The second was a reflex pathway in which tension receptors detect muscular activity and code the information for processing by internuncial synaptic circuits. The internuncial circuits then transform the information into organized commands which activate the motor innervation of the epithelium.

Dr Davison concluded by pointing out that, intuitively, it makes sense for motor and secretory activity to be co-ordinated by the nervous system. Nevertheless, he was careful to point out the dearth of solid supporting evidence for existence of parallel co-ordinating pathways. He expressed confidence that the questions of neural integration of motility and secretion were approachable experimentally and that future research would clarify the mechanisms of integration.

INTESTINAL NEUROIMMUNE INTERACTIONS

G. Castro's lecture was introduced with the statement that the gastrointestinal neurobiologists chauvinistically flaunt the ENS as possessing as many neurons as the spinal cord; whereas, the gastrointestinal immunologist can boast that the GI tract contains as many immune cells as the remainder of the body. Professor Castro presented new discoveries in the rapidly advancing area of chemical communication between the enteric nervous and immune systems.

He described his longstanding interest in the mechanisms by which the intestine develops resistance to invasion by the parasite *Trichinella spiralis*. Resistance involves the development of immunity to antigens in the traditional sense, as well as changes in secretory function of the intestinal mucosa in concert with alterations in motility. Exposure of mucosal preparations in Ussing chambers to antigen from the parasite evokes a distinctive Cl^-/H_2O secretory response. If the antigen is introduced into the intestinal lumen *in vivo*, it evokes a characteristic propulsive motor response reminiscent of 'giant migrating contractions' that are propulsive and clear the lumen of secretions and solid material. The motor response still occurs in the intestine removed from sensitized guinea-pigs and studied *in vitro*.

The antigenically induced epithelial and muscular responses are blocked by tetrodotoxin, suggesting that they are neurally mediated. Histaminergic and serotonergic antagonists also influence the effector responses to present-ation of the antigen. Dr Castro presented evidence that these are immune mediators that are probably released from intestinal mast cells during antigenic challenge.

The results from Prof. Castro's model suggests communication between the intestinal immune system and the ENS. Behaviour of the immune system is like a sensory system that detects and identifies foreign antigens in the lumen and transfers the specific information to the intestinal nervous system. The nervous system responds to the immune signals by organizing musculo- and secretomotor responses that are co-ordinated for elimination of the noxious material from the lumen. This aspect of gastrointestinal investigation represents a relatively unexplored new frontier important for both basic physiology and abnormalities such as intestinal allergies and inflammatory disease. The author of this summary has for several years touted the ENS as an accessible model for investigation of cellular and network neurophysiology. Professor Castro's work foresees the intestine as a valuable model for investigation of neuroimmune communication.

Section IV
Brain–Gut Interaction

Introduction to brain–gut interaction

J.H. WALSH AND D.L. WINGATE

The enteric nervous system and the central nervous system constantly communicate with each other. Sensory information from the gut is transmitted to the brain, processed and integrated with other information in the CNS. Efferent messages from the CNS are transmitted to the ENS, leading to a variety of physiological and sometimes pathophysiological effects. The pathways for this exchange of information are the parasympathetic and sympathetic nerves. Processing of information occurs in various nuclei of the brain, the spinal cord, the sympathetic ganglia and the ganglia of the ENS. The chapters in this section explore the anatomical, pharmacological and physiological pathways and mechanisms responsible for brain–gut interactions. Special emphasis is given to new knowledge about the nature and role of neuropeptides as mediators of brain–gut information exchange and to the function of the peripheral autonomic sensory nervous system in reflex responses involving gastrointestinal motility.

The first three chapters set the stage for the later ones. They describe the anatomical basis and the likely transmitters involved in gut–brain–gut reflexes. Yvette Tache describes five peptides that are likely to act as central neurotransmitters to alter efferent autonomic pathways. Thyrotropin-releasing hormone site of action is located in the region of the dorsal vagal complex and activates vagal excitatory outflow. Microinjection of this peptide into the cerebrospinal fluid or appropriate sites in the brainstem stimulates gastric acid, pepsin and serotonin secretion, mucosal blood flow, motility and emptying, and can cause gastric ulcertaion. This substance may be a critical mediator involved in the pathogenesis of stress ulcers. Several other peptides, including gastrin releasing peptide and corticotrophin releasing factor (CRF), are potent inhibitors of gastric acid secretion, motility and emptying in rats and dogs when injected centrally, especially in parts of the hypothalamus. These peptides activate spinal-sympathetic outflow that leads to inhibition of gastric acid secretion and can prevent gastric ulceration. The pathways and mechanisms for these actions have been elucidated more clearly than their physiological significance. However, recent development of CRF antagonist and antibodies that specifically antagonize these neuropeptides promises to provide the tools needed to reveal the physiological roles of specific central and peripheral neuropeptides. Examples of successful use of CRF antagonist is found in some chapters of this section.

The types of sensory information transmitted from the gut to the brain include mechanical, thermal, chemical, osmotic, painful and nutritional signals. Most of this information passes along sensory fibres in the vagus nerves that project to the nucleus of the solitary tract, where information is mingled with signals carried via the sensory cranial nerves. Two techniques have been especially useful in characterizing the activities in the sensory system: one is the extracellular recording of action potentials in single nerve fibres; the other is immunohistochemical tracing of nerve fibres and pathways containing specific neuropeptides. Wendy Ewart points out the progress that has been made by use of these techniques in defining the simplest pathways involving peripheral sensory receptors, vagal sensory fibres, the nucleus of the solitary tract and activation of efferent signals from the dorsal motor nucleus to complete a refle arc from gut to brain to gut. She also points out the complexities of integration of information between the brainstem and higher centres in the brain. Herman and Rogers provide us with a detailed description of the connections between the nucleus of the solitary tract and the dorsal motor nucleus with the cortex, hypothalamus, stria terminalis, amygdala and medullary reticular area. These higher central sources of neural input influence the basic vagovagal reflex pathways. They point out the need for intracellular recording techniques to determine the role of specific neurochemical mediators such as peptides in modulation of the activity of these systems.

The remaining chapters analyse neural regulation of various aspects of gastrointestinal motility. Blackshaw and Grundy have studied the electrical activity in the vagal efferent fibres during emesis. Their data are consistent with the concept of a trigger mechanism resulting from afferent information that indicates the presence of a noxious stimulus in the gastrointestinal mucosa followed, after a relatively long latency, by a sudden increase in vagal efferent elecltrical activity. Scratchard and co-workers have obtained evidence for difference types of gastric reflexes induced by distension of the corpus and of the antrum of the stomach. Distension of the corpus causes the antrum to contract, but distension of the antrum inhibits contraction of the corpus. Both of these activities are likely to involve vagovagal reflexes. Janing and Koltzenburg have reviewed in detail the visceral pathways that signal gastrointestinal pain. There do not appear to be specific pain receptors in the colon. Rather, an increased frequency of signals is perceived as pain. However, the possibility of a subset of neurons that might be selectively activated in the presence of painful pathological conditions has not been excluded. Sarr and co-workers have analysed the extent to which the ENS interacts with external nervous impulses and with hormonal stimulation by motilin to regulate interdigestive motility. Various types of selective denervation of the small intestine and stomach lead to different degrees of disruption of intrinsic cyclical patterns of motility. After complete denervation, the stomach retains a dependence upon circulating motilin for initiation of motility complexes, but the autotransplanted small intestine functions completely independently from the remaining gut.

Specific peptide mediators of reflex activities are examined by several symposium authors. Gue and Bueno utilized specific antagonists of corticotrophin-releasing factor to demonstrate that this peptide is involved in the enhancement of gastric emptying in mice caused by acoustic stress or by cold stress. Peripheral injection of antiserum against this peptide or central nervous injection of an antagonist blocked the effects on gastric emptying. Burks and co-workers demonstrated that different opioid receptor subtypes act in the brain and spinal cord to influence gastrointestinal motility and secretion. Green, Dimaline and Dockray have utilized specific cholecystokinin octapeptide (CCK) antagonists to determine reflex mechanisms by which specific nutrients inhibit gastric emptying in the conscious rat and utilize CCK as a peripheral sensory mediator. They found that destruction of sensory nerves with capsaicin or administration of a CCK such as peptone or protease antagonists but did not alter the inhibition of gastric emptying caused by duodenal acidification. The most convenient explanation of these findings is that nutrients that release CCK utilize this peptide to initiate an inhibitory vagovagal reflex that slows gastric emptying, while duodenal acidification slows gastric emptying by an hormonal mechanism probably involving secretin.

Identification of pathways between and within the brain and gut that are involved in reflex regulation of gastrointestinal activities has set the stage for a new era of pharmacological manipulations to investigate the involvement of specific neuropeptides as mediators of specific responses. This section anticipates much more work that will follow as investigators use new tools for receptor blockade and electrical recording to investigate mediators of brain–)gut reflexes.

25
Peptidergic activation of brain–gut efferent pathways

Y. TACHE

INTRODUCTION

The functional link between the brain and gastrointestinal secretory and motor function has been established experimentally since the beginning of this century[1,2]. During the last decade, the use of electrophysiological and axoplasmic tracing techniques and the characterization of biologically active peptides in the brain and the gut renewed interest in the elucidation of brain afferent and efferent pathways and neurochemical substrata involved in brain–gut interactions. New findings with potential important physiological implications came from neuropharmacological studies demonstrating that the brain is a target site of action for peptides to influence gastrointestinal function. Several peptides were found to act in the brain to alter gastric acid secretion (acid, pepsin, mucus, bicarbonate, serotonin), mucosal blood, emptying, motility and ulcer formation and intestinal and colonic transit and motility[3-5]. Further studies have established that their brain sites of action are localized in hypothalamic and medullary nuclei regulating autonomic function. This chapter reviews experimental evidence on CNS action of thyrotropin-releasing factor (TRH), corticotropin-releasing factor (CRF), bombesin, calcitonin and calcitonin gene-related peptide (CGRP) to alter gastrointestinal secretion, transit and motility and the role of the efferent autonomic pathways in mediating such responses. The central action of other peptides influencing gut function such as opioid peptides and somatostatin is addressed in the Chapters 27 and 33 by Hermann and Rogers and Burks et al.

TRH: POTENT CENTRALLY ACTING STIMULANT OF GASTROINTESTINAL FUNCTION AND GASTRIC ULCERATION THROUGH ACTIVATION OF PARASYMPATHETIC EFFERENT TO THE GUT

TRH is a tri-amino acid hypothalamic-releasing factor first established to play a physiological role in the regulation of pituitary TSH secretion. Further studies rapidly revealed that the peptide was localized in brain sites unrelated to the regulation of pituitary hormone secretion and exerts a vast spectrum of CNS-mediated actions independently from its endocrine effects[6]. Horita et al.[7] were the first to report that TRH can influence gut function in particular colonic motility by acting on central vagal efferent pathways. TRH was also the first peptide established to elicit a CNS-mediated stimulation of gastric acid secretion[8]. Further studies investigating the gastrointestinal responses to central injection of TRH, its mechanisms and brain sites of peptide action have broadened these observations[4,9,10].

Injection of TRH into the cerebrospinal fluid stimulates in the rat, cat, rabbit or sheep[4,10] gastric acid[8,11], pepsin[11,12] and serotonin[13] secretion, mucosal blood flow[11,14], motility[15], emptying[16] and ulcer formation[17-21], intestinal transit and motor activity[22-24], colonic transit, motility and fluid accumulation[7,24-26] and faecal water excretion[25,27]. The efferent pathways through which central injection of TRH exerts its stimulatory effects on gut function have been elucidated. The sympathetic outflow to the stomach assessed by the eletrical activity of the gastric branch of the splanchnic nerve was inhibited by central injection of TRH, whereas the adrenal sympathetic activity was increased as shown by the enhanced nerve activity of the adrenal branch of the splanchnic nerve[28] and the elevated levels of circulating epinephrine and norepinephrine[29]. However, these alterations of sympathetic outflow to the adrenals and stomach do not seem to contribute to TRH actions on the gut since blockade of sympathetic nervous system by adrenalectomy, adrenergic antagonists or cervical cord transection did not alter gastrointestinal responses to central injection of the peptide[12,19,23,24,30]. Convergent information indicates that TRH acts through vagal and cholinergic pathways. Intracisternal or intracerebroventricular injection of TRH or the stable TRH analogue, RX77368, stimulates vagal efferent discharges recorded from fibres of cervical[31] (Figure 1) or anterior gastric branches[28]. Moreover vagotomy[7,8,23-25,32-35] or atropine[8,11,16-20,23,25] completely blocked TRH- or RX77368-induced stimulation of gastrointestinal secretion, transit, motility, blood flow and ulcer formation, with the exception of the enhanced colonic transit. The latter effect appears expressed through vagal serotoninergic mechanisms since it was reversed by vagotomy combined with sacral cord transection and antiserotoninergic drugs, but not by atropine at a dose inhibiting colonic motility[25]. The fact that central TRH-induced stimulation of gut function is primarily mediated through stimulation of vagal efferent pathways was further substantiated by mapping studies of brain sites of action of the peptide. The most responsive sites eliciting increase in gastric acid secretion, motility, blood flow and ulceration upon microinjection with TRH or the stable TRH analogue, RX77368, in rats or cats, were localized in the dorsal vagal complex and nucleus ambiguus[14,33-42], sites of origin of vagal preganglionic neurons to the stomach[43-45], and the raphé pallidus (Ishikawa and Taché, unpublished observations) which sends direct projectins to the dorsal motor nucleus[46]. Microinjection into other medullary or hypothalamic nuclei or intrathecal injection did not alter gastric acid secretion or motility in the rat[33,36,39,40,42]. The cellular mechanisms of action of TRH on gastric vagal preganglionic neurons are still to be investigated.

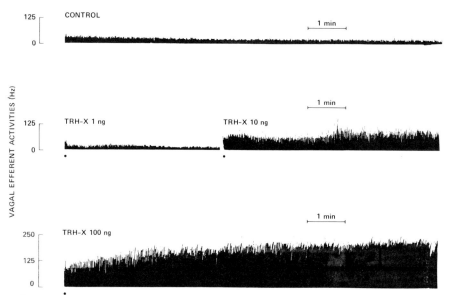

Figure 1 Dose-related stimulation of vagal efferent activity recorded from the cervical branch of the vagus induced by intracisternal injection of TRH-X (TRH analogue, RX 77368), in urethane-anaesthetized rats. Dots represent time of the intracisternal injection of saline (control) or step doses of TRH analogue which were performed at 30 min intervals

These neuropharmacological findings are well correlated with the presence of TRH-immunoreactivity and receptors in the brainstem. In particular, 65% of total medullary TRH is concentrated in the dorsal motor nucleus of the vagus, nucleus tractus solitarius and nucleus raphé. This represents the highest content of TRH in specific extrahypothalamic area[47,48]. Immunohistochemical techniques have revealed that TRH immunoreactivity in the dorsal vagal complex is located in nerve fibres and terminals that arise mostly from the raphé nuclei whereas the hypothalamus does not contribute to the TRH innervation of the medulla[48]. TRH receptors are also abundantly distributed in the dorsal vagal complex[49,50]. Moreover endogenous release of brain TRH by exposing rats to cold[51,52] mimics the effects of exogenous TRH injection since it increases gastric contractility[53-56], emptying[57,58], acid secretion[59] and ulceration[60,61] and watery faecal excretion[62,63].

The lack of TRH receptor antagonist has hampered further demonstration of the physiological role of medullary TRH in the regulation of the parasympathetic outflow to the gut in particular during the cephalic phase of gastric secretion, vagovagal reflex elicited by gastric distension, or the ulcerogenic response to cold exposure. While waiting further establishment of its physiological relevance, TRH and the stable TRH analogue, RX 77368, appear as useful tools to investigate further the stimulation of gastrointestinal function by activation of the parasympathetic outflow and to elucidate the underlying cellular mechanisms through which TRH influences gastric preganglionic neuronal activity.

CENTRAL ACTION OF PEPTIDES TO ALTER GASTROINTESTINAL FUNCTION THROUGH MODULATION OF THE EFFERENT AUTONOMIC NERVOUS SYSTEM

The central action of TRH on gut function is homogeneous (Table 1) in terms of both the functional response throughout the gastrointestinal tract (only stimulation) and the mechanism of action (solely mediated by vagal excitatory efferent). By contrast, all the other peptides, including bombesin, CRF, opioid peptides, calcitonin or CGRP acting in the brain to alter gut function induce heterogeneous patterns of gastrointestinal changes (inhibition of certain functions along with stimulation of others). Moreover, the neural mechanisms through which these effects are expressed are also heterogeneous (sympathetic and/or parasympathetic) depending upon the function (secretory vs. motor), its location (stomach vs. intestine) or the peptides initiating the response (Table 2).

Table 1 Summary of CNS-mediated TRH actions on gastrointestinal function and mediation through vagal   pathways in the rat

Efferent autonomic activity	Intact	Vag-X	Atropine	Cervical cord-X	Adr-X
Gastric vagal activity	S				
Gastric splanchnic activity	I				
Adrenal splanchnic activity	S				
Plasma norepinephrine	S				
Plasma epinephrine	S				
Gastric function					
Acid	S	0	0		S
Pepsin	S				
Gastrin	0				
Serotonin	S	0	0		S
Emptying	S	0	0		
Motility	S	0	0		
Ulceration	S		0		
Mucosal blood flow	S	0	0		
Intestinal function					
Small intestine:					
Transit	S	0	0	S	
Motility	S	0	0		
Large intestine:					
Transit	S	0	S	S	
Motility	S	0	0		
Fluid accumulation	S	0			
Faecal output	S	0			

I: inhibition; S: stimulation; 0: no effect; Vag-X: vagotomy; Cord-X: cord transection; Adr-X: adrenalectomy.

Table 2 Summary of CNS actions of peptides on gastrointestinal function and mediation through efferent pathways in the rat

Efferent autonomic activity	Bombesin				CRF				CGRP				Calcitonin		
	Intact	Vag-X	Cord-X	Adr	Intact	Vag-X	Adr	Symp-X	Intact	Vag-X	Adr	Symp-X	Intact	Vag-X	Symp-X
Gastric vagal	I														
Gastric splanchnic	I														
Adrenal splanchnic	IS														
Plasma norepinephrine	S				S										
Plasma epinephrine	SS				0										
Gastric function															
Acid	I		0	I	I	IO	0	0	I	0	I	I	I	I	I
Pepsin	I														
Gastrin	S														
Emptying	I				I	OI	I	0	I	0	OI	OI			
Motility	I								I		OI	I			
Ulceration	I								I						
Mucosal blood flow									S	0					
Intestinal function															
Small intestine:															
Transit	I				I	0	I	I	I	0	I	I	I	I	I
Motility	S				I		I	I	I	0	I	I		0	
Large intestine:															
Transit	S				S	0	0	0	0						
Faecal output	S				S	0	0	0	0						

I: inhibition; S: stimulation; 0: no effect; Vag-X: vagotomy; Cord-X: cervical cord transection; Adr: adrenalectomy; Symp-X: sympathectomy

Bombesin

Bombesin is a 14 amino acid peptide originally characterized from the amphibian skin and, later on, isolated from mammalian gut as a 27 amino acid peptide named gastrin releasing peptide (GRP). GRP shares full structural homology with the C-terminal biologically active fragment of bombesin and similar spectrum of activity[64]. The first evidence that bombesin acts in the brain to alter gastric function arises from observations of its preventative effect against stress-induced gastric ulcerations upon intracerebroventricular injection[65]. This was followed by the report of its potent inhibitory effect on gastric acid secretion when injected intracisternally but not intravenously in the rat[66]. The CNS-mediated actions of bombesin to influence gastrointestinal secretory and motor function as well as ulceration has been reviewed in detail previously[4,5,67] (Table 2).

Bombesin injected into the CSF inhibits gastric acid and pepsin secretion[66,68,69], emptying[70], and ulcer formation[65,71-73], and increases gastric bicarbonate and mucus secretion[66,73,74], gastric tonic and phasic intraluminal pressure[75] in rats or dogs[4,69]. Central bombesin inhibits gastrointestinal transit in rats and mice[76-78], delays small intestinal transit and stimulates small intestinal contractility[79,80] and large intestinal transit and faecal excretion in rats[70]. Several studies have been conducted to elucidate whether these changes are related to alterations of the efferent autonomic nervous system activity.

Intracerebroventricular injection of bombesin suppressed both the sympathetic and parasympathetic outflow to the stomach assessed by electrophysiological recording of nerve activity[28] and stimulated adrenal sympathetic outflow, as evidenced by the dramatic increase in plasma levels of epinephrine which is completely suppressed by adrenalectomy[81,82]. Bombesin has little effect on plasma norepinephrine except at high doses[82]. The inhibition of gastric parasympathetic activity may contribute to the inhibition of vagally stimulated gastric acid secretion. Bombesin microinjected concomitantly with TRH into the dorsal vagal complex completely prevented the stimulatory effect of TRH[37] (Figure 2). Intracisternal injection of bombesin inhibited gastric acid secretion elicited by electrical or chemical (2-deoxy-D-glucose, insulin, or baclofen) vagal stimulation[69,83]. However, the inhibitory effect of bombesin on acid secretion involved additional mechanisms unrelated to alteration of vagal efferent. Vagotomy did not alter the inhibition of pentagastrin-stimulated gastric acid secretion in rats and dogs[84-86]. Moreover, microinjection of bombesin into the dorsal vagal complex is less efficient than intracisternal injection to inhibit pentagastrin-stimulated gastric acid secretion[37]. The role of the sympathetic nervous system has been investigated using various surgical or pharmacological manipulations. CSF injection of bombesin-induced inhibition of gastric acid secretion was either not modified or was slightly reduced by bilateral adrenalectomy, chemical (6-hydroxydopamine) or surgical (removal of coeliac and mesenteric ganglia) sympathectomy or ganglionic blockade by hexamethonium[66,83,86,87], was significantly reduced by cervical cord transection or bilateral cutting of the greater splanchnic nerve[83,84] and was abolished by adrenalectomy combined with

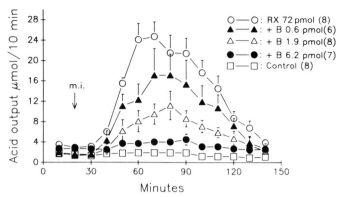

Figure 2 Stimulation of gastric acid output by microinjection (m.i.) of the stable TRH analogue, RX 77368, into the dorsal vagal complex and dose-related inhibition of the stimulatory effect of TRH analogue by concomitant microinjection of bombesin in urethane-anaesthetized rats. Each point represents the mean ± SE of number of rats indicated in parenthesis

chemical sympathectomy[83]. These data indicate that the central effect of bombesin to inhibit acid secretion may be expressed primarily through spinal pathways modulating preganglionic fibres of the splanchnic activity to both the adrenals and stomach; to a lesser extent the decrease in gastric parasympathetic outflow may also contribute. The central bombesin-induced increase in the amount of mucus coating the gastric wall and inhibition of gastrointestinal transit are adrenal dependent since they are completely blocked by adrenalectomy[74,76]. A vagal-dependent pathway has been demonstrated for intracerebroventricular bombesin-induced delay in gastric emptying of a liquid non-caloric meal[70]. The stimulatory effect of bombesin on gastric motility elicited by microinjection of bombesin into the nucleus tractus solitarius was shown neurally mediated without establishing the respective role of the sympathetic vs. parasympathetic nervous system[75].

The physiological role of bombesin in the central regulation of gastrointestinal function has not been investigated due to the lack of a specific, non-toxic antagonist. However, the presence of bombesin-like immunoreactivity and specific receptors in the paraventricular nucleus or dorsal vagal complex[88,89], along with the localization of bombesin sites of action in these nuclei[75,90,91] are compatible with a possible physiological role of central bombesin-like peptides.

Corticotropin-releasing hormone (CRF)

CRF is a 41 amino acid peptide, characterized in 1981 and established to play a physiological role in the regulation of pituitary ACTH secretion[92]. The demonstration that central CRF is involved in mediating partly the endocrine, behavioural, cardiovascular and autonomic responses to stress[93-95] has triggered interest in its possible role in mediating stress-related effects on gastrointestinal function[96]. Neuropharmacological studies have demonstrated that CRF induces a specific CNS-mediated pattern of gastrointestinal alterations in rats or dogs, including inhibition of gastric acid[97,98] and pepsin secretion[99], emptying[100-102] and motility[103,104], stimulation of gastric bicarbonate secretion[99] and prevention of gastric lesions elicited by cold restraint stress[105,106]. CSF injection of CRF also reduced intestinal transit and stimulated colonic transit and faecal output[101,102]. The central actions of CRF are mediated by the autonomic nervous system and not secondary to alteration of pituitary hormone secretion since CRF actions are not altered in hypophysectomized rats[97,101]. Central injection of CRF markedly increases sympathetic outflow to the adrenal medulla and peripheral noradrenergic terminals, as shown by the elevation of circulating levels of both epinephrine and norepinephrine, although central CRF is more potent in elevating plasma levels of norepinephrine that epinephrine in the rat[107-109]. Changes in parasympathetic outflow to the gut following central injection of CRF have not been directly assessed. Indirect evidence indicates that the stimulation of sympathetic nervous activity is associated with concurrent inhibition of vagal activity to the heart[110]. CRF-induced inhibition of gastric acid secretion is completely prevented by ganglionic blockade in rats and dogs[109,111], blockade of the sympathetic nervous system using bretilium[111], adrenalectomy[97,111] (Figure 3) or spinal cord transection[112]. Vagotomy was found to decrease the antisecretory effect in the rat or the dog[109] in one study[97] but not in another[111]. The inhibition of gastric emptying and small intestinal transit and the stimulation of colonic transit elicited by CRF in

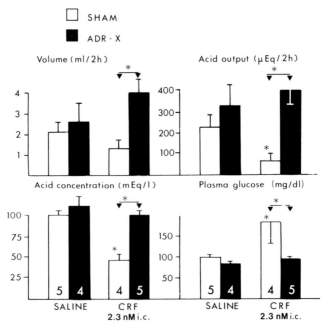

Figure 3 Reversal by adrenalectomy (adr-x) of intracisternal (i.c.) CRF-induced inhibition of gastric acid secretion in conscious pylorus ligated rats. Gastric secretion were collected 2 h after CRF injection and pylorus ligation

the rat are reversed by chlorisondamine and vagotomy and unaltered by adrenalectomy, demonstrating that CRF actions on gastrointestinal transit is mediated by parasympathetic efferent pathways[100,101]. By contrast, another study found that the CNS action of CRF to delay gastric emptying is not vagal dependent but rather involves the sympathetic noradrenergic nervous system and partly opioid receptors[101]. The role of the autonomic nervous system in mediating the central action of CRF on bicarbonate secretion, ulcer prevention or motility has not yet been explored.

Preliminary evidence suggests a possible role of central CRF in the gastrointestinal response to stress. First, neuroanatomic data substantiate the presence of CRF-like immunoreactivity and receptors in hypothalamic and medullary nuclei regulating visceral function[113–115]. Secondly, central injection of CRF and most stressors, excluding cold exposure in rats, produced a similar pattern of alterations of gut function (inhibiting gastric acid secretion, gastric and small intestinal transit and motility and stimulation of colonic transit and fecal excretion)[59]. Lastly, the CRF antagonist, α-helical CRF9-41, injected intracerebroventricularly at doses that antagonized the effects of central CRF on gastric secretion and gastrointestinal transit, completely prevented restraint or surgery-induced inhibition of gastric acid secretion and emptying and restraint-induced increase in large intestinal transit[41,102,116]. The stimulation of faecal pellet output elicited by restraint stress was also significantly diminished by central injection of CRF antagonist[102,116]. However, central CRF does not appear to be involved in the ulcerogenic response to stress since central injection of CRF did not cause gastric erosions[17] and prevented the formation of gastric pathology induced by cold restraint[105,106]. Moreover the CRF antagonist did not alter the development of gastric ulceration induced by cold restraint stess[105].

CGRP

CGRP is a 37 amino acid peptide which was first identified by prediction of the processing of the calcitonin gene in the neural tissue[117]. CGRP-immunoreactivity as well as specific receptors have been localized in discrete population of neurons in the hypothalamus and brain stem nuclei regulating visceral function[118,119].

CGRP acts centrally to suppress gastric acid secretion[120–122], emptying[123,124], motility[123] and ulcer formation (unpublished observations) and to stimulate gastric mucosal blood flow[122]. Alterations of intestinal function by central injection of CGRP include decrease in small intestinal transit[124] and restoration of fasted MMC pattern in fed rat[125], whereas large intestinal transit is not modified[124]. Although central CGRP has been shown selectively to elevate plasma norepinephrine[126], most of the gastrointestinal alterations elicited by central CGRP are exerted via vagal efferent pathways. The inhibition of gastric acid secretion and small intestinal transit elicited by CSF injection of CGRP are abolished by vagotomy but not altered by adrenalectomy alone or combined with chemical sympathectomy[120,121,124]. The delay in gastric emptying in response to CSF injection of CGRP is completely blocked by adrenalectomy and partly by vagotomy or surgical sympathectomy[123] whereas, in another study, it was found mediated by vagal pathways and unaltered by adrenalectomy or chemical sympathectomy[124].

Calcitonin

Growing evidence indicates that calcitonin, a 32 amino acid peptide hormone involved in the regulation of calcium, may also act as neurotransmitter in the brain. Specific binding sites are localized in high concentrations in the hypothalamus[119]. Potent CNS-mediated actions of the peptide on gastrointestinal function include inhibition of gastric acid secretion[127,128], emptying[124,129] and ulceration[127,129], and small intestinal transit[124] and restoration of fasted MMC pattern in fed rats[130]. Central injection of calcitonin did not alter gastric mucosal blood flow or large intestinal transit[122,124]. Although the pattern of gastrointestinal response exhibited by central calcitonin is very similar to that elicited by central CGRP, the efferent mechanisms through which these effects are mediated differ. Ganglionic blockade abolished the inhibitory effect of central calcitonin on gastric acid secretion, emptying and intestinal transit, whereas neither vagotomy nor chemical sympathectomy or adrenalectomy alter peptide action in the rat[124,131]. By contrast, the central effect of calcitonin on intestinal motility was found reversed by vagotomy[130]. Since recent molecular studies do not support the formation of calcitonin from the calcitonin gene present in neural tissue[117], the presence of an endogenous ligand for calcitonin receptors in the brain and the physiological significance of these observations are still to be elucidated.

SUMMARY

Several peptides including TRH, CRF, bombesin, calcitonin and CGRP act centrally to induce a specific pattern of gastrointestinal response and appear as new probes to gain insight on brain sites and efferent pathways involved in the central regulation of gut function. TRH and the stable TRH analogue, RX 77368, stand as the only peptides eliciting stimulation of gastrointestinal secretion, transit, motility, blood flow and ulcer formation through activation of vagal efferent to the gut in the rat, cat or rabbit[4,9,10]. Anatomical, neuropharmacological and biological evidence suggest that TRH-like immunoreactivity and receptors located in the dorsal vagal complex may have physiological relevance in stimulating vagal excitatory outflow to the gut.

The pattern of gastrointestinal response to central injection of the other peptides is less homogeneous. Central CRF inhibited gastric acid and pepsin secretion, but stimulated bicarbonate secretion and reduced cold restraint stress-induced ulceration. It also delayed gastric and small intestinal transit and motility but enhanced large intestinal transit and faecal output in the rat or the dog. These effects are not secondary to the alteration of pituitary–adrenal secretion but appear mainly vagally mediated (inhibition of gastric emptying, small intestinal transit and stimulation of large intestinal transit) or partly vagally mediated along with adrenal dependent mechanisms (acid secretion). The reversal by central CRF antagonist of restraint or surgical stress-induced delay in gastric emptying and acid secretion and stimulation of large intestinal transit along with other neuroanatomical and functional studies support a role of endogenous brain CRF in triggering some of the stress-related alterations of gastrointestinal function. However, there is no evidence that central CRF is involved in mediating the ulcerogenic response to stress[4,96].

Bombesin was found to be a potent centrally acting inhibitor of gastric acid and pepsin secretion, emptying, ulcer formation and gastrointestinal transit and stimulant of gastric bicarbonate and mucus secretion. The efferent mechanisms through which bombesin acts involve either vagal (inhibition of gastric emptying) or sympathetic pathways (inhibition of gastric acid secretion and stimulation of mucus secretion). CGRP and calcitonin act centrally to inhibit gastric acid secretion, ulceration, emptying and motility and small intestinal transit and motility, but have no effect on large intestinal function. CGRP action on gastric secretion and gastrointestinal motility and transit is vagally mediated, whereas calcitonin acts through non-vagal, non-cholinergic autonomic efferent[124].

These findings indicate that a number of peptides act centrally to elicit a specific pattern of gastrointestinal response which is mostly mediated by vagal efferent pathways, conveying both stimulatory or inhibitory output on gastrointestinal secretory and motor function (Table 2). Further challenges will be to elucidate the central and peripheral cellular mechanisms through which these peptides act, as well as the establishment of their physiological relevance in relation with the extrinsic regulation of gut function in health and disease.

Acknowledgements

The author thanks David Claus for helping in the preparation of the manuscript. The author's work cited in the review was supported by the National Institute of Mental Health, Grant MH-00663 and the National Institute of Arthritis Metabolism and Digestive Disease, Grants DK 33061, 30110 and AM 17238.

References

1. Cannon, W. B. (1929). *Bodily Changes in Pain, Hunger, Fear and Rage.* (New York: Appleton)
2. Pavlov, I (1910). In *The Work of the Digestive Glands.* (English transl. by W. H. Thompson. London: C. Criffin)
3. Taché, Y. (1988). CNS peptides and regulation of gastric acid secretion. *Annu. Rev. Physiol.,* **50**, 19–39
4. Taché, Y. (1988). Central control of gastrointestinal transit and motility by brain–gut peptides. In Snape, W. J. (ed.) *Pathogenesis of Functional Bowel Disease.* (New York: Plenum Press). (In press)

5. Taché, Y. (1989). Central nervous system action of neuropeptides to influence experimental gastroduodenal ulcerations. In Szabo, S. and Pfiefer, C. J. (eds.) *Ulcer Disease: New Aspects of Pathogenesis and Pharmacology.* Ch. 16. (CRC Press: Boca Raton, F)

6. Yarbrough, G. G. (1979). On the neuropharmacology of thyrotropin releasing hormone (TRH). *Prog. Neurobiol.,* **12**, 291–312

7. Smith, J. R., LaHann, T. R., Chesnut, R. M., Carino, M. A. and Horita, A. (1977). Thyrotropin-releasing hormone: stimulation of colonic activity following intracerebroventricular administration. *Science,* **196**, 660–1

8. Taché, Y., Vale, W. and Brown, M. (1980). Thyrotropin-releasing hormone-CNS action to stimulate gastric acid secretion. *Nature,* **287**, 149–51

9. Taché, Y., Maeda-Hagiwara, M., Goto, Y. and Garrick, T. (1988). Central nervous system action of TRH to stimulate gastric function and ulceration. *Peptides,* **9**, (Suppl.1), 9–13

10. Taché, Y., Stephens, R. L. and Ishikawa, T. (1989). Central nervous system action of TRH to influence gastrointestinal function and ulceration. *Ann. N Y Acad. Sci.* **553**

11. Takagi, A., Mizuta, K., Moriga, M., Aono, M. and Uchino, H. (1982). Effects of gut hormones on gastric mucosal blood flow in rats. In Kasuya, Y., Tsuchiya, M., Nagao, F. and Matsuo, Y. (eds.) *Gastrointestinal Function Regulation and Disturbances,* pp. 139–44. (Amsterdam: Excerpta Medica)

12. Taché, Y., Lesiege, D., Vale, W. and Collu, R. (1985). Gastric hypersecretion by intracisternal TRH: dissociation from hypophysiotropic activity and role of central catecholamine. *Eur. J. Pharmacol.,* **107**, 149–55

13. Stephens, R. L. and Taché, Y. (1989). Intracisternal injection of TRH analogue, RX 77368, stimulates serotonin release into the gastric lumen in the rat. *Am. J. Physiol.* (In press)

14. Okuma, Y., Osumi, Y., Ishigawa, T. and Mitsuma, T. (1987). Enhancement of gastric acid output and mucosal blood flow by tripeptide thyrotropin releasing hormone microinjected into the dorsal motor nucleus of the vagus in rats. *Jpn. J. Pharmacol.,* **43**, 173–8

15. Garrick, T., Buack, S., Veiseh, A. and Taché, Y. (1987). Thyrotropin-releasing hormone (TRH) acts centrally to stimulate gastric contractility in rats. *Life Sci.,* **40**, 649–57

16. Maeda-Hagiwara, M. and Taché, Y. (1987). Central nervous system action of TRH to stimulate gastric emptying in rats. *Regul. Pept.,* **17**, 199–207

17. Goto, Y. and Taché, Y. (1985). Gastric erosions induced by intracisternal thyrotropin-releasing hormone (TRH) in rats. *Peptides,* **6**, 153–6

18. Maeda-Hagiwara, M., Watanabe, H. and Watanabe, K. (1983). Enhancement by intracerebroventricular thyrotropin-releasing hormone of indomethacin-induced gastric lesions in the rat. *Br. J. Pharmacol.,* **80**, 735–9

19. Maeda-Hagiwara, M. and Watanabe, H. (1985). Intracerebroventricular injection of a TRH analogue, y-butyrolactone-y-carbonyl-L-histidyl-prolinamide, induces gastric lesions and gastric acid stimulation in rats. *Naunyn-Schmiedeberg's Arch Pharmacol.,* **330**, 142–6

20. Nakane, T., Kanie, N., Audhya, T. and Hollander, C. S. (1985). The effects of centrally administered neuropeptides on the development of gastric lesions in the rat. *Life Sci.,* **36**, 1197–1203

21. Basso, N., Bagarani, M., Pekary, E. Genco, A. and Materia, A. (1988). Role of thyrotropin-releasing hormone in stress ulcer formation in the rat. *Dig. Dis. Sci.,* **33**, 819–23

22. Carino, M. A. and Horita, A. (1988). Localization of TRH-sensitive sites in rat brain mediating intestinal transit. *Life Sci.,* **41**, 2663–7

23. Tonoue, T. and Nomoto, T. (1979). Effect of intracerebroventricular administration of thyrotropin-releasing hormone upon the electroenteromyogram of rat duodenum. *Eur. J. Pharmacol.,* **58**, 369–77

24. LaHann, T. R. and Horita, A. (1982). Thyrotropin releasing hormone: centrally mediated effects on gastrointestinal motor activity. *J. Pharmacol. Exp. Ther.,* **222**, 66–70

25. Horita, A. and Carino, M. A. (1982). Centrally administered thyrotropin-releasing hormone (TRH) stimulates colonic transit and diarrhea production by a vagally mediated serotonergic mechanism in the rabbit. *J. Pharmacol. Exp. Ther.,* **222**, 367–71

26. Horita, A., Carino, M. A. an Pae, Y.-S. (1985). Blockade by naloxone and naltrexone of the TRH-induced stimulation of colonic transit in the rabbit. *Eur. J. Pharmacol.,* **108**, 289–93

27. Beleslin, D. B., Jovanovic Micic, D., Samardzic, F. and Terzic, B. (1987). Studies of thyrotropin-releasing hormone (TRH)-induced defecation in cats. *Pharmacol. Biochem. Behav.,* **26**, 639–41

28. Somiya, H. and Tonoue, T. (1984). Neuropeptides as central integrators of autonomic

nerve activity: effects of TRH, SRIF, VIP and bombesin on gastric and adrenal nerves. *Regul. Pept.*, **9**, 47–52

29. Brown, M.R. (1981). Thyrotropin releasing factor: a putative CNS regulator of the autonomic nervous system. *Life Sci.*, **28**, 1789–95

30. Maeda-Hagiwara, W., Watanabe, H. and Watanabe, K. (1984). Inhibition by central alpha-2 adrenergic mechanism of thyrotropin-releasing hormone-induced gastric acid secretion in the rat. *Jpn. J. Pharmacol.*, **36**, 131–6

31. Taché, Y., Goto, Y., Hamel, D., Pekary, A. and Novin, D. (1985). Mechanisms underlying intracisternal TRH-induced stimulation of gastric acid secretion in rats. *Regul. Pept.*, **13**, 21–30

32. Taché, Y., Goto, Y., Lauffenburger, M. and Lesiege, D. (1984). Potent central nervous system action of p-Glu-His-(3,3'-dimethyl)-Pro NH_2, a stabilized analog of TRH, to stimulate gastric secretion in rats. *Regul. Pept.*, **8**, 71–8

33. Stephens, R.L., Ishikawa, T., Weiner, H., Novin, D. and Taché, Y. (1988). TRH analog, RX 77368, injected into the dorsal vagal complex stimulates gastric secretion in rats. *Am. J. Physiol.*, **254**, G639–43

34. Jakobsen, L.J., Raybould, H.E., Taché, Y. and Novin, D. (1987). Alteration of gastric motility by picomole quantities of glutamic acid and TRH in the dorsal complex (DVC) in rats. *Soc. Neurosci.*, **13**, 736 (Abstract)

35. Rogers, R.C. and Hermann, G.E. (1987). Oxytocin, oxytocin antagonist, TRH, and hypothalamic paraventricular nucleus stimulation effects on gastric motility. *Peptides*, **8**, 505–13

36. Rogers, R.C. and Hermann, G.E. (1985). Dorsal medullary oxytocin, vasopressin, oxytocin antagonist, and TRH effects on gastric acid secretion and heart rate. *Peptides*, **6**, 1143–8

37. Ishikawa, T. and Taché, Y. (1989). Bombesin microinjected into the dorsal vagal complex inhibits vagally stimulated gastric acid secretion in the rat. *Regul. Pept.* **24**, 187–94

38. Lynn, R.B., Han, J., Feng, H.-S. and Brooks, F. (1988). TRH injection into the dorsal motor nucleus of the vagus (DMV) increases gastric acid output and the force of gastric contractions in anesthetized cats. *Gastroenterology*, **94**, A274 (Abstract)

39. Garrick, T., Stephens, R., Ishikawa, T., Sierra, A., Yosephian, A., Weiner, H. and Taché, Y. (1988). TRH-analogue, RX 77368, microinjected into the dorsal vagal complex and nucleus ambiguus stimulates gastric contractility in the rat. *Am. J. Physiol.* (In press)

40. Rossiter, C.D., Pineo, S.V., Norman, W.P., Benjamin, S., Hornby, P. and Gillis, R.A. (1988). Effects of microinjections of thyrotropin releasing hormone into the dorsal motor nucleus of the vagus on gastrointestinal motility, blood pressure and heart rate in the cat. *Gastroenterology*, **94**, A622 (Abstract)

41. Stephens, R.L., Yang, H., Rivier, J. and Taché, Y. (1988). Intracisternal injection of CRF antagonist blocks surgical stress-induced inhibition of gastric secretion in the rat. *Peptides* **9**, 1067–6

42. Ishikawa, T., Yang, H. and Taché, Y. (1988). Medullary sites of action of the TRH analogue, RX 77368, to stimulate gastric acid secretion in the rat. *Gastroenterology* **95**, 1470–6

43. Neuhuber, W.L. and Sandoz, P.A. (1986). Vagal primary afferent terminals in the dorsal motor nucleus of the rat: are they making monosynaptic contacts on preganglionic efferent neurons? *Neurosci. Lett.*, **69**, 126–30

44. Shapiro, R.E. and Miselis, R.-R. (1985). The central organization of the vagus nerve innervating the stomach of the rat. *J. Comp. Neurol.*, **238**, 473–88

45. Gwyn, D.G., Leslie, R.A. and Hopkins, D.A. (1985). Observations on the afferent and efferent organization of the vagus nerve and the innervation of the stomach in the squirrel monkey. *J. Comp. Neurol.*, **239**, 163–75

46. Rogers, R.C., Kita, H., Butcher, L.L. and Novin, D. (1980). Afferent projections to the dorsal motor nucleus of the vagus. *Brain Res. Bull.*, **5**, 365–73

47. Kubek, M.J., Rea, M.A., Hodes, Z.I. and Aprison, M.H. (1983). Quantitation and characterization of thyrotropin-releasing hormone in vagal nuclei and other regions of the medulla oblongata of the rat. *J. Neurochem.*, **40**, 1307–13

48. Palkovits, M., Mezey, E., Eskay, R.L. and Brownstein, M.J. (1986). Innervation of the nucleus of the solitary tract and the dorsal vagal nucleus by thyrotropin-releasing hormone-containing raphe neurons. *Brain Res.*, **373**, 246–51

49. Mantyh, P.W. and Hunt, S.P. (1985). Thyrotropin-releasing hormone (TRH) receptors. Localization by light microscopic autoradiography in rat brain using [^{3}H][3-Me-

His[2]]TRH as the radioligand. *J. Neurosci.*, **5**, 551–61

50. Manaker, S., Winokur, A., Rostene, W. H. and Rainbow, T. C. (1985). Autoradiographic localization of thyrotropin-releasing hormone receptors in the rat central nervous system. *J. Neurosci.*, **5**, 167–74

51. Arancibia, S., Tapia-Arancibia, L., Assenmacher, I. and Astier, H. (1983). Direct evidence of short-term cold-induced TRH release in the median eminence of unanesthetized rats. *Neuroendocrinology*, **37**, 225–8

52. Arancibia, S. and Assenmacher, I. (1987). Sécrétion de TRH dans le troisième ventricle cérébral lors de l'exposition aigue au froid chez le rat non anesthésie. Effect des drogues adrénergiques. *C.R. Soc. Biol. (Paris)*, **181**, 323–31

53. Yano, S., Akahane, M. and Harada, M. (1978). Role of gastric motility in development of stress-induced gastric lesions of rats. *Jpn. J. Pharmacol.*, **28**, 607–15

54. Koo, M. W. L., Cho, C. H. and Ogle, C. W. (1986). Effect of cold-restraint stress on gastric ulceration and motility in rats. *Pharmacol. Biochem. Behav.*, **25**, 775–9

55. Garrick, T., Buack, S. and Bass, P. (1986). Gastric motility is a major factor in cold restraint-induced lesion formation in rats. *Am. J. Physiol.*, **250**, G191–9

56. Yano, S., Matsukura, H., Shibata, M. and Harada, M. (1982). Stress procedures lowering body temperature augment gastric motility by increasing the sensitivity to acetylcholine in rats. *J. Pharmacobiodyn.*, **5**, 582–92

57. Taché, Y., Ishikawa, T., Stephens, R. and Hagiwara, M. (1988). Stressor specific alterations of gastric function in rats: role of brain TRH and CRF. *Gastroenterology*, **94**, 452 (Abstract)

58. Koo, M. W. L., Ogle, C. W. and Cho, C. H. (1985). The effect of cold-restraint stress on gastric emptying in rats. *Pharmacol. Biochem. Behav.*, **23**, 969–72

59. Taché, Y., Stephens, R. L. and Ishikawa, T. (1988). Stress-induced alterations of gastrointestinal function: involvement of brain CRF and TRH. In Weiner, H., Florin, I., Hellhammer, D. and Murison, M. (eds.) *IV. New Frontiers of Stress Research*, pp. 1–11. *Hans Huber*)

60. Robert, A., Lancaster, C., Kolbasa, K. P., Olafsson, A. and Lum, J. (1986). Cold sensitizes to ulcer formation by aspirin, but not to gastric injury by ethanol or taurocholate. *Gastroenterology*, **90**, 1605 (Abstract)

61. Senay, E. C. and Levine, R. J. (1967). Synergism between cold and restraint for rapid production of stress ulcers in rats. *Proc. Soc. Exp. Biol. Med.*, **124**, 1221–3

62. Barone, F. C., Deegan, J. F., Fowler, P. J., Fondacaro, J. D. and OrmSbee III, H. S. (1986). Stress-induced diarrhea is not associated with abnormal gut secretion. *Gastroenterology*, **90**, 13372

63. Williams, C. L., Villar, R. G., Peterson, J. M. and Burks, T. F. (1988). Stress-induced changes in intestinal transit in the rat: a model for irritable bowel syndrome. *Gastroenterology*, **94**, 611–21

64. McDonald, T. J., Jornvall, H., Nilsson, G., Vagne, M., Ghatei, M., Bloom, S. R. and Mutt, V. (1979). Characterization of a gastrin releasing peptide from porcine non-antral gastric tissue. *Biochem. Biophys. Res. Commun.*, **90**, 227–33

65. Taché, Y., Simard, P. and Collu, R. (1979). Prevention by bombesin of cold-restraint stress induced hemorrhagic lesions in rats. *Life Sci.*, **24**, 1719–25

66. Taché, Y., Vale, W., Rivier, J. and Brown, M. (1980). Brain regulation of gastric secretion: influence of neuropeptides. *Proc. Natl. Acad. Sci. USA*, **77**, 5515–19

67. Taché, Y., Ishikawa, T., Gunion, M. and Raybould, H. (1988). Central nervous system action of bombesin to influence gastric secretion and ulceration. *Ann. N.Y. Acad. Sci.* **247**, 183–93

68. Taché, Y., Brown, M. and Collu, R. (1982). Central nervous system actions of bombesin-like peptides. In Collu, R., Ducharme, J. R., Barbeau, A. and Tolis, G. (eds.) *Brain Neurotransmitters and Hormones*, pp. 183–196. (New York: Raven Press)

69. Taché, Y. and Gunion, M. (1985). Central nervous system action of bombesin to inhibit gastric acid secretion. *Life Sci.*, **37**, 115–23

70. Porreca, F. and Burks, T. F. (1983). Centrally administered bombesin affects gastric emptying and small and large bowel transit in the rat. *Gastroenterology*, **85**, 313–17

71. Hernandez, D. E., Burke, J. D., Orlando, R. C. and Prange, A. J. (1986). Differential effects of intracisternal neurotensin and bombesin on stress- and ethanol-induced gastric ulcers. *Pharmacol. Res. Commun.*, **18**, 617–27

72. Hernandez, D. E., Nemeroff, C. B., Orlando, R. C. and Prange, A. J. Jr. (1983). The effect of centrally administered neuropeptides on the development of stress-induced gastric ulcers

in rats. *J. Neurosci. Res.*, **9**, 145–57

73. Hagiwara, M., Watanabe, H. and Kanaoka, R. (1985). Effects of intracerebroventricular bombesin on gastric ulcers and gastric glycoproteins in rats. *J. Pharmacobiodyn.*, **8**, 864–7

74. Taché, Y. (1982). Bombesin: central nervous system action to increase gastric mucus in rats. *Gastroenterology*, **83**, 75–80

75. Spencer, S. E. and Talman, W. T. (1987). Centrally administered bombesin modulates gastric motility. *Peptides*, **8**, 887–91

76. Gmerek, D. E. and Cowan, A. (1984). Pituitary-adrenal mediation of bombesin-induced inhibition of gastrointestinal transit in rats. *Regul. Pept.*, **9**, 299–304

77. Koslo, R. J., Gmerek, D. E., Cowan, A. and Porreca, F. (1986). Intrathecal bombesin-induced inhibition of gastrointestinal transit: requirement for an intact pituitary-adrenal axis. *Regul. Pept.*, **14**(3), 237–42

78. Koslo, R. J., Burks, T. F. and Porreca, F. (1986). Centrally administered bombesin affects gastrointestinal transit and colonic bead expulsion through supraspinal mechanisms. *J. Pharmacol. Exp. Ther.*, **238**, 62–7

79. Porreca, F., Burks, T. F. and Koslo, R. .J (1985). Centrally-mediated bombesin effects on gastrointestinal motility. *Life Sci.*, **37**, 125–34

80. Porreca, F., Fulginiti, J. T. and Burks, T. F. (1985). Bombesin stimulates small intestinal motility after intracerebroventricular administration to rats. *Eur. J. Pharmacol.*, **114**, 167–73

81. Brown, M., Taché, Y. and Fisher, D. (1979). Central nervous system action of bombesin: mechanism to induce hyperglycemia. *Endocrinology*, **105**, 660–5

82. Brown, M. R. and Fisher, L. A. (1984). Brain peptide regulation of adrenal epinephrine secretion. *Am. J. Physiol.*, **247**, E41–6

83. Okuma, Y., Yokotani, K. and Osumi, Y. (1987). Sympatho-adrenomedullary system mediation of the bombesin-induced central inhibition of gastric acid secretion. *Eur. J. Pharmacol.*, **139**, 73–8

84. Taché, Y., Lesiege, D. and Goto, Y. (1986). Neural pathways involved in intracisternal bombesin-induced inhibition of gastric secretion in rats. *Dig. Dis. Sci.*, **31**, 412–17

85. Pappas, T., Hamel, D., Debas, H., Walsh, J. H. and Taché, Y. (1985). Cerebroventricular bombesin inhibits gastric acid secretion in dogs. *Gastroenterology*, **89**, 43–8

86. Lenz, H. J., Klapdor, R., Hester, S. E., Webb, V. J., Galyean, R. F., Rivier, J. E. and Brown, M. R. (1986). Inhibition of gastric acid secretion by brain peptides in the dog. Role of the autonomic nervous system and gastrin. *Gastroenterology*, **91**, 905–12

87. Taché, Y., Vale, W., Rivier, J. and Brown, M. (1981). Brain regulation of gastric acid secretion in rats by neurogastrointestinal peptides. *Peptides*, **2**(2), 51–5

88. Zarbin, M. A., Kuhar, M. J., O'Donohue, T. L., Wolf, S. S. and Moody, T. W. (1985). Autoradiographic localization of (125I-Tyr4) bombesin-binding sites in rat brain. *J. Neurosci.*, **5**, 429–37

89. Moody, T. W., O'Donohue, T. L. and Jacobowitz, D. M. (1981). Biochemical localization and characterization of bombesin-like peptides in discrete regions of rat brain. *Peptides*, **2**, 75–9

90. Gunion, M. W. and Taché, Y. (1987). Bombesin microinfusion into the paraventricular nucleus suppresses gastric acid secretion in the rat. *Brain. Res.*, **411**, 156–61

91. Okuma, Y., Yokotani, K. and Osumi, Y. (1987). Central site of inhibitory action of bombesin on gastric acid secretion. *Jpn. J. Pharmacol.*, **45**, 129–33

92. Rivier, C. L. and Plotsky, P. M. (1986). Mediation by corticotropin releasing factor (CRF) of adenohypophysial hormone secretion. *Ann. Rev. Physiol.*, **48**, 475–94

93. Rivier, J., Rivier, C. and Vale, W. (1984). Synthetic competitive antagonists of corticotropin-releasing factor: effect on ACTH secretion in the rat. *Science*, **224**, 889–91

94. Brown, M. R., Gray, T. S. and Fisher, L. A. (1986). Corticotropin-releasing factor receptor antagonist: effects on the autonomic nervous system and cardiovascular function. *Regul. Pept.*, **16**, 321–9

95. Krahn, D. D., Gosnell, B. A., Grace, M. and Levine, A. S. (1986). CRF antagonist partially reverses CRF- and stress-induced effects on feeding. *Brain Res. Bull.*, **17**, 285–9

96. Taché, Y., Gunion, M. M. and Stephens, R. (1988). CRF: Central nervous system action to influence gastrointestinal function and role in the gastrointestinal response to stress. In De Souza, E. B. and Nemeroff, C. B. (eds.) *Corticotropin-releasing Factor: Basic and Clinical Studies of a Neuropeptide.* (In press)

97. Taché, Y., Goto, Y., Gunion, M. W., Vale, W., Rivier, J. and Brown, M. (1983). Inhibition of gastric acid secretion in rats by intracerebral injection of corticotropin-releasing factor. *Science*, **222**, 935–7

98. Lenz, H. J., Hester, S. E. and Brown, M. R. (1985). Corticotropin-releasing factor mechanisms to inhibit gastric acid secretion in conscious dogs. *J. Clin. Invest.*, **75**, 889–95

99. Gunion, M. W., Kauffman, G. L. and Taché, Y. (1988). Intrahypothalamic microinfusion of corticotropin-releasing factor elevates gastric bicarbonate secretion and protects against cold-stress ulceration in rats. *Am. J. Physiol.* (In press)

100. Taché, Y., Maeda-Hagiwara, M. and Turkelson, C. M. (1987). Central nervous system action of corticotropin-releasing factor to inhibit gastric emptying in rats. *Am. J. Physiol.*, **253**, G241–5

101. Lenz, H. J., Burlace, M., Raedler, A. and Greten, H. (1988). Central nervous system effects of corticotropin-releasing factor on gastrointestinal transit in the rat. *Gastroenterology*, **94**, 598–602

102. Williams, C. L., Peterson, J. M., Villar, R. G. and Burks, T. F. (1987). Corticotropin-releasing factor directly mediates colonic responses to stress. *Am. J. Physiol.*, **253**, G582–6

103. Garrick, T., Veiseh, A., Sierra, A., Weiner, H. and Taché, Y. (1988). Corticotropin-releasing factor acts centrally to suppress stimulated gastric contractility in the rat. *Regul. Pept.*, **21**, 173–81

104. Bueno, L. and Fioramonti, J. (1986). Effects of corticotropin-releasing factor, corticotropin and cortisol on gastrointestinal motility in dogs. *Peptides*, **7**, 73–7

105. Krahn, D. D., Wright, B., Billington, C. J. and Levine, A. S. (1986). Exogenous corticotropin-releasing factor inhibits stress-induced gastric ulceration. *Soc. Neurosci.*, **12**, 1063 (Abstract)

106. Gunion, M. W. and Taché, Y. (1986). Gastric mucosal damage is inhibited by intraventromedial hypothalamic corticotropin releasing factor. *Soc. Neurosci.*, **12**, 644 (Abstract)

107. Brown, M. R., Fisher, L. A., Spiess, J., Rivier, C., Rivier, J. and Vale, W. (1932). Corticotropin-releasing factor: Action on the sympathetic nervous system and metabolism. *Endocrinology*, **111**, 928–31

108. Brown, M. R., Fisher, L. A., Rivier, J., Spiess, J., Rivier, C. and Vale, W. (1982). Corticotropin-releasing factor: effects on the sympathetic nervous system and oxygen consumption. *Life Sci.*, **30**, 207–10

109. Lenz, H. J., Raedler, A., Greten, H. and Brown, M. R. (1987). CRF initiates biological actions within the brain that are observed in response to stress. *Am. J. Physiol.*, **252**, R34–9

110. Fisher, L. A. and Brown, M. R. (1984). Corticotropin-releasing factor and angiotensin II: comparison of CNS actions to influence neuroendocrine and cardiovascular function. *Brain Res.*, **296**, 41–7

111. Druge, G., Raedler, A., Greten, H. and Lenz, H. J. (1989). Pathways mediating XRF-induced inhibition of gastric acid secretion in rats. *Am. J. Physiol.*, **256**, 6214–19

112. Taché, Y., Hamel, D. and Gunion, M. (1984). Inhibition of gastric acid secretion in rats by intracisternal or intrathecal injection of rat corticotropin releasing factor (rCRF). *Dig. Dis. Sci.*, **29**, 86S

113. Swanson, L. W., Sawchenko, P. E., Rivier, J. and Vale, W. W. (1983). Organization of ovine corticotropin-releasing factor immunoreactive cells and fibers in the rat brain: an immunohistochemical study. *Neuroendocrinology*, **36**, 165–86

114. Merchenthaler, I. (1984). Corticotropin releasing factor (CRF)-like immunoreactivity in the rat central nervous system: extrahypothalamic distribution. *Peptides*, **5**, 53–69

115. De Souza, E. B. (1987). Corticotropin-releasing factor receptors in the rat central nervous system: characterization and regional distribution. *J. Neurosci.*, **7**, 88–100

116. Lenz, H. J., Raedler, A., Greten, H., Vale, W. W. and Rivier, J. E. (1988). Stress-induced gastrointestinal secretory and motor responses in rats are mediated by endogenous corticotropin-releasing factor. *Gastroenterology*, **95**, 1510–17

117. Rosenfeld, M. G., Mermod, J.-J., Amara, S. G., Swanson, L. W., Sawchenko, P. E., Rivier, J., Vale, W. W. and Evans, R. M. (1983). Production of a novel neuropeptide encoded by the calcitonin gene via tissue-specific RNA processing. *Nature*, **304**, 129–35

118. Amara, S. G., Arriza, J. L., Leff, S. E., Swanson, L. W., Evans, R. M. and Rosenfeld, M. G. (1985). Expression in brain of a messenger RNA encoding a novel neuropeptide homologous to calcitonin gene-related peptide. *Science*, **229**, 1094–7

119. Goltzman, D. and Mitchell, J. (1985). Interaction of calcitonin and calcitonin gene-related

peptide at receptor sites in target tissues. *Science*, **227**, 1343–6

120. Taché, Y., Gunion, M., Lauffenberger, M. and Goto, Y. (1984). Inhibition of gastric acid secretion by intracerebral injection of calcitonin gene related peptide in rats. *Life Sci.*, **35**, 871–8

121. Lenz, H. J., Mortrud, M. T., Rivier, J. E. and Brown, M. R. (1985). Central nervous system actions of calcitonin gene-related peptide on gastric acid secretion in the rat. *Gastroenterology*, **88**, 539–44

122. Bauerfeind, P., Cucala, M., Hof, R. P., Emde, C., Hof, A., Fischer, J. and Blum, A. L. (1987). Calcitonin gene-related peptide mediates CNS regulation of gastric secretion and blood flow. *Gastroenterology*, **92**, 1311 (Abstract)

123. Raybould, H. E., Kolve, E. and Taché, Y. (1988). Central nervous system action of calcitonin-gene related peptide to inhibit gastric emptying in the conscious rat. *Peptides*, **9**, 735–7

124. Lenz, H. J. (1988). Calcitonin and CGRP inhibit gastrointestinall transit via distinct neuronal pathways. *Am. J. Physiol.*, **254**, G920–4

125. Fargeas, M. J., Fioramonti, J. and Bueno, L. (1985). Calcitonin gene-related peptide: brain and spinal action on intestinal motility. *Peptides*, **6**, 1167–71

126. Fisher, L. A., Kikkawa, D. O., Rivier, J. E., Amara, S. G., Evans, R. M., Rosenfeld, M. G., Vale, W. W. and Brown, M. R. (1983). Stimulation of noradrenergic sympathetic outflow by calcitonin gene-related peptide. *Nature*, **305**, 534–6

127. Morley, J. E., Levine, A. S. and Silvis, S. E. (1981). Intraventricular calcitonin inhibits gastric acid secretion. *Science*, **214**, 671–3

128. Okimura, Y., Chihara, K., Abe, H., Kaji, H., Kita, T., Kashio, Y. and Fujita, T. (1986). Effect of intracerebroventricular administration of rat calcitonin gene-related peptide (CGRP), human calcitonin and [Asul,7]-eel calcitonin on gastric acid secretion in rats. *Endocrinol. Jpn.*, **33**, 273–7

129. Taché, Y., Kolve, E., Maeda-Hagiwara, M. and Kauffman, G. (1987). CNS action of calcitonin to alter experimental gastric ulcers in rats. *Gastroenterology*, **41**, 651–5

130. Bueno, L., Ferre, J. P., Fioramonti, J. and Honde, C. (1983). Effects of intracerebroventricular administration of neurtensin, substance P and calcitonin on gastrointestinal motility in normal and vagotomized rats. *Regul. Pept.*, **6**, 197–205

131. Hughes, J. J., Gosnell, B. A., Morley, J. E., Levine, A. S., Krahn, D. D. and Silvis, S. E. (1985). The localization and mechanism of the effect of calcitonin on gastric acid secretion in rats. *Gastroenterology*, **88**, 1424 (Abstract)

26
Gut–brain–gut: action or reaction?

W. R. EWART

INTRODUCTION

In the early days of physiology, at the turn of the century, it was common to explain the complexities of the nervous system in terms of action and reaction. Behaviour could be reduced to a hierarchical system of reflexes, each one of which defined a specific response to an individual stimulus. This 'reactive' concept goes a long way towards explaining how the somatosensory system might operate but, when applied to the relationship between the gastrointestinal tract and the central nervous system (CNS), it falls somewhat short as a total explanation of this powerful interrelationship. The principal reason for this failure is the presence in the gut of an equally sophisticated control system, the enteric nervous system (ENS). The existence of the ENS endows the gastrointestinal tract with a degree of autonomy which may be said to diminish the influence of the CNS and augment the importance of peripheral control mechanisms in the control of the gastrointestinal tract (Figure 1).

As a consequence, investigation of the gut–brain axis must involve a certain duality and must address both aspects of neural control; this is a difficult requirement to meet. However, many of the precepts originally established to explain the somatic nervous system may be retained and applied to the gut–brain axis, for example, the existence of clearly defined inputs to the brain either from the periphery (sensory receptors and visceral afferents) or from other areas of the brain (stress or behavioural drives such as hunger and satiety). To some extent the output from the brain may also be clearly defined, for example, in terms of the effect of activation of motor nerves on motility and even secretion and absorption. Less easy to describe is the internal circuitry responsible for the modulation of basic behavioural drives, such as hunger and the control of food intake. In every facet of gut–brain interaction there remains a certain imponderable—the extent to which the ENS remains independent of central control. Despite this limitation, advances in this field in recent years have allowed considerable progress towards understanding the intricate relationship between the gut and the brain.

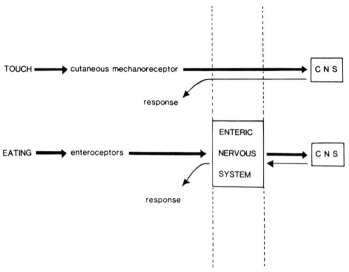

Figure 1 Schematic comparison between somatic sensation and sensation in the gastrointestinal tract. The principal difference is the presence in the gastrointestinal tract of an independent intrinsic nervous system, the 'enteric' nervous system (reproduced, with permission, from Ewart)

GUT–BRAIN REACTION

Sensation in the gastrointestinal tract

Only in the last 30 years have technical advances allowed the definitive recording of single extracellular action potentials in nerve filaments. This elegant experimental technique has been put to good use in exploring the nature and properties of the sensory receptors in the abdominal cavity (enteroceptors). If recordings are made of single unit activity of vagal afferent neurons, the responses of these neurons to physiological stimulation of the GI tract allows the different classes of enteroceptors to be characterized. In this way receptors have been identified which transduce information not only about touch and movement (mechanoreceptors) but also about temperature and the chemical constituents of the luminal contents (thermo and chemoreceptors). In the stomach, mechanoreceptors have been identified in the mucosa and epithelia[1–6]. These receptors respond dynamically to light touch and stroking movements; however, there is evidence that these receptors are polymodal in that they have also been shown to respond to pH changes and the osmotic challenge of hypotonic and hypertonic solutions. There is also evidence of thermoreceptors and chemoreceptors in the stomach[7]. There is, however, some doubt as to the specificity of some of these 'classes' of surface enteroceptors in the stomach. Further down the GI tract there is convincing evidence that there are indeed specific intestinal glucoreceptors[8,9].

The receptors located in the layers of the muscle walls are a considerably more homogeneous population. Only one type of sensory receptor has been localized to the muscle wall; these receptors have been identified as mechanoreceptors responding to muscle tension changes brought about principally by distension[10,11], a property thought to be of great value in signalling the mechanical consequences of food ingestion. The different types of enteroceptors currently identified have been recently reviewed by Mei[12], and shown diagrammatically in Figure 2.

It is worth noting that the majority of sensation from the GI tract is carried in vagal afferents; only a small proportion of sensory information is relayed in the sympathetic nerves and this is largely restricted to a relatively weak input from splanchnic gastromechanoreceptors[54]. These may well be a similar population of receptors to those reported by Morrison[14] which were identified as originating from the serosa near the mesenteric attachment of the small and large intestines. In general, it has been assumed that the function of these 'splanchnic' receptors is to detect the position and gross movement of the viscera or, indeed, to report on abnormally vigorous movement such as vomiting.

This diversity of enteroceptors enables a wealth of sensory information to be transmitted to the brain about the quality and quantity of the stimuli presented to the GI tract. It is a system well adapted to the particular discontinuous pattern in which the gut has to operate between the metabolic opposites of fed and fasting.

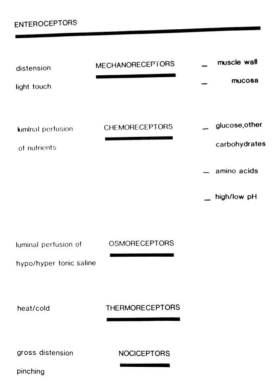

Figure 2 Summary of receptors found in the gastrointestinal tract; for complete review see Mei[12] (reprinted, with permission, from Ewart)

Central projection of visceral afferents

It has been clearly demonstrated that over 70% of the fibres in the vagus are afferent[15]; this is perhaps a surprising finding in view of the historical importance accorded the motor components of this nerve. These unmyelinated afferent fibres project almost exclusively to the nucleus of the solitary tract (NTS). The arrival of visceral sensory information in this brainstem nucleus is therefore the first point at which post-synaptic interaction may occur. The NTS also receives input from the glossopharyngeal, facial and trigeminal nerves[16] and a second-order relay via the spinosolitary tract[17].

Within the nucleus there is evidence of crude somatotopy, with axons from the oral region (gustatory and somatosensory) projecting to the rostral areas of NTS, while visceral afferents tend to terminate in the more caudal regions[18]. Consistent with these anatomical observations, electrophysiological experiments have failed to demonstrate convergence between visceral and gustatory information in the NTS[19], although convergence of information from the abdominal viscera has indeed been demonstrated in this region of the brain[20]. There is an abundance of anatomical evidence using a variety of tracer techniques to show a specific gastric vagal afferent projection to the medial subnuclei of the NTS[21,22]. There also appears to be extremely close apposition between the site of the incoming gastric vagal afferents and either the dendritic field of vagal motoneurons or even the cell bodies of the motoneurons themselves[23,24,60]. This is not perhaps surprising as the NTS lies adjacent to the dorsal (motor) nucleus (DMN), the location of the vagal preganglionic motoneurons.

This area of the brainstem therefore presents an ideal anatomical substrate for the functional integration of activities associated not only with the mainstream role of the GI tract; that is, motility, secretion and absorption but also with behavioural expressions such as the control of food intake.

In recent years immunocytochemical techniques have been used most effectively in this region of the brain to bring together the 'wiring diagram' predicted by anatomical experiments, with functional correlates provided by the localization of biologically active peptides. Peptides such as cholecystokinin octapeptide (CCK) have been shown to be present in vagal afferent neurons and in the brainstem[25]; more recently, bombesin (BBS) has also been shown to be present in both afferent cranial nerves and brainstem nuclei[26]. Intense bombesin-like immunoreactivity has been shown to occur in fibre bundles of the nucleus of the trigeminal nerve and in the fibres connecting this nucleus with the mediolateral NTS[27]. These findings allow speculation that peptides such as BBS are neuromodulators that mediate convergence of afferent information in the brainstem. As peptides such as CCK and BBS have also been shown to be highly active as behavioural agents of satiety[28–30], it is to be hoped that progress is being made towards understanding the contribution which the brainstem makes to the control of the GI tract, beyond its anatomical status as the primary relay station for visceral sensation.

Further processing of sensory information may well take place at the level of the medulla utilizing clearly defined pathways within this part of the brain[31,32]. This intrinsic circuitry thus provides widespread reflex channels for mechanisms controlling not only the GI tract but also the cardiovascular and respiratory systems. Physiological co-activation of these vital functions has already been demonstrated[33,34]. Of course, the flow of sensory information does not end at this level of the CNS; rather, there are well-established central projections from both the more rostral areas of NTS (relaying principally gustatory information) and also the more caudal portion of NTS (relaying abdominal visceral information)[35]. These central projections travel via the parabrachial nucleus in the forebrain, where there is ample opportunity for synaptic interaction between these sensory modalities[36]. Not surprisingly, the hypothalamus is the main destination for vagal afferent information. Anatomical observations have been supported and given a functional correlate by electrophysiological studies which demonstrate the hypothalamic representation of physiological activation of gastric mechanoreceptors[37]. Thus there is, in part, both an anatomical and a physiological explanation of how the hypothalamus may be able to play its role as the prime co-ordinator of basic behaviour drives such as hunger and satiety.

The end-point of the central projection of visceral afferent information has recently been demonstrated. Studies in humans, using recordings of evoked cerebral cortical potentials, have shown that sensation originating in the distal region of the GI tract does indeed reach the thalamocerebrocortical areas[38,39].

Beyond the apparently straightforward anatomical projection of visceral afferent information described necessarily somewhat simplistically in this context, there is obviously a degree of organizational complexity which has not been unravelled. At each level of central processing it is clear that there must be a multitude of reciprocal connections and 'downward' traffic which remains to be elucidated. At the very least it is clear that, with the exception of the cranial nuclei, all the areas receiving input from the NTS project back to this nucleus or the DMN and so are in a position to modulate the vagal motor outflow[32].

Functional interpretation of afferent information from the GI tract

Although there is an immense amount of information on the physiological and anatomical description of the afferent input from the GI tract to the brain, it would not be totally unfair to suggest that beyond this we have not progressed very far in understanding the functional interpretation of this sensory information. There has been a diverse experimental approach to this problem. On one side are the reductionist protocols of recording the responses of either single or small groups of neurons responses to stimulation of the GI tract. Using these techniques, a number of investigators have attempted to characterize the central representation of enteroceptor activation. It has been found that patterns of neuronal activity closely follow the dynamics of receptor activation. Following gastric distension, dramatic changes in firing rate (both excitation and inhibition) have been observed in single neurons recorded in the region of the NTS and DMN[40-44]. It is interesting to note that these central gastric distension responses are almost identical to those recorded in primary vagal afferents, indicating little modulation of the afferent information at the second order (at least) neurons.

Behavioural experiments have used a more holistic approach where observation of specific activities such as feeding and fasting have been used to explain the neural and hormonal mechanisms which underlie them. There is, however, considerable common ground between these two approaches, a number of workers use both types of experimental approach as complementary resources. For example, the study of the control of food intake has utilized a whole spectrum of experimental techniques to look at both the neural and hormonal control of ingestive behaviour.

It is well established that systemic administration of peptides such as CCK and BBS exert a behaviourally specific satiety effect[28-30]. Equally, it has been clearly shown that these peptides have a potent effect when locally applied to neurons in areas of the CNS known to have a part to play in visceral autonomic control[42,45]. This has led to the question of whether the satiety effect of such peptides is mediated peripherally or centrally, and to what extent vagal sensation is a crucial mediator. Certainly, the satiety effect of CCK is vagally mediated, whereas, the same effect of BBS appears to be independent of the vagus[46,61]. In a similar vein it has been shown that gastric preload, and consequent distension of the stomach, attenuates the satiety effect of systemically administered CCK[47]. It may be inferred from this finding that gastric distension and the peripheral effect of CCK have a common, vagal route to the CNS. More recently it has been shown that capsaicin treatment, which selectively destroys a subpopulation of vagal sensory neurons, concomitantly dissociates the central neuronal response to gastric distension and the response to close arterial injection of CCK, indicating that at least gastric distension and CCK have a pharmacologically separable route to the brain[48]. Perhaps not surprisingly, as the satiety effect of BBS does not appear to be mediated through a vagal route, the same treatment with capsaicin does not affect central responses to peripherally applied BBS and the central response to gastric distension[13]. Of course, BBS has been shown to have other very powerful effects on the GI tract[49], not least of which is the well-documented agonist effect on gastric motility. This raises the possibility, therefore, that BBS's behavioural satiety effect may be mediated through responses to this peptide neuromodulator in the GI tract which are non-specific, perhaps reflecting the general post prandial state of the gut, rather than the individual indices of satiety. The role of a selective 'vagal' satiety agent may be the exclusive domain of CCK.

Summary

In reviewing the above material on the 'gut–brain' axis one is led to the inescapable conclusion that, at least on the input side there is a continuum between the ENS and the CNS. The afferent information available to the CNS spans the breadth of different sensory modality. This sensory information travels to the brainstem principally in vagal afferent fibres. There is opportunity for integration and modulation of sensory information in the brainstem, not only through post-synaptic interaction but also through the intervention of regulatory peptides, which have been shown to be able to exert their potent effects in this area of the CNS. Beyond the brainstem there is clearly a role for the hypothalamus and thalamocortical areas in the processing of sensation from the GI tract; however, the exact contribution of these 'higher' centres remains to be understood fully.

BRAIN–GUT REACTION

In terms of the control of the GI tract, the 'brain–gut' axis infers the direct neural control mediated through the effects of the vagal motoneurons whose cell bodies are located in the brainstem. The effects of stimulation of the vagus nerve have been exceptionally well documented—increased motility, gastric acid and pancreatic secretion and so on. Similarly, autonomic neurotransmitters are a rarity in the neuroscience world in that their identity is known and accepted. However, in recent years the clear picture of neural control of the gut has become quite hazy; peptides known and accepted simply as humoral agents have now gained increasing respectability as neurotransmitters. The intricate complexity of the ENS has been discovered, giving to the gut a degree of 'smartness' hitherto reserved for the CNS itself. Thus the extent to which the GI tract is autonomous in its control has become a major issue in this field.

The effectiveness of the vagal efferent outflow relies heavily on a number of vagovagal reflexes; these have been most carefully studied using electrophysiological techniques to record from single efferent fibres[50]. When physiological stimulation is applied to activate enteroceptors by gastric distension or luminal perfusion, the reflex response of the efferent limb of these reflexes can be studied and the role of the central processing component indirectly inferred. It is interesting to note that in a number of reflexes thus investigated the latency of the response was short and the nature of the stimulus faithfully reflected, indicating a relatively small degree of central processing[51-54]. Gastric distension, in particular, has been shown to account for a number of reflex target organ responses including receptor relaxation[55], increases in antral motility[56], gastric and pancreatic secretion and the change from a fasted[57] to a fed pattern[58] (Figure 3). Although vagovagal reflexes appear relatively 'hardwired' at their central end, direct application of gut peptides to the cerebral ventricles bordering the brainstem has shown that the target organ responses are indeed suseptible to central peptide modulation[45,59]. It is therefore possible that there may be some degree of descending influence from 'higher' centres on the basic pattern of vagovagal response.

When the effects of the brain–gut output are absent, as for example, following truncal vagotomy, this is not without serious consequence. Decreased gastric motility resulting from the lack of vagal 'tone' delays emptying of the solid phase of a meal from the stomach. Similarly, deficient receptive relaxation may lead to premature sensation of satiety and, finally,

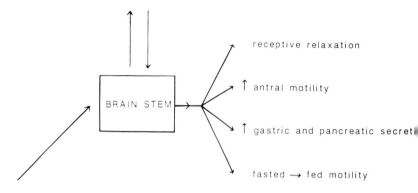

GASTRIC DISTENSION

Figure 3 Gastric distension has been shown to be responsible for a variety of reflex target organ responses, mediated at the level of the medulla. Although these 'vagovagal' reflexes appear relatively hardwired, local appliation of regulatory peptides has shown that they are susceptible to modulation, possibly from areas such as the hypothalamus and cerebral cortex Ch27 legends

impaired sensing of the nutrient load arriving in the duodenum can lead to early abolition of post-prandial motility patterns.

CONCLUSIONS

In conclusion, the pattern of gut neural control appears to be a hybrid between autonomous peripheral mechanisms operating through the ENS and the close integration of both afferent and efferent connections to the brain. This unique arrangement allows not only 'action', such as complex patterns of motor control such as peristalsis and the migrating myoelectric complex; but also, 'reaction', sophisticated reflex responses mediated through all levels of the central nervous system, which allow the GI tract to respond promptly and appropriately to changes in the internal environment. In this way when presented with a meal, the gut is largely able to recognize the quantity and composition of the input and is able to execute the appropriate endocrine and motor responses which maximize the nutrient value of the meal.

References

1. Clarke, G. D. and Davison, J. S. (1978). Mucosal receptors in the gastric antrum and small intestine of the rat with afferent fibres in the cervical vagus. *J. Physiol.*, **284**, 55–67
2. Davison, J. S. (1972). Response of single vagal afferent fibres to mechanical and chemical stimulation of the gastric and duodenal mucosa in cats. *Q. J. Exp. Physiol.*, **57**, 405–16
3. Harding, R. and Leek, B. F. (1972). Gastro-duodenal receptor responses to chemical and mechanical stimuli, investigated by a single fibre technique. *J. Physiol.*, **222**, 139–40

4. Harding, R. and Leek, B.F. (1972). Rapidly adapting mechanoreceptors in the reticulo-rumen which also respond to chemicals. *J. Physiol.*, **223**, 32–3

5. Iggo, A. (1957). Gastric mucosal chemoreceptors with vagal afferent fibres in the cat. *Q. J. Exp. Physiol.*, **42**, 398–409

6. Paintal, A.S. (1957). Responses from mucosal mechanoreceptors in the small intestine of the cat. *J. Physiol.*, **139**, 353–68

7. El Ouazzani, T. (1984). Thermoreceptors in the digestive tract and their role. *J. Aut. Nerv. Syst.*, **10**, 246–54

8. Hardcastle, J., Hardcastle, P.T. and Sandford, P.A. (1978). Effect of actively transported hexoses on afferent nerve discharge from rat small intestine. *J. Physiol.*, **285**, 71–84

9. Mei, N. (1978). Vagal glucoreceptors in the small intestine of the cat. *J. Physiol.*, **282**, 485–506

10. Iggo, A. (1955). Tension receptors in the stomach and the urinary bladder. *J. Physiol.*, **128**, 593–607

11. Paintal, A.S. (1954). A study of gastric stretch receptors. Their role in the peripheral mechanisms of satiation of hunger and thirst. *J. Physiol.*, **12**, 255–70

12. Mei, N. (1983). Sensory structures in the viscera. In Ottoson, D. (ed.) *Progress in Sensory Physiology*, Vol. 4, pp. 1–42. (Berlin: Springer-Verlag)

13. Primi, M.-P., Ewart, W.R. and Jones, M.V. (1988). Bombesin: a central indicator of gastric motility? *Hepato-gastroenterology*, **35**, 192–3

14. Morrison, J.B.F. (1973). Splanchnic slowly adapting mechanoreceptors with punctate receptive fields in the mesentery and gastrointestinal tract of the cat. *J. Physiol.*, **233**, 349–61

15. Gabella, G. and Pearse, H.L. (1973). Number of axons in the abdominal vagus of the rat. *Brain Res.*, **58**, 465–9

16. Nauta, W.J.H. and Freitag, M. (1986). *Fundamental Neuroanatomy.* (New York: Freeman)

17. Torvik, A. (1956). Afferent connections to the sensory trigeminal nuclei, the nucleus of the solitary tract and adjacent structures. *J. Comp. Neurol.*, **106**, 51–141

18. Hamilton, R.B. and Norgren, R. (1984). Central projections of gustatory nerves in the rat. *J. Comp. Neurol.*, **222**, 560–77

19. Hermann, G.E., Kohlerman, N.J. and Rogers, R.C. (1983). Hepatic–vagal and gustatory afferent interactions in the brainstem of the rat. *J. Aut. Nerv. Syst.*, **9**, 477–95

20. Appia, F., Ewart, W.R., Pittam, B.S. and Wingate, D.L. (1986). Convergence of sensory information from abdominal viscera in the rat brain stem. *Am. J. Physiol.*, **251**, G169–79

21. Leslie, R.A., Gwyn, D.G. and Hopkins, D.A. (1982). The central distribution of the cervical vagus nerve and gastric afferent and efferent projections in the rat. *Brain Res. Bull.*, **8**, 37–43

22. Norgren, R. and Smith, G.P. (1983). The central distribution of vagus subdiaphragmatic branches in the rat. *Soc. Neurosci. Abstr.*, **9**, 611

23. Ewart, W.R., Jones, M.V. and King, B.F. (1988). Localisation and distribution of brainstem efferent neurones projecting to the rat stomach. *J. Physiol.* **401**, 65p

24. Kalia, M. and Sullivan, J.M. (1982). Brainstem projections of sensory and motor components of the vagus nerve in the rat. *J. Comp. Neurol.*, **211**, 248–64

25. Dockray, G.J., Desmond, H., Gayton, R.H., Jonsson, A-C., Raybould, H., Sharkey, K.A., Varro, A. and Williams, R.G. (1985). Cholecystokinin and gastrin forms in the nervous system. *Ann. N.Y. Acad. Sci.*, **448**, 32–43

26. Panula, P., Yang, H.-Y.T. and Costa, E. (1982). Neuronal location of bombesin-like immunoreactivity in the central nervous system of the rat. *Regul. Peptides*, **4**, 275–83

27. King, B.F., Jones, M.V. and Ewart, W.R. (1988). Immunocytochemical localisation of a bombesin-like peptide in afferent cranial nerves and brain stem nuclei in rat. *Ann. N.Y. Acad. Sci.* (In press)

28. Gibbs, J., Fauser, D.J., Rowe, E.A., Rolls, B.J., Rolls, E.T. and Maddison, S.P. (1979). Bombesin suppresses feeding in rats. *Nature*, **282**, 208–10

29. Gibbs, J., Kulkowsky, P.J. and Smith, G.P. (1981). Effects of peripheral and central bombesin on feeding behaviour of rats. *Peptides*, **2**, 179–83

30. Gibbs, J., Young, R.C. and Smith, G.P. (1973). Cholecystokinin decreases food intake in rats. *J. Comp. Physiol. Psychol.*, **84**, 488–95

31. Norgren, R. (1983). Afferent connections of cranial nerves involved in ingestion. *J. Autonom. Nerv. Syst.*, **9**, 67–77

32. Sawchenko, P. E. (1983). Central connections of the sensory and motor nuclei of the vagus nerve. *J. Aut. Nerv. Syst.*, **9**, 13–26
33. Grundy, D. and Davison, J. S. (1981). Cardiovascular changes elicited by vagal gastric afferents in the rat. *Q. J. Exp. Physiol.*, **66**, 307–10
34. Pittam, B. S., Ewart, W. R., Appia, F. and Wingate, D. L. (1988). Cardiovascular reflexes elicited by gastric distension or portal vein infusion. *Am. J. Physiol.* **255**, G319–28
35. Norgren, R. (1978). Projections from the nucleus of the solitary tract in the rat. *Neuroscience*, **3**, 207–18
36. Hermann, G. E. and Rogers, R. C. (1985). Convergence of vagal and gustatory afferent input within the parabrachial nucleus of the rat. *J. Aut. Nerv. Syst.*, **13**, 1–17
37. Jeanningros, R. (1984). Modulation of lateral hypothalamic single unit activity by gastric and intestinal distension. *J. Aut. Nerv. Syst.*, **11**, 1–11
38. Frieling, T., Enck, P., Lubke, J. H., Bilharz, M., Pause, M., Karaus, M., Erckenbrecht, J. and Wienbeck, M. (1987). Cerebral responses evoked by electrical stimulation of the rectosigmoid in humans. *Dis. Dig. Sci.*, **32**(8), 911
39. Meunier, P., Collet, L., Duclaux, R. and Chery-Croze, S. (1987). Cerebral evoked potentials after endo-rectal mechanical stimulation in humans. *Dig. Dis. Sci.*, **921**, A22
40. Barber, W. D. and Burks, T. F. (1983). Brain stem response to phasic gastric distension. *Am. J. Physiol.*, **245**(8), G242–48
41. Ewart, W. R. and Wingate, D. L. (1983). Central representation and opioid modulation of gastric mechanoreceptor activity in the rat. *Am. J. Physiol.*, **244**, G27–32
42. Ewart, W. R. and Wingate, D. L. (1983). Cholecystokinin-octapeptide and the central representation of gastric mechanoreceptor activity in the rat. *Am. J. Physiol.*, **244**, G613–17
43. Harding, R. and Leek, B. F. (1971). The locations and activities of medullary neurones associated with ruminant forestomach motility. *J. Physiol.*, **219**, 587–610
44. Harding, R. and Leek, B. F. (1972). The effects of peripheral and central nervous influences on gastric centre neuronal activity in sheep. *J. Physiol.*, **225**, 309–38
45. Porreca, F. and Burks, T. F. (1983). Centrally administered bombesin affects gastric emptying and small and large bowel transit in the rat. *Gastroenterology*, **85**, 313–17
46. Smith, G. P., Jerome, C. and Norgren, R. (1986). Afferent axons in abdominal vagus mediate satiety effect of cholecystokinin in rats. *Am. J. Physiol.*, **249**, R638–41
47. Ritter, R. C. and Ladenheim, E. E. (1985). Capsaicin pretreatment attenuates suppression of food intake by cholecystokinin. *Am. J. Physiol.*, **248**, R501–4
48. Ritter, S., Ritter, R. C., Ewart, W. R. and Wingate, D. L. (1987). Hindbrain single unit responses to gastric distension and cholecystokinin in normal and capsaicin treated rats. *Soc. Neurosci. Abstr.* **13**, (2), 881
49. Walsh, J. H. (1987). Bombesin/GRP peptides. In Martin, J. B., Brownstein, M. J. and Krieger, D. T. (eds.) *Brain Peptides Update*, pp. 193–214. (: Wiley)
50. Davison, J. S. and Grundy, D. (1978). Modulation of single vagal efferent fibre discharge by gastrointestinal afferents in the rat. *J. Physiol.*, **284**, 69–82
51. Andrews, P. L. R. and Lawes, I. N. C. (1982). The role of vagal and intramural inhibitory reflexes in the regulation of intragastric pressure in the ferret. *J. Physiol.*, **326**, 435–51
52. Blackshaw, L. A., Grundy, D. and Scratcherd, T. (1987). Vagal afferent discharge from gastric mechanoreceptors during contraction and relaxation of the ferret corpus. *J. Aut. Nerv. Sys.*, **18**, 19–24
53. Blackshaw, L. A., Grundy, D. and Scratcherd, T. (1987). Involvement of gastrointestinal mechano- and intestinal chemoreceptors in vagal reflexes: an electrophysiological study. *J. Aut. Nerv. Syst.*, **18**, 255–234
54. Ranieri, F., Mei, N. and Crousillat, J. (1973). Les afférences splanchniques provenant des mécanorecepteurs gastrointestinaux et péritoneaux. *Exp. Brain Res.*, **16**, 276–90
55. Abrahamsson, H. and Janssen, G. (1973). Vago-vagal gastro-gastric relaxation in the cat. *Acta Physiol. Scand.*, **88**, 289–95
56. Andrews, P. L. R., Grundy, D. and Scratcherd, T. (1980). Reflex excitation of antral motility induced by gastric distension in the ferret. *J. Physiol.*, **298**, 79–84
57. Blair, E. L., Brown, J. C., Harper, A. A. and Scratcherd, T. (1966). A gastric phase of pancreatic secretion. *J. Physiol.*, **184**, 812–824
58. Code, C. F. and Marlett, J. A. (1975). The interdigestive myoelectric complex of the stomach and small bowel of dogs. *J. Physiol.*, **246**, 289–309

59. Pappas, T., Hamel, D., Debas, H., Walsh, J. and Taché, Y. (1985). Cerebroventricular bombesin inhibits gastric acid secretion in dogs. *Gastroenterology*, **89**, 43–8
60. Shapiro, R. E. and Niselis, R. R. (1986). The central organization of the vagus nerve innervating the stomach of the rat. *J. Comp. Neurol.*, **238**, 473–88
61. Smith, G. P., Jerome, C. and Gibbs. J. (1981). Abdominal vagotomy does not block the satiety effect of bombesin in the rat. *Peptides*, **2**, 409–11

27
Extrinsic neural control of brainstem gastric vagovagal reflex circuits

G. E. HERMANN AND R. C. ROGERS

The basic central neural circuitry which controls gastric function involves the vagovagal interconnections of the nucleus of the solitary tract (NST), the dorsal motor nucleus of the vagus (DMN)[1] and the nucleus ambiguus (NA)[2-5]. The NST receives first-order sensory input from the special and general visceral divisions of the cranial nerves VII, IX and X[6]. Of interest to this review is the fact that vagal chemosensory and mechanosensory afferent axons terminate in a region of the NST which lies directly above the gastric division of the DMN[7,8]. This area of the NST projects, in turn, to the subjacent gastric-DMN[9,10]. The final common pathway to the stomach emanates primarily from the medial part of the DMN[11]. This vagal–NST–DMN connection probably carries viscerogastric vagovagal reflexes[7]. A similar reflexive connection between the NST and NA has been demonstrated anatomically[9,12].

It has been known for some time that higher centres in the brain exert substantial control over the stomach by activating vagal efferent neurons of the dorsal motor nucleus of the vagus (DMN) (for reviews see refs. 1,13,14). The hypothalamus and limbic system are responsible for integrating inputs from a vast array of internal and external sensory receptors[15]. The result of this high-level integration is reflected in regulatory and control processes that maintain the *milieu intérieur* in response to internal and external perturbations. Thus, basic gastric functions can be maintained by vagovagal reflexes localized within the brainstem. However, these reflexes can be modulated to a considerable degree by forebrain input to these medullary neural connections.

Three structures in the ventral forebrain—the paraventricular nucleus of the hypothalamus (PVH), the central nucleus of the amygdala (CNA) and the bed nucleus of the stria terminalis (BST)—all send a considerable number of axons *directly* to the vagal medullary region which contains the NST as

345

well as the DMN and NA[16-21]. Detailed anatomical studies have revealed that the PVH, CNA and BST together form a continuous interconnected band of 'prevagal' neurons. This band extends laterally from the PVH through the dorsal part of the lateral hypothalamus[19,22]. This lateral extension of the PVH is continuous with the CNA which, in turn, merges medially with the BST[19,22]. These recent anatomical observations indicate that the entire dorsal half of the lateral hypothalamus is thought to belong to this band of forebrain, prevagal neurons[19,22]; this area has long been associated with the regulation of gastric function (e.g. ref. 14). Thus, this interconnected band of three limbic–hypothalamic structures may alter gastric function by its synaptic projections directly to the DMN or it may change the gain of viscerogastric vagovagal reflexes by its direct synaptic connections with the NST[10,17].

A number of investigators have recently demonstrated that injection of endogenous neuropeptides into cerebral nuclei or the ventricular system can greatly affect gastric function (for review, see refs. 15,23). As a result of these studies, it is now thought that the central neural regulation of gastric function involves a delicate balancing of the concentrations of a number of interacting neuropeptides within the synaptic circuitry of the limbic system and the hypothalamus[15]. The advent of advanced immunocytochemical methods has provided support for this view in that those limbic and hypothalamic areas thought to regulate gastrointestinal functions are replete with the brain–gut peptides. Further, some of these forebrain areas make direct connections to neurons within brainstem nuclei that represent the final common path for central control over gastric events.

Our electrophysiological studies have demonstrated that both the paraventricular nucleus of the hypothalamus (PVH) and the central nucleus of the amygdala (CNA) maintain direct connections with the dorsal medullary vagal complex (DVC, i.e. the nucleus of the solitary tract (NST) and the dorsal motor nucleus of the vagus (DMN))[24-26]. The purpose of these ongoing experiments has been to examine the physiological role that these connections may play in the regulation of gastric function and to determine the neurochemicals involved in this communication.

INFLUENCE OF PARAVENTRICULAR NUCLEUS OF THE HYPOTHALAMUS ON GASTRIC FUNCTIONS

Earlier electrophysiological studies have shown that neurons of the NST which receive sensory input from the stomach via the vagus may also receive direct input from the PVH[25,27]. Similar electrophysiological evidence indicates an interaction between descending PVH neurons and vagal motor neurons of the DMN[28]. Microstimulation of the PVH enhances neuronal responses of NST neurons to gastric inflation (Figures 1 and 2), while destruction of the PVH sharply reduces the sensitivity of the vagovagal reflex which controls acid secretion (Figure 3). Thus, the PVH is in position to control gastric function by controlling the basic medullary reflex vagovagal sensitivity.

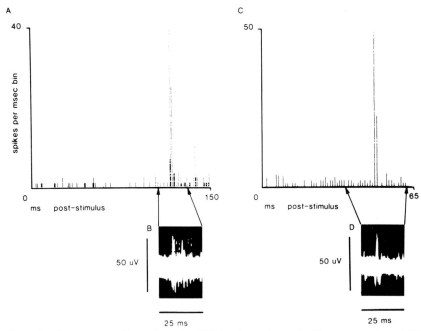

Figure 1 Convergence of input from the PVH and gastric vagal afferent onto single NST neurons. **A**: Post-stimulus histogram response profile of single NST neuron following stimulation of ventral gastric branch of vagus nerve (0.5 Hz, 1 ms, 200 μA, 100 trials). **B**: Oscilloscope record of same NST unit as in (A) responding to stimulation of vagal branch: 10 superimposed sweeps. Record correlates with the histogram in time indicated by the arrows. **C**: Post-stimulus histogram response profile of same NST unit illustrated in (A) and (B) following microstimulation of PVH (0.5 Hz, 0.1 ms, 20 μA, 100 trials). **D**: Parallel oscilloscope traces of same NST unit responding to stimulation of PVH; 10 superimposed sweeps. Though the constancy of the NST response to PVH stimulation is suggestive of antidromic invasion of the NST, this neuron failed to follow PVH stimulation greater than a few Hz, indicating orthodromic activation of this NST unit by the PVH. (From *J. Auton. Nerv. Sys.* (1985), **14**:351–363)

Immunohistochemistry has revealed that this PVH–DVC pathway contains several peptides, including oxytocin and, possibly, TRH[5,20,29,30,31]. Our studies[32–34] indicate that oxytocin is a very likely neuroeffector candidate in the regulation of gastric function by the PVH. Specifically, microstimulation of the PVH evokes increased gastric acid secretion and enhanced, phasic gastric contractions, superimposed on a reduction of circular smooth muscle activity (Figures 4 and 8). Picomolar injections of oxytocin into the DVC mimics the increased acid secretion and decreased tone seen following PVH stimulation (Figures 5 and 6). These PVH-stimulation effects are blocked by picomolar injections of an oxytocin antagonist into this same brainstem site (Figures 7 and 8). *In vitro* studies by Dreifuss and colleagues have revealed that oxytocin has direct excitatory effects on neurons in the DMN[35,36].

TRH may also be involved in the communication between the PVH and DVC. Picomolar injections of TRH into the DVC mimics the increased gastric secretion and enhanced phasic contractions (superimposed on the

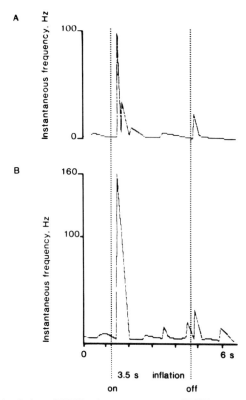

Figure 2 Microstimulation of PVH enhances responses of NST neurons to gastric inflation. A: Instantaneous frequency plot of the activity of a single medial NST neuron responding to rapid gastric inflation and deflation. Gastric inflation (3 ml air injected rapidly, held for 3.5 s and withdrawn via indwelling catheter; max. inflation pressure of 10 cm H_2O) was delivered by digital linear actuator-based pump. Note phasic activation pattern of NST neuron activity. **B**: Instantaneous frequency plot of same NST cells as in (A) now responding to gastric inflation (as above) during simultaneous PVH microstimulation background. Half-threshold PVH stimulation (2 Hz, 0.1 ms, 10 uA) was initiated 1 min prior to the onset of gastric inflation. Note the approximate 60% increase in instantaneous firing rate compared to the control condition in (A). (From *J. Auton. Nerv. Sys.* (1985), **14**:351–362)

reduced tone) seen following PVH stimulation (Figures 5, 6 and 8). Recent *in vitro* and *in situ* neurophysiological studies in our laboratory indicate that TRH has direct excitatory effects on identified DMN neurons, as well as apparently direct inhibitory effects on NST neurons (Figures 9 and 10)[37]. It should be noted, however, that recent studies[38,39] now question whether a direct, TRH-containing projection exists between the PVH and the dorsal medulla.

NUCLEUS RAPHE OBSCURUS

A likely source of TRH (and serotoninergic) input to the DVC is the nucleus raphe obscurus. Indeed, serotonin (5HT) and thyrotropin releasing hormone

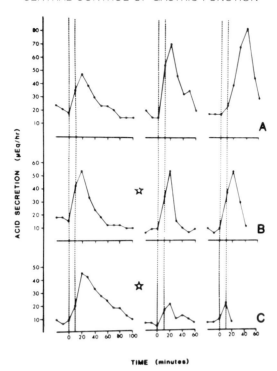

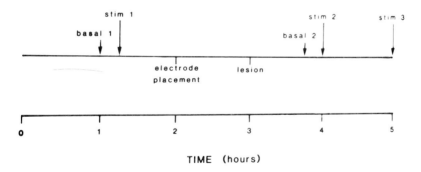

Figure 3 Destruction of PVH sharply reduces sensitivity of vagovagal reflex involved in gastric acid secretion. **Upper**: Gastric acid secretion evoked by vagal afferent stimulation. Secretion results presented left to right occurred following vagal stimulation delivered at points 1, 2, and 3 as depicted in time line. panel A no lesion control—acid secretion following vagal afferent stimulation; panel B extra-PVH lesion control—acid secretion in response to vagal afferent stimulation before and after control lesion; panel C PVH lesion—acid secretion in response to vagal afferent stimulation before and after PVH lesion (*denotes time of lesion). **Lower**: Time-line representation of experimental stimulation sequence; two lesion groups (PVH and extra-PVH control) were prepared for electrode placement and lesion during hours 2–3; all animals were exposed to three vagal afferent stimulation periods at the times indicated. Vagal stimulation parameters: 5 V, 2 ms, 10 s ON, 10 s OFF) (From *J. Auton. Nerv. Sys.* (1985), **13**:191–199)

349

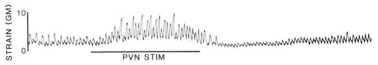

Figure 4 Microstimulation of paraventricular nucleus of the hypothalamus (20 Hz, 50 μA, 0.3 ms for 5 min; stimulation on at 'PVN STIM' bar) evokes enhanced phasic gastric contractions. Note modest reduction in post-stimulus motility (From *Peptides* (1987), **8**:505–513)

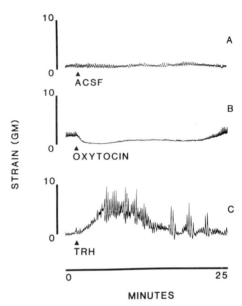

Figure 5 Effects on gastric motility following nanolitre injections of ACSF, oxytocin, or TRH into the DMN. **A**: ACSF (2 nanolitres); **B**; oxytocin (4 pmol in 2 nl); **C**: TRH (4 pmol in 2 nl) (From *Peptides* (1987), **8**:505–513)

(TRH) have been reported to be co-localized within cell bodies of the nucleus raphe obscurus[39–41]. This medullary nucleus sends direct projections to the DVC[10]. The raphe nuclei, in general, appear to be involved in the transition between sleep and wakefulness[42]. Such changes in arousal are highly correlated with gross changes in gastrointestinal motility[43,44]. Thus, it is possible that the raphe nuclei control the transitions from sleep and waking as well as the associated changes in gastrointestinal function appropriate to the arousal state.

Recent studies from our laboratory[45] have demonstrated that when serotonin alone is micropressure injected into the DMN, a modest increase in gastric motility and circular muscle tone can be elicited (Figure 11). As shown earlier, application of TRH evokes a massive increase in both gastric motility and tone which lasts approximately 20 min. If serotonin is applied to the DMN well after the primary effects of TRH on these motility indices have subsided, this subsequent exposure to serotonin results in greatly

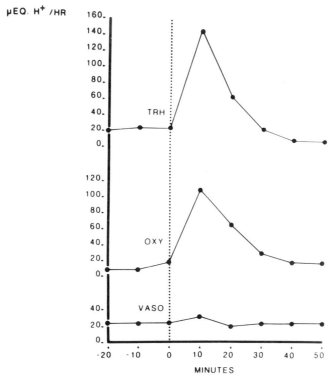

Figure 6 Typical time course of the gastric secretory responses following central application of TRH (11 pmol), oxytocin (11 pmol), or vasopressin (11 pmol) injected into the DMN area at time '0'. (From *Peptides* (1985), **6**:1143–1148)

amplified effects on gastric function. This amplification of serotonin's effect by TRH is quite longlasting, in the order of several hours. Although the mechanism by which TRH enhances the effects of serotonin is not known, longlasting intracellular changes in a second messenger cascade have been observed after TRH administration to cultured pituitary cells[46]. It is tempting to speculate that the excitability level of neurons within the vagal nuclei can be adjusted by one neurochemical (e.g. TRH) such that the efficacy of another neurochemical (e.g. 5HT) can be regulated. The understanding of this mechanism may be significant to elucidating the causes of the arousal related onset of irritable bowel syndrome[43,44].

Intracellular recording techniques will be required to verify whether TRH is capable of changing excitability levels of vagal neurons in a manner similar to that seen with several neurochemical agents in the ENS, e.g. histamine, serotonin, adenosine and opioid peptides. Wood and colleagues (for review see ref. 47) have demonstrated that these neurochemical agents in the ENS can alter the excitability level of those neural networks. Their observations suggest a mechanism by which different gastrointestinal activity patterns can be elicited from the same population of enteric neurons. Specifically, a

351

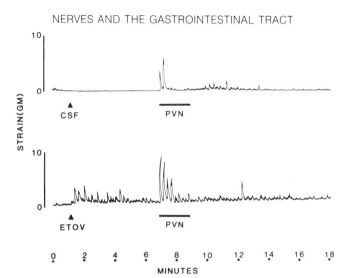

Figure 7 PVN-stimulation effects are blocked by picomolar injections of oxytocin antagonist (ETOV) into the DMN. **Upper**: (control) effect of PVN stimulation (20 Hz, 50 µA, 0.3 ms for 2 min) on gastric motility following a control injection of artificial CSF (2 nl) into the DMN. **Lower:** effect of PVN stimulation (as above) on gastric motility following an ETOV (2 nl x 4 pmol) injection into the DMN. Note the immediate increase in motility following the central injection of the oxytocin antagonist, as well as the augmented effect PVN stimulation has on motility. (From *Peptides* (1985), 7:695–700.)

subpopulation of enteric neurons may be dormant until a particular neurochemical agent is present which, in turn, arouses this specific subset of the neuronal population to produce a particular pattern of intestinal activity appropriate for the digestive state[47].

CENTRAL NUCLEUS OF THE AMYGDALA

Amygdalar involvement in the control of autonomic function has been known for some time[48-54]. In particular, the central portion of the amygdala (CNA) has been associated with augmentation of gastric acid secretion and gastric motility[13,23,51,55]. Until recently, the control of the stomach by the CNA had been explained in terms of complex interactions involving limbic, hypothalamic, reticular, and autonomic preganglionic nuclei[13]. However, anatomical data have since indicated that direct reciprocal connections exist between the CNA and regions of the DVC[19,21,56-58]. Such reciprocal connections between these nuclei could put this limbic structure in a position to process internal visceral sensory cues; it could then alter a variety of autonomic functions by changing the setpoint or gain of autonomic reflexes by altering the excitability of NST or DMN neurons in a similar manner as that described for the PVH–DVC pathway[25,27].

Recent electrophysiological studies confirmed that the CNA does maintain direct connections with the medullary DVC[24,48]. In our experiments, NST neurons were identified by their response to cervical vagal stimulation. In

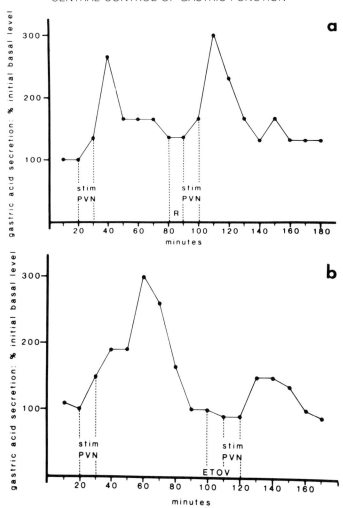

Figure 8 Oxytocin antagonist (ETOV) blocks effect of PVN microstimulation. **A**: Typical control case illustrating the effect of PVN microstimulation on gastric acid output. The first PVN stimulation, at 20–30 min (10 Hz, 50 μA, 0.3 ms for 10 min at 'stim PVN'), evokes a substantial rise in acid production. An injection of artificial CSF (5 nl; at 'R') into the ipsilateral DMN has no effect on the acid output evoked by a second, identical PVN stimulation (stim PVN' at 90–100 min). **B**: Typical case illustrating the effect of the oxytocin antagonist, ETOV, on PVN stimulation-evoked gastric acid production. Though the initial PVN stimulation (same parameters as above 'stim PVN') evokes a large increase in gastric acid output, injection of ETOV (25 pmol in 5 nl artificial CSF) into the DMN greatly reduces the response to the second PVN stimulation (From *Peptides* (1985), **7**:695–700.)

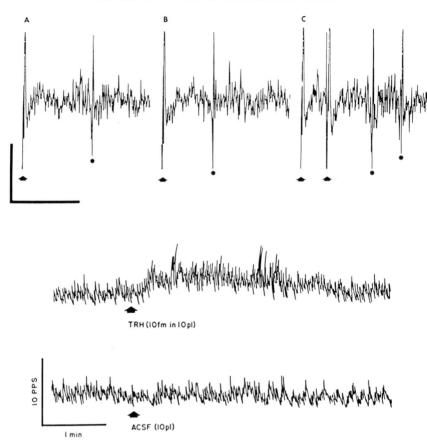

Figure 9 Excitatory effects of TRH on DMN neurons. **Upper**: Antidromic identification of a DMN neuron; **A**, antidromic response at 32 ms; **B**, 'collision' with a spontaneously occurring spike; **C**, response following at high-frequency (100 Hz) vagal stimulations. Antidromic spike at*. Scale bars = $100\,\mu$V/32 ms. **Middle**: Rate-meter plot of the activity of the DMN cell identified above. Cell firing rate doubled following the micropressure injection of TRH (10 fmol in 10 pl) into the DMN region. **Lower**: Rate-meter plot of the activity of the same DMN cell following control microinjection of artificial CSF (10 pl) into the DMN region.

turn, CNA neurons were antidromically identified following stimulation of the identified NST population; demonstrating that a monosynaptic CNA–NST projection exists. Conversely, approximately 15% of identified NST cells were orthodromically activated by CNA stimulation. These NST neurons were thus receiving convergent input from the vagus and CNA.

A substantial number of somatostatin-containing neurons exist in the CNA and these cells appear to maintain a long, descending connection with neurons in the dorsal vagal complex[18,21,24,56,58,59]. It seems reasonable to suspect, therefore, that the central nucleus of the amygdala may directly influence gastric function by activating a descending somatostatinergic pathway to the DVC region. This hypothesis is generally supported by the

354

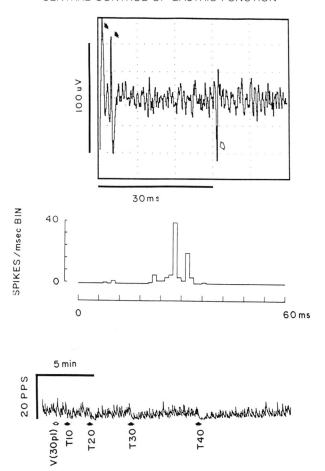

Figure 10 Inhibitory effects of TRH on NST neurons. **Upper**: Orthodromically identified NST neuron's response to vagal stimulation; note failure to follow high frequency vagal stimulation pulses (arrows). **Middle**: Peristimulus histogram of the same NST neuron responding to 100 vagal stimulations. Note typical orthodromic, i.e. irregular latency, pattern of activation of the unit following vagal stimulation. **Lower**: Effects of TRH on activity pattern of the NST neuron identified above. T10–T40 = 10–40 fmol of TRH applied by micropressure injection in volumes from 10–40 pl, respectively. Artificial CSF (V30 pl = 30 pl) injection had no effect on unit activity

observation that intracerebroventricular injections of somatostatin evoke increases in duodenal motility[60].

If a somatostatinergic path between the CNA and dorsal medulla is responsible for increases in gastric motility, then the injection of small amounts of somatostatin into the DMN area should markedly increment gastric motility. Also, if a CNA–dorsal medullary somatostatinergic path controls gastric motility, then increases in motility induced by microstimulation of the CNA should be blocked by an antagonist of somatostatin action[61] i.e. cyclo[7-aminoheptanoyl-Phe-d-Trp-Lys-Thr(oBzl)] or CPP1,

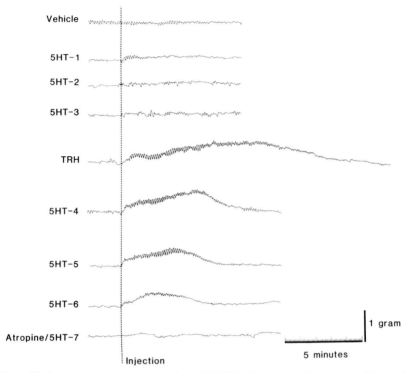

Figure 11 Interaction between serotonin and TRH in the control of gastric motility by the dorsal medulla. TRH appears to augment the effectiveness of 5HT-evoked changes in gastric motility. **Vehicle**: effects on gastric motility following injection of artificial CSF (4 nanolitres) into the DMN; **5HT-1 to 3**: injection of serotonin (5HT; 8 picomoles in 4 nanolitres) into the DMN at intervals of 20 minutes between the end of the record and the beginning of the next injection. **TRH**: application of TRH (1 nmol in 1 ml) onto the dorsal medulla. **5HT-4 to 6**: injection of serotonin (8 pmol in 4 nl) into the DMN beginning 20 min after the end of the TRH record. **Atropine/5HT-7**: atropine methyl nitrate (1 mg/kg, s.c.) completely suppresses the gastric response to subsequent injections of 5HT into the DMN

from Bachem Labs).

Microinjection of somatostatin (SST; 5 pmol) into the DMN region evokes phasic gastric contractions. This increase in gastric motility can be mimicked by microstimulation of the CNA and can be completely abolished by pretreatment with atropine methyl nitrate. Similar injections of SST also evoke significant elevations in gastric acid secretion (Figures 12–15). Additionally, when the SST antagonist, CPP1, is injected into the DMN prior to CNA microstimulation, subsequent CNA-induced changes in gastric motility are reduced (Figure 17). Thus, these data suggest that a somatostatinergic projection between the limbic forebrain and the dorsal vagal nuclei may play a role in regulating parasympathetic input to the stomach[62].

The precise mechanism of somatostatin effects on the dorsal medullary neurons which control gastric function are unknown. The issue is confused

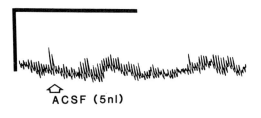

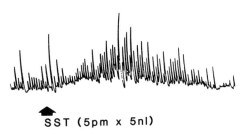

Figure 12 Effects on gastric motility following injection of artificial CSF (vehicle control; 5 nanolitres) and somatostatin (SST; 5 pmol in 5 nl) into the DMN. Scale bars = 2 gm/10 min

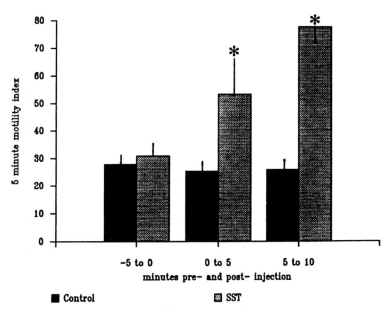

■ Control   ▨ SST

Figure 13 Injection of somatostatin (SST; 5 pmol in 5 nl) into the DMN evokes a significant increase in gastric motility relative to the motility seen following injection of artificial CSF (5 nl) (* = $p \leqslant 0.05$, Sign test)

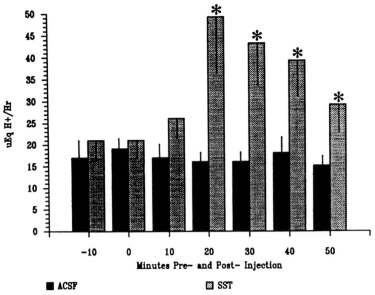

Figure 14 Injection of somatostatin (SST; 5 pmol in 5 nl) into the DMN evokes a marked increase in gastric acid secretion relative to secretion levels seen after injection of artificial CSF (5 nl). (* = $p \leqslant 0.05$, Sign test)

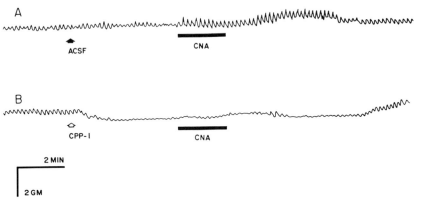

Figure 15 Effects on gastric motility following microstimulation of central nucleus of the amygdala. **A**: Changes in gastric motility and circular muscle tone evoked by injection of artificial CSF (ACSF; 5 nl) into the DMN; followed 5 min later by electrical stimulation of the central nucleus of the amygdala (CNA; 25 Hz, 50 μA, 0.3 ms for 2 min). **B**: Reduction in gastric tone and motility evoked by injection of somatostatin antagonist (CPP-1; 5 pmol, in 5 nl) into the DMN also suppresses motility increases normally elicited by microstimulation of CNA

by a number of reports which demonstrate seemingly contradictory roles for somatostatin as a central effector substance. For example, somatostatin has been observed both to increase[63,64] and decrease[65,66] the excitability of central neurons through a variety of mechanisms. Thus, an apparent increase in parasympathetic outflow to the stomach may be the result of (a) direct, excitatory action on the efferent vagal neurons; (b) indirect presynaptic facilitation; or (c) disinhibition. Intracellular recordings will be required to determine which mechanism is responsible for this change in parasympathetic efferent activity.

BED NUCLEUS OF THE STRIA TERMINALIS

As mentioned above, anatomical studies have revealed that the PVH, CNA and the bed nucleus of the stria terminalis (BST) together form a continuous interconnected band of 'prevagal' neurons[16,19,22,57]. Like the PVH and CNA, the BST makes direct projections to the nuclei of the DVC[16]. It is reasonable to suspect that this nucleus may also be involved in the potential modulation of vagally mediated gastric function.

Preliminary work from our laboratory indicates that microstimulation of the BST elicits an increase in contractility and/or tone of the gastric musculature. This increase in gastric activity can be mimicked by micropressure injections of glutamate into the BST and can be abolished following systemic administration of atropine methyl nitrate[67].

Immunohistochemical studies on the distribution of neuropeptides reveals that cell bodies and fibres in the BST contain somatostatin, enkephalin and corticotropin-releasing factor, as well as fibres which contain TRH and bombesin[29,68-72], oxytocin and vasopressin[73,74]. These neurochemicals have also been localized to terminal endings within the NST and DMN[29,30, 68-74]. It remains to be seen, however, which of these neurochemical candidates from the BST may be responsible for modulating gastric functions and how.

CEREBRAL CORTEX

Cortical influence on autonomic systems has been known for some time[75-78]. It has long been recognized that emotions and stress have a powerful influence on gastrointestinal motility. For example, gastrointestinal activity is normally drastically reduced in response to fear-inducing stimulation[79,80]. Data from electrical stimulation and lesion studies suggest that the cortex exerts an inhibitory influence on ongoing gastrointestinal activity[81-86].

Anatomical studies have recently indicated the existence of direct projections from the infralimbic and insular cortex (also referred to as the 'visceral sensory and motor' cortex[87,88]) to the medullary dorsal vagal complex[21, 87-90]. Given that this area of the medial frontal cortex is considered to be part of the limbic system[88], its direct connections with the medullary DVC provides a conduit through which various emotions may attenuate ongoing gastrointestinal function and, ultimately, may be responsible for stress-induced gastric ulcers[91].

SUMMARY

Nuclei of the dorsal vagal complex, i.e. the nuclei of the solitary tract and dorsal motor nuclei of the vagus, are primary components responsible for the direct autonomic control of gastrointestinal functions. These brainstem nuclei receive direct input from cortex, paraventricular nucleus of the hypothalamus, bed nucleus of the stria terminalis, central nucleus of the amygdala and nucleus raphe obscurus of the medullary reticular area. Thus, the basic vagovagal reflex of the DVC is influenced as a result of these extrinsic sources of neural input which contain a bewildering array of mediator substances. This diversity of input may provide a large repertoire of possible response mechanisms for the DVC. This chapter has given a few examples of how different putative neurochemical agents contained in the central projections to the DVC can modify or attenuate the basic vagovagal reflexes involved in controlling gastric function. Given that these DVC neurons are also involved in the control of other autonomic functions, it is tempting to speculate that the delicate balancing of various interacting neurochemicals within the synaptic microenvironment of the DVC may be responsible for orchestrating the full array of parasympathetically controlled automatic functions.

References

1. Grijalva, C. V., Lindholm, E. and Novin, D. (1980). Physiological and morphological changes in the gastrointestinal induced by hypothalamic intervention: an overview. *Brain Res. Bull.*, **5**(1) , 19–31
2. Coil, J. and Norgren, R. (1979). Cells of origin of motor axons in the subdiaphraghmatic vagus of the rat. *J. Auton. Nerv. Syst.*, **1**, 203–10
3. Kalia, M. and Mesulam, M. M. (1980). Brainstem projections of sensory and motor components of the vagus complex in the cat. II. Laryngeal, tracheobronchial, pulmonary, cardiac and gastrointestinal branches. *J. Comp. Neurol.*, **193**, 467–508
4. Pagani, F. D., Norman, W. P., Kasbekar, D. K. and Gillis, R. A. (1985). Localization of sites within the dorsal motor nucleus of the vagus that affect gastric motility. *Am. J. Physiol.*, **249**, G73–84
5. Zimmerman, E. A., Nilaver, G., Hou-Ya, A. and Silverman, A. J. (1984). Vasopressinergic and oxytocinergic pathways in the central nervous system. *Fed. Proc.*, **43**, 91–6
6. Contreras, R. J., Beckstead, R. M., Norgren, R. (1982). Central projections of trigeminal, facial glossopharyngeal, and the vagus nerves: an autoradiographic study in the rat. *J. Auton. Nerv. Syst.*, **6**, 303–22
7. Barber, W. D. and Burks, T. F. (1983). Brainstem response to phasic gastric distension. *Am. J. Physiol.*, **245**, G242–8
8. Rogers, R. C. and Hermann, G. E. (1983). Central connections of the hepatic branch of the vagus nerve: a horseradish peroxidase study. *J. Auton. Nerv. Syst.*, **7**, 165–74
9. Norgren, R. (1978). Projections from the nucleus tractus solutions in the rat. *Neuroscience*, **3**, 207–18
10. Rogers, R. C., Kita, H., Butcher, L. L. and Novin, D. (1980). Afferent projections to the dorsal motor nucleus of the vagus. *Brain Res. Bull.*, **5**, 365–73
11. Fox, E. A. and Powley, T. L. (1985). Longitudinal columnar organization within the dorsal motor nucleus represents separate branches of abdominal vagus. *Brain Res.*, **341**, 269–82
12. Beckstead, R. M., Morse, J. R. and Norgen, R. (1980). The nucleus tractus solitarius in the monkey: projections to the thalamus and brainstem. *J. Comp. Neurol.*, **190**, 259–82
13. Henke, P. G. (1979). The hypothalamus–amygdala axis and experimental gastric ulcers. *Neurosci. Biobehav. Rev.*, **3**, 75–82

14. Kadekaro, M., Timo-Iaria, C. and Vincenti, . de L. M. (1977). Control of gastric secretion by the central nervous system. In Brooks and Evers (eds.) *Nerves and the Gut*, p. 377–429

15. Morley, J. E., Levine, A. S. and Silvis, S. E. (1982). Minireview: Central regulation of gastric acid secretion: The role of neuropeptides. *Life Sci.*, **31**, 399–410

16. Holstege, G., Meiners, L. and Tan, K. (1985). Projections of the bed nucleus of the stria terminalis to the mesencephalon, pons, and medullar oblongata in the cat. *Exp. Brain Res.*, **58**, 379–91

17. Luiten, P. G. M., ter Horst, G. J., Karst, H. and Steffens, A. B. (1985). The course of paraventricular hypothalamic efferents to autonomic structures in medulla and spinal cord. *Brain Res.*, **329**, 374–8

18. Schwaber, J. S., Kapp, B. S. and Higgins, G. (1980). The origin and extent of direct amygdala projections to the region of the dorsal motor nucleus of the vagus and the nucleus of the solitary tract. *Neurosci. Lett.*, **20**, 15–20

19. Schwaber, J. S., Kapp, B. S., Higgins, G. A. and Rapp, P. R. (1982). Amygdaloid and basal forebrain connections with the nucleus of the solitary tract and the dorsal motor nucleus. *J. Neurosci.*, **2**, 1424–38

20. Sofroniew, M. V. and Schrell, U. (1981). Evidence for a direct projection from oxytocin and vasopressin neurons in hypothalamic paraventricular nucleus to the medullar oblongata: immunohistochemical visualization of both the horseradish peroxidase transported and the peptide produced by the same neurons. *Neurosci. Lett.*, **22**, 211–17

21. van der Kooy, D., Koda, L., McGinty, J. F., Gerfen, C. R. and Bloom, F. (1984). The organization of projections from the cortex, amygdala and hypothalamus to the nucleus of the solitary tract in rat. *J. Comp. Neurol.*, **224**, 1–24

22. Swanson, L. W. and Kuypers, H. G. J. M. (1980). The paraventricular nucleus of the hypothalamus: cytoarchitectonic subdivisions and the organization of projections to the pituitary, the dorsal vagal complex and spinal cord as demonstrated by retrograde fluorescence double-labelling methods. *J. Comp. Neurol.*, **194**, 555–70

23. Gillis, R. A., Quest, J. A., Pagani, F. D. and Norman, W. P. (1988). Control centers in the central nervous system for regulating gastrointestinal motility. In Wood, J. D. (ed.), *Handbook of Physiology*. (Bethesda, MD: American Physiological Society). (In press)

24. Rogers, R. C. and Fryman, D. L. (1988). Direct connections between the central nucleus of the amygdala and the nucleus of the solitary tract: an electrophysiological study in the rat. *J. Auton. Nerv. Sys.*, **22**, 83–7

25. Rogers, R. C. and Hermann, G. E. (1985). Gastric vagal solitary neurons excited by paraventricular nucleus microstimulation. *J. Auton. Nerv. Sys.*, **14**, 351–62

26. Rogers, R. C. and Nelson, D. O. (1984). Neurons of the vagal division of the solitary nucleus activated by the paraventricular nucleus of the hypothalamus. *J. Auton. Nerv. Sys.*, **10**, 193–7

27. Rogers, R. C. and Hermann, G. E. (1985). Vagal afferent stimulation-evoked gastric secretion suppressed by paraventricular nucleus lesion. *J. Auton. Nerv. Sys.*, **13**, 191–9

28. Lawrence, D. and Pittman, Q. J. (1985). Interaction between descending paraventricular neurons and vagal motor neurons. *Brain Res.*, **332**, 158–60

29. Elde, R. and Hokfelt, T. (1979). Localization of hypophysiotrophic peptides and other biologically active peptides within the brain. *Annu. Rev. Neurosci.*, **41**, 587–602

30. Hokfelt, T., Fuxe, K., Johansson, O., Jeffcoate, S. and White, N. (1975). Thyrotropin-releasing hormone (TRH) containing nerve terminals in certain brainstem nuclei and in the spinal cord. *Neurosci. Lett.*, **1**, 133–9

31. Swanson, L. W. and Sawchenko, P. E. (1983). Hypothalamic integration: organization of the paraventricular and supraoptic nuclei. *Ann. Rev. Neurosci.*, **6**, 269–325

32. Rogers, R. C. and Hermann, G. E. (1985). Dorsal medullary oxytocin, vasopressin and TRH effects on gastric secretion and heart rate. *Peptides*, **6**, 1143–48

33. Rogers, R. C. and Hermann, G. E. (1986). Hypothalamic paraventricular nucleus stimulation-induced gastric acid secretion and bradycardia suppressed by oxytocin antagonist. *Peptides*, **7**, 695–700

34. Rogers, R. C. and Hermann, G. E. (1987). Oxytocin, oxytocin antagonist, TRH and hypothalamic paraventricular nucleus stimulation effects on gastric motility. *Peptides*, **8**, 505–13

35. Charpak, S., Armstrong, W. E., Muhlethaler, M. and Dreifuss, J. J. (1984). Stimulatory action of oxytocin on neurones of the dorsal motor nucleus of the vagus nerve. *Brain Res.*, **300**,

83–9

36. Dreifuss, J. J., Ragenbass, M., Charpak, S., Dubois-Dauphin, M. and Tribollet, E. (1987). A role of central oxytocin in autonomic functions: its action in the motor nucleus of the vagus nerve. *IBRO Proc.* (In press)

37. Rogers, R. C., McCann, M. J. and Hermann, G. E. (1988). TRH effects on physiologically-identified neurons in the dorsal vagal complex: in vivo and in vitro studies. *Neurosci. Abs.* **14**, 538

38. Lechan, R. M., Snapper, S. B. and Jackson, I. M. D. (1983). Evidence that spinal cord TRH is independent of the paraventricular nucleus of the hypothalamus. *Neurosci. Letters*, **43**, 61–5

39. Palkovits, M., Mezey, E., Eskay, R. L. and Brownstein, M. J. (1986). Innervation of the nucleus of the solitary tract and dorsal vagal nucleus by thyrotropin-releasing hormone containing raphe neurons. *Brain Res.*, **373**, 246–51

40. Eskay, R. L., Long, R. T. and Palkovits, M. (1983). Localization of immunoreactive thyrotropin-releasing hormone in the lower brainstem of the rat. *Brain Res.*, **277**, 159–62

41. Kubek, M. J., Rea, M. A., Hodes, Z. I. and Aprison, M. H. (1983). Quantitation and characterization of thyrotropin releasing hormone in vagal nuclei and other regions of the medullar oblongata of the rat. *J. Neurochem.*, **40**, 1307–13

42. Hobson, J. A. and Scheibel, A. B. (1980). The brainstem core: sensorimotor integration and behavioural state control. *Neurosci. Res. Prog. Bull.*, **18**, 173

43. Kellow, J. E., Gill, R. C. and Wingate, D. L. (1987). Proximal gut motor activity in irritable bowel syndrome: patients at home and at work. *Gastroenterology*, **92**, (Part 2), 1463

44. Kumar, D. and Wingate, D. L. (1985). The irritable bowel syndrome: a paroxysmal motor disorder. *Lancet*, **2**, 973–7

45. McCann, M. J., Hermann, G. E. and Rogers, R. C. (1988). Thyrotropin-releasing hormone (TRH) potentiates the gastric responses evoked by dorsal medullary serotonin (5HT). *Neurosci. Abs.* **14**, 538

46. Barker, J. L., Dufy, B., Harrison, N. L., Owen, D. G. and MacDonald, J. F. (1987). Signal transduction mechanisms in cultured CNS neurons and clonal pituitary cells. *Neuropharmacology*, **26**, 941–55

47. Wood, J. D. (1987). Signal transduction in intestinal neurons. In Szurszewski (ed.) *Proceedings of Xth International Symposium on Gastrointestinal Motility*, pp.55–69. (Amsterdam: Elsevier)

48. Cox, G. E., Jordan, D., Moruzzi, P., Schwaber, J. S., Spyer, K. M. and Turner, S. A. (1986). Amygdaloid influences on brainstem neurons in the rabbit. *J. Physiol.*, **381**, 135–48

49. Gebber, G. L. and Klevans, L. R. (1972). Central nervous system control of cardiovascular reflexes. *Fed. Proc.*, **31**, 1245–52

50. Grijalva, C. V., Taché, Y., Gunion, M. W., Walsh, J. H. and Geiselman, P. J. (1986). Amygdaloid lesions attenuate neurogenic gastric mucosal erosions but do not alter gastric secretory changes induced by intercisternal bombesin. *Brain Res. Bull.*, **16**, 55–61

51. Henke, P. G. (1982). The telecephalic limbic system and experimental gastric pathology: a review. *Neurosci. Biobehav. Rev.*, **6**, 381–90

52. Kapp, B. S., Gallagher, M., Underwood, M. D., McNall, C. L. and Whitehorn, D. (1982). Cardiovascular responses elicited by electrical stimulation of the amygdala central nucleus in the rabbit. *Brain Res.*, **234**, 251–62

53. Loewy, A. D. and McKellar, S. (1980). The neuroanatomical basis of central cardiovascular control. *Fed. Proc.*, **39**, 2495–503

54. Smith, O. A. and de Vito, J. L. (1984). Central neural integration for the control of autonomic responses associated with emotion. *Ann. Rev. Neurosci.*, **7**, 43–65

55. Smith, G. P. and McHugh, P. R. (1967). Gastric secretory response to amygdaloid or hypothalamic stimulation in monkeys. *Am. J. Physiol.*, **213**, 640–4

56. Cassell, M. D., Gray, T. S. and Kiss, J. Z. (1986). Neuronal architecture in the rat central nucleus of the amygdala: a cytological, hodological and immunocytochemical study. *J. Comp. Neurol.*, **246**, 478–99

57. Ricardo, J. A. and Koh, E. T. (1978). Anatomical evidence of direct projections from the nucleus of the solitary tract to the hypothalamus, amygdala and other forebrain structures in the rat. *Brain Res.*, **153**, 1–26

58. Veening, J. G., Swanson, L. W. and Sawchenko, P. E. (1982). The organization of projections from the central nucleus of the amygdala to brainstem sites in central autonomic regulation: a combined retrograde transport-immunohistochemical study. *Brain Res.*, **303**, 337–57

59. Kawai, Y., Inagaki, S., Shiosaka, S., Senba, E., Hara, Y., Sakanaka, M., Takatsuki, K. and Tohyama, M. (1982). Long descending projections from amygdaloid somatostatin containing cells to the lower brain stem. *Brain Res.*, **239**, 603–7

60. Bueno, L. and Ferre, J. P. (1982). Central regulation of intestinal motility by somatostatin and cholecystokinin and octapeptide. *Science*, **216**, 1427–9

61. Fries, J. L., Murphy, W. A., Suerias-Diaz, J. and Coy, D. H. (1982). Somatostatin antagonist analog increases GH, insulin and glucagon release in the rat. *Peptides*, **3**, 811–14

62. Hermann, G. E. and Rogers, R. C. (1987). Dorsal medullary somatostatin causes an increase in gastric acid secretion. *Neurosci. abs.*, **17**, 737

63. Mancillas, J. R., Siggins, G. R. and Bloom, F. E. (1986). Somatostatin selectively enhances acetylcholine-induced excitations in the rat hippocampus and cortex. *Proc. Natl. Acad. Sci.*, **83**, 7518–21

64. Mueller, A. L., Kunkel, D. D. and Schwartzkroin, P. A. (1986). Electrophysiological actions of somatostatin in hippocampus: and in vitro study. *Cell Mol. Neurobiol.*, **6**, 363–79

65. Pittman, Q. J. and Siggins, G. R. (1981). Somatostatin hyperpolarizes hippocampal pyramidal cells in vitro. *Brain Res.*, **221**, 402–8

66. Watson, T. W. and Pittman, Q. J. (1987). Mechanism of action of somatostatin in the hippocampal slice. *Proc. West. Pharmac. Soc.*, **30**, 361–3

67. Hermann, G. E., McCann, M. J. and Rogers, R. C. (1988). Bed nucleus of stria terminalis influence over gastric function. *Neurosci. Abs.* (In press)

68 Atweh, S. F., Murrin, L. C. and Kuhar, M. J. (1978). Presynaptic localization of opiate receptors in vagal and accessory optic systems: an autoradiographic study. *Neuropharmacol.*, **17**, 65–71

69. Schwaber, J. S., Wray, S., Higgins, G. A. and Hoffman, G. (1981). The central nucleus of the amygdala: descending autonomic connections and neuropeptide systems in the rat. *Anat. Res.*, **199**, 228A

70. Swanson, L. W., Sawchenko, P. E., Rivier, J. and Vale, W. W. (1985). Organization of ovine corticotropin-releasing factor immunoreactive cells and fibers in the rat brain: an immunohistochemical study. *Neuroendocrin.*, **36**, 165–86

71. Villarreal, J. A. and Brown, M. R. (1978). Bombesin-like peptide in hypothalamus: chemical and immunological characterization. *Life Sci.*, **23**, 2729–33

72. Wray, S., Schwaber, J. S. and Hoffman, G. (1981). Neuropeptide localization in the rat central nucleus of the amygdala. *Anat. Rec.*, **199**, 282A

73. Caffe, A. R. and Van Leeuwen, F. W. (1983). Vasopressin-immunoreactive cells in the dorsomedial hypothalamic region, medial amygdaloid nucleus and locus coeruleus of the rat. *Cell Tissue Res.*, **233**, 23–33

74. Van Leeuwen, F. and Caffe, R. (1983). Vasopressin-immunoreactive cell bodies in the bed nucleus of the stria terminalis of the cat. *Cell Tissue Res.*, **228**, 525–34

75. Kaada, B. R., Pribram, K. H. and Epstein, J. A. (1949). Respiratory and vascular responses in monkeys from temporal pole, insula, orbital surface, and cingulate gyrus. *J. Neurophysiol.*, **12**, 347–56

76. Lofving, B. (1961). Cardiovascular adjustments induced from the rostral cingulate gyrus. *Acta Physiol. Scand.*, (Suppl. 53), 1841–84

77. Smith, W. K. (1945). The functional significance of the rostral singular cortex as revealed by its response to electrical stimulation. *J. Neurophysiol.*, **8**, 241–55

78. Ward, A. A., Jr. (1948). The cingulate gyrus: area 24. *J. Neurophysiol.*, **11**, 13–23

79. Cannon, W. B. (1909). The influence of emotional states on the functions of the alimentary canal. *Am. J. Med. Sci.*, **137**, 480–7

80. Wolf, S. and Wolf, H. G. (1943). *Human Gastric Function: An Experimental Study of Man and His Stomach.* (New York: Oxford University Press)

81. Babkin, B. P. and Speakman, T. J. (1950). Cortical inhibition of gastric motility. *J. Neurophysiol.*, **13**, 55–63

82. Eliasson, S. (1952). Cerebral influence on gastric motility in cat. *Acta Physiol. Scand.*, **26** (Suppl.95), 1–70

83. Hoffman, B. L. and Rasmussen, T. (1953). Stimulation studies of insular cortex of *macaca mulatta*. *J. Neurophysiol.*, **16**, 343–51

84. Sheehan, D. (1957). The effect of cortical stimulation on gastric movements in the monkey. *J. Physiol.*, **83**, 177–84

85. Spiegel, E. A., Weston, K. and Oppenheimer, M. J. (1943). Postmotor foci influencing the

363

gastrointestinal tract and their descending pathways. *J. Neuropath. Exp. Neurol.*, **2**, 45–53
86. Strom, G. and Uvnas, B. (1950). Motor responses of gastrointestinal tract and bladder to topical stimulation of frontal lobe, basal ganglia and hypothalamus in cat. *Acta Physiol. Scand.*, **21**, 90–104
87. Hurley-Guis, K. M. and Neafsay, E. J. (1986). The medial frontal cortex and gastric motility: microstimulation results and their possible significance for the overall pattern of organization of rat frontal and parietal cortex. *Brain Res.*, **365**, 241–8
88. Terreberry, R. R. and Neafsay, E. J. (1983). Rat medial frontal cortex: a visceral motor region with a direct projection to the solitary nucleus. *Brain Res.*, **278**, 245–9
89. Saper, C. B. (1982). Convergence of autonomic and limbic connections in the insular cortex of the rat. *J. Comp. Neurol.*, **210**, 163–73
90. Shipley, M. T. (1982). Insular cortex projection to the nucleus of the solitary tract and brainstem visceromotor regions in the mouse. *Brain Res. Bull.*, **8**, 138–48
91. Hencke, P. G. and Savoie, R. J. (1982). The cingulate cortex and gastric paathology. *Brain Res. Bull.*, **8**, 489–92

28
Vagal efferent discharge during vomiting

L. A. BLACKSHAW AND D. GRUNDY

INTRODUCTION

The act of vomiting may be triggered by a wide variety of stimuli ranging from those which may be considered appropriate, such as ingested toxins and bowel obstruction, to more inappropriate and quite bizarre stimuli such as space motion sickness and pregnancy.

Associated with vomiting are visceral responses, including reverse peristalsis and gastric relaxation[1], which serve to confine luminal contents in the upper gastrointestinal tract prior to their elimination by powerful contractions of the diaphragm and abdominal musculature. The vagus has an important role to play both in the initiation of vomiting by gastrointestinal stimuli[2] and in the control of visceral events associated with vomiting[1,3] (see also Poster 44, this volume). The latter appears to be the same for both central and peripherally induced emesis and may be the result of a programmed output from the brainstem circuitry responsible for co-ordinating the visceral and somatic components. Although the involvement of vagal preganglionic neurons in visceral emetic responses is well established, the nature of the vagal efferent signals to the gastrointestinal tract are unknown. In continuing electrophysiological studies of vagal efferent control mechanisms in the ferret, vomiting was an occasional response to chemical perfusions of the stomach and duodenum aimed to activate gastrointestinal mucosal afferents. This afforded the opportunity to record directly the discharge of vagal efferent fibres during emesis and it is their characteristic responses that are reported here.

METHODS

Ferrets were anaesthetized with urethane (1.5 g/kg i.p.) after an overnight fast. The gastrointestinal tract was cannulated to enable either the whole stomach or separated corpus and antrum to be distended or perfused; while in some experiments a 15 cm loop of intestine, starting immediately below the pylorus, was similarly prepared to permit perfusion or distension of the duodenum. Intraluminal pressures were recorded under isovolumetric conditions from either the whole stomach or isolated antrum and corpus and also from the duodenum.

For single-unit recordings of vagal efferent fibres, the vagus was dissected away from the adjacent carotid artery on one side (usually the right), and a paraffin pool made in the neck. The vagus was supported on a dissecting platform, the nerve sheath split, and fine strands of efferent fibres teased from the main vagal trunk. Single-unit recordings were then achieved as previously described[4].

RESULTS

Efferent responses to gastrointestinal distension

One hundred and eighty-eight vagal efferent units were recorded during the course of this study. All showed a low-frequency (<10 Hz), irregular spontaneous discharge which was unrelated to respiratory or cardiovascular inputs. This discharge was modified in 89% of units by gastric or duodenal distension with isotonic saline (50 ml—whole stomach; 20 ml—corpus; 4 ml—antrum; 4 ml—duodenum). These responses occurred as either excitation or inhibition of firing (Figure 1), with approximately equal numbers of units showing excitation and inhibition to the range of mechanical stimuli used. The main characteristics of efferent responses to gastrointestinal distension were: short latency (<1 s), powerful excitation or inhibition, slow adaptation throughout the stimulus, and rapid return to predistension frequency on deflation. These efferent units therefore received a powerful input from

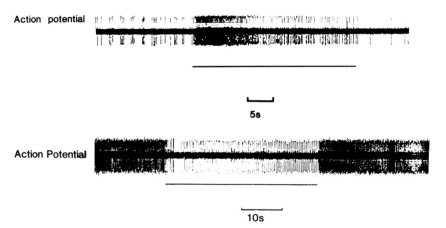

Figure 1 **Upper trace**: Response of a single vagal efferent unit to duodenal distension with 4 ml of isotonic saline (bar). The unit was powerfully excited throughout the period of distension. **Lower trace**: Response of another efferent unit to the same stimulus. The slightly higher spontaneous discharge in this unit was strongly inhibited by distension in this case

gastrointestinal mechanoreceptors. Vomiting did not occur during these moderate levels of distension.

Efferent responses to luminal chemical perfusions

The antrum or duodenum could also be perfused with isotonic saline at 12 ml/min which was substituted with any of a range of chemical solutions, including isotonic HC1, D-glucose, L-tryptophan, 50–1000 mM NaOH, distilled water, or hypertonic saline (308, 500 or 100 mM). These stimuli were chosen on the grounds of their ability to activate vagal mucosal chemoreceptors as found in previous studies in several species[5]. In response to these perfusions, efferent units showed generally weak, long-latency, poorly maintained, poorly reproducible responses with only 14% of units showing clear-cut responses (Figure 2). The criteria for determining clear-cut responses is described elsewhere[4]. Acid in the duodenum and alkali in the antrum were found to give rise to the majority of these responses.

Efferent discharge during vomiting

Emetic responses were associated with acidification, alkalinization or increasing osmolarity of the luminal contents and were manifested as a long latency (usually > 1.5 min), sudden fall in intrastric pressure which was coincident with the onset of lip-licking and rhythmic jaw movements. These are characteristic prodromata of vomiting and on 22/24 occasions retching ensued shortly afterwards, with the prodromata alone occurring on two occasions. On 17 occasions efferent discharge showed a characteristic pattern during emetic responses. A sudden (244 ± 125%; mean ± SEM) increase in

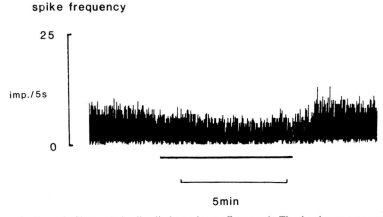

spike frequency

Figure 2 Record of integrated spike discharge in an efferent unit. The duodenum was perfused with isotonic saline, and distilled water was substituted for the period indicated by the bar. This resulted in a clear-cut (25%) reduction in efferent discharge. The response was gradual in onset, reaching a plateau after 2 min and recovering over a similar timecourse on reintroduction of saline (from ref. 4 with kind permission)

discharge was seen after a mean latency of 141 s from the onset of perfusion which was coincident with or slightly preceded gastric relaxation. A further rapid increase in firing (732 ± 269%; mean ± SEM) over control levels was seen during retching, being manifested as either a phasic modulation with each individual retch (Figure 3), or as a tonic high frequency discharge (Figure 4). It is possible that the phasic modulation of discharge was due to activation of visceral mechanoreceptors during large excursions of intra-abdominal pressure.

Retching occurred on five occasions during duodenal HC1 perfusion and also, somewhat surprisingly on four occasions after reintroduction of isotonic saline into the duodenum following a period of perfusion with distilled water. This phenomenon was taken to indicate that a sudden increase in luminal osmolarity may cause an emetic response. Indeed, switching perfusions from isotonic to 308 mM saline resulted in retching with an associated efferent response in three of 14 units tested (Figure 3). Despite the large movements during the retching episodes in only four cases did it result in the loss of recording.

On two occasions retching did not actually take place, but the prodromata of vomiting, including lip-licking and gastric relaxation were evident, accompanied by a slight elevation in discharge (Figure 5).

Unlike duodenal perfusions, isotonic HC1 and 308 mM saline, when perfused in the antrum were ineffective as emetic stimuli. On the other hand

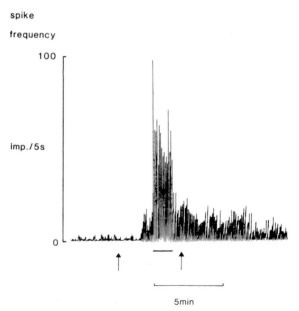

Figure 3 Response of an efferent unit to duodenal perfusion of hypertonic saline (308 mM), introduced at the first arrow. After 90 s there was an increase in discharge followed by a further phasic increase during retching (bar). On reintroduction of isotonic saline (second arrow), discharge gradually fell to its original level over a 15 min period (from ref. 4 with kind permission)

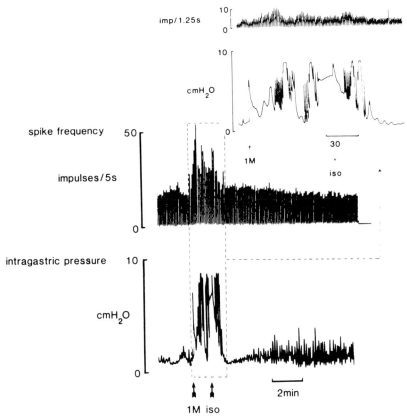

Figure 4 Integrated record of efferent unitary discharge. After the duodenum had been perfused with 500 mM saline, 1 M saline was introduced into the antrum, which resulted in a short latency increase in firing coincident with the onset of retching. Discharge was tonically increased, showing no modulation with individual retches, as can be seen from the inset of the retching period itself. In this example an antral stimulus is required in addition to the duodenal perfusion to reach threshold for retching to be triggered

1 M saline and 50–100 mM NaOH, caused retching with an associated efferent response on ten occasions (Figure 4).

In contrast to non-emetic responses to mechanical and chemical stimuli, no inhibitory effects on vagal efferent discharge were seen during retching and related phenomena. When the behaviour of efferent units showing emetic responses is assessed during mechanical stimuli, no pattern emerges (Table 1).

DISCUSSION

These data on the characteristics of vagal efferent fibre discharge during chemical stimulation of the gastrointestinal mucosa provide some insight

spike

frequency

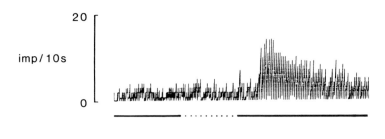

20

imp/10s

0

5min

Figure 5 Integrated record of efferent unitary discharge. The duodenum was perfused with isotonic saline and distilled water was substituted for the period indicated by the dotted line. Approximately 2 min after the reintroduction of isotonic saline the unit became excited coincident with lip-licking but vomiting, which was commonly associated with this type of response, did not occur (from ref. 4 with kind permission)

Table 1 Responses of 17 units to gastrointestinal distension—these all showed powerful excitation during retching

Response type	+	-	0
Gastric distension	10	5	2
Duodenal distension	4	8	1

into the role of the vagus nerve in both the genesis of emesis and the mediation of the visceral emetic response. The present data are consistent with the concept of a trigger mechanism for the initiation of vomiting and its prodromata[2]. The efferent units do not show a gradual build-up of discharge prior to the emetic response. Instead, vagal efferent responses occurred suddenly after a relatively long latency and in most cases were shortly followed by retching. This has the functional advantage that vomiting only proceeds if the emetic stimulus is persistent and therefore valuable nutrients are not unnecessarily voided. It also appears that there is a thin divide between the threshold for initiation of prodromata and that for the full-blown emetic response as only twice were the prodromata alone observed. Comparable differences in threshold were also observed in previous studies in the conscious dog[1]. As only 22 bouts of vomiting occurred in over 200 experiments it is also apparent that thresholds for triggering retching are widely variable in the anaesthetized ferret.

Chemical stimuli as a whole were more effective in causing retching when perfused in the duodenum than in the antrum in this study. This would fit well with a 'last-ditch stand' role, as emetogenic stimuli arriving in the stomach may be rendered less harmful by gastric digestion and dilution, whereas if they were allowed access to the small intestine absorption would be their most likely fate, where the substance may prove harmful.

Vagal efferent units showing characteristic responses before and during retching were all affected by gastric or duodenal distension. This indicates that the direct reflex effects of mechanical and chemical stimuli on gastrointestinal function and the drive for visceral correlates of vomiting share common motor pathways in the vagus. While this might seem reasonable for corpus relaxation which occurs during both receptive relaxation and vomiting, the way in which the vagus is able to convert the normal aboral progression of motor activity to the pre-emetic pattern of retroperistalsis is unclear. There is some evidence that the orad progression of retrograde contractions is achieved by sequential activation by the vagus nerves of ascending regions of gastrointestinal musculature (see Poster 44, this volume). However, in the present study, efferent units did not show a discrete burst of discharge in a way consistent with sequential activation of individual vagal fibres. It is interesting, though, that units showing both inhibition and excitation in response to distension and luminal perfusions in the non-emetic situation were exclusively excited during emetic responses. Thus, during normal reflex control of the gastrointestinal tract the vagal excitatory and inhibitory motor pathways may be reciprocally activated[5]. Since only excitation was observed in efferent units before and during retching, it is possible that, by increasing firing along all efferent fibres, the vagus is providing a discordant pattern of control to the enteric nervous system, which it interprets as a signal for the initiation of retroperistalsis and relaxation.

References

1. Lang, I. M., Sarna, S. K. and Condon, R. E. (1986). Gastrointestinal motor correlates of vomiting in the dog. *Gastroenterology*, **90**, 40–7
2. Borison, H. L. and Wang, S. C. (1953). Physiology and pharmacology of vomiting. *Pharmacol. Rev.*, **5**, 193–230
3. Miolan, J. P., Lajard, A. M., Rega, P. and Roman, C. (1984). Vagal control of the gastrointestinal tract during vomiting. In Roman, C. (ed.) *Gastrointestinal Motility*, pp. 167–76. (Lancaster: MTP Press)
4. Blackshaw, L. A., Grundy, D. and Scratcherd, T. (1987). Involvement of gastrointestinal mechano- and intestinal chemoreceptors in vagal reflexes: an electrophysiological study. *J. Auton. Nerv. Syst.*, **18**, 225–34
5. Grundy, D. (1988). Vagal control of gastrointestinal function. *Baillières Clinical Gastroenterology*, **2**(1), 23–43

29
Reflex control of gastric motility by stimuli acting from within the stomach

T. SCRATCHERD, D. GRUNDY, L. RUDGE, J. S. BALL AND R. G. CLARK

INTRODUCTION

Gastric emptying is controlled in such a way as to limit the amount of food entering the intestine from the stomach and it is generally accepted that this is achieved by negative feedback regulation from the duodenum and the small intestine. The receptors responsible respond to osmolytes, acid, volume, fats and fatty acids, certain amino acids and the calorific value of the meal[1,2]. Both neural and humoral mechanisms have been implicated. Except for the receptive relaxation which can occur when a meal enters the stomach[3], most stimuli which act from within the stomach are regarded as excitatory[4]. The possible participation in the control of gastric motility by reflexes which originate in the stomach and are inhibitory in nature, was originally proposed by Abrahamsson[5]. He described that distension of the antrum of the anaesthetised cat caused reflex relaxation and inhibition of motility of the corpus-fundus region of the stomach, which persisted after the injection of atropine and/or guanethidine, with both vagal and sympathetic pathways.

Afferent discharge in vagal fibres from the corporofundic region monitors the volume of the meal with a discharge which is directly proportional to the volume of the content of that region. Afferent discharge from the antrum on the other hand is phasic and the receptors here respond in a manner which monitors the presence and force of every peristaltic wave[6]. Whereas the role of the discharge from the proximal stomach is understandable, that from the antrum is less clear. Evidence is presented in this chapter that the stomach has within its walls the means of regulating its own activity, at least in terms of volume, which is independent of the duodenum and small intestine and which is likely to be mediated by these two forms of neural activity.

METHODS

Experiments were performed on four retriever dogs (19.5–25 kg weight) which had previously been prepared with the antrum separated from the corpus, care being taken to leave the innervation as intact as possible. Stainless steel cannulae were inserted into the antrum and into the most dependent part of the corpus and brought to the exterior on each side of the midline. Gastrointestinal continuity was re-established by an enterstomy between the corpus and the first part of the jejunum. The details of the surgical procedures and the care of the animals has been published previously[7].

Experimental protocol

At least four weeks were allowed for recovery before any experiments were carried out. The dogs were denied food, but not water for 18–24 h before an experiment. They were placed in slings on a Pavlov table in which they were able to rest comfortably. The cannula caps were removed and any food debris cleared. A balloon prepared from a condom was tied to the end of a plastic catheter and gently inserted through the cannula into the antrum and corpus respectively. The dead space of tubes was filled with warm water. The plastic catheters were each attached to pressure transducers (Elcomatic EM 750), the output from which was amplified and recorded on magnetic tape, a flat bed recorder and a BBC Master Microcomputer[8].

The characteristic spontaneous contractile activity of each dog was determined before any experimental work was carried out. The recording periods were divided into 5 min periods. Distensions were carried out by the slow injection of warm water at body temperature, usually over 30 s periods for small volumes (5–30 ml) or over 1–2 min for volumes greater than this, mimicking the time the dog would eat a meal of meat of that size.

Analysis of the motor patterns in both antrum and corpus were carried out using a program developed for the BBC Master Microcomputer[8]. The recordings were divided into 5 min periods. Peak heights of the contractions were measured and expressed in kilopascals (kPa) above atmospheric pressure. To measure the integrated activity over 5 min periods the area under the contraction curve was measured and the results expressed as kPa/min.

Statistical analysis

The mean data from each dog was computed and used to calculate group means and standard errors. Statistical differences were assessed using both paired and unpaired sample t-test.

RESULTS

Resting motility patterns

When isometric recordings were made simultaneously from both the proximal and distal stomach, periods of activity separated by periods of quiescence were observed similar to the migrating motor complexes seen in the intact organ. In two dogs this activity was investigated in detail with activity occurring in the proximal stomach over an average period of 45.7 ± 3.9 min and a quiescent period of 34.2 ± 3.0 min, giving a total cycle time of 79.9 ± 5.4 min for 10 cycles. The corresponding figures for the second dog were 36.2 ± 4.0, 36.4 ± 4.3 and 68.8 ± 3.6 min respectively.

The response of the pyloric antrum to distension of the body of the stomach

Distending the body of the stomach in a quiescent phase, with volumes ranging from 100 to 400 ml initiated reflex contractions of the pyloric antrum. However, the effect was inconsistent when the antrum contained no fluid.

When the antral balloon contained fluid, i.e. there was some minimal distension then reflex activity could be consistently induced; in general, the greater the antral volume the bigger was the antral response. The response was also dependent upon the degree of distension of the corpus. The response increasing as the distension was increased from 100 to 300 ml, further increases above the latter distending volume were only rarely observed (Figure 1).

The influence of the volume of the proximal stomach on the response of the antrum to distension

The antrum was distended every 5 min in 5 ml increments up to a total volume of 30 ml, after which the fluid was withdrawn from the antral balloon. The body of the stomach was then inflated with volumes which ranged from 100 to 300 ml, after which the antrum was reinflated in steps of 5 ml as before. It was observed that after corporal (proximal stomach) inflation the antral response was potentiated and the effect was statistically significant up to volumes of 20 ml in all experiments. Above this volume, no significant differences were found in the group as a whole (Figure 2).

From these experiments it is concluded that corpus distension will initiate reflex antral contractions, an effect which is more consistent if the antrum is partially distended. The magnitude of the response is also determined by the degree to which the corpus is distended. It is interpreted that antral activity can be initiated by a vagovagal reflex originating from stretch receptors in the corpus wall and that this vagal action may also play a permissive role by augmenting local reflex action of stimuli acting from within the antrum.

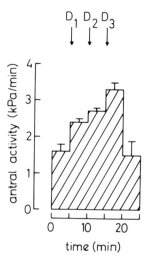

Figure 1 The effect on antral motility when the corpus was distended at D_1 with 100 ml, at D_2 with 200 ml and at D_3 with 300 ml of fluid. The antral balloon contained 5 ml fluid

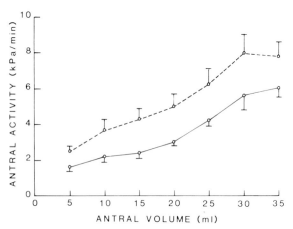

Figure 2 The effect on antral motility when the antrum was distended in 5 ml increments, before distension of the corpus (continuous line) and after distension (interrupted line). there was a highly significant differences ($p > 0.05$) when the antrum was distended with volumes of 20 ml and less. Corpus distension was between 100 and 300 ml (nine experiments in four animals)

The action of the antrum on the corpus

When the corpus is distended with volumes greater than about 50 ml a reflex increase in motility is observed which will continue for hours unabated. If during this activity or if activity of a migrating complex is present, the antrum is sufficiently distended, then a prompt inhibition of corporal contractions occurs (Figure 3). When isotonic recordings are made this inhibition of contractile activity is accompanied by a profound loss in tone.

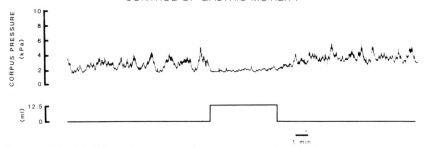

Figure 3 The inhibition of corporal activity (upper curve) when the pyloric antrum was distended with a volume of 12.5 ml (signal on lower curve). Corpus activity was stimulated in the quiescent phase by inflation with 100 ml

The degree of inhibition was found to be related to the volume of distension. With all stimuli there was an immediate cessation of all corporal contractions with the duration of the effect being determined by the distending volume. Volumes greater than 10 ml were effective and at 50 ml the inhibition outlasted the stimulus by as long as 30 min or more in many instances. Even in the case of a moderate stimulus the inhibition was not transient but continued, so long as the distending stimulus was present (Figure 4).

Is the inhibition of corporal activity secondary to passage of acid into the jejunum?

As the corpus was connected to the jejunum by an anastomosis it might be conceivable that the inhibition of motility was due to the action of acid stimulated by gastrin release or from the pyloro-oxyntic reflex[9]. This would seem to be unlikely as the gastric cannula was in the most dependent part of the stomach and left open so that acid drained to the exterior. Also the

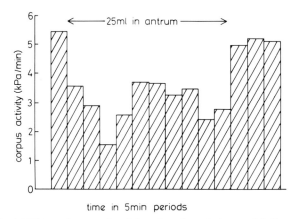

Figure 4 The inhibition of corporal activity when the pyloric antral balloon was distended with a volume of 25 ml. Note that the inhibition persisted for the duration of the application of the stimulus, which in this experiment was 50 min

latency of the motility inhibition was of the order of a few seconds. Finally, when acid secretion was surpressed by the H_2 blocking agent cimetidine (8.75 mg/kg) the inhibitory response was unaffected (Figure 5).

Excitatory influences on the corpus from stimuli in the antrum

Excitatory influences as well as inhibitory influences can be brought to bear on the corpus. It was observed that either lightly stroking the mucosa with the smooth end of plastic catheter or directing a jet of warm water or saline against the mucosa, caused contractions which were either single or in pairs to be produced by the corpus. These contractions could be graded and often were as high as 10 kPa.

DISCUSSION

Distension of the corporal fundic region of the stomach is an effective stimulus in causing contractions of the pyloric antrum. It probably represents in the conscious animal what has been demonstrated before in the anaesthetized ferret a corporo-antral reflex[4] and is the major driving force for gastric emptying. Distension of the antrum causes an increase in its own activity probably by both a vagovagal reflex and also a local reflex in the wall of the antrum. Again this is a similar phenomenon previously described by Grundy et al.[10], also in the anaesthetized ferret. In the latter work evidence was presented for permissive role by the vagus. From the present work the fact that an increase in motor activity of the antrum could not be consistently demonstrated until the antrum was partially distended also argues in favour of a permissive role.

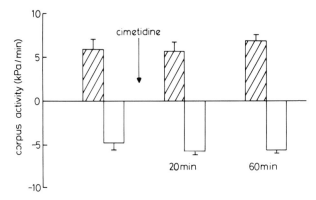

Figure 5 The absence of an effect of the H_2 blocking agent cimetidine on the antro-corporal inhibitory reflex. Hatched columns represent corporal activity as the result of corporal distension with a volume of 100 ml. Open columns represent integrated corporal activity in the 5 min period immediately after distension of the antrum with a volume of 25 ml: on the left before the i.v. injection of cimetidine, on the right 20 and 60 min after its injection. Cimetidine suppressed acid secretion

A long vagovagal reflex with receptors in the body of the stomach and an efferent limb to the antrum is supported by the evidence that increasing volumes of fluid in the corporal balloon caused an increase in antral activity. The afferent and efferent discharge in the vagus nerves which are probably the basis of such reflex effects have been previously described[6,11,12]. The inhibitory effects on corpus motility and tonus on distension of the antrum could be obtained by quite small volumes well within the physiological range. Such a reflex was first described on the anaesthetized cat[5]. As in the cat, this reflex has at least a vagovagal component as it persists after adrenergic blockage and guanethidine. Atropine abolished all contractile events but did not abolish the fall in corpus tone as a result of antral distension suggesting that non-adrenergic, non-cholinergic neurons may also be involved. Acid passing into the small intestine is unlikely to be the mediator of the response as it persisted after cimetidine and for reasons discussed in the text. The pathways for the two reflexes described would seem to lie in the vagus nerves by analogy with the experiments observed in the cat and ferret and is also in keeping with the current state of knowledge about the function of the vagus. Harper et al.[13] first demonstrated a reflex pathway in the vagus nerves which evoked gastric relaxation and confirmed later by Abrahamsson and Jannson[14]. They also demonstrated that there were pathways for an excitatory reflex component[13]. However, final proof that in the dog these are reflex effetcts mediated by vagovagal reflexes must await the denervation experiments to be carried out on these animals. It is interesting to observe that although this is the first time to our knowledge that these reflexes have been described in the conscious dog, the work confirms that already published on the much-criticized anaesthetized animal, proving the value of at least exploratory work on such preparations.

What is the likely physiological importance of these observations? First, they demonstrate that the stomach has the means to control its own activity from receptors within the stomach and does not rely entirely on a braking mechanism from the duodenum. A scenario of action could proceed as follows. When a meal enters the stomach and receptive relaxation complete, the stretch receptors in the wall of the proximal stomach will be stimulated and three events take place. The initiation of motor activity locally, which will propel some of the more liquid food into the antrum and a reflex increase in antral motility.

The first food entering the antrum will make contact with the mucosa and reflexly excite the corpus to contract further. As the contents of the antrum begin to accumulate, local reflex activity will increase and this in its turn is potentiated by reflex activity in the vagus which would be proportional to the size of the meal. However, such a sequence of events could not continue indefinitely, the stomach would begin to empty and the volume within the antrum would grow, increasing the tension within the wall with every peristaltic wave generated. Once threshold pressure was reached, feedback inhibition would be imposed on the proximal stomach causing peristaltic activity to reduce and relaxation to occur until the antrum had emptied sufficiently to allow antral pressure to fall and thereby cause disinhibition of the proximal stomach with the sequence of events repeating. This mechanism would allow the antrum to function without overloading the duodenum in terms of volume. Such an explanation would make good physiological sense and afford a reason why the antrum monitors every contractile event within its wall and signals the information back to the medulla. These prepyloric receptors are exquisitely sensitive and are more strategically placed than those in the duodenum which are post-pyloric and not in an ideal site to play a defensive role. A direct comparison can be made with the control of gastrin release.

SUMMARY

The motor responses of the surgically separated antrum and corpus were studied in four conscious dogs, when the corpus was distended, when the antrum was distended and when no stimuli were applied. In the absence of any distending stimulus migrating motor complexes were recorded in corpus and antrum.

Distending the corpus volumes from 50 to 300 ml caused contractions of the corpus, probably reflex in origin, which persisted for as long as the distending stimulus was applied. These were blocked by atropine. Similar distension of the corpus initiated antral contractions which were greater if the antrum was moderately distended and greater with a larger corporal distending volume.

The contractile response of the antrum to graded 5 ml inflations was potentiated when the corpus of the stomach was inflated. The potentiation was only statistically significant for antral volumes below 25 ml.

Distension of the antrum with 10 to 50 ml caused complete inhibition of corporal contractions both during a migrating complex or when stimulated by corporal inflation. The degree of inhibition was proportional to the distending stimulus and was present for the duration of the applied distension. For larger antral volumes the inhibition persisted for a variable time after the stimulus was withdrawn.

The inhibition was still effective after blocking acid secretion with cimetidine, which eliminates spillage of acid into the jejunum as a cause of the inhibition.

It is concluded that the stomach has the means of controlling its own activity, from receptors within the stomach wall, which is independent of the duodenum and small intestine.

Acknowledgements

We wish to acknowledge the help given to us by the Medical Research Council and the Wellcome Trust in support of the research reported here.

References

1. Meyer, J. H. (1987). Motility of the stomach and gastroduodenal junction. In Johnson, L. R., Christensen, J., Jackson, M. J., Jacobson, E. D. and Walsh, J. H. (eds.) *Physiology of the*

Gastrointestinal Tract, 2nd edn., pp. 613–29. (New York: Raven Press)

2. Thomas, J. E. (1957). Mechanics and regulation of gastric emptying. *Physiol. Rev.*, **37**, 453–74

3. Jansson, G. (1969). Extrinsic nervous control of gastric motility. An experimental study in the cat. *Acta Physiol. Scand.*, **326** (Suppl), 1–42

4. Andrews, P. L. R., Grundy, D. and Scratcherd, D. (1980). Reflex excitation of antral motility induced by gastric distension in the ferret. *J. Physiol. (Lond.)*, **298**, 79–84

5. Abrahamsson, H. (1973). Vagal relaxation of the stomach induced from the gastric antrum. *Acta Physiol. Scand.*, **89**, 406–14

6. Andrews, P. L. R., Grundy, D. and Scratcherd, T. (1980). Vagal afferent discharge from mechanoreceptors in different regions of the ferret stomach. *J. Physiol. (Lond.)*, **298**, 513–24

7. Bull, J. S., Grundy, D. and Scratcherd, T. (1987). Disruption of the jejunal motor migrating complex by gastric distension and feeding in the dog. *J. Physiol. (Lond.)*, **394**, 381–92

8. Scratcherd, T. and Scratcherd, T. J. (1987). A data acquisition and analysis package for empirical waveforms. *J. Physiol. (Lond.)*, **386**, 2P

9. Debas, H. T., Konturek, S. J., Walsh, J. H. and Grossman, M. I. (1974). Proof of a pyloro-oxyntic reflex for stimulation of acid secretion. *Gastroenterology*, **66**, 526–32

10. Grundy, D., Hutson, D. and Scratcherd, T. (1986). A permissive role for the vagus nerves in the genesis of antro-antral reflexes in the anesthetised ferret. *J. Physiol.*, **381**, 377–84

11. Grundy, D., Salih, A. A. and Scratcherd, T. (1981). Modulation of vagal efferent discharge by mechanoreceptors in the stomach, duodenum and colon of the ferret. *J. Physiol. (Lond.)*, **319**, 43–52

12. Andrews, P. L. R., Fussey, I. V. and Scratcherd, T. (1980). The spontaneous discharge in abdominal vagal efferents in dog and ferret. *Pflügers Arch.*, **387**, 55–60

13. Harper, A. A., Kidd, C. and Scratcherd, T. (1959). Vago-vagal reflex effects on gastric and pancreatic secretion and gastrointestinal motility. *J. Physiol. (Lond.)*, **148**, 417–36

14. Abrahamsson, H. and Jansson, G. (1973). Vago-vagal gastro-gastric relaxation in the cat. *Acta Physiol. Scand.*, **88**, 289–95

30
The neural basis of consciously perceived sensations from the gut

W. JÄNIG AND M. KOLTZENBURG

NATURE OF GASTROINTESTINAL SENSATIONS

It has been the experience of surgeons operating on their patients without general anaesthesia that many forms of direct trauma which are painful to the skin, such as cutting or burning, are not consciously perceived when applied to the gut[1-3]. Yet, a variety of sensations can be elicited from the gastrointestinal tract, including feelings of fullness, the desire to defaecate and, probably most important, many forms of acute visceral pain. Visceral sensibility in general, and pain in particular, is vague and ill-localized. The difference of these sensations from those elicited from skin may suggest the existence of different neural mechanisms encoding the sensations from both body domains.

Increases of intracolonic volume and pressure that raise gut wall tension are an adequate natural stimulus for the extrinsic primary afferent innervation. The distension of bowel segments may evoke non-painful and painful sensations, regulatory reflexes and pseudoaffective responses in humans and animals[4-17]. Although such brief stimuli are good tools to study the basis of visceral sensations, they clearly do not simulate clinically relevant pathophysiological states that are rather characterized by continuing tenderness, pathological tissue changes and longlasting reflex disturbances. Sensory stimuli may affect the normal, healthy gastrointestinal tract quite differently from the diseased one.

The pioneering study of Wolff and Wolff[18,19] on their patient Tom who had a chronic gastric fistula showed that the pain threshold for distension dropped dramatically during inflammation. They made the remarkable observation that the healthy mucosa is largely insensitive to touch and could only very crudely detect stronger pressure stimuli. However, when it became engorged, oedematous or inflamed following trauma or experimental irritation, its sensitivity was so much increased that even light touch would elicit pain.

Studies on the neurobiological substrates of gastrointestinal sensations have nearly exclusively concentrated on the extrinsic primary afferent innervation under healthy conditions with mechanical stimuli. Unfortunately our knowledge is very limited about the changes occurring during pathophysiological states.

NEUROANATOMICAL BASIS OF GASTROINTESTINAL SENSATIONS

The extrinsic afferent innervation of the viscera passes along the vagal nerves to the brain stem and via splanchnic nerves to the spinal cord (Figure 1). The cell somata of these afferents lie in the nodose and jugular ganglion or in thoracolumbar and sacral dorsal root ganglia respectively.

Peripheral pathways mediating sensations

Although the exact contribution of vagal afferents to consciously perceived sensations is somewhat unclear[20], there are good reasons to assume that pain below the diaphragm is not communicated by these nerve fibres. This assumption is based on the complete abolition of pain following the selective disruption of spinal afferents[21-25] and the absence of pain in tetraplegic patients after spinal cord injury at a cervical level[26]. Furthermore, severe visceral pain can be elicited in conscious humans by electrical stimulation of the splanchnic nerves[27], but not of the vagi below the diaphragm[21]. Although textbook dogma maintains that painful sensations are only mediated by visceral afferents travelling in thoracolumbar splanchnic nerve trunks, it has been repeatedly proved that this is a dated, erroneous concept[28,29]. In fact, the afferent impulse activity evoking pain from the pelvic organs projects predominantly through the pelvic nerve to the CNS[6,16,22-25,28,29]. Both the sacral and thoracolumbar visceral afferent supply can be identified in all mammalian species including humans, the only difference being a rostrocaudal shift of the segmental levels[11,30] (Figure 1). The present review will focus on the properties of the spinal afferent innervation of the gut projecting into the lumbar splanchnic and pelvic nerves. Most studies were done in the cat using the colon as a model.

Quantitative estimates of the extrinsic afferent innervation

Electron microscopy shows that nearly all extrinsic afferents supplying the abdominal and pelvic viscera have thin myelinated or unmyelinated axons[31-33]. Numerical analysis of the lumbar afferent innervation of the feline colon using quantitative neuroanatomical tracing techniques have found some 2100 neurons projecting from the segments L_2–L_4 via the lumbar splanchnic and lumbar colonic nerves to the hindgut[34]. There is a yet unstudied population of colonic afferents travelling in the hypogastric nerve (unpublished observations), but neither detailed anatomical nor neurophysiol-

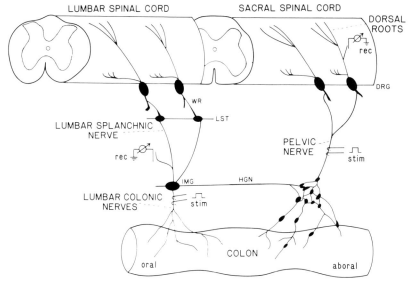

Figure 1 Schematic drawing of the afferent extrinsic innervation of the cat hindgut. All neurons have their cell somata in the dorsal root ganglia (DRG). The lumbar afferents run in the lumbar colonic nerves, bypass the inferior mesenteric ganglion (IMG) and travel with the lumbar splanchnic nerves and the white rami (WR) of the lumbar sympathetic trunk (LST) to the spinal cord. Some lumbar colonic afferents run also in the hypogastric nerve (HGN). The sacral supply projects via the pelvic nerve to the spinal cord. In the electrophysiological studies neural activity was recorded from single axons (rec) in fine filaments that were microdissected from a lumbar splanchnic nerve a sacral or spinal root. Using electrical stimulation (stim) the axons could be identified and from the latency of the responses the conduction velocity could be determined.

ogical data are available at present. Quantitative measures for the sacral afferent innervation of the distal colon are less accurate, as the pelvic nerves contain also the afferents supplying the genitourinary tract. A rough estimate of the colonic supply would calculate 1500–2000 dorsal root ganglion cells in the segments S_1–S_3 of both sides[35]. This number includes the visceral innervation of the anus which does not receive a lumbar afferent supply. In general, the afferent innervation of the colon increases aborally with the highest density in the anal canal that, besides its visceral supply, also receives a portion of afferents from the pudendal nerve.

The extrinsic visceral afferents make only a small contribution of 2.5% or less to the total number of spinal afferents[29]. The relatively few afferents supplying the colon are scattered over many spinal segments and innervate a relatively large peripheral target. This low density of the peripheral innervation and its spatially widely scattered central representation may explain the ill-defined localization of colonic sensations. Nevertheless, this small population of afferents can have strong effects on the CNS as evidenced by the intensity of visceral pain and autonomic reflexes.

385

NEUROPHYSIOLOGICAL BASIS OF GASTROINTESTINAL SENSATIONS

Evidence about the functional properties of extrinsic primary afferents has mainly been obtained from neurophysiological recordings of single neurons. These afferents were studied with standard electrophysiological techniques. The afferent axons were isolated by repeatedly splitting small bundles from the peripheral nerves (lumbar splanchnic nerve, white rami) or spinal roots until single or few conducting axons remained in those strands. The conduction velocities of the axons were determined from the latencies of the responses to electrical stimulation of lumbar colonic or pelvic nerve (Figure 1). Once a suitable filament had been selected it could then be tested with natural adequate stimuli using a series of graded isotonic colonic distensions or by inflation of intracolonic balloons and by observing the neural response during subsequent isovolumetric contractions. Some studies used close intra-arterial injections of algesic chemicals, notably bradykinin or capsaicin, to stimulate afferents through their vascular supply.

Most neurophysiological studies have focused on the lumbar portion and there is relatively little information about the sacral supply, although the latter is of greater biological importance for the control of continence and defaecation. A point of major interest for the understanding of the principles of visceral sensation is whether specific subpopulations of afferents can be classified that could be related to distinct sensations of the hindgut or autonomic reflex behaviours. Of particular interest for the insight of visceral pain states is whether specific nociceptors can be found. The question is whether painful gastrointestinal events are encoded by an entirely separate set of visceral nociceptors that are different from those receptors signalling non-painful experiences.

Mechanosensitivity of lumbar afferents

Lumbar splanchnic afferents responded to passive distensions and active contractions of the colon. Some two-thirds of the afferents displayed ongoing activity in the order of 0.5 Hz. The units were reproducibly excited by increases of intracolonic pressure. The majority (70%) had their thresholds in the innocuous range around 25 mmHg or less, but the distribution tailed off at higher pressure intensities where few units started to respond at 50–75 mmHg[36]. The afferent units showed graded responses to progressive increases of gut distension. Depending on the degree of a more phasic or more tonic component of the afferent response it was possible to differentiate these afferents into four further subcategories[36]. Yet, it is still unclear whether this is an inherent quality of the receptors or whether this difference can, what seems to be more likely to us, be attributed to the location of the receptive fields.

The receptive fields of these lumbar visceral units were small mechanosensitive spots located in the mesentery of the gut rather than in the colon proper (Figure 2A). Thus spinal afferents seem to be different in this respect from mechanosensitive vagal ones whose receptive field are presumably located

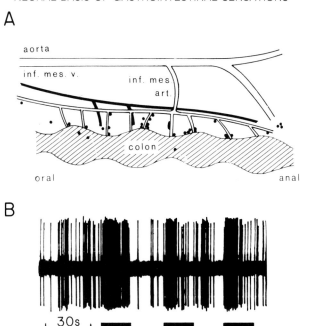

Figure 2 Localization of the receptive fields of lumbar colonic afferents (A). Receptive fields were mechanosensitive spots (.) that were mainly found in the mesentery along the tributaries of the inferior mesenteric artery (inf. mes. art.) and were not associated with the branches of the inferior mesenteric vein (inf. mes. v.). (B): Probing of the receptive field (bars) elicited a tonic or phasic discharge (modified with permission from ref. 36)

in the muscle wall of the organ[20,37–39]. Probing of the receptive field with a glass rod elicited mostly slowly and rarely rapidly adapting discharges in splanchnic afferents[36,39–42] (Figure 2B). Local thresholds were usually less than $10 \, mN$[29]. These types of receptive field are found for the majority of abdominal viscera and they tend to be associated with small arteries. However, for approximately half the afferent units responding to increase of colon wall tension the receptive field could not be found, probably due to methodological reasons. Since afferents responded both to contraction and distension it had—in analogy to the Golgi tendon organs of skeletal muscle— been suggested that the extrinsic afferents of the gut were arranged *in series* to the smooth muscle cells[43,44]. As mentioned above this functional description does not have an appropriate morphological correlate.

Although quantitative differences of the receptor properties have been found, it has not been possible to subclassify these afferents qualitatively. The high threshold afferents that were discovered were not distinctly different in terms of resting activity, conduction velocity or responses to mechanical or chemical stimuli (*vide infra*). It seems more plausible that they were the tail-off of the distribution, particularly if one takes into account that the receptive endings of some units might have been stimulated at some distance. Even receptors supplying the aorta, mesenteric artery or retroperitoneal space could at times be stimulated with colon distension[45] and it would seem to us inappropriate to label them solely on the basis of an inadequate test as colonic nociceptors.

Chemosensitivity of lumbar afferents

To overcome some of the ambiguities of mechanical tests, algesic chemicals were used to search for putative nociceptors. Intraperitoneal or intra-arterial injections of bradykinin elicit pain in humans[46,47] and pseudoaffective responses in animals[46,48]. Close arterial injections into the vascular supply of the colon appear to be the stimulus of choice to activate the spinal afferents of the colon that evoke pain. Indeed, small quantitites of bradykinin are a potent excitant for afferents (Figure 3). Regardless of their mechanosensitive properties most units responded to this algesic chemical and no additional neurons were recruited[49]. The response pattern was fairly uniform: afferents started to fire within 15 s of the injection and reached a dose-dependent maximal frequency, usually below 30 Hz, shortly thereafter. The response usually lasted for under 90 s, although there were frequently after-discharges, occasionally occurring in intermittent bursts.

Essentially very similar results have recently been obtained from an *in vitro* study of these receptors in the small intestine of the rat[31] using a variety of stimulants including bradykinin, substance P and capsaicin. As there were also concomitant contractions of the smooth muscle during chemical stimulation it could be argued that this action might have been an indirect one[50]. This possibility has been excluded, however. First, some afferents started to fire before there was an appreciable rise in intracolonic pressure[31]. Secondly, bradykinin was equipotent before and after paralysing the colon with loperamide[49] (Figure 3) or during an occasional adynamic ileus that had occurred spontaneously in some experiments[49]. Finally, the topical application of irritants onto the receptive endings in the mesentery could elicit vigorous firing without affecting gut motility[49].

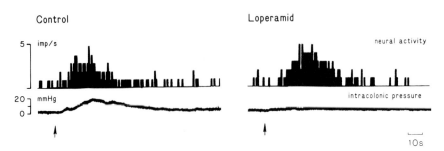

Figure 3 Response of a single lumbar colonic afferent unit to bradykinin. In the control the close intra-arterial injection of bradykinin (6.5 μg bolus injected at the arrow) stimulated the afferent unit, but there was a concomitant increase of the intracolonic pressure. The direct chemical excitation was demonstrated by the administration of loperamide (20 mg close intra-arterially) that paralysed the gut. Although the increase of intracolonic pressure was attenuated the afferent response was not affected (modified with permission from ref. 49)

Thus it appears that specific nociceptors cannot be found for lumbar afferents of the gut and that under normal conditions visceral pain is encoded by the discharge intensity of a homogenous population of afferents. Similar neural mechanisms of visceral nociception may in fact apply to many other abdominal and pelvic organs[29].

Response of lumbar afferents to ischaemia of the colon

It was furthermore interesting to monitor the response of primary afferent neurons under pathophysiological conditions that are known to produce severe pain in patients. Ischaemia of the gut is such a powerful noxious stimulus[51]. Several afferents were studied over many hours following the partial or complete occlusion of the arterial supply[49]. The baseline level of ongoing activity increased steadily after the reduction of mesenteric blood flow. With a latency of 30–60 min these neurons now started to fire intermittently with high-frequency bursts (Figure 4). During ischemia the receptors were sensitized to mechanical stimuli and distension of the colon led to a dramatic increase of the evoked neural activity. Thus, lumbar afferents can encode clinically relevant pain states by their discharge intensity. It is tempting to suggest that the high-frequency bursts are the neurophysiological basis for the intermittent bouts of pain experienced by patients.

Mechanosensitivity of sacral afferents of the colon

Far less is known about the sacral afferents supplying the hindgut, even though they are biologically more important in controlling continence and defaecation. Only recently have quantitative neurophysiological studies been carried out[52] (H.-J. Häbler, W. Jänig, M. Koltzenburg, in preparation). In contrast to their lumbar companions, the sacral afferents did not discharge spontaneously when the colon was empty. Units were stimulated by series

RESPONSE TO ISCHEMIA

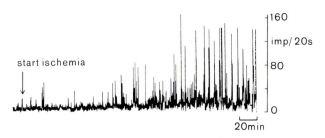

Figure 4 Response of a single lumbar colonic afferent unit to ischaemia. The afferent unit displayed some ongoing activity before partially arresting colonic blood flow by clamping the vascular supply. With some latency there was a dramtic increase in afferent firing (modified with permission from ref. 49)

of graded distension delivered by separate 10 cm-long balloons to the oral (12–22 cm proximal to the anus) or aboral (2–12 cm proximal to the anus) segments of the colon. The thresholds were generally around 20–30 mmHg and only occasionally did units require up to 40 mmHg of intracolonic pressure for activation. Further increases of intracolonic pressure led to a proportionate rise of neural activity (Figure 5). Most units appeared to respond tonically to distension of the colon and some were more phasically activated during filling of the colon (Figure 6). Some afferents were excited by the distension of one bowel segment only, but the majority responded to the distension of both balloons. Here, the units displayed different response

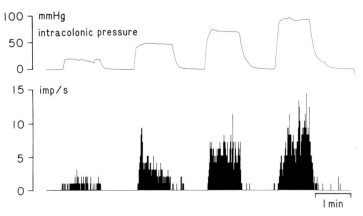

Figure 5 Response of a single sacral afferent unit to graded increases of intracolonic pressure. Note the proportionate afferent activation (H.-J. Häbler, W. Jänig and M. Koltzenburg, unpublished observation)

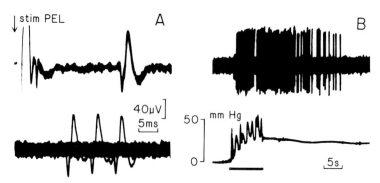

Figure 6 Response of an unmyelinated sacral afferent unit isolated from the dorsal root S_2. **A**: Identification of the unit that was excited by the electrical stimulation (upper trace) of the pelvic nerve with single electrical pulses (stim PEL) and by distension of the colon (lower trace; both traces are several times superimposed). **B**: Inflation of a balloon in the distal colon (bar) increased intracolonic pressure (lower trace) and evoked a phasic response of the afferent unit (upper trace). The fast oscillations of the intracolonic pressure are a technical artefact (H.-J. Häbler, W. Jänig and M. Koltzenburg unpublished observation)

characteristics and thresholds. This again illustrates the difficulties to adequately stimulate the receptors. Afferents that would discharge vigorously at low intracolonic presure delivered to the aboral segment of the bowel could require high and potentially noxious intensities when the oral part was stimulated or vice versa. Thus the extrinsic sacral afferents of the colon appear to be a homogeneous group of afferents. On the basis of the mechanical stimuli we did not obtain any evidence for specific colonic nociceptors. So far, algesic chemicals or other noxious agents have not been tried on this population of afferents.

Stimulation response characteristics

Stimulation response curves were calculated for afferents with tonic properties. The mean stimulation response curves lend further support to the idea that innocuous and noxious messages from the hindgut are encoded by the intensity of afferent firing enabling the CNS to extract the information from this discharge (Figure 7). As the slope of the stimulation response curve for the sacral afferents is steeper, these neurons appear to be better suited to signal the tension of the hindgut than the lumbar ones. Since most sacral afferents innervate the aboral parts of the hindgut and as the lumbar supply is largely confined to more oral parts, the findings are in agreement with psychophysiological investigations showing more accurate perception in the aboral parts of the hindgut.

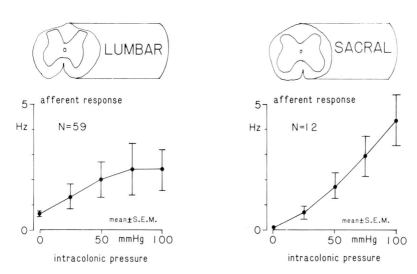

Figure 7 Stimulation response curves of 59 lumbar and 12 sacral single colonic afferents to graded distension of the colon. (Data from ref. 36 and unpublished data from H.-J. Häbler, W. Jänig and M. Koltzenburg)

Mechanosensitive afferents supplying the anus

A subpopulation of extrinsic afferents supplying the anal canal are distinctly different from units innervating the aboral parts of the colon. These anal afferents were usually not spontaneously active nor did they respond to increases of intracolonic pressure. Only rarely were they phasically excited at the onset or end of an intracolonic pressure stimulus of high intensity usually exceeding 50 mmHg. However, these units were vigorously activated by innocuous craniocaudal mechanical shearing stimuli applied to the mucosa of the anal canal (Figure 8) that was used to simulate the passage of faeces. The peak discharge frequency could be as high as 20 Hz and the response was rapidly adapting. Circular shearing stimuli were always less effective suggesting that the units could be involved in signalling defaecation[52].

Ventral root afferents

In the sacral segments of the cat there is a small population of primary afferent neurons that project with their central process into the ventral root[53–58]. Receptive fields were found in the colon and anal canal and their properties are conspicuously similar to their dorsal root companions. At the moment, it is not known whether this anatomical separate group subserves different functions or, indeed, whether they enter the spinal cord at all[54,55,58,59].

Conduction velocities

As predicted by the anatomical studies the conduction velocity of afferents from the hindgut was low. Axons conducting at less than 2.5 m/s are thought

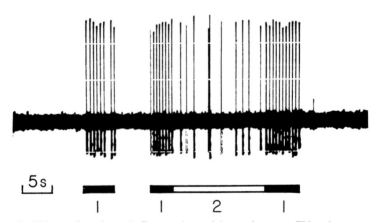

Figure 8 Thin myelinated sacral afferent unit supplying anal mucosa. This unit was not excited by distension of the colon, but by an innocuous mechanical shearing stimulus applied to the anal mucosa. Craniocaudal shearing (bar 1) is more effective than circular one (bar 2) (modified with permission from reference 52)

to be unmyelinated and the majority of colonic afferents fall into this category (Figure 9). There is a gradual increase in the mean conduction velocity from the oral to the aboral parts of the hindgut. The median of the conduction velocity of colonic afferents increased from 0.9 m/s for the axons travelling to the lumbar segments to 2.2 m/s for sacral afferents. Nearly all anal afferents are thin myelinated and conduct significantly faster ($p < 0.01$; U-test) than the afferents supplying the colon.

DO SPINAL GASTROINTESTINAL AFFERENTS HAVE MULTIPLE ROLES?

There exists an interesting difference between the neurophysiological and morphological studies on the colonic afferents. Some two-thirds of the thin myelinated or unmyelinated axons isolated in the lumbar splanchnic nerves could be excited by mechanical stimuli. This included practically all axons that had ongoing activity. The remaining axons are thought to be antidromically activated sympathetic post-ganglionic efferents and this assumption is supported by quantitative neuroanatomical tracing studies[34]. However, neuroanatomical studies on the peripheral nerve terminals of the gastrointestinal tract show that many extrinsic spinal afferents supply the organ wall[60,61] rather than the mesentery where most receptive fields were found in neurophysiological experiments.

This could mean that neurophysiological experiments could, for technical reasons, not find the receptive endings of tension receptors in the organ walls. Although we cannot disprove this possibility we are sceptical about it. First, afferents for which a receptive field was found, did not behave

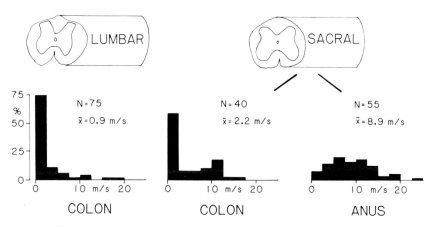

Figure 9 Distributions of the conduction velocities of lumbar and sacral colonic afferents and sacral afferents supplying the anal mucosa. The first left column of each panel shows the percentage of unmyelinated afferents. The median of the conduction velocity of afferents of both colonic populations is significantly different ($p < 0.01$, U-test) from the median conduction velocity of the anal afferents (data from refs. 36, 52 and unpublished data from H.-J. Häbler, W. Jänig and M. Koltzenburg)

differently to colon distension from those afferents without an identified receptive field. Secondly, it has to be kept in mind that the search for receptive fields is a difficult and laborious task for an organ as large and flexible as the feline colon. Thirdly, large parts of the organ including its mesentery are inaccessible during the electrophysiological recordings. Finally, the tension receptors of the vagus, which innervate the gastrointestinal tract and which have similar response characteristics as spinal afferents during distension of the gut, can be located more easily in the organ wall[20,37-39, 43,44,62].

One explanation of this paradox would be that the spinal afferents that are excited at a sensitive spot in the mesentery have multiple effects. The afferent impulse travelling in the central branch would impinge on the spinal cord, but activity would also sweep distally and could release neuroactive or trophic factors at their mucosal or muscular endings. As part of a nocifensive response this could affect blood flow or proliferation and integrity of the different tissue layers. Beside an action on peripheral non-neuronal tissues it is known that the afferents can significantly modulate integrative functions in prevertebral ganglia[63] or possibly even in the enteric plexuses[64].

IS THERE A POPULATION OF YET UNSTUDIED AFFERENTS?

While the multiple roles for the spinal afferents are reasonably supported by experimental evidence, this final section is somewhat more speculative. We want to suggest that the discrepancy between anatomical and electrophysiological studies could reside in the inadequate testing of fine afferents and this may be particularly relevant for the sacral innervation of the colon.

We have recorded from more than 200 unmyelinated afferents in the sacrodorsal roots that had large, clearly discernible action potentials (cf. Figure 6) with stable latencies and an all-or-nothing characteristic upon stimulation with single electrical pulses applied to the pelvic nerve. Yet, only 5% of these fibres were activated by colonic distension (H.-J. Häbler, W. Jännig and M. Koltzenburg, in preparation). Similar results were also obtained based on several hundred other unmyelinated afferents tested with innocuous and noxious stimulation of the lower urinary tract. Less than 2.5% of the unmyelinated afferents were activated by such stimulus[65]. Thus the properties of some 90% of the unmyelinated afferents projecting into the pelvic nerve remain obscure. However, using the urinary bladder as a model, we have recently shown that an acute inflammation of this viscus can activate a novel population of unmyelinated visceral afferents that do not respond to mechanical stimulation of the urinary bladder prior to inflammation[65]. If the same applies to the colon, a class of colonic afferents may exist that start only to respond in the presence of a pathological event. Very limited information is available about this hitherto unstudied afferent population that has also been described for the joint[66,67] and skin[68,69]. In these three organs this novel type of afferent is silent and does not respond to acute noxious mechanical stimuli. However, the receptors may 'lie in wait' continuously 'tasting' their environment; they would remain dormant as long as there is no pathophysiological change within the environment. But, once a lesion has occurred in the tissue, it would then be recruited, thus greatly increasing the primary afferent input to the CNS. If such receptors exist in the gastrointestinal tract, they could severely aggravate the tenderness, pain and autonomic reflex disturbances that seem to be so typical for inflamed tissues.

Acknowledgements

This work was supported by the Deutsche Forschungsgemeinschaft.

References

1. Lennander, K. G. (1902). Beobachtungen über die Sensibilität in der Bauchhöhle. *Mitt. a. d. Grenzgeb. d. Med. u. Chir.*, **10**, 39–104
2. Lennander, K. G. (1904). Weiter Beobachtungen über Sensibilität in Organ und Geweben und über lokale Anästhesie. *Dtsch. Zeitschr. f. Chir.*, **73**, 297–350
3. Mackenzie, J. (1909). *Symptoms and their Interpretation* (London: Shaw)
4. Bentley, F. H. and Smithwick, R. H. (1940). Visceral pain produced by balloon distension of the jejunum. *Lancet*, **2**, 389–91
5. Bloomfield, A. L. and Polland, W. S. (1931). Experimental referred pain from the gastrointestinal tract. Part II. Stomach, duodenum and colon. *J. Clin. Invest.*, **10**, 453–73
6. Goligher, J. C. and Hughes, E. S. R. (1951). Sensibility of the rectum and colon: it's role in the mechanism of anal continence. *Lancet*, **1**, 543–8
7. Hertz, A. F. (1911). The sensibility of the alimentary canal in health and disease. Lectures I–III. *Lancet*, **1**, 1051–6, 1119–24, 1187–93
8. Jänig, W. (1985). Organisation of the lumbar sympathetic outflow to skeletal muscle and skin of the cat hindlimb and tail. *Rev. Pharmacol. Biochem. Physiol.*, **102**, 119–213
9. Jänig, W. (1986). Spinal cord integration of visceral sensory systems and sympathetic nervous system reflexes. In Cervero, F. and Morrison, J. F. B. (eds.) *Visceral Sensation. Progress in Brain Research*, Vol. 67, pp. 255–77. (Amsterdam: Elsevier)
10. Jänig, W. (1988). Integration of gut function by sympathetic reflexes. In Grundy, G. and Read, N. W. (eds.) *Bailière's Clinical Gastroenterology: Gastrointestinal Neurophysiology*, Vol. 2, No. 1, pp. 45–62. (London: Baillière Tindall)
11. Jänig, W. and McLachlan, E. M. (1987). Organization of lumbar spinal outflow to distal colon and pelvic organs. *Physiol. Rev.*, **67**, 1332–404
12. Lipkin, M. and Sleisinger, M. H. (1958). Studies of visceral pain: measurements of stimulus intensity and duration associated with the onset of pain in esophagus, ileum and colon. *J. Clin. Invest.*, **37**, 28–34
13. Morley, J. (1928). Abdominal pain as exemplified in acute appendicitis. *Br. Med. J.*, **1**, 887–90
14. Morley, J. (1931). *Abdominal Pain.* (Edinburgh: Livingstone)
15. Müller, L. R. (1908). Ueber die Empfindungen in unseren inneren Organen. *Mitt. a. d. Grenzgeb. d. Med. u. Chir.*, **18**, 600–41
16. Ness, T. J. and Gebhart, G. F. (1988). Colorectal distension as a noxious visceral stimulus: physiological and pharmacological characterization of pseudaffective reflexes in the rat. *Brain Res.*, **450**, 153–69
17. Zimmermann, R. (1909). Experimentelle Untersuchungen über die Empfindungen in der Schlundröhre und im Magen, in der Harnröhre und in der Blase und im Enddarm. *Mitt. a. d. Grenzgeb. d. Med. u. Chir.*, **20**, 445–57
18. Wolf, S. (1965). *The Stomach.* (New York: Oxford University Press)
19. Wolf, S. and Wolff, H. G. (1943). Pain arising from the stomach and mechanisms underlying gastric symptoms. *Res. Publ. Ass. Nerv. Ment. Dis.*, **23**, 289–98
20. Andrews, P. L. R. (1986). Vagal innervation of the gastrointestinal tract. In Cervero, F. and

Morrison, J. F. B. (eds.) *Visceral Sensation. Progress in Brain Research*, Vol. 67, pp. 65–86. (Amsterdam: Elsevier)

21. Foerster, O. (1927). *Die Leitungsbahnen des Schmerzgefühls und die chirurgische Behandlung der Schmerzzustände*. (Berlin: Urban und Schwarzenberg)

22. Ruch, T. C. (1979). Pathophysiology of pain. In Ruch, T. and Patton, H. D. (eds.) *Physiology and Biophysics I: The Brain and Neural Function*, pp. 272–324. (Philadelphia: Saunders)

23. White, J. C. (1943). Sensory innervation of the viscera. *Res. Publ. Ass. Nerv. Ment. Dis.*, **23**, 373–90

24. White, J. C., Smithwick, R. H. and Simeone, F. A. (1952). *The Autonomic Nervous System: Anatomy, Physiology and Surgical Applications*, 3rd Edn. (New York: Macmillan)

25. White, J. C. and Sweet, W. H. (1969). *Pain and the Neurosurgeon: A Forty Year Experience*. (Springfield: C.C. Thomas)

26. Guttmann, L. (1976). *Spinal Cord Injuries*, 2nd Edn. (Oxford: Blackwell)

27. Leriche, R. (1939). *Surgery of Pain*. (London: Ballière Tindall)

28. Jänig, W. (1987). Neuronal mechanisms of pain with special emphasis on visceral and deep somatic pain. *Acta Neurochirurgica Suppl.*, **38**, 16–32

29. Jänig, W. and Morrison, J. F. B. (1986). Functional properties of spinal visceral afferents supplying abdominal and pelvic organs with special emphasis on visceral nociception. In Cervero, F. and Morrison, J. F. B. (eds.) *Visceral Sensation. Progress in Brain Research*, Vol. 67, pp. 87–114. (Amsterdam: Elsevier)

30. Morrison, J. F. B. (1988). The neural control of pelvic viscera. In Grundy, G. and Read, N. W. (eds.) *Bailière's Clinical Gastroenterology: Gastrointestinal Neurophysiology*, Vol. 2, No. 1, pp. 63–84. (London: Baillière Tindall)

31. Cervero, F. and Sharkey, K. A. (1988). An electrophysiological and anatomical study of intestinal afferent fibres in the rat. *J. Physiol. (Lond.)*, **401**, 381–97

32. Hulsebosch, C. and Coggeshall, R. E. (1982). An analysis of the axon populations in the nerve of the pelvic viscera in the rat. *J. Comp. Neurol.*, **211**, 1–10

33. Kuo, D. C., Yang, G. C. H., Yamasaki, D. S. and Krauthamer, G. M. (1982). A wide field electron microscopic analysis of the fibre constituents of the major splanchnic nerve in the cat. *J. Comp. Neurol.*, **210**, 49–58

34. Baron, R., Jänig, W. and McLachlan, E. M. (1985). The afferent and sympathetic components of the lumbar spinal outflow to the colon and pelvic organs in the cat. III. The colonic nerves, incorporating an analysis of all components of the lumbar prevertebral outflow. *J. Comp. Neurol.*, **238**, 158–68

35. deGroat, W. C. (1986). Spinal cord projections and neuropeptides in visceral afferent neurons. In Cervero, F. and Morrison, J. F. B. (eds.) *Visceral sensation: Progress in Brain Research*, Vol. 67, pp. 165–87. (Amsterdam: Elsevier)

36. Blumberg, H., Haupt, P., Jänig, W. and Kohler, W. (1983). Encoding of visceral noxious stimuli in the discharge pattern of visceral afferent fibres from the colon. *Pflügers Arch.*, **398**, 33–40

37. Leek, B. F. (1977). Abdominal and pelvic visceral receptors. *Br. Med. Bull.*, **33**, 163–8

38. Mei, N. (1983). Sensory structures of the viscera. In Autrum, H., Ottoson, D., Perl, E. R., Schmidt, R. F., Shimazu, H. and Willis, W. D. (eds.) *Progress in Sensory Physiology*, Vol. 4, pp. 1–42. (Berlin: Springer)

39. Morrison, J. F. B. (1977). The afferent innervation of the gastrointestinal tract. In Brooks, F. P. and Evers, P. W. (eds.) *Nerves and the Gut*, pp. 297–322. (New York: Charles Slack)

40. Floyd, K. and Morrison, J. F. B. (1974). Splanchnic mechanoreceptors in the dog. *Q. J. Exp. Physiol.*, **59**, 359–64

41. Floyd, K., Hick, V. E. and Morrison, J. F. B. (1976). Mechanosensitive afferent units in the hypogastric nerve of the cat. *J. Physiol. (Lond.)*, **259**, 457–71

42. Morrison, J. F. B. (1973). Splanchnic slowly adapting mechanoreceptors with punctate receptive fields in the mesentery and gastrointestinal tract of the cat. *J. Physiol. (Lond.)*, **233**, 349–61

43. Iggo, A. (1955). Tension receptors in the stomach and the urinary bladder. *J. Physiol. (Lond.)*, **128**, 593–607

44. Iggo, A. (1986). Afferent C-fibres and visceral sensation. In Cervero, F. and Morrison, J. F. B. (eds.) *Visceral Sensation. Progress in Brain Research*, Vol. 67, pp. 29–36. (Amsterdam: Elsevier)

45. Bahns, E., Ernsberger, U., Jänig, W. and Nelke, A. (1986). Discharge properties of

mechanosensitive afferents supplying the retroperitoneal space. *Pflügers Arch.*, **407**, 519–25

46. Lim, R. K. S. (1970). Pain. *Annu. Rev. Physiol.*, **32**, 269–88
47. Lim, R. K. S., Miller, D. G., Guzman, F., Rodgers, D. W., Rogers, R. W., Wang, S. K., Chao, P. Y. and Shih, T. Y. (1967). Pain and analgesia evaluated by the intraperitoneal bradykinin-evoked pain method in man. *Clin. Pharmacol. Ther.*, **8**, 521–42
48. Guzman, F., Braun, C. and Lim, R. K. S. (1962). Visceral pain and pseudoaffective response to intra-arterial injection of bradykinin and other algesic agents. *Arch. Int. Pharmacodyn.*, **86**, 353–84
49. Haupt, P., Jänig, W. and Kohler, W. (1983). Response pattern of visceral afferent fibres supplying the colon upon chemical and mechanical stimuli. *Pflügers Arch.*, **398**, 41–7
50. Floyd, K., Hick, V. E., Koley, J. and Morrison, J. F. B. (1977). The effects of bradykinin on afferent units in intra-abdominal sympathetic nerve trunks. *Q. J. Exp. Physiol.*, **62**, 19–25
51. LaMont, J. T. and Isselbacher, K. J. (1983). Diseases of the small and large intestine. In Petersdorf, R. G., Adams, R. D., Braunwald, E., Isselbacher, K. J., Martin, J. B. and Wilson, J. D. (eds.) *Harrisons's Principles of Internal Medicine*, 11th Edn., pp. 1752–65. (Auckland: McGraw-Hill)
52. Bahns, E., Halsband, U. and Jänig, W. (1987). Responses of sacral visceral afferents from the lower urinary tract, colon and anus to mechanical stimulation. *Pflügers Arch.*, **410**, 296–303
53. Clifton, G. L., Coggeshall, R. E., Vance, W. H. and Willis, W. D. (1976). Receptive fields of unmyelinated ventral root afferent fibres in the cat. *J. Physiol. (Lond.)*, **256**, 573–600
54. Coggeshall, R. E. (1980). Law of separation of function of the spinal roots. *Physiol. Rev.*, **60**, 716–55
55. Coggeshall, R. E. (1986). Nonclassical features of dorsal root ganglion cell organization. In Yaksh, T. L. (ed.) *Spinal Afferent Processing*, pp. 83–96. (New York: Plenum Press)
56. Coggeshall, R. E. and Ito, H. (1977). Sensory fibres in ventral roots L_7 and S_1 in the cat. *J. Physiol. (Lond.)*, **267**, 215–35
57. Floyd, K., Koley, J. and Morrison, J. F. B. (1976). Afferent discharges in the sacral ventral roots of cats. *J. Physiol. (Lond.)*, **259**, 37–8P
58. Jänig, W., Häbler, J., Koltzenburg, M., McMahon, S. and Lobenberg-Khosravi, N. (1987). Evidence that unmyelinated ventral root afferents are not branches or loops of dorsal root afferents. *Neurosci. Lett. Suppl.*, **29**, S61
59. Risling, M., Hildebrand, C. and Dalsgaard, C.-J. (1987). Unmyelinated axons in spinal ventral roots and motor cranial nerves. Do these fibres have a role in somatovisceral sensation? In Schmidt, R. F., Schaible, H.-G. and Vahle-Hinz, C. (eds.) *Fine Nerve Fibers and Pain*, pp. 35–4. (Weinheim: VCH)
60. Dockray, G. J. and Sharkey, K. A. (1986). Neurochemistry of visceral afferent neurones. In Cervero, F. and Morrison, J. F. B. (eds.) *Visceral Sensation. Progress in Brain Research*, Vol. 67, pp. 133–48. (Amsterdam: Elsevier)
61. Furness, J. B. and Costa, M. (1987). *The Enteric Nervous System.* (Edinburgh: Churchill Livingstone)
62. Paintal, A. S. (1973). Vagal sensory receptors and their reflex effects. *Physiol. Rev.*, **53**, 159–227
63. Szurszewski, J. H. (1981). Physioloy of mammalian prevertebral ganglia. *Annu. Rev. Physiol.*, **43**, 53–68
64. Fändriks, L. and Delbro, D. (1985). Non-nicotinic, non-adrenergic excitatory motor fibres in the preganglionic sympathetic supply of the feline colon. An axon reflex arrangement associated to thin sensory neurons, involving substance P? *Acta Physiol. Scand.*, **123**, 273–84
65. Häbler, H.-J., Jänig, W. and Koltzenburg, M. (1988). A novel type of unmyelinated chemosensitive nociceptor in the acutely inflamed urinary bladder. *Agents and Actions*, **25**, 219–21
66. Grigg, P., Schaible H.-G. and Schmidt, R. F. (1986). Mechanical sensitivity of group III and IV afferents from posterior articular nerve in normal and inflamed cat knee. *J. Neurophysiol.*, **55**, 635–43
67. Schaible, H.-G. and Schmidt, R. F. (1988). Direct observation of the sensitization of articular afferents during an experimental arthritis. In Dubner, R., Gebhart, G. F. and Bond, M. R. (eds.) *Proceedings of the Vth World Congress on Pain. Pain Research and Clinical Management,*

Vol. 3, pp. 44–50. (Amsterdam: Elsevier)
68. LaMotte, R. H., Simone, D. A., Baumann, T. K., Shain, C. N. and Alreja, M. (1988). Hypothesis for novel classes of chemoreceptors mediating chemogenic pain and itch. In Dubner, R., Gebhart, G. F. and Bond, M. R. (eds.) *Proceedings of the Vth World Congress on Pain. Pain Research and Clinical Management*, Vol. 3, pp. 529–35. (Amsterdam: Elsevier)
69. Meyer, R. A. and Campbell, J. N. (1988). A novel electrophysiological technique for locating cutaneous nociceptive and chemospecific receptors. *Brain Res.*, **441**, 81–6

31
Control of interdigestive motility patterns of the stomach and jejunum: Neural vs. hormonal

M. G. SARR, M. P. SPENCER, N. S. HAKIM,
J. A. VAN LIER RIBBINK, J. A. DUENES AND A. R. ZINSMEISTER

INTRODUCTION

Control of cyclic, interdigestive motor patterns of the upper gut remains controversial[1]. Initiation of the migrating motor complex (MMC) in the stomach, in the duodenum and in the jejunoileum may be controlled by neural factors (extrinsic or intrinsic innervation), by hormonal factors (peptides such as motilin), by local enteric factors (mechanical distension, luminal nutrients, enteric content) or by a complex interplay of all these factors. Experimental evidence suggests that these proposed controlling factors may be of different importance in the stomach versus the small intestine.

The present study was designed to address the roles of extrinsic innervation and intrinsic neural continuity with the remainder of the gut, specifically in the stomach and jejunum. We utilized selective surgical denervations of each region (stomach, jejunum) in the dog to examine the role of neural factors in controlling initiation and migration of the MCC. Our findings support the concept of hormonal control as the principal regulator of gastric motor patterns, while jejunal motor patterns appear to be controlled by the intrinsic nerves (the ENS).

METHODS

Preparation of dogs

Eight groups of four dogs each were prepared as follows (Figures 1 and 2). Groups 1–4 addressed control of gastric motility, while Groups 5–8 addressed control of jejunal motility. Group 1 (gastric controls) were neurally intact dogs. Group 2 (gastric intrinsic transection) underwent transection and re-anastomosis of the proximal duodenum immediately distal to pylorus to

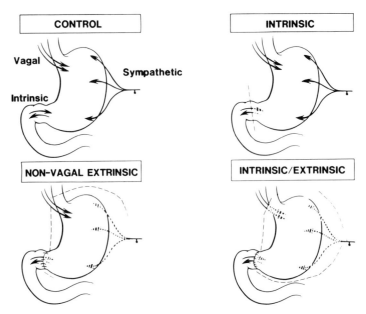

Figure 1 Gastric denervations. Neurally intact controls (Group 1); transection of intrinsic neural continuity with duodenum (Group 2); transection of intrinsic and non-vagal extrinsic neural continuity (Group 3); and transection of *all* intrinsic and extrinsic continuity to stomach (Group 4)

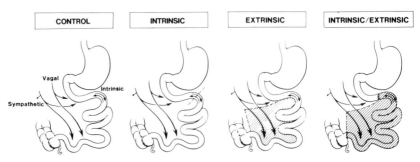

Figure 2 Jejunal denervations. Neurally intact controls (Group 5); transection of intrinsic neural continuity with duodenum (Group 6); transection of extrinsic innervation to jejunoileum (Group 7); and transection of *all* intrinsic and extrinsic neural continuity to jejunoileum (Group 8)

interrupt intrinsic neural continuity between stomach and duodenum. Group 3 (gastric non-vagal extrinsic transection) underwent a modification of a model of gastric autotransplantation[2] which involved transection of *all* extrinsic innervation and intrinsic neural continuity with the remainder of the gut except that the vagal nerve trunks were carefully preserved intact; vagal integrity was confirmed by a positive gastric motor and secretory response to insulin-induced hypoglycaemia. Group 4 (gastric intrinsic/

extrinsic transection) underwent the same model of gastric autotransplant-ation as in Group 3 but with *all* extrinsic and intrinsic neural continuity to the stomach transected. Dogs in Groups 1–4 had antral manometry catheters and monopolar serosal Ag/AgCl electrodes positioned along the small intestine for recording of motility.

Group 5 (jejunal controls) were neurally intact dogs. Group 6 (jejunal intrinsic transection) underwent transection and reanastomosis of the distal duodenum to interrupt intrinsic neural continuity of jejunum with duodenum. Group 7 (jejunal extrinsic transection) underwent transection of all extrinsic innervation to the entire jejunoileum as in a previous study[3], but without disruption of intrinsic neural continuity by duodenal transection. Group 8 (jejunal intrinsic/extrinsic transection) underwent a model of autotransplant-ation of the entire jejunoileum as described previously[4] which necessitated disruption of all intrinsic and extrinsic neural continuty to jejunoileum. Dogs in Groups 5–8 had serosal electrodes positioned along duodenum and jejunum.

Conduct of studies

All dogs were allowed 1–2 weeks to recover and were studied after a fast of ⩾ h. All recordings were completed within 3–6 weeks of operation. Record-ings were obtained in conscious dos resting comfortably in a Pavlov sling. Contractile and myoelectric activity was recorded on Grass Model 7D or Gould Model 360 recorders with alternating current amplifiers and a time constant of one second.

Analysis of data

Motility recordings were analysed by visual inspection. Contractile activity in the stomach was used in preference to myoelectric activity because we have found that gastric contractile activity better delineates motility patterns. In contrast, myoelectric activity is easier to record in the small intestine and delineates patterns equally well. The MMC was evaluated according to the criteria of Code and Marlett[5] using control Groups 1 and 5 as the reference groups. The mean periods of cyclic motor activity in the stomach and of the MMC in the duodenum were measured between consecutive phase III-like bursts of large amplitude contractions ($> 50\,mmHg$) for each dog in Groups 1–4. Similarly, the median periods of the duodenal and jejunal MMC and their respective interquartile ranges were measured between consecutive phase IIIs in Groups 5–8.

Co-ordination of motility patterns between regions

Gastroduodenal co-ordination, i.e. co-ordination of cyclic MMC-like motor activity in the stomach with the duodenal MMC, in the groups which had undergone gastric denervations (Groups 1–4) was evaluated by determining the mean time window $\pm$ 2SD (standard deviations) between gastric phase III activity and duodenal phase III in the dogs in control Group 1. Using this time window, we determined the percentage of gastric phase III-like activities in Groups 2–4 which were followed by duodenal phase III within this time window. Duodenojejunal co-ordination in the groups with jejunal denervations (Groups 5–8) was evaluated in several ways.

First, using duodenal phase III as the index event, the time until the start of the next jejunal phase III was determined. When inspecting the distributions of these intervals and of the periods of the MMC, we noted that they were not normally distributed and therefore analysed them with non-parametric methods. A summary of the distribution of time intervals for dogs in Groups 5–8 was based on the median value and the interquartile range for each dog. Secondly, using control Group 5 as the reference, the intervals until the next jejunal Phase III were determined, again using each duodenal Phase III as the index event. A time window corresponding to the 95th percentile in the control dogs in Group 5 was then determined. Using this time window as a cut-off, dogs in Group 6–8 were evaluated for the percentage of their respective intervals that fell within this time window. Multiple comparisons of values were made between Group 5 (controls) and test Groups 6, 7 and 8 using a Wilcoxein rank sum test for three tests. Data below will be as the mean $\pm$ SEM, unless stated otherwise.

RESULTS

General health of dogs

All dogs remained healthy for the duration of the study. Two dogs in Group 4 (gastric intrinsic/extrinsic transection) were able to eat only a blenderized diet because of endoscopically documented oesophageal strictures. Although no formal tests of gastric emptying were performed, there were no signs of delayed gastric emptying or gastric stasis, and the stomach appeared normal at the time of autopsy. Dogs in Group 7 (jejunal extrinsic transection) and Group 8 (intrinsic/extrinsic transection) all developed a profuse watery diarrhoea which lasted from 6–12 weeks, and they lost $12 \pm 2\%$ and $11 \pm 1\%$ of preoperative weight, respectively. At autopsy, the bowel appeared normal grossly in all dogs.

Gastric denervations (Groups 1–4)

Patterns of motility

The characteristic gastric MMC occurred in the neurally intact dogs in Group 1 (control) (Figure 3). A very similar, cyclic pattern of motor activity also persisted in the stomach and small bowel in all dogs in Group 2 (intrinsic transection), Group 3 (non-vagal extrinsic transection), and Group 4 (intrinsic/extrinsic transection) (Figures 4–6). Consecutive phases of motor quiescence (Phase I-like), intermittent low-amplitude contractions (Phase II-

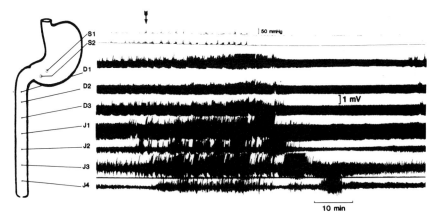

Figure 3 Interdigestive motility in neurally intact controls (Group 1). Arrow denotes onset of Phase III; note temporal co-ordination of gastric and duodenal Phase III activity. S = manometry (pressure) catheters, D and J = serosal electrodes on duodenum and jejunum, respectively

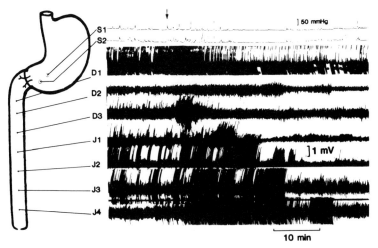

Figure 4 Interdigestive motility after transection of intrinsic neural continuity with the duodenum. Note maintenance of temporal co-ordination of Phase III activity between stomach and duodenum

like), a burst of clustered large-amplitude contractions ($> 50 \, \mathrm{mmHg}$) lasting about 15 min (Phase III-like), and finally, a short transition of intermittent contractions (Phase IV-like) reverting back to motor quiescence (Phase I-like) were immediately obvious in each dog. The characteristics of this cyclic motor activity are outlined in Table 1. The periods of this cyclic motor pattern were similar in all groups, and Phase III-like activity in Groups 2–4 occurred as a series of several groups of two to five large amplitude contractions as in Group 1. The overall pattern of contractions in each phase of activity was similar, but Groups 3 and 4 often had a longer Phase IV-

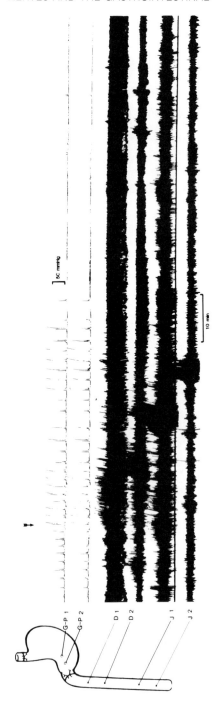

Figure 5 Interdigestive motility after transection of intrinsic and non-vagal extrinsic innervation to stomach. Note maintenance of temporal co-ordination of Phase III-like activity between stomach and duodenum. P = gastric manometric (pressure) catheters

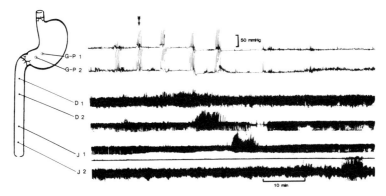

Figure 6 Interdigestive motility after transection of *all* intrinsic and extrinsic neural continuity to the entire stomach. Note maintenance of temporal co-ordination of Phase III-like activity between stomach and duodenum

Table 1 Characteristics of cyclic gastric motor activity during fasting

Parameter[a]	Group 1[b] Control	Group 2[c] Intrinsic transection	Group 3[d] Non-vagal extrinsic transection	Group 4[e] Intrinsic/ extrinsic transection
Period of cycle	97 ± 4	112 ± 26	113 ± 8	117 ± 9
Duration				
Phase I-like	53 ± 5	51 ± 12	44 ± 6	39 ± 7
Phase II-like	23 ± 7	38 ± 7	47 ± 5	39 ± 9
Phase III-like	18 ± 1	13 ± 2	21 ± 3	18 ± 6
Phase IV-like	6 ± 1	9 ± 1	1 ± 1	24 ± 1

[a]$\bar{x}$ ± SEM; minutes, $n = 4$ dogs.
[b]Controls.
[c]Trasection of intrinsic neural continuity to stomach.
[d]Transection of extrinsic non-vagal innervation to stomach.
[e]Transection of intrinsic and extrinsic neural continuity to stomach.

like activity (Figures 5 and 6) and often had a few low-amplitude contractions during the PhaseI-like interval of motor quiescence. The periods of the cyclic astric MMC-like pattern and the duodenal MMC were similar in each group (Table 1).

Gastroduodenal co-ordination

In the control dogs in Group 1, all gastric Phase IIIs were temporally associated with Phase III activity in the duodenum. The interval (mean ± 2SD) between the starts of Phase III in each region was 6.8 ± 11.7 min. In Groups 2, 3 and 4, all gastric Phase III-like activities were also temporally associated with duodenal Phase III, and 93%, 100% and 91%, respectively, of the gastric Phase III-like activities occurred within the time window defined in Group 1. Thus, co-ordination of the gastric and duodenal MMCs was preserved in all four groups.

Jejunal denervations (Groups 5–8)

Patterns of motility

The characteristic MMC persisted in the duodenum and in the jejunum in all groups (Groups 5–8) (Figures 7–10). The periods (median values) of the duodenal MMC tended to be greater and to have significantly ($p < 0.05$) larger variations (interquartile ranges) for Group 6 (intrinsic transection), for Group 7 (extrinsic transection), and for Group 8 (intrinsic/extrinsic transection). Although the periods of the duodenal MMCs were not different statistically, the interquartile ranges in Groups 7 and 8 were significantly greater ($p < 0.05$) than in Group 5 (jejunal controls). The periods of the jejunal MMCs were similar to the duodenal MMC within each group except in Group 6 (intrinsic transection) where the period of the jejunal MMC was shorter (78 ± 13 min) than in the duodenum (126 ± 30 min). However, the period of the jejunal MMC did differ between the four groups ($p < 0.05$). When each of Groups 6, 7 and 8 was compared with control Group 5, the median period of jejunal Phase III in Group 7 and the interquartile range

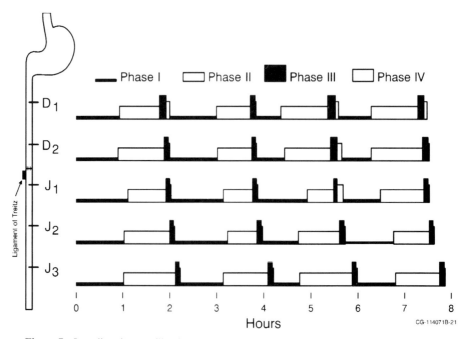

Figure 7 Interdigestive motility in neurally intact control dogs (Group 5). Note intimate temporal co-ordination of duodenal and jejunal MMCs. D = duodenal serosal electrodes, J = jejunal serosal electrodes. Because of duration of recordings (8 h), actual tracings are reproduced graphically.

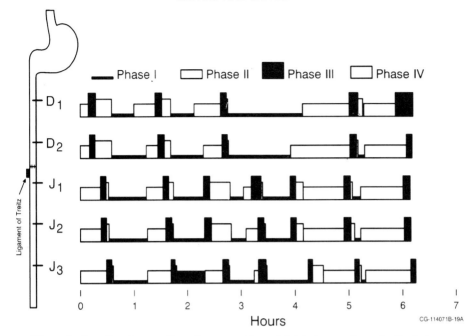

Figure 8 Interdigestive motility after transection of intrinsic neural continuity between duodenum and jejunum (Group 6). Note overall temporal co-ordination of jejunal Phase IIIs with duodenal Phase IIIs and 'ectopic' jejunal Phase IIIs (3rd and 4th jejunal Phase IIIs)

in Group 8 were greater than in control Group 5 ($p < 0.05$). The durations of the individual phases of the MMC in both duodenum and jejunum, as shown in Table 2, were not markedly different. The MMC in the duodenum and in the jejunum in Group 8 (intrinsic/extrinsic transection) did not occur as regularly as in the other groups, as indicated by the very large interquartile ranges. There were intervals when the duodenal MMC cycled but the jejunal MMC was absent, and vice versa. Occasionally, the MMC would be replaced by a non-cyclic pattern of intermittent spike potentials for 4–6 h despite continued fasting.

Duodenojejunal co-ordination

All duodenal Phase IIIs in the control dogs in Group 5 were intimately co-ordinated in time with a jejunal Phase III (Figure 7). The median time interval ($\bar{x} \pm$ SEM minutes) between the starts of Phase III in duodenum and in jejunum was 8 ± 1 minutes (Table 3). The values for Groups 6, 7 and 8 were 8 ± 2, 8 ± 1, and 61 ± 21, respectively. Thus, the jejunal MMCs remained co-ordinated overall with the duodenal MMC in Groups 6 (intrinsic transection) and 7 (extrinsic transection) but were not as tightly linked and had greater interquartile ranges. In contrast, the jejunal and duodenal MMCs in Group 8 (intrinsic/extrinsic transection) were not temporally co-ordinated and cycled independently in each region; the interquartile range was as large

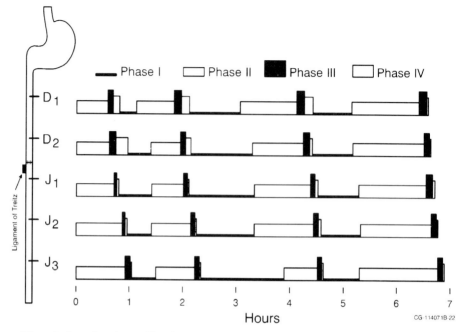

Figure 9 Interdigestive motility after transection of extrinsic innervation to jejunoileum (Group 7). Note overall maintenance of temporal co-ordination of MMCs between duodenum and jejunum

as the period of the jejunal MMC. When analysed differently by using Group 5 (controls) to define a time window between the start of Phase III and the onset of jejunal Phase III which included 95% of the control values, the percentage of 'co-ordinated' jejunal Phase IIIs that fell within the time window in Groups 6, 7 and 8 were 60%, 83% and 21%, respectively (Table 3). In Groups 6 (intrinsic transection) and 7 (extrinsic transection), all the jejunal Phase IIIs that fell outside of this time window were evaluated. Invariably, the index duodenal Phase IIIs were preceded immediately (within 15 min) by a jejunal Phase III; the next consecutive jejunal Phase III then occurred after a long interval which approximated the period of the jejunal MMC. In contrast, this relationship did not occur in Group 8 (intrinsic/extrinsic transection). In Group 6 (intrinsic transection), there were many 'ectopic' Phase IIIs that had no relationship to duodenal Phase IIIs (Figure 8). These ectopic MMC cycles accounted for the shorter overall period of the jejunal MMC in this group.

DISCUSSION

This study shows that cyclic, interdigestive motor patterns of the stomach continue after in vivo 'neural-isolation' of the stomach and remain temporally co-ordinated with the duodenal MMC, suggesting that interdigestive gastric

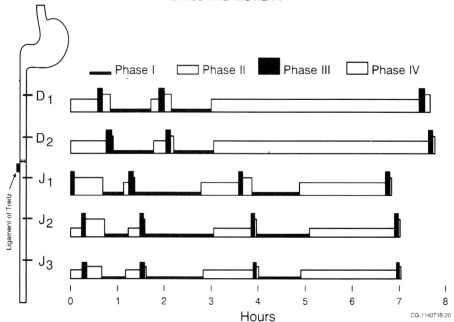

Figure 10 Interdigestive motility after transection of *all* intrinsic and extrinsic innervation to entire jejunoileum (Group 8). Note lack of temporal co-ordination between duodenal and jejunal MMCs and irregular period durations in each region

motility is controlled by hormonal factors. In contrast, characteristic jejunal patterns of fasting motility also persist after *in vivo* neural isolation of the jejunoileum, but cycle independently from the duodenal MMC. This suggests that jejunal MMCs are controlled by the intrinsic nervous system of the gut. Although this study does not imply that other factors (neural, hormonal, enteric or mechanical) do not modulate the control of motility, it does support the concept that interdigestive motility patterns in different regions of the upper gut may be controlled and initiated by different mechanisms.

Control of interdigestive gastric motility has remained controversial[1]. Early studies utilized selective surgical denervations (vagotomy[6] or sympathectomy[7]) and found that the characteristic MMC persisted with only minor alterations in regularity and duration. Motility patterns in Heidenhain[8] or autotransplanted gastric pouches[9] also demonstrated a cyclic activity co-ordinated with the remainder of the upper gut, suggesting that hormonal factors, and not extrinsic innervation, control cyclic interdigestive motility in the stomach. However, several recent studies have questioned this concept. Diamont and colleagues[10,11] have developed a canine model which allows study of gastrointestinal motility patterns during transient, reversible inhibition of vagal innervation to and from the gut (by cooling of the cervical vagus).

During vagal blockade, the gastric MMC was disrupted, suggesting vagal control (or modulation) of the gastric MMC. Also, Sarna *et al.*[12] found that

Table 2 Characteristics of MMC myoelectric activity during fasting[a]

Parameter[a]	Group 5[b] Control		Group 6[c] Intrinsic transaction		Group 7[d] Extrinsic transaction		Group 8[e] Intrinsic/extrinsic transaction	
	Duodenum	Jejunum	Duodenum	Jejunum	Duodenum	Jejunum	Duodenum	Jejunum
Median cycle duration (min)[f]	104 ± 5	102 ± 5	126 ± 30	78 ± 13	145 ± 10	142 ± 13*	128 ± 6	123 ± 17
Median interquartile range (min)[f]	20 ± 5	22 ± 3	81 ± 24	30 ± 14	62 ± 8*	58 ± 15	110 ± 29*	108 ± 45*
Duration (min)								
Phase I	38 ± 8	48 ± 4	52 ± 12	38 ± 6	63 ± 8	64 ± 8	48 ± 11	43 ± 9
Phase II[f]	46 ± 3	46 ± 7	63 ± 16	30 ± 6	57 ± 7	55 ± 6	72 ± 17	71 ± 10
Phase III	8 ± 1	5 ± 1	7 ± 1	5 ± 1	7 ± 1	5 ± 1	6 ± 1	5 ± 1
Phase IV	7 ± 2	2 ± 1	5 ± 1	6 ± 1	9 ± 2	5 ± 2	7 ± 1	5 ± 1

[a] Mean $\pm$ SEM; $n = 4$ dogs/group.
[b] Controls.
[c] Transection of intrinsic neural continuity to jejunoileum.
[d] Transection of extrinsic innervation to jejunoileum.
[e] Transection of intrinsic and extrinsic neural continuity to jejunoileum.
[f] Overall group differences for median cycle duration in jejunum ($p < 0.05$), for interquartile range values in duodenum ($p < 0.05$) and jejunum ($p < 0.05$), and for duration of Phase II in jejunum ($p < 0.05$).
* Different from value in control Group 5; $p < 0.05$ (adjusted for 3 tests).

410

Table 3 Temporal co-ordination of duodenal and jejunal MMCs[a]

Parameter[a]	Group 5[b] Control	Group 6[c] Intrinsic transection	Group 7[d] Non-vagal extrinsic transection	Group 8[e] Intrinsic/ extrinsic transection
Median interval[b] (min)	8 ± 1	8 ± 2	8 ± 1	61 ± 21*
Interquartile range (min)	4 ± 1	36 ± 11*	16 ± 11	115 ± 46*
Percentage[c] of intervals < 12 min	96%	60%*	83%	21%*

[a]Mean $\pm$ SEM; $n = 4$ dogs/group.
[b]Time between start of duodenal Phase III and start of next sequential jejunal Phase III.
[c]Percentage of jejunal Phase IIIs that occur within a time interval following duodenal Phase III; time window (12 min) defined by Group 5 (controls) that includes 95% of Group 5's values.
*Different from value in control Group 5; $p < 0.05$ (adjusted for 3 tests).

the gastric MMC did not occur after a model of subtotal gastric denervation, also suggesting that the gastric MMC was controlled by neural factors. In contrast, our observations in a model of complete 'neural isolation' of the entire stomach *in vivo* (Group 4—intrinsic/extrinsic transection), in which the entire stomach was in effect 'autotransplanted' by transecting *all* extrinsic and intrinsic neural continuity to the stomach, unquestionably demonstrate the persistence of a cyclic pattern of motility. Moreover, this cyclic motility pattern remained temporally co-ordinated with the small intestinal MMC and closely resembled the characteristic gastric MMC in the neurally intact control dogs (Group 1). These observations demonstrate that cyclic interdigestive gastric motility patterns occur in the absence of direct neural input from outside the stomach and strongly implicate hormonal factors in this control. While it is possible that a cyclic motility is generated by the intrinsic neural system of the stomach, it is unlikely that this cyclic motility would remain so well co-ordinated in time with the cyclic MMC in the duodenum unless it were controlled by some external (hormonal) signal such as the putative regulatory peptide hormone, motilin. This concept is supported by our observations that plasma motilin concentration also cycles in association with Phase III-like activity in the neurally isolated stomach and that exogenous motilin induces a premature series of large amplitude, gastric contractions associated with initiation of a premature intestinal MMC[2]. 'Recruitment' of the gastric MMC[13] by cycling of plasma motilin concentration is also supported by experiments in which immunoneutralization of plasma motilin[14,15] or total duodenectomy[16], both of which decrease plasma motilin concentration and prevent any cycling of plasma motilin, are associated with the absence of a cyclic pattern of gastric motility. Other factors, neural, hormonal and mechanical, may modulate gastric motility, but interdigestive control of cyclic gastric motility appears to be dependent on hormonal factors.

Control of interdigestive motility of the small intestine is also controversial. A number of studies have attempted to address selectively the role of intrinsic nerves, extrinsic nerves and hormonal factors in this control. Weisbrodt and

411

colleagues[17] and Carlson et al.[18] studied interdigestive motility patterns in Thiry–Vella loops of jejunum. Their observations led them to conclude that the MMC in the loop remained temporally co-ordinated with the remainder of the upper gut, suggesting that intrinsic myoneural continuity was not necessary for orderly migration of the MMC along the small bowel, provided extrinsic innervation remained intact. However, several groups have re-examined this concept with similar Thiry–Vella preparations and found that migration of the MMC (and thus temporal co-ordination with the intact gut) was disrupted, either completely[19] or partially[20,21]. This sugested that both intrinsic and extrinsic nerves played a role in this control. Sarna and colleagues[22,23] approached this topic by giving test substances via close intra-arterial injection to a jejunal segment and showed that agents which disrupt cholinergic transmission (atropine, hexamethonium) or inhibit neural activity (tetrodotoxin) block migration of the MMC[22]. Similarly, simple surgical transections of the intestine also appeared to block migration across the site of transection initially ($<$ 6 weeks) cycled independently and without apparent temporal co-ordination[23]. They concluded that enteric mechanisms within the intrinsic neural plexus of the gut control migration of the MMC. In contrast, Bueno and colleagues[20] found that overall temporal co-ordination of the MMC persisted after simple intestinal transection two-thirds of the time, but that there was a delay in migration of 8–20 min across the anastomosis. They interpreted their observations by suggesting that migration of Phase III was indeed disrupted at the site of intestinal transection, but that it was reorganized or re-initiated distally, possibly via mediation by the intact extrinsic innervation.

Studies utilizing selective extrinsic denervation of intestinal segments with maintenance of intrinsic myoneural continuity have shown little or no effect on migration of the MMC[3,24], while complete autotransplantation (disruption of both intrinsic and extrinsic neural continuity with intact gut) of either jejunal segments[25,26,27] or the entire jejunoileum[4] led to complete disruption of temporal co-ordination of motility patterns between the innervated and denervated segments. Pertinent to these observations, the potential importance of hormonal factors in the control of interdigestive motility patterns in the jejunum, unlike in the duodenum, seems improbable in view of the independent cycling of the MMC in the duodenum and jejunum after autotransplantation of the jejunoileum. Indeed, Sarr et al.[27] have shown that plasma motilin concentration cycles with the duodenal MMC but has no relationship to MMC cycles in an autotransplanted jejunal loop.

Our findings in the present study after selective denervations of the jejunoileum support much of the above work. The method of analysis seems to be very important when analysing the effects of transection of intrinsic neural continuity with the proximal gut (Group 6—intrinsic transection). We noted that conventional parametric analysis would be inappropriate because the data was not normally distributed. When analysed by several non-parametric techniques, we found that transection of either intrinsic or extrinsic neural continuity to the jejunoileum did alter migration of the MMC across the site of denervation, but did not disrupt the overall temporal co-ordination of the MMC patterns between the duodenum and the jejunum. After these two specific types of denervation, duodenal Phase III activity was usually associated with Phase III occurring in the jejunum either immediately beforehand or afterwards. Actual migration of duodenal Phase III across the anastomosis seems unlikely because, although the median intervals between the onset of duodenal and jejunal Phase III were similar in Groups 5, 6 and 7, the interquartile ranges of the latter two groups were much larger, showing that many jejunal Phase IIIs preceded duodenal Phase III, which did not occur in the controls. However, Phase IIIs in each region were usually associated in time. Our interpretation of these findings is that continuity of the intrinsic nerves controls the orderly migration of the MMC along the bowel wall. Extrinsic nerves serve as another mechanism to co-ordinate temporally the patterns of motility between regions of the upper small intestine.

The role of hormonal factors in co-ordinating motility patterns is uncertain. Plasma motilin concentration cycles in temporal association with the gastric and duodenal MMC[28-30]. We know that exogenous motilin will initiate a premature Phase III in the intact gut[31,32] and also in the jejunum distal to an intestinal transection[33]. However, experimental evidence suggests that motilin may act via a mechanism located outside the wall of the duodenum[34]. Further support for this concept comes from preliminary studies in which motilin was unable to initiate Phase III activity after autotransplantation of the jejunoileum, where the extrinsic innervation to the jejunum had been transected[35]. The relative maintenance of temporal co-ordination of jejunal Phase III activity with duodenal Phase III in Group 6 (intrinsic transection) may be related to the peaking of plasma motilin concentration which then acts to initiate Phase III in the jejunum via the extrinsic nerves. Similarly, the frequent 'ectopic' jejunal Phase IIIs (Figure 8) have been noted previously by others after transection of intrinsic myoneural continuity with the duodenum[23]. This may be secondary to loss of a descending inhibitory 'brake' on the jejunum by the duodenum[16], allowing the jejunum frequently to escape from a strict temporal co-ordination.

In contrast, in Group 8 (intrinsic/extrinsic transection), the lack of either intrinsic or extrinsic neural continuity with the jejunum prevents a neural mechanism from co-ordinating motor patterns. Moreover, the loss of extrinsic innervation prevents the cycling of plasma motilin from initiating Phase III activity in the jejunum at or near the time of initiation of Phase III in the duodenum. Thus, the continued independent cycling of the MMC in the jejunum virtually eliminates the possibility of a hormonal control and implicates the intrinsic nerves of the jejunum as possessing the ability to generate the MMC. Control of the jejunal MMC appears, therefore, to arise within the intrinsic nervous system of the gut. Other factors, such as extrinsic innervation and hormonal factors may modulate the cycling of the MMC and thereby co-ordinate motor patterns between regions, but the underlying control mechanism lies within the intrinsic nerves.

References

1. Sarna, S. K. (1985). Cyclic motor activity; migrating motor complex: 1985. *Gastroenterology*, **89**, 894–913
2. VanLierRibbink, J. A. and Sarr, M. G. (1988). Autotransplantation of the stomach: motility is controlled by hormonal factors. *Curr. Surg.* (In press)
3. Heppell, J., Kelly, K. A. and Sarr, M. G. (1983). Neural control of canine small intestinal interdigestive myoelectric complexes. *Am. J. Physiol.*, **244**, G95–100
4. Sarr, M. G., Tanaka, M. and Duenes, J. A. (1987). Jejunoileal autotransplantation: effects on small intestinal motility. *Surg. Forum.*, **38**, 160–2
5. Code, C. F. and Marlett, J. A. (1975). The interdigestive myo-electric complex of the stomach and small bowel of dogs. *J. Physiol.*, **246**, 289–309
6. Weisbrodt, N. W., Copeland, E. M., Moore, E. P., Kearley, R. W. and Johnson, L. R. (1975). Effect of vagotomy on electrical activity of the small intestine of the dog. *Am. J. Physiol.*, **228**, 650–4
7. Marlett, J. A. and Code, C. F. (1979). Effects of celiac and superior mesenteric ganglionectomy on interdigestive myoelectric complex in dogs. *Am. J. Physiol.*, **237**, E432–6
8. Itoh, Z., Takayanagi, R., Takeuchi, S. and Isshiki, S. (1978). Interdigestive motor activity of Heidenhain pouches in relation to main stomach in conscious dogs. *Am. J. Physiol.*, **234**, E333–8
9. Thomas, P. A., Kelly, K. A. and Go, V. L. W. (1979). Does motilin regulate canine interdigestive gastric motility? *Am. J. Dig. Dis.*, **24**, 577–82
10. Hall, K. E., El-Sharkawy, T. Y. and Diamant, N. E. (1982). Vagal control of migrating motor complex in the dog. *Am. J. Physiol.*, **243**, G270–84
11. Diamant, N. (1984). Neurological control of the interdigestive migrating motor complex. In Poitras, P. (ed.) *Small Intestinal and Colonic Motility*, pp. 3–14. (Montreal: Jouveinal Laboratories Inc.)
12. Sarna, S. K., Matsumoto, T., Condon, R. E. and Cowles, V. E. (1985). Does stomach have an independent spontaneous cyclic motor activity? *Gastroenterology*, **88**, 1571
13. Tanaka, M. and Sarr, M. G. (1987). Total duodenectomy: effect on canine gastrointestinal motility. *J. Surg. Res.*, **42**, 483–93
14. Poitras, P. (1984). Motilin is a digestive hormone inducing the Phase III of the interdigestive migrating complex (IDMC) of the small intestine in dog. *Dig. Dis. Sci.*, **29**, 66S
15. Lee, K. Y., Chang, T. M. and Chey, W. Y. (1983). Effect of rabbit antimotilin serum on myoelectric activity and plasma motilin concentration in fasting dog. *Am. J. Physiol.*, **245**, G547–53
16. Tanaka, M. and Sarr, M. G. (1988). The role of duodenum in the control of canine gastrointestinal motility. *Gastroenterology*, **94**, 622–9
17. Weisbrodt, N. W., Copeland, E. M., Thor, P. J., Mukhopadhyay, A. K. and Johnson, L. R. (1974). Nervous and humoral factors which govern the fasted and fed patterns of intestinal myoelectric activity. In *Proceedings of the Vth International Symposium on Gastrointestinal Motility*, pp. 82–7. (Herentals, Belgium: Typoff Press)
18. Carlson, G. M., Bedi, B. S. and Code, C. F. (1972). Mechanism of propagation of interdigestive myoelectric complex. *Am. J. Physiol.*, **222**, 1027–30
19. Pearce, E. A. N. and Wingate, D. L. (1980). Myoelectric and absorptive capacity in the transected canine small bowel. *J. Physiol.*, **302**, 11–12
20. Bueno, L., Praddaude, F. and Ruckebusch, Y. (1979). Propagation of electrical spiking activity along the small intestine: intrinsic versus extrinsic neural influences. *J. Physiol.*, **292**, 15–26
21. Ormsbee, H. S., III, Telford, G. L., Suter, C. M., Wilson, P. D. and Mason, G. R. (1981). Mechanism of propagation of canine migrating motor complex—a reappraisal. *Am. J. Physiol.*, **240**, G141–6
22. Sarna, S., Stoddard, C., Belbeck, L. and McWade, D. (1981). Intrinsic nervous control of migrating myoelectric complexes. *Am. J. Physiol.*, **241**, G16–23
23. Sarna, S., Condon, R. E. and Cowles, V. (1983). Enteric mechanisms of initiation of migrating myoelectric complexes in dogs. *Gastroenterology*, **84**, 814–22
24. Ruckebusch, Y. and Bueno, L. (1975). Electrical activity of the ovine jejunum and changes due to disturbances. *Am. J. Dig. Dis.*, **20**, 1027–34

25. Aeberhard, P. F., Magnenat, L. D. and Zimmerman, W. A. (1980). Nervous control of migrating myoelectric complex of the small bowel. *Am. J. Physiol.*, **238**, G102–8
26. Sarr, M. G. and Kelly, K. A. (1981). Myoelectric activity of the autotransplanted canine jejunoileum. *Gastroenterology*, **81**, 303–10
27. Sarr, M. G., Kelly, K. A. and Go, V. L. W. (1983). Motilin regulation of canine interdigestive intestinal motility. *Dig. Dis. Sci.*, **28**, 249–56
28. Lee, K. Y., Chey, W. Y., Tai, H. H., Wagner, D. and Yajima, H. (1977). Cyclic changes in plasma motilin levels and interdigestive myoelectric activity of canine antrum and duodenum. *Gastroenterology*, **72**, 1162
29. Lee, . Y., Kim, M. S. and Chey, W. Y. (1980). Effects of a meal and gut hormones on plasma motilin and duodenal motility in dog. *Am. J. Surg.*, **238**, G280–3
30. Poitras, P., Steinbach, J. H., VanDeventer, G., Code, C. F. and Walsh, J. H. (1980). Motilin-independent ectopic fronts of the interdigestive myoelectric complex in dogs. *Am. J. Physiol.*, **239**, G215–20
31. Wingate, D. L., Ruppin, A., Thompson, H. H., Green, W. E. R., Domschke, W., Wunsch, E., Demling, L. and Ritchie, H. D. (1977). The gastrointestinal myoelectric response to 13-Nle-Motilin infusion during interdigestive and digestive states in the conscious dog. *Acta Hepato-Gastroenterol.*, **24**, 278–87
32. Itoh, Z., Honda, R., Hiwatashi, K., Takeuchi, S., Aizawa, I., Takayanagi, R. and Couch, E. F. (1976). Motilin-induced mechanical activity in the canine alimentary tract. *Scand. J. Gastroenterol.*, **11** (Suppl. 39), 93–110
33. Matsumoto, T., Sarna, S. K., Condon, R. E., Cowles, V. E. and Frantzides, C. (1986). Differential sensitivites of morphine and motilin to initiate migrating motor complex in isolated intestinal segments: regeneration of intrinsic nerves. *Gastroenterology*, **90**, 61–7
34. Sarr, M. G., Duenes, J. A. and Tanaka, M. (1986). Mechanism of action of motilin in mediating fasting motor activity. *Surg. Forum.*, **37**, 136–40
35. Hakim, N. S. and Sarr, M. G. (1988). Humoral induction of migrating motor complex (MMC): role of extrinsic innervation. *Gastroenterology*, **94**, A166

32
Involvement of CNS corticotropin-releasing factor in the genesis of stress-induced gastric motor alterations

M. GUE AND L. BUENO

INTRODUCTION

It is well established that centrally acting stressful stimuli induces changes in gastrointestinal motility in humans[1-3], in dogs[4] and in rats[5-9]. Evidence for humoral pathways on gastrointestinal disorders induced by stress is supported by the release of β-endorphin and catecholamines into the peripheral circulation during stress[10-13]. In agreement with such hypothesis, naloxone or a combination of α- and β-adrenergic blockers abolishes the inhibition of gastric motility induced by cold pain in humans. However, they have no effect on the migrating duodenal burst of activity induced by labyrinthine stimulation[14,15] in humans *or* on acoustic, stress-induced inhibition of gastric motility in fasted dogs[16]. This suggests that other humoral factors may be involved in the mediation of gastrointestinal motor disturbances induced by centrally acting stimuli. The acoustic stress-induced gastric motor inhibition in dogs is abolished by previous treatment with benzodiazepine or GABA agonist substances[16] which have been shown to alter CRF release in hypothalamic cell culture[17]. Accordingly, it has also been shown that various types of stressors cause a release of corticotropin-releasing factor (CRF) and that intracerebroventricular (ICV) administration of CRF mimics the motor, behavioural, metabolic and haemodynamic responses to such stimuli in animals[18-20].

However, in anaesthetized rodents, pinching of the skin is accompanied by gastric motor inhibition[8], whereas an increased motility and an acceleration on gastric emptying is observed during the early phase of restraint stress in rats[7].

Consequently, the present work was designed first to evaluate the effect of acoustic versus cold stress on gastric emptying and intestinal transit in

417

mice and to test the antagonistic effect of several drugs shown to be active on disorders induced by stress, namely, diazepam, muscimol, propranolol and naloxone; and, secondly to establish the role of the central release of CRF in the genesis of such gastrointestinal motor alterations by using treatment with antiserum against rat (r) CRF and ICV administration of α-helical CRF_{9-41}.

MATERIALS AND METHODS

Gastric emptying and transit evaluation

Gastric emptying and intestinal transit of a test meal were evaluated in male NMRI mice (20–30 g) that had been fasted for 12 h, using a technique described by Porreca and Burks[21], and adapted to nutritive meals. The test meal consisted of 0.5 ml of reconstituted milk (1 g of milk powder in 3 ml of water containing 1 μCi/ml of [^{51}Cr] sodium chromate). Thirty minutes after the test meal, the animals were sacrificed by cervical dislocation and the stomach and bowel removed. These organs were placed on a ruled template and the intestine was cut into 10 segments of equal length. The stomach, the intestinal segments and the proximal colon were then placed into individual test tubes and counted in a gamma radiation counter for 2 min. Gastric emptying (GE) was calculated from the counter values as the percentage of total counts found in the small intestine and the colon. Intestinal transit was evaluated by the described geometric centre (GC) technique[21] according to the equation

$$GC = \Sigma \; [(\text{fraction of counts in each segment}) \times (\text{segment number})].$$

Experimental procedure

In a first series of experiments, 10 min after the test meal (0.5 ml of milk), three groups of animals were placed in a closed box equipped with loudspeakers and were subjected either to acoustic stress (AS) produced by continuously playing taped music ($\leqslant$ 90 dB) with the box at room temperature (20° $\pm$ 2°C) or to cold stress (CS) by lowering of the box temperature to 10 $\pm$ 1°C. A similar procedure, without music and at room temperature was used for the controls. Each group of animals (six subjects) was sacrificed either 15, 30 or 60 min after the test meal.

In a second series of experiments, 10–15 min before the test meal, the animals were injected intraperitoneally with diazepam (0.5 mg/kg), muscimol (0.5 mg/kg), propranolol (1 mg/kg) or naloxone (0.2 mg/kg) and, as in the first series, the animals were divided in three groups. One group received AS, one CS and the third group served as control. All the animals were killed 30 min after the meal.

In a third series of experiments, 30 min before the test meal and under light ether anaesthesia, one group received intracerebroventricularly[22] rat corticotropin-releasing factor (rCRF) (5 μg/kg) diluted in distilled water.

Another control group was injected intracerebroventricularly with water alone.

The four other groups were injected i.p. 10–15 minutes before the test meal with rCRF (5 μg/kg), ACTH (12.5 mUI/kg), corticosterone (10 μg/kg) or their vehicle (0.1% alcohol solution). All the animals were sacrificed 30 min after the test meal.

In a fourth series of experiments, 30 min before the meal, the animals were injected either i.p. with 5 μl of diluted (1/10) rabbit antiserum against (human/rat) CRF provided from CRB (Cambridge, UK) or i.c.v. with α-helical CRF$_{9-41}$ (200 ng). Then, the animals were submitted as in 1st series to AS, CS or to the i.c.v. administration of rCRF as in the third series.

Values of gastric emptying and geometric centre were compared by analysis of variance followed by a Student's t-test when ANOVA was significant.

RESULTS

In control (no stress) mice at room temperature (20 ± 2°C), the volume of the meal emptied after 30 min represented 42.5 ± 6.5% of the total meal (Figure 1) and the value of the intestinal geometric centre was 6.03 ± 0.74. Measured 15 and 60 min after the meal, the percentage of meal emptied was respectively 34.5 ± 10.3 and 48.4 ± 12.9%. When AS was applied from 10

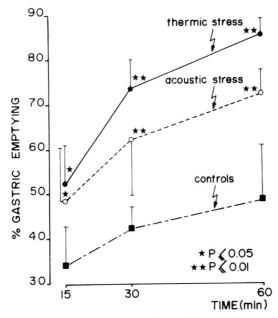

Figure 1 Comparative time-related influence of acoustic and cold stress on gastric emptying of a radiolabelled test meal in mice. Experiments were performed at 20 ± 2°C for control and acoustic stress groups and at 10°C ± 1°C for cold stress, stress sessions beginning 10 min after test meal ($t = 0$). Values are mean ± SD; $n = 6$, $p < 0.05$ and $p < 0.01$ compared with controls

to 30 min after the meal the volume emptied was $62.8 \pm 15.5\%$, i.e. a 47.7% increase in gastric emptying compared to controls. Similarly, exposure to CS also increased the rate of gastric emptying by 65.6% (Figure 1) and there was a significant ($p < 0.01$) aboral displacement of the intestinal geometric centre.

Influence of various drugs on the effects of AS and CS

Diazepam administered intraperitoneally (0.5 mg/kg) completely abolished the effects of both AS and CS on GE while it had no effect *per se* either on GE or on GC (Figure 2). Furthermore, diazepam also abolished the CS-induced aboral displacement of the geometric centre (Figure 3). Intraperitoneal administration of muscimol (0.5 mg/kg) produced a slowing of GE in mice compared to those receiving saline intraperitoneally (Figure 2). Muscimol also delayed significantly the intestinal transit. Despite its slowing effect on GE, muscimol abolished the effects of CS on GE and intestinal GC but did not reduce the increase in GE induced by AS (Figure 2).

Propranolol given alone (1 mg/kg i.p.) did not affect GE and intestinal transit. It completely abolished the effects of AS and CS on both gastric emptying and intestinal transit.

When naloxone (0.2 mg/kg) was given alone, 15 min before the meal, the volume emptied was increased from 42.5 ± 5.9 to $51.9 \pm 6.2\%$. However,

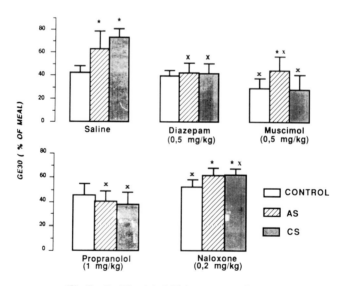

*Significantly different (p<0,05) from corresponding control values.
xSignificantly different (p<0,05) from corresponding saline values.

Figure 2 Comparative influence of diazepam, muscimol, propranolol and naloxone on gastric emptying in mice submitted to AS and CS. Values are means $\pm$ = SD for $n = 6$; gastric emptying was determined 30 min after the test meal, AS, acoustic stress; CS, cold stress

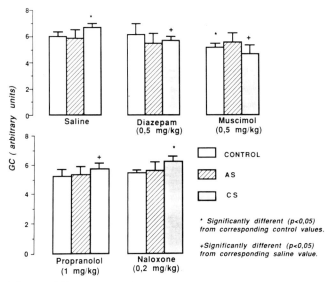

Figure 3 Influence of diazepam, muscimol, propranolol and naloxone on AS and CS-induced changes in intestinal transit in mice. Values are means ± SD for $n = 6$ mice. Value of the geometric centre determined 30 min after test meal; AS, acoustic stress; CS, cold stress

naloxone did not reduce the CS-induced enhancement of GE as well as the increase of the geometric centre (Figure 3).

Influence of i.c.v. administration of CRF

Intracerebroventricular administration of rCRF (5 µg/kg) increased the gastric emptying 30 min after the test meal by 52.1% compared with the controls (Figure 2) without affecting the intestinal geometric centre (Figure 4). Such an effect is not reproduced by i.p. administration of rCRF at the same dosage (5 µg/kg). Furthermore, neither ACTH (12.5 mUI/kg) nor corticosterone (10 µg/kg)-injected i.p. affected the volume of meal emptied after 30 min (Table 1).

AntiCRF serum (5 µl of 1/10 dilution) injected intraperitoneally 30 min

Table 1 Comparative influence of ACTH, corticosterone and rat corticotropin-releasing factor (rCRF) administered intraperitoneally on gastric emptying and intestinal transit of a milk test meal in mice (mean ± SD, $n = 6$); no significant ($p \geqslant 0.05$) difference compared to control paired t-test

	Gastric emptying (% test meal)	Geometric centre (arbitrary units)
Vehicle (0.1 ml/i.p.)	45.3 ± 4.2	5.66 ± 0.61
ACTH (12.5 mUI/kg)	40.6 ± 7.1	5.29 ± 0.84
Corticosterone (10 µg/kg)	47.1 ± 6.8	4.32 ± 0.45
rCRF (5 µg/kg)	39.2 ± 6.3	5.66 ± 1.2

before the test meal did not significantly change the gastric emptying (44.9 ± 8.7 vs. $42.5 \pm 6.5\%$) and the values of the geometric centre measured at $t = 30$ min but it abolished the effects of both AS and CS (Figure 4). Similarly, α-helical CRF_{9-41} administered i.c.v. at a dose of 200 ng/mice did not affect *per se* the gastric emptying but completely abolished the increase induced by AS, CS and i.c.v. administration of rCRF (Figure 4).

DISCUSSION

This work shows that in mice both AS and CS increase the gastric emptying of a milk meal for a period of at least one hour. The intestinal transit was not affected by AS while it is increased with CS, as judged by an aboral displacement of the intestinal centre. The effects of these two stressors on GE accord with previous observations performed in rats showing that cold restraint-stress increased GE rate in the first hour of application[7].

Nevertheless, the stimulatory effect of stress on GE observed in rats and our results in mice contrast with the slowing of GE and the concomitant inhibition of gastric motility[23] observed in humans after repeated immersions of a hand into cold water[2]. This stress-induced increased GE may be related to an early increased gastric motility as previously described during acute stress in rats[5,6,9].

Several findings have led us to speculate that the central release of CRF is involved in the gastrointestinal motor alterations associated with stressful stimuli. In dogs, intracerebroventricular administration of CRF suppresses the cyclic gastric migrating myoelectric complexes[24] as well as acoustic stress[4]. This effect is not related to adrenocroticotropin and cortisol release[24], suggesting that CRF acts directly on brain structures controlling gastric motility. The motor alterations induced by AS in dogs are blocked by diazepam[16] and muscimol which are thought to have a direct central

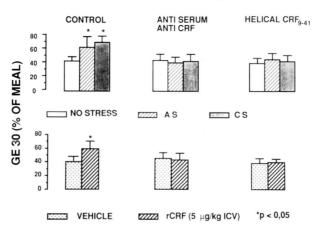

Figure 4 Influence of pretreatment with antiserum against rCRF and α-helical $CRF_{(9-41)}$ on the effects of AS, CS and i.c.v. administration of rCRF on GE in mice (mean $\pm$ SD; $n = 6$), t-test. GE was measured 30 min after a test meal comprising 0.5 ml of reconstituted milk

inhibitory effect on stress-induced CRF release in dogs[25].

In this study, diazepam and propranolol were able to suppress the effects of both AS and CS on GE, whereas muscimol selectively blocked the effects of CS. In contrast, naloxone, which increased GE when given alone, did not antagonize such effect. Diazepam is known for its anxiolytic action, reducing heart rate, blood pressure and plasma cortisol increase associated with stress[25]. It also blocks the increase in colonic motility in humans[26] during exposure to stressful situations. A central inhibitory effect on stress-induced CRF release has been proposed[25]. Muscimol, a GABAergic agonist, also has an antagonistic effect on stress-induced CRF or adrenocorticotropin release[17,27]. In the present study, the selective inhibition of the effects of CS by muscimol suggests that the effects of somatosensory (but not auditory) stimulation are mediated through pathways modulated by GABA.

Propranolol is also able to block the effects of both AS and CS on GE, suggesting the involvement of central and/or peripheral β-adrenergic receptors and/or pathways in their mediation. This hypothesis is supported by observation showing that a β-adrenergic antagonist, atenolol, but not α-blockers, reduce the CS-induced acceleration of the orocaecal transit in humans[23].

The second part of our work shows that the stress-induced alterations of GE in mice are abolished by immunoneutralization of circulating CRF and by i.c.v. administration of the CRF antagonist: α-helical CRF_{9-41} conforming that CRF is well involved in the gastrointestinal motor alterations induced by both AS and CS. The efficiency of the immunoneutralization technique used is confirmed by blockade of the effects of i.c.v. administration of rCRF on gastric emptying.

Furthermore, CRF seems to act directly on the supraspinal structures controlling the gastric and intestinal motility and not through a stimulation of the HPA system, as systemic administration of ACTH or corticosterone does not increase gastric emptying. Absence of alterations in gastric emptying following systemic administration of rCRF reinforces the hypothesis of a CNS origin. This result is also in agreement with previous data showing that in dogs, the gastrointestinal motor effects induced by picomolar doses of CRF administered centrally are not reproduced by i.v. or i.c.v. ACTH or cortisol[24,28]. Several other findings have also suggested that the behavioural effects of supraspinal administration CRF are independent of its effects on the pituitary gland. The inhibition of gastric acid secretion by CRF also persisted after hypophysectomy or adrenalectomy[29,30]. In rats, as in dogs, several peptides administered centrally are able to affect the gastrointestinal motility; these effects depend on the digestive status and are mediated through different neural or hormonal pathways[31-33]. Central administration of CRF modulates the parasympathetic outflow from the brain regulating gastric functions[34]; similarly stressful stimuli are known to produce vagal excitation and both the i.c.v. administration of CRF and AS-induced inhibition of gastric motility in dogs[4,28] as well as the central CRF-induced inhibition of gastric secretion in rats[30] are blocked by bilateral vagotomy. All this information supports the major role of CRF in initiating centrally the gastric motor disturbances observed during stressful situations through an increase of the vagal parasympathetic outflow to the stomach.

Finally, our present data demonstrate first that, in mice, both AS and CS alter GE; secondly that CRF released in response to these stressful stimuli is directly responsible for alteration in gastrointestinal motility.

Acknowledgements

The authors are indebted to C. Dargelos and C. Delrio for their skilful technical assistance, A. Cortes for preparing the manuscript, and Institut National de la Recherche Agronomique for its financial support.

References

1. McRae, S., Younger, K., Thompson, D. G. and Wingate, D. L. (1982). Sustained mental stress alters human jejunal motor activity. *Gut*, **23**, 404–9
2. Thompson, D. G., Richelson, J. R. and Malagelada, J. R. (1983). Perturbation of upper gastrointestinal function by cold stress. *Gut*, **24**, 277–83
3. Valori, R. M., Kumar, D. and Wingate, D. (1986). Effects of different types of stress and of 'prokinetic' drugs on the control of the fasting motor complex in humans. *Gastroenterology*, **90**, 1890–1900
4. Gue, M., Fioramonti, J., Frexinos, J., Alvinerie, M. and Bueno, L. (1987). Influence of acoustic stress by noise on gastrointestinal motility in dogs. *Dig. Dis. & Sci.*, **32**(12), 1411–17
5. Brodie, D. A. (1962). Ulceration of the stomach produced by restraint in rats. *Gastroenterology*, **43**, 107–9
6. Fioramonti, J. and Bueno, L. (1980). Gastrointestinal myoelectric activity disturbances in gastric ulcer disease in rats and dogs. *Dig. Dis. & Sci.*, **25**, 875–900
7. Koo, M., Ogle, C. and Cho, C. (1985). The effect of cold-restraint stress on gastric emptying in rats. *Pharm. Biochem. Behav.*, **23**, 969–72
8. Sato, Y. and Terui, N. (1976). Changes in duodenal motility produced by noxious mechanical stimulation of the skin in rats. *Neurosci. Lett.*, **2**, 189–93
9. Watanabe, K. (1966). Some pharmacological factors involved in formation and prevention of stress ulceration in rats. *Chem. Pharm. Bull.*, **14**, 101–7
10. Bortz, W. M., Angwin, P., Mefford, I. N., Boarder, M. R., Noyce, N. and Barchas, J. D. (1982). Catecholamines, dopamine and endorphin levels during extreme exercise. *N. Engl. J. Med.*, **1305**, 466–7
11. Cohen, M., Pickar, D., Dubois, M., Roth, Y. F., Naber, D. and Bunney, W. E. (1981). Surgical: stress and endorphins. *Lancet*, **1**, 213–14
12. Kalin, N. H. (1985). Behavioral effects of ovine corticotropin-releasing factor administered to rhesus monkey. *Federation Proc.*, **44**, 249–53
13. Kopin, K. J., Lake, R. C. and Ziegler, M. (1978). Plasma levels of norepinephrine. *Ann. Intern. Med.*, **88**, 671–80
14. Stanghellini, V., Malagelada, J. R., Zinsmeister, A. R., Go, V. L. and Kao, P. C. (1983). Stress-induced gastroduodenal motor disturbances in humans: possible humoral mechanisms. *Gastroenterology*, **85**, 83–91
15. Stanghellini, V., Malagelada, J. R., Zinsmeister, A. R., Go, V. L. and Kao, P. C. (1984). Efects of opiate and adrenergic blockers on the gut motor response to centrally acting stimuli. *Gastroenterology*, **87**, 1104–13
16. Gue, M. and Bueno, L. (1986). Diazepam and muscimol blockade of the gastrointestinal motor disturbances induced by acoustic stress in dogs. *Eur. J. Pharmacol.*, **131**, 123–7
17. Ramade, F. and Bayle, J. D. (1985). Influence du muscimol (GABA-agoniste) sur une boucle de régulation thalamo-hypothalamique à efference corticotrope (modèle thalamique). *CR Soc. Biol.*, **179**, 383–8
18. Brown, M. C., Fischer, L. A., Spiess, J., Rivier, C. and Wale, W. (1982). Corticotropin-

releasing factor: effects on the sympathetic nervous system and oxygen consumption. *Life Sci.*, **30**, 207–10

19. Rivier, C., Rivier, J. and Vale, W. (1982). Inhibition of adrenocroticotropic hormone secretion in the rat by immunoneutralisation of corticotropin releasing factor. *Science*, **218**, 377–9

20. Sutton, R. E., Koob, G. G., Lemoal, M., Rivier, J. and Vale, W. (1982). Corticotropin releasing factor produces behavioral activation in rats. *Nature*, **297**, 331–3

21. Porreca, F. and Burks, T. F. (1983). The spinal cord as a site of opioid effects on gastrointestinal transit in the mouse. *J. Pharmacol. Exp. Ther.*, **227**, 22–7

22. Pedigo, N. W., Dewey, W. L. and Harris, L. S. (1975). Determination of the antinociceptive activity of intraventricularly administered acetylcholine in mice. *J. Pharmacol. Exp. Ther.*, **193**, 845–52

23. O'Brien, J. D., Thompson, D. G., Day, S., Burnham, W. R. and Walker, E. (1985). Stress induced disturbances of human postprandial antroduodenal motility and orocaecal transit. The contribution of adrenergic pathways. *Dig. Dis. Sci.*, **30**, 785A

24. Bueno, L. and Fioramonti, J. (1986). Effects of corticotropin-releasing factor, corticotropin and cortisol on gastrointestinal motility in dogs. *Peptides*, **7**, 73–7

25. Ninan, D. J., Insel, T. M., Cohen, R. M., Cook, J. M., Skolnick, P. and Paul, S. M. (1982). Benzodiazepine receptor-mediated experimental 'anxiety' in primates. *Science*, **218**, 1332–34

26. Narducci, F., Snape, W. J., Battle, W. M., London and Cohen, S. (1985). Increased colonic motility during exposure to stressful situation. *Dig. Dis. Sci.*, **30**, 40–44

27. Buckingham, J. C. and Hodges, J. R. (1979). Hypothalamic receptors influencing the secretion of corticotrophin releasing hormone in the rat. *J. Physiol. (Lond.)*, **290**, 421–31

28. Bueno, L., Fargeas, M. J., Gue, M., Peeters, T. L., Bormans, V. and Fioramonti, J. (1986). Effects of corticotropin-releasing factor on plasma motilin and somatostatin levels and gastrointestinal motility in dogs. *Gastroenterology*, **91**, 884–9

29. Britton, D. R., Varela, M., Garcia, A. and Rivier, J. (1984). Behavioral effects of intracerebral CRF are independent of effects at the pituitary. *Soc. Neurosci. Abstr.*, **10**, 178

30. Tache, Y., Goto, Y., Gunion, M., Rivier, J. and Debas, H. (1984). Inhibition of gastric acid secretion in rats and dogs by corticotropin releasing factor. *Gastroenterology*, **86**, 281–6

31. Bueno, L. and Ferre, J. P. (1982). Central regulation of intestinal motility by somatostatin and cholecystokinin octapeptide. *Science*, **216**, 1427–9

32. Fargeas, M. J., Fioramonti, J. and Bueno, L. (1984). Prostaglandin E2: a neuromodulator in the central control of gastrointestinal motility and feeding behavior by calcitonin. *Science*, **225**, 1050–2

33. Bueno, L., Fioramonti, J., Honde, C., Fargeas, M. J. and Primi, M. P. (1985). Central and peripheral control of gastrointestinal and colonic motility by endogenous opiates in conscious dogs. *Gastroenterology*, **88**, 549–56

34. Brown, M. R., Fischer, L. A., Spiess, J., Rivier, C. and Wale, W. (1982). Corticotropin-releasing factor: actions on the sympathetic nervous system and metabolism. *Endocrinology*, **111**, 928–32

33
Central nervous system neuropeptide regulation of gastrointestinal motility and secretion

T. F. BURKS, C. L. WILLIAMS, D. A. FOX, J. E. SHOOK AND F. PORRECA

The mammalian gastrointestinal tract is subject to regulatory control arising from supraspinal and spinal influences, peripheral autonomic ganglia, enteric plexuses, locally generated autacoids and circulating hormones. The diversity of regulatory influences reflect the central importance of digestive function to the survival of the organism; the variety of storage, motor, secretory and absorptive functions served by the gastrointestinal tract; its complex structure; and the critical interplay between components of the alimentary canal required for optimal digestive activity. One of the last regulatory frontiers to be explored is the reciprocal interactions between the central nervous system (CNS) and the gastrointestinal tract. Current knowledge is both providing answers to longstanding questions about CNS–gut interactions and, of even greater importance, is sharpening the focus of questions which now demand answers.

One of the developments with positive impact on understanding CNS–gut interactions has been increasing availability of pharmacological tools with which to explore the anatomy, physiology and biochemistry of regulatory influences on gastrointestinal function. Definite progress, for example, has been achieved in those areas in which specific and selective receptor agonists and antagonists are available. The influence of opioid regulatory influences probably best exemplifies the great utility of receptor-selective activating and blocking drugs with sufficient biological stability *in vivo* to allow convenient use in intact animals.

OPIOIDS

It is now well established that endogenous opioid peptides in mammals arise from three types of precursor peptides containing sequences with opioid

427

activity[1]. The large precursor peptides or their identified processing fragments occur in brain, spinal cord, and enteric and other peripheral neurons, and in adrenal medulla, pancreas and pituitary gland[2]. An array of peptides formed by enzymatic cleavage at different amide bonds in the parent peptides or intermediate peptides has been identified[3]. Different tissues, cells or subcellular fractions are capable of processing opioid peptides differently or at different rates.

In vivo and *in vitro* studies of opioid actions have resulted in identification of multiple types of opioid receptors. Among the receptors postulated, three types occur regularly in mammalian species: μ, δ and κ. These receptors are acted upon by agonists during certain physiological states to regulate or modulate many different functions, including gastrointestinal functions.

It was previously assumed that some fundamental correspondence between specific endogenous opioids and specific types of opioid receptors would be identified. Thus, the pentapeptide enkephalins were thought to represent endogenous ligands for δ-opioid receptors and dynorphin-related peptides could be ligands for κ-opioid receptors. As with most endogenous transmitters/modulators that are released in close anatomical proximity to their sites of action and thereby often achieve specificity, endogenous opioid peptides are usually not selective for particular types of receptors. For example, native [Met^5]enkephalin and [Leu^5]enkephalin are not selective for δ-opioid receptors, but act also at other types, particularly at μ receptors. The natural enkephalins are δ-preferring ligands, but can be non-discriminatory especially in high concentrations. Similarly, dynorphin-(1–17) and several dynorphin-related peptides appear to be κ-preferring ligands, but can act at μ- and δ-opioid receptors[4]. No convincing candidate for the endogenous μ-opioid ligand has been put forward, partially because many natural opioids possess activity at μ-opioid sites. In addition, endogenous substances with regulatory functions, such as opioid neuropeptides, are usually unstable in biological tissues, an advantage in moment-to-moment regulation but a disadvantage from the experimental point of view.

A number of receptor-selective, biologically stable ligands for opioid receptors has become available for use as pharmacological tools. Examples include [D-Ala^2,NMePhe^4,Gly^5-ol]enkephalin (DAGO)[5] and Tyr-Pro-NMe-Phe-D-Pro-NH$_2$ (PLO17)[6] as agonists as μ receptors, cyclic [D-Pen^2,D-Pen^5]enkephalin (DPDPE)[7] as an agonist at δ-opioid receptors, and trans-3,4-dichloro-N-methyl-N-(2-(1-pyrrolidinyl)cyclohexyl)benzeneacetamine (U-50,488H)[8] as an agonist at κ-opioid receptors.

Transit and motility

Intracerebroventricular (i.c.v.) injection of morphine in unanaesthetized rats simultaneously inhibits intestinal transit and decreases contractions of the intestine[9]. In rats and other rodents, the antitransit effects of morphine appear to result from decreases in intestinal propulsive contractions. In other mammalian species, opioid inhibition of transit may be associated with increased contractions of intestinal smooth muscle[10], presumably resulting in increased resistance to flow and inhibition of aborally moving propulsive contractions.

To determine the roles of specific types of opioid receptors in regulation of gastrointestinal transit, highly selective opioid agonists were administered i.c.v. to unanaesthetized rats: DAGO (μ-agonist), DPDPE (δ-agonist) and U-50,488H (κ-agonist)[11]. DAGO, but not DPDPE or U-50,488H, produced dose-related inhibition of gastrointestinal transit, whereas all three opioid agonists induced significant analgesic responses. Similar results were obtained in unanaesthetized mice[12]: only μ-agonists given i.c.v. inhibited gastrointestinal transit, whereas μ-, δ- and κ-opioid agonists induced analgesia. As morphine had previously been shown to act at chemosensitive sites in the spinal cord to inhibit gastrointestinal transit[13], receptor-selective agonists were also evaluated for transit effects after intrathecal (i.t.) injection[12]. Interestingly, both DAGO and DPDPE, but not U-50,488H, inhibited transit after i.t. administration. When administered peripherally[14], only μ-opioid agonists (PLO17 and DAGO) inhibited intestinal transit in mice. Identity ot the types of opioid receptors responsible for supraspinal and spinal antitransit effects has been confirmed by use of highly selective μ- and δ-opioid receptor antagonists[15,16]. The gastrointestinal transit effects of receptor-selective opioid agonists are summarized in Table 1.

Gastric secretion

Several neuropeptides are known to act in the CNS to alter gastric acid secretion[17]. The effects of receptor-selective opioid agonists on gastric secretion in rats have been recently examined[18]. When given by i.c.v. injection in unanaesthetized rats, μ-agonists (DAGO, PLO17) produced dose-related decreases in acid output, whereas δ- and κ-agonists had no significant effects. When administered intravenously, U-50,488H produced a large, dose-related increase in acid output, whereas δ- and μ-agonists had no effect in doses that did not cross the blood–brain barrier. These data indicate that brain μ-receptors are linked to inhibition of acid secretion, while peripheral κ-opioid receptors may be linked to stimulation of acid secretion by the stomach.

Table 1 Effects of opioid agonists on gastrointestinal transit in mice

Agonists	Type of receptor	Site of action		
		Brain	Spinal cord	Peripheral
DAGO, PLO17	μ	$\downarrow$?	$\downarrow$	$\downarrow$
DPDPE	δ	0	$\downarrow$	0
U-50,488H	κ	0	0	0

$\downarrow$ = decrese in gastrointestinal transit
0 = no significant effect on transit

BOMBESIN

When administered in the brain, bombesin, a tetradecapeptide originally isolated from amphibian skin, produces a variety of behavioural and gastro-intestinal effects. Centrally administered bombesin inhibits gastric secretion[19] and increases gastric mucus production[20]. Bombesin also has been found to alter gastrointestinal motility and transit by actions in the brain and spinal cord.

After i.c.v. injection in unanaesthetized rats, bombesin produced an increase in the frequency of contractions in the duodenum and, usually, in the jejunum[21]. Intraperitoneal (i.p.) administration of bombesin, at doses 200-fold higher than those given centrally, failed to alter intestinal motility in the duodenum or jejunum. Interestingly, i.c.v. administration of bombesin slows gastric emptying, inhibits small intestinal transit and transiently increases colonic transit in rats[22]. Unlike morphine, bombesin centrally directed antitransit effects in the small intestine are associated with an increase, not a decrease, of intestinal contractions.

Bombesin also inhibits small intestinal transit after i.t. administration[23] and colonic transit is consistently decreased. When given i.c.v., bombesin was 13.5 times more potent than by i.t. injection in inhibiting gastrointestinal transit and some 3400 times more potent than by i.p. injection. Studies were undertaken to determine the anatomical pathways involved in brain and spinal gastrointestinal actions of bombesin. Subdiaphragmatic vagotomy was found to prevent the inhibitory effects of i.c.v. bombesin on gastric emptying, but not on small intestinal transit in rats[22]. In mice, transection of the spinal cord at the level of the second thoracic vertebra eliminated the small intestinal and colonic antitransit effects of bombesin given i.t., but not antitransit effects of bombesin given i.c.v.[24] These results indicate that bombesin given intrathecally acts at chemosensitive sites associated with ascending neural pathways that require intact spinal cord–brain connections for expression of gastrointestinal motility effects. By contrast, the antitransit effects of i.t. morphine were not blocked by T_2 spinal cord transection[24], indicating that the opioid can act in descending neural pathways to influence gastrointestinal motility.

CORTICOTROPIN-RELEASING FACTOR

Corticotropin-releasing factor (CRF) is a 41 amino acid peptide that serves as the principal regulator of pituitary adrenocorticotropic hormone (ACTH) release[25]. CRF has also been shown to exert numerous extrapituitary actions after exogenous administration[26]. When administered i.c.v. to unanaesthetized rats, CRF produced dose-related decreases in gastric emptying and small intestinal transit, but dose-related increases in colonic transit and faecal excretion[27]. The CRF-induced inhibition of small intestinal transit and stimulation of colonic transit were both antagonized by α-helical CRF-(9-41), a CRF receptor antagonist[28].

Because certain models of stress also inhibit small intestinal transit yet stimulate colonic transit and increase faecal excretion[29], the ability of the CRF antagonist to modify gastrointestinal responses to stress was evaluated. CRF was administered i.c.v. in doses that produced changes in transit and elevations in plasma ACTH levels comparable to those obtained with stress[27]. α-helical CRF_{9-41} was found to block the increase in colonic transit and increase in faecal excretion associated with stress or CRF, but not the stress-induced inhibition of small bowel transit. These results indicated that the effects of stress on colonic motility may be mediated centrally by CRF^{27}.

CONCLUSIONS

Neuropeptides may act at chemosensitive sites in the brain and spinal cord to regulate gastrointestinal motility and propulsion as well as influence gastric secretion. It is clear that the brain and spinal cord represent distinct regulatory sites for neuropeptide actions. Likewise, neuropeptides acting in the brain and spinal cord may produce quite different effects on different portions of the gastrointestinal tract. For example, CRF decreases small intestinal transit but increases colonic transit after i.c.v. administration. Multiple types of peptide receptors may be linked differently to gastrointestinal regulatory mechanisms. For example, μ-opioid receptors in the brain, spinal cord and periphery are linked to inhibition of gastrointestinal transit, while κ-opioid receptors seem not to be involved in opioid transit effects. It is also evident that transit and motility or contractile activity of the intestine are related in a complex manner. Given i.c.v., both morphine and bombesin inhibit small intestinal transit, but morphine inhibits contractions whereas bombesin stimulates contractions.

The recent availability of biologically stable, highly receptor-selective peptide agonists and antagonists is permitting detailed exploration of neuropeptide-mediated CNS–gastrointestinal interactions.

Acknowledgements

This work was supported by USPHS grants DA-02163, DK-36289 and DK-33547.

References

1. McDowell,J. and Kitchen, I. (1987). Development of opioid systems: peptides, receptors and pharmacology. *Brain Res. Rev.*, **12**, 397–421
2. Watson, S. J., Akil, H., Khachaturian, H., Young, E. and Lewis, M. E. (1984). Opioid systems: anatomical, physiological and clinical perspectives. In Hughes, J., Collier, H. O. J., Rance, M. J. and Tyers, M. D. (eds.) *Opioids Past Present and Future*, pp. 145–78. (London: Taylor and Francis)
3. Burks, T. F., Galligan, J. J., Hirning, L. D. and Porreca, F. (1987). Brain, spinal cord and peripheral sites of action of enkephalins and other endogenous opioids on gastrointestinal motility. *Gastroenterol. Clin. Biol.*, **11**, 44B–51B
4. James, I. F. and Goldstein, A. (1984). Site-directed alkylation of multiple opioid receptors. I. Binding selectivity. *Molec. Pharmacol.*, **25**, 337–42
5. Handa, B. K., Lane, A. C., Lord, J. A. H., Morgan, B. A., Rance, M. J. and Smith, C. F. C. (1981). Analogues of B-LPH$_{61-64}$ possessing selective agonist activity at μ-opiate receptors. *Eur. J. Pharmacol.*, **70**, 531–40
6. Chang, K.-J., Wei, E. T., Killian, A. and Chang, J.-K. (1983). Potent morphiceptin analogs:

structure-activity relationships and morphine-like activities. *J. Pharmacol. Exp. Ther.*, **227**, 403–8

7. Mosberg, H. I., Hurst, R., Hruby, V. J., Gee, K., Yamamura, H. I., Galligan, J. J. and Burks, T. F. (1983). *Bis*-penicillamine enkephalins possess highly improved specificity toward delta opioid receptors. *Proc. Natl. Acad. Sci. USA*, **80**, 5871–4

8. VonVoigtlander, P. F., Lahti, R. A. and Ludens, J. H. (1983). U-50,448: a selective and structurally novel non-mu (kappa) opioid agonist. *J. Pharmacol. Exp. Ther.*, **224**, 7–12

9. Galligan, J. J. and Burks, T. F. (1983). Centrally mediated inhibition of small intestinal transit and motility by morphine in the rat. *J. Pharmacol. Exp. Ther.*, **226**, 356–61

10. Vaughan Williams, E. M. (1954). The mode of action of drugs upon intestinal motility. *Pharmacol. Rev.*, **6**, 159–90

11. Galligan, J. J., Mosberg, H. I., Hurst, R., Hruby, V. J. and Burks, T. F. (1984). Cerebral delta opioid receptors mediate analgesia but not the intestinal motility effects of intracerebroventricularly administered opioids. *J. Pharmacol. Exp. Ther.*, **229**, 641–8

12. Porreca, F., Mosberg, H. I., Hurst, R., Hruby, V. J. and Burks, T. F. (1984). Roles of mu, delta and kappa opioid receptors in spinal and supraspinal mediation of gastrointestinal transit effects and hot-plate analgesia in the mouse. *J. Pharmacol. Exp. Ther.*, **230**, 341–8

13. Porreca, F. and Burks, T. F. (1983). The spinal cord as a site of opioid effects on gastrointestinal transit in the mouse. *J. Pharmacol. Exp. Ther.*, **227**, 22–7

14. Shook, J. E., Lemcke, P. K., Gehrig, K., Hruby, V. J. and Burks, T. F. (1987). Supraspinal mu and delta receptors and peripheral mu, delta and kappa receptors, posses antidiarrheal activity in mice. *Intl. Narcotic Res. Conf.*, **18**, 56 (Abstract)

15. Shook, J. E., Pelton, J. T., Lemcke, P. K., Porreca, F., Hruby, V. J. and Burks, T. F. (1987). Mu opioid antagonist properties of a cyclic somatostatin octapeptide in vivo: identification of mu receptor-related functions. *J. Pharmacol. Exp. Ther.*, **242**, 1–7

16. Heyman, J. S., Williams, C. L., Burks, T. F., Mosberg, H. I. and Porreca, F. (1988). Dissociation of opioid antinociception and central gastrointestinal propulsion in the mouse: studies with naloxonazine. *J. Pharmacol. Exp. Ther.*, **245**, 238–43

17. Morley, J. E., Levine, A. S. and Silvia, S. E. (1982). Central regulation of gastric acid secretion: the role of neuropeptides. *Life Sci.*, **31**, 339–410

18. Fox, D. A. and Burks, T. F. (1988). Roles of central and peripheral mu, delta and kappa opioid receptors in the mediation of gastric acid secretory effects in the rat. *J. Pharmacol. Exp. Ther.*, **244**, 456–62

19. Tache, Y. and Collu, R. (1982). CNS mediated inhibition of gastric secretion by bombesin: independence from interaction with brain catecholaminergic and serotinergic pathways and pituitary hormones. *Peptides*, **3**, 51–9

20. Tache, Y. (1982). Bombesin: central nervous system action to increae gastric mucus in rats. *Gastroenterology*, **83**, 75–80

21. Porreca, F., Fulginiti, J. T. and Burks, T. F. (1985). Bombesin stimulates small intestinal motility after intracerebroventricular administration to rats. *Eur. J. Pharmacol.*, **114**, 167–73

22. Porreca, F. and Burks, T. F. (1983). Centrally-administered bombesin affects gastric emptying and small and large bowel transit in the rat. *Gastroenterology*, **85**, 313–17

23. Porreca, F., Burks, T. F. and Koslo, R. J. (1985). Centrally-mediated bombesin effects on gastrointestinal motility. *Life Sci.*, **37**, 125–34

24. Koslo, R. J., Burks, T. F. and Porreca, F. (1986). Centrally-administered bombesin affects gastrointestinal transit and colonic bead expulsion through supraspinal mechanisms. *J. Pharamacol. Exp. Ther.*, **238**, 62–7

25. Rivier, C., Browstein, M., Spiess, J., Rivier, J. and Vale, W. (1982). *In vivo* corticotropin-releasing factor-induced secretion of adrenocorticotropin, β-endorphin, and corticosterone. *Endocrinology*, **110**, 272–8

26. Brown, M. R., Fisher, L. A., Spiess, J., Rivier, C., Rivier, J. and Vale, W. (1982). CRF: actions on the sympathetic nervous system and metabolism. *Endocrinology*, **111**, 928–31

27. Williams, C. L., Peterson, J. M., Villar, R. G. and Burks, T. F. (1987). Corticotropin-releasing factor directly mediates colonic responses to stress. *Am. J. Phisiol.*, **253**, G582–656

28. Rivier, J., Rivier, C. and Vale, W. (1985). Synthetic competitive antagonists of corticotropin-releasing factor-induced ACTH secretion in the rat. *Science (Washington)*, **224**, 889–91

29. Williams, C. L., Villar, R. G., Peterson, J. M. and Burks, T. F. (1988). Stress-induced changes in intestinal transit in the rat: a model for irritable bowel syndrome. *Gastroenterology*, **94**, 611–21

34
Neuroendocrine control mechanisms of gastric emptying in the rat

T. GREEN, R. DIMALINE AND G. J. DOCKRAY

INTRODUCTION

The rate at which liquids empty from the stomach is a function of the pressure difference between the body of the stomach and the duodenum, and the resistance to flow across the pylorus[1,2]. A variety of factors including the volume, osmolarity, viscosity, pH and composition of a meal are known to influence gastric emptying[3,4,5]. The role of duodenal osmoreceptors in particular is well known, but the subsequent pathways are less clearly understood, and both nervous and hormonal mechanisms are thought to be involved.

In humans, dog and rat, the intestinal hormone cholecystokinin (CCK) is a potent inhibitor of gastric emptying of liquid test meals[6-13]. Cholecystokinin is released by protein and fat and this type of meal is also known to slow gastric emptying. On this basis, therefore, it is reasonable to postulate that CCK has a physiological role in the control of gastric emptying. Until recently, however, it has not been possible to test this idea directly. In the last two years potent specific CCK antagonists have become available and these have greatly facilitated studies of the physiology of CCK[14]. We shall review here recent evidence using CCK antagonists which suggests that endogenous CCK regulates gastric emptying in the conscious rat, and we shall discuss the mechanisms involved. The mechanisms appear to be distinct from those mediating the effects of acid and hyperosmolal solutions on gastric emptying.

EXPERIMENTAL APPROACHES

Animal preparations

The emptying of liquid test meals in conscious gastric fistula rats were studied, using surgical (coeliac ganglionectomy) and chemical (capsaicin) nerve-lesioning techniques to destroy afferent and efferent nerve pathways to the stomach. Administration of the sensory neurotoxin, capsaicin ($50 \, mg \, kg^{-1}$) to neonatal rats destroys virtually all small diameter afferent fibres[15]; a high proportion of gastric vagal and spinal afferents are known to be unmyelinated[16,17] so there is substantial visceral deafferentation in capsaicin-treated rats. Removal of the coeliac-superior mesenteric ganglion complex destroys splanchnic afferents which pass through the ganglion to the terminal regions in the stomach, as well as sympathetic efferent post-ganglionic neurons, but leaves intact most gastric vagal fibres. Gastric emptying of liquid meals has been studied in the past by recovery of test meals following intragastric instillation using non-absorbable dilution markers, e.g. charcoal or phenol red[3,7]. We have used this approach in rats fitted with an in-dwelling stainless steel gastric cannula[18]. At least two weeks recovery is needed after installing the cannula before experiments are started. In the case of nerve-lesioned rats three months recovery was allowed. The rats are trained to stand in a Bollman-type cage before experiments are started. Repeated measurements have been made in the same group of animals, two or three times a week for several months. We used a physiological saline test meal (pH 7.4, 300 m.osmol/kg) as a control, and liquid test meals of meat peptone, protease inhibitors, hydrochloric acid and hypersmolal saline. With the exception of the latter, all solutions were made iso-osomolal with physiological saline.

Peripheral CCK-receptor antagonists

A number of CCK antagonists, e.g. proglumide, CR1409, asperlicin have been available for some years[19,20,21] and some of these have been used in studies of the action of CCK on gastric emptying[22,23]. For the most part these antagonists either have poor oral bioavailability or do not discriminate between different subclasses of CCK receptors. The recent development of a new class of potent and highly selective peripheral CCK-receptor antagonists related to the benzodiazepines[14] has provided a valuable tool with which to investigate the physiology of CCK. One of these compounds, L-364,718 is orally active, lacks any CCK-agonist properties, and in radioligand-binding studies is a specific antagonist for the peripheral type of CCK receptor found on the gallbladder, pylorus and pancreas[24]. We have used doses of 0.01– 1 mg in methylcellulose given into the gastric fistula[25]. This blocks the action of exogenous CCK within 30 min, and the effect lasts for several hours. No deleterious effects have been noted in rats receiving L-364,718 two or three times a week for several months.

INHIBITORY ACTION OF DIFFERENT LIQUID TEST MEALS

Physiological saline empties rapidly from the stomach. Approximately 50% of the initial solution empties in the first 30 s, and after 8 min only about 5% of the test meal remains (Figure 1). In contrast, acid, peptone and

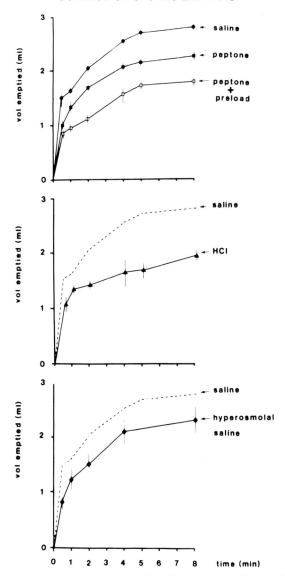

Figure 1 Gastric emptying of physiological saline (300 m.osmol.kg^{-1}) and 4.5% meat peptone II (upper panel), HCl (middle), and 900 m.osmol.kg^{-1} saline (lower panel) in the conscious gastric fistula rat. In the middle and lower panels the emptying of physiological saline is shown as a broken line. Note peptone, HCl and hyperosmolal saline all delay emptying compared with physiological saline. In the case of peptone, the inhibition of emptying is increased by administration of an additional peptone test meal five min before the emptying trial (identified in the upper panel as peptone plus preload)

hyperosmolal solutions all delay gastric emptying. Each initially empties rapidly, but after 30 s the rate of emptying is decreased compared with physiological saline and this persists over the following 8 min. Of these test meals 50 mM HCI produced the greatest inhibition of emptying. The action of peptone was dose dependent; the greatest inhibition was caused by a 4.5% solution of meat peptone II, while an iso-osmotic solution of 1.13% was scarcely different to saline. The effects of a 4.5% peptone meal on gastric emptying were markedly enhanced by a preload of 4.5% peptone given 6 min earlier and allowed to remain in the stomach for 5 min, and then drained for 1 min before starting a second peptone trial.

Evidence for the action of endogenous CCK on gastric emptying

The CCK antagonist L-364,718 is reported to antagonize the effects of exogenous CCK on gastric emptying in mouse, rat and dog, and pancreatic secretion in cat, dog and rat[26-29]. In our hands intravenous infusion of 400 pmol/kg/h or CCK8 delayed the emptying of a physiological saline meal by about the same degree as 4.5% peptone test meal. This action of exogenous CCK was reversed by L-364,718. Intragastric administration of L-364,718 in doses up to 1 mg reversed the effects of peptone (Figure 2). Even at the high dose of antagonist, however, there remained a small response to peptone.

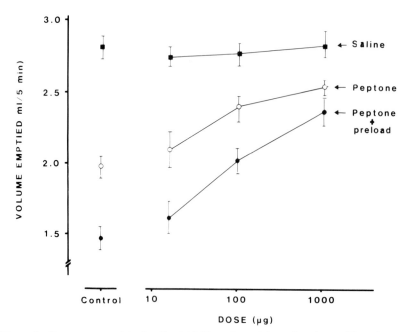

Figure 2 Dose-response data for the inhibition of emptying of peptone, either alone, or following a peptone preload, by the peripheral CCK antagonist L-364,718. At the left is shown the control rates of emptying; note that L-364,718 depresses the effect of peptone in inhibiting gastric emptying, but has no effect on the emptying of saline

The ED50 reported by Lotti et al.[26] for antagonism of exogenous CCK on gastric emptying in rats was 140 μg/kg and this is consistent with our findings. The inhibitory effects of the acid and hyperosmolal test meals were not significantly affected by L-364,718 which provides evidence for the specificity of L364,718 *in vivo* against CCK (Figure 3). The results indicate protein-rich meals are able to release sufficient amounts of CCK to inhibit gastric emptying and, in consequence, this action is likely to be physiological. This conclusion is compatible with analogous studies in humans, in which plasma CCK concentrations were measured[12]; inhibition of gastric emptying was associated with similar plasma concentrations of exogenous and endogenous peptide.

Action of protease inhibitors

A variety of protease inhibitors are reported to release CCK[30-34]. The mechanism of action is still uncertain; though it seems that luminal proteases depress CCK release and protease inhibitors reverse the effect[35]. One possibility is that an endogenous CCK-releasing peptide normally binds trypsin or other proteases and can be displaced by either protease inhibitors or protein substrates. The free CCK-releasing peptide then acts to increase circulating hormone concentrations[36].

The protease inhibitor FOY-305 (Camostate mesilate) has been shown to induce a rise in serum CCK following oral administration[33,34]. This release of CCK appears to be sufficient to cause pancreatic growth and hypersecretion, and these effects can be blocked by L-364,718[37]. We have shown that FOY-305 inhibits gastric emptying in the conscious rat[25]. A similar compound, FOY-007 (Gabexate mesilate) also acts to delay gastric emptying in the conscious rat, but is about four times less potent than FOY-

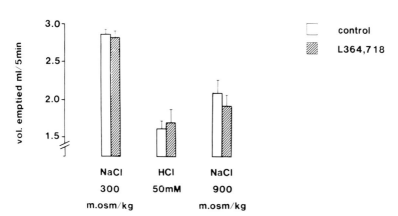

Figure 3 Gastric emptying of NaCl (300 or 900 m.osmol.kg^{-1}) and HC1 in control rats after either vehicle (methylcellulose: open bars) or L-364,718 (1 mg, hatched bars). The volume emptied in 5 min is shown. Note that the CCK antagonist does not change the inhibition of emptying produced by hyperosmolal solutions or HCl

305. Aprotinin and the natural protease inhibitors, soyabean trypsin inhibitor and potato trypsin inhibitor also delay gastric emptying, although the effects are less striking than those of FOY-305. The effects of protein inhibitors on gastric emptying were reversed after treatment with L-364,718 (Table 1). This action of protease inhibitors provides a specific means for investigating the effects of CCK release on gastric emptying since it is known that, while proteins are potent releasers of CCK, they also have a variety of other gastrointestinal effects on secretion and motility that are not attributable to CCK release.

LESIONING EXPERIMENTS

Chronic coeliac ganglionectomy

After chronic coeliac ganglionectomy, the gastric emptying of peptone (whether alone or following a peptone preload) is similar to that in control animals; the response was reproduced by intravenous infusion of exogenous CCK, and in both cases inhibited by L-364,718 (Figure 4; Table 2). HCl also delayed gastric emptying after coeliac ganglionectomy, but the inhibitory effect of hyperosmolal saline on gastric emptying was markedly depressed.

Capsaicin

In rats that had been treated with the sensory neurotoxin, capsaicin, a peptone meal emptied faster than in control animals. The action of HCl on gastric emptying still persisted in these animals, but that of hyperosmolal saline was reduced (Figure 5). The CCK antagonist L-364,718 had no effect on the emptying of peptone. Both we and others[38] have found exogenous CCK also failed to delay the emptying of a saline meal in capsaicin-treated rats (Table 2). In these animals, the pathway through which CCK acts to delay gastric emptying appears, therefore, to be blocked.

MECHANISMS OF ACTION OF CCK

The results reviewed above provide direct evidence that endogenous CCK in the rat mediates the action of protein-rich meals, and protease inhibitors,

Table 1 Emptying of 0.14 M saline (3 ml) containing protease inhibitors

	Volume emptied (ml/5 min)	
	Vehicle (n = 5)	L-364,718 (1 mg/rat) (n = 5)
0.14 M NaCl control	2.81 ± 0.15	2.75 ± 0.05
10 mg/ml FOY-305	2.13 ± 0.24	2.70 ± 0.16*
10 mg/ml FOY-007	2.48 ± 0.28	2.75 ± 0.05
1.17 mg/ml Aprotinin	2.16 ± 0.14	2.68 ± 0.12*

*$p < 0.05$, t-test

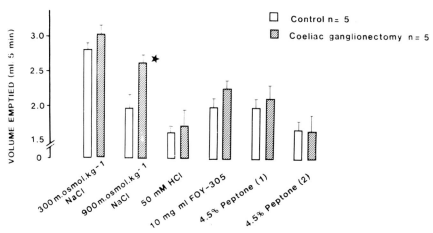

Figure 4 Emptying of a variety of test meals in control (open bars) and coeliac ganglionecto-mized rats (hatched bars). Note that over 5 min the emptying of 300 m.osmol.kg^{-1} NaCl, peptone (either alone, identified as '1', or after a preload, identified as '2') and HCl is similar in control and coeliac ganglionectomized rats. The inhibition of emptying by hyperosmolal saline is significantly reduced in the coeliac ganglionectomized rats (t-test, $p < 0.05$)

Table 2 Effects of exogenous CCK8s on gastric emptying of 0.14 M NaCl (3 ml)

	Volume emptied (ml/5 min)	
	Saline (i.v.)	CCK8s (400 pmol/kg/h i.v.)
Control rats (n = 6)	2.67 ± 0.14	1.99 ± 0.12*
Coeliac ganglionectomy (n = 5)	2.87 ± 0.15	2.12 ± 0.08*
Capsaicin treated (n = 5)	2.55 ± 0.09	2.53 ± 0.15

*$p < 0.05$, t-test

in delaying gastric emptying. Similar results have recently been reported by Dektor et al. with respect to the emptying of semi-solid mixed meals[28]. The availability of potent, specific orally active CCK antagonists has been of decisive importance in this work, since they have made it possible to examine directly the idea first proposed by Debas et al.[7] that CCK might have a physiological role in the control of gastric emptying. The data is presently strongest for the action of protein-rich meals in releasing CCK. It is often thought that fat is also a releaser of CCK which again might explain its action in delaying gastric emptying. However, studies using L–364,718 in the dog have so far failed to provide evidence that the action of fat in delaying gastric emptying is mediated by CCK[27]. There may, in any case, be differences between dog and rat in the factors that release CCK; Liddle et al. have reported that, whereas protein and protease inhibitors increase plasma CCK

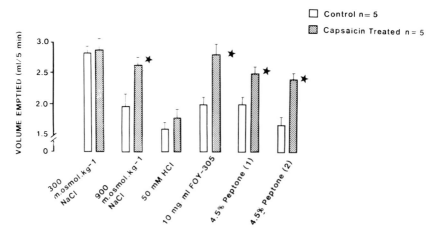

Figure 5 Emptying of a variety of test meals in control (open bars) and capsaicin-treated rats (hatched bars). For further details see legend to Figure 4. Capsaicin (50 mg.kg^{-1}) had been given to neonatal rats, that were studied when 300–400 g. Note that the inhibitory action of hyperosmolal saline and peptone on gastric emptying, but not that of HCl, was decreased in capsaicin-treated rats

in the rat, amino acids and fat do not[39]. These observations accord with our own experience in studying the action of amino acids, protein and protease inhibitors on gastric emptying in the rat.

There are several possible sites at which circulating CCK could act to delay gastric emptying. These include a decrease in intragastric pressure, an increase in duodenal pressure and an increase in resistance to flow at the pylorus[1,2]. Yamagishi and Debas[8] have shown that both the proximal and distal stomach contribute to the action of exogenous CCK in delaying gastric emptying in the dog. In the rat there is also evidence that CCK might increase duodenal pressure[23]. Further evidence in support for an action of CCK on the pylorus comes from the finding that (1) there are abundant CCK binding sites on pyloric smooth mucle, and (2) CCK contracts the pylorus[40,41]. In the rat, the latter effect is mediated by both direct actions on the smooth muscle and indirect effects mediated by the release of noradrenaline[42]. It would appear, however, that sympathetic noradrenergic mediation might not be important physiologically, since coeliac ganglionec-tomy does not reduce the action of endogenous or exogenous CCK on gastric emptying in conscious rats. In general, moreover, the pylorus is thought to have a relatively minor role in controlling the emptying of liquid test meals, and for reasons discussed below we think that CCK acts mainly by control of pressure in the body of the stomach.

In the anaesthetized rat, intravenous CCK decreases intragastric pressure by relaxing the body of the stomach[43]. This effect is reduced by section of either the cervical vagi or the splanchnic nerves, and is abolished by section of both. The vagal pathway is sensitive to hexamethonium and the splanchnic pathway is adrenergic. It would seem that, since coeliac ganglionectomy did not reduce the action of exogenous or endogenous CCK on gastric emptying in the conscious rat, the sympathetic pathway does not make an important contribution to the normal control of gastric emptying. Nevertheless, the action of CCK on gastric emptying was decreased in rats treated with capsaicin, indicating that small diameter extrinsic afferents are required. Taken together with the results in coeliac ganglionectomized rats, it appears that CCK might act through a vagal afferent pathway. It is well established that there are vagovagal reflex mechanisms that relax the body of the stomach[44]. The afferent arm of the reflex is evoked by stimulation of gastric mechanoreceptors the properties of which have been fairly extensively studied by electrophysiological recording from vagal afferent fibres[45-49]. The efferent arm probably involves both increased discharge of preganglionic parasympathetic vagal fibres that terminate on non-adrenergic, non-cholinergic (probably VIP-containing) gastric neurons which directly relax the stomach[50], and decreased discharge of vagal efferent excitatory fibres which terminate on cholinergic post-ganglionic neurons in the stomach[51]. Two lines of evidence suggest that CCK might act directly on vagal afferents to mimic the effect of gastric distension (Figure 6).

First, electrophysiological recordings from neurons in the brainstem with an input from the stomach and from vagal afferents, suggest that CCK and gastric distension produce identical responses and that the effects of CCK are not secondary to changes in gastric motility[52-54]. Secondly, there is autoradiographic evidence for the presence of CCK-binding sites on vagal fibres, including the subdiaphragmatic projection[55,56]. Taken as a whole, these findings raise the interesting possibility that the hormonal action of CCK on gastric emptying is exerted in the first place by a direct action on vagal afferents that otherwise mediate gastric mechanoreceptor discharge.

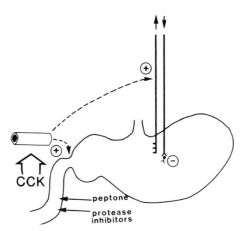

Figure 6 Schematic representation of the pathway mediating the action of CCK on gastric emptying in the rat. The combined results of capsaicin-treated and coeliac ganglionectomy suggest that CCK might act via small-diameter vagal afferents. Electrophysiological evidence suggests it could act directly on those afferents that mediate gastric mechanoreceptor discharge to produce vagovagal reflex relaxation of the stomach

CCK, hyperosmolal solutions and HCl activate different mechanisms

In both capsaicin-treated and coeliac ganglionectomized rats, the delaying action of hyperosmolal saline on gastric emptying was reduced. These observations are consistent with a role for small-diameter afferents in mediating the action of hyperosmolal solutions. Further work will be needed to establish the precise mechanism of action but three fairly obvious possible pathways are worth identifying at the present time. These are (1) a vagal afferent route and sympathetic, presumably adrenergic, efferent pathway; (2) a spinal afferent and sympathetic efferent pathway; and (3) a spinal afferent and vagal efferent pathway. Electrophysiological recordings from efferent fibres as well as afferents suggest that all pathways ought at least to be considered[16,17,57]. There are, however, other possibilities which should not be rejected. The spinal afferents to the upper gastrointestinal tract are rich in calcitonin gene-related peptide and substance P and these peptides are transported to peripheral afferent terminals[58,59]. Afferent stimulation by hyperosmolal solutions would release CGRP and substance P locally within the gut. Substance P is known to have excitatory effects both directly on gut smooth muscle and on myenteric neurons, and CGRP has inhibitory effects on gut motility possibly by acting on non-adrenergic, non-cholinergic myenteric neurons[50] (See also Dockray et al., Chapter 10. this volume). One possibility is that afferent stimulation activates axon reflexes mediated by these or other peptides which in turn delay gastric emptying.

Finally, it appears that the action of HCl on gastric emptying does not depend on the same extrinsic nervous pathways that are utilized by CCK or hyperosmolal solutions. The mechanisms mediating the action of HCl remain to be established: they could include other hormonal mechanisms, e.g. secretin, or intrinsic nervous pathways.

SUMMARY

CCK has a physiological role in mediating the inhibition of gastric emptying caused by protein meals in the conscious rat. This action of CCK appears to require an intact vagal afferent pathway, suggesting that the mechanism might involve vagovagal reflex relaxation of the body of the stomach. This would decrease intragastric pressure and so delay gastric emptying. The action of hyperosmolal stimuli on gastric emptying in the conscious rat appears to depend on the splanchnic innervation, whereas HCl requires neither the splanchnic nor small-diameter afferents in general.

Acknowledgements

We are grateful to the University of Liverpool for a research studentship and to the MRC for financial support. The help of Christine Carter in preparing this manuscript is also gratefully acknowledged. Samples of FOY-

305, and L-364,718 were kindly donated by Ono Pharmaceuticals, and Merck, Sharpe and Dohme, respectively.

References

1. Kelly, K.A. (1980). Gastric emptying of liquids and solids: roles of proximal and distal stomach. *Am. J. Physiol.*, **239**, G71–6
2. Kelly, K.A. (1981). Motility of the stomach and gastroduodenal junction. In Johnson, L.R. (ed.) *Physiology of the Gastrointestinal Tract.* pp. 393–410. (New York: Raven Press)
3. Hunt, J.N. and MacDonald, I. (1954). The influence of volume on gastric emptying. *J. Physiol.*, **126**, 459–74
4. Hunt, J.N. and Stubbs, D.F. (1975). The volume and energy content of meals as determinants of gastric emptying. *J. Physiol.*, **245**, 209–25
5. Barker, G.R., Cochrane, G.McL., Corbett, G.A., Hunt, J.N. and Roberts, S.K. (1974). Actions of glucose and potassium chloride on osmoreceptors slowing gastric emptying. *J. Physiol.*, **237**, 183–6
6. Chey, W.Y., Hitanant, S., Hendricks, J. and Lorber, S.H. (1970). Effect of secretin and cholecystokinin on gastric emptying and gastric secretion in man. *Gastroenterology*, **58**, 820–7
7. Debas, H.T., Farooq, O. and Grossman, M.I. (1975). Inhibition of gastric emptying is a physiological action of cholecystokinin. *Gastroenterology*, **68**, 1211–17
8. Yamagishi, T. and Debas, H.T. (1978). Cholecystokinin inhibits gastric emptying by acting on both proximal stomach and pylorus. *Am. J. Physiol.*, **234**, E375–8
9. Anika, M.S. (1982). Effects of cholecystokinin and caerulein on gastric emptying. *Eur. J. Pharmacol.*, **85**, 195–9
10. Mangel, A.W. and Koegel, A. (1984). Effects of peptides on gastric emptying. *Am. J. Physiol.*, **246**, G342–5
11. Valenzuela, J.E. and Defilippi, C. (1981). Inhibition of gastric emptying in humans by secretin, the octapeptide of cholecystokinin, and intraduodenal fat. *Gastroenterology*, **81**, 898–902
12. Liddle, R.A., Morita, E.T., Conrad, C.K. and Williams, J.A. (1986). Regulation of gastric emptying in humans by cholecystokinin. *J. Clin. Invest.*, **77**, 992–6
13. McHugh, P.R. and Moran, T.H. (1986). The stomach, cholecystokinin and satiety. *Fed. Proc.*, **45**, 1384–90
14. Evans, B.E., Bock, M.G., Rittle, K.E., DiPardo, R.M., Whitter, W.L., Veber, D.F., Anderson, P.S. and Freidinger, R.M. (1986). Design of potent, orally effective, nonpeptidal antagonists of the peptide hormone cholecystokinin. *Proc. Natl. Acad. Sci. USA*, **83**, 4918–22
15. Jancso, G., Kiraly, E. and Jancso-Gabor, A. (1977). Pharmacologically induced selective degeneration of chemosensitive primary sensory neurones. *Nature*, **270**, 741–3
16. Andrews, P.L.R. (1986). Vagal afferent innervation of the gastrointestinal tract. *Prog. Brain Res.*, **67**, 65–86
17. Janig, W. and Morrison, J.F.B. (1986). Functional properties of spinal visceral afferents supplying abdominal and pelvic organs, with special emphasis on visceral nociception. *Prog. Brain Res.*, **67**, 87–114
18. Dimaline, R., Carter, N. and Barnes, S. (1986). Evidence for reflex adrenergic inhibition of acid secretion in the conscious rat. *Am. J. Physiol.*, **251**, G615–18
19. Hahne, W.F., Jensen, R.T., Lemp, G.F. and Gardner, J.D. (1981). Proglumide and benzotript: Members of a different class of cholecystokinin receptor antagonists. *Proc. Natl. Acad. Sci. USA*, **78**, 6304–8
20. Chang, R.S.L., Lotti, V.J., Monaghan, R.L., Birnbaum, J., Stapley, E.O., Goetz, M.A., Albers-Schonberg, G., Patchett, A.A., Liesch, J.M., Hensens, O.D. and Springer, J.P. (1985). A potent nonpeptide cholecystokinin antagonist selective for peripheral tissues isolated from *Aspergillus alliaceus. Science*, **230**, 177–9
21. Makovec, F., Chiste, R., Bani, M., Revel, L., Setnikar, I. and Rovati, A.L. (1986). New glutamic and aspartic derivatives with potent CCK-antagonistic activity. *Eur. J. Med.*

Chem., **21**, 9–20

22. Lotti, V. J., Cerino, D. J., Kling, P. J. and Chang, R. S. L. (1986). A new simple mouse model for the *in vivo* evaluation of cholecystokinin (CCK) antagonists: comparative potencies and durations of action of nonpetide antagonists. *Life Sciences*, **39**, 1631–38

23. Shillabeer, G. and Davison, J. S. (1987). Proglumide, a cholecystokinin antagonist, increases gastric emptying in rats. *Am. J. Physiol.*, **252**, R353–60

24. Chang, R. S. L. and Lotti, V. J. (1986). Biochemical and pharmacological characterization of an extremely potent and selective nonpeptide cholecystokinin antagonist. *Proc. Natl. Acad. Sci. USA*, **83**, 4923–6

25. Green, T., Dimaline, R., Peikin, S. and Dockray, G. J. (1988). The action of cholecystokinin antagonist, L-364,718 on gastric emptying of liquid meals in the conscious rat. *Am. J. Physiol.*, **255**, G685–9

26. Lotti, V. J., Pendleton, R. G., Gould, R. J., Hanson, H. M., Chang, R. S. L. and Clineschmidt, B. V (1987). *In vivo* pharmacology of L-364,718, a new potent nonpeptide peripheral cholecystokinin antagonist. *J. Pharm. Expt. Therapeut.*, **241**, 103–9

27. Pendleton, R. G., Bendesky, R. J., Schaffer, L., Nolan, T. E., Gould, R. J. and Clineschmidt, B. V. (1987). Roles of endogenous cholecystokinin in biliary, pancreatic and gastric function: studies with L-364–718, a specific cholecystokinin receptor antagonist. *J. Pharm. Expt. Therapeut.*, **241**, 110–16

28. Decktor, D. L., Pendleton, R. G., Elnitsky, A. T., Jenkins, A. M. and McDowell, A. P. (1988). Effect of metoclopramide, bethanchol and cholecystokinin receptor antagonist, L-364,718 on gastric emptying in the rat. *Eur. J. Pharmacol.*, **147**, 313–16

29. Anderson, L. and Dockray, G. J. (1988). The cholecystokinin antagonist L-364,718 inhibits the action of cholecystokinin but not bombesin on rat pancreatic secretion *in vivo*. *Eur. J. Pharmacol.*, **146**, 307–11

30. Chernick, S. S., Lepkovsky, S. and Chaikoff, I. L. (1948). A dietary factor regulating the enzyme content of the pancreas: changes induced in size and proteolytic activity of the chick pancreas by the ingestion of raw soybean meal. *Am. J. Physiol.*, **155**, 33–41

31. Green, G. M. and Lyman, R. L. (1972). Feedback regulation of pancreatic enzyme secretion as a mechanism for trypsin inhibitor-induced hypersecretion in rats. *Proc. Soc. Exp. Biol. Med.*, **140**, 6–12

32. Lyman, R. L., Wilcox, S. S. and Monsen, E. R. (1962). Pancreatic enzyme secretion produced in the rat by trypsin inhibitors. *Am. J. Physiol.*, **202**, 1077–82

33. Rausch, U., Adler, G., Weidenbach, H., Weidenbach, F., Rudolff, D., Koop, I. and Kern, H. F. (1987). Stimulation of pancreatic secretory process in the rat by low-molecular weight proteinase inhibitor I. Dose-response study on enzyme content and secretion, cholecystokinin release and pancreatic fine structure. *Cell Tiss. Res.*, **247**, 187–93

34. Rausch, U., Weidenbach, H., Adler, G. and Kern, H. F. (1987). Stimulation of pancreatic secretory process in the rat by low-molecular weight proteinase inhibitor II. Regulation of total protein and individual enzyme biosynthesis. *Cell Tiss. Res.*, **249**, 63–7

35. Owyang, C., Louie, D. S. and Tatum, D. (1986). Feedback regulation of pancreatic enzyme secretion: suppression of cholecystokinin release by trypsin. *J. Clin. Invest.*, **77**, 2042–7

36. Iwai, K., Fukuoka, S.-I., Fushiki, T., Tsujikawa, M., Hirose, M., Tsunasawa, S. and Sakiyama, F. (1987). Purification and sequencing of a trypsin-sensitive cholecystokinin-releasing peptide from rat pancreatic juice. *J. Biol. Chem.*, **262**, 8956–59

37. Wisner, J. R., Jr., McLaughlin, R. E., Rich, K. A., Ozawa, S. and Renner, I. G. (1988). Effects of L-364,718, a new cholecystokinin receptor antagonist, on camostate-induced growth of the rat pancreas. *Gastroenterology*, **94**, 109–13

38. Raybould, H. E. and Taché, Y. (1988). Cholecystokinin inhibits gastric motility and emptying via a capsaicin-sensitive vagal pathway in rats. *Am. J. Physiol.*, **255**, G242–6

39. Liddle, R. A., Green, G. M., Conrad, C. K. and Williams, J. A. (1986). Proteins, but not amino acids, carbohydrates, and fats stimulate cholecystokinin secretion in the rat. *Am. J. Physiol.*, **251**, G243–8

40. Smith, G. T., Moran, T. H., Coyle, J. T., Kuhar, M. J., O'Donahue, T. L. and McHugh, P. R. (1984). Anatomic localization of cholecystokinin receptors to the pyloric sphincter. *Am. J. Physiol.*, **246**, R127–30

41. Fisher, R. S., Lipshutz, E. and Cohen, S. (1973). The hormonal regulation of pyloric sphincter function. *J. Clin. Invest.*, **52**, 1289–96

42. Scheurer, U., Varga, L., Drack, E., Burki, H.-R. and Halter, F. (1983). Mechanism of action

of cholecystokinin octapeptide on rat antrum, pylorus and duodenum. *Am. J. Physiol.*, **244**, G266–72

43. Raybould, H. E., Roberts, M. E. and Dockray, G. J. (1987). Reflex decreases in intragastric pressure in response to cholecystokinin in rats. *Am. J. Physiol.*, **253**, G165–70
44. Abrahamsson, H. (1973). Studies on the inhibitory nervous control of gastric motility. *Acta Physiol. Scand. Suppl.*, **390**, 1–38
45. Paintal, A. S. (1973). Vagal sensory receptors and their reflex effects. *Physiol. Rev.*, **53**, 159–227
46. Iggo, A. (1955). Tension receptors in the stomach and the urinary bladder. *J. Physiol.*, **128**, 593–607
47. Niijima, A. (1967). Afferent impulses in the gastric and oesophageal branch of the vagal nerve of toad. *Physiol. and Behav.*, **2**, 1–4
48. Leek, B. F. (1977). Abdominal and pelvic visceral receptors. *Brit. Med. Bull.*, **33**, 163–8
49. Scratcherd, T. and Grundy, D. (1982). Nervous afferents from the upper gastrointestinal tract which influence gastrointestinal motility. In Wienbech, M. (ed.) *Motility of the Digestive Tract*, pp. 7–17. (New York: Raven Press)
50. Dockray, G. J. (1987). Physiology of enteric neuropeptides. In Johnson, L. R. (ed.) *Physiology of the Gastrointestinal Tract, 2nd Edn.*, pp.41–66. (New York: Raven Press)
51. Azpiroz, F. and Malgelada, J.-R. (1986). Vagally mediated gastric relaxation induced by intestinal nutrients in the dog. *Am. J. Physiol.*, **251**, G727–35
52. Raybould, H. E., Gayton, R. J. and Dockray, G. J. (1985). CNS effects of circulating CCK8: involvement of brainstem neurones responding to gastric distension. *Brain Res.*, **342**, 187–90
53. Raybould, H. E., Gayton, R. J. and Dockray, G. J. (1988). Mechanisms of action of peripherally administered cholecystokinin octapeptide on brainstem neurons in the rat. *J. Neurosci.*, **8**, 3018–24
54. Davison, J. S. (1986). Response of vagal gastric mechanoreceptors to circulating cholecystokinin and adrenaline in the rat. *Can. J. Physiol. Pharm.*, Suppl. 44
55. Zarbin, M. A., Wamsley, J. K., Innis, R. B. and Kuhar, M. J. (1981). Cholecystokinin receptors: Presence and axonal flow in the rat vagus nerve. *Life Sciences*, **29**, 697–705
56. Moran, T. H., Smith, G. P., Hostetler, A. M. and McHugh, P. R. (1987). Transport of cholecystokinin (CCK) binding sites in subdiaphragmatic vagal branches. *Brain Res.*, **415**, 149–52
57. Grundy, D., Salih, A. A. and Scratcherd, T. (1981). Modulation of vagal efferent fibre discharge by mechanoreceptors in the stomach, duodenum and colon of the ferret. *J. Physiol.*, **319**, 43–52
58. Green, T. and Dockray, G. J. (1988). Characterisation of the peptidergic afferent innervation of the stomach in the rat, mouse and guinea pig. *Neuroscience*, **25**, 181–93

35
Integration of gustatory and gut afferent activity in the brainstem

R. NORGREN

INTRODUCTION

The process of digestion originates with ingestive behaviour. Signals arising during digestion eventually terminate the ingestive behaviour, thus defining the primary unit of feeding behaviour—the meal. The importance of feedback from the gut can be demonstrated dramatically in animals prepared with gastric cannulas. With such a cannula closed, so that food or fluid remains in the stomach and reaches the duodenum, a deprived rat will ingest at most 20–30 ml of a liquid diet. With the cannula open, so that most or all of the food drains from the stomach, the same animal will ingest hundreds of millilitres of the same stimulus without pause[1]. Although this observation may appear trivial, the physiological mechanisms through which food in the gut terminates ingestive behaviour remain at issue.

The system is rich in determinants and so, to make the problem tractable, its complexity must be artificially limited. First, feeding behaviour is temporally controlled—not only meal size, but also intermeal intervals and long-term body weight, are regulated. Secondly, animals can regulate intake of macronutrients, as well as calories, and thus must have the sensory apparatus required to evaluate sources of carbohydrates, fats and protein as they pass through the oral cavity and the gut. Finally, the interaction of oral afferent activity and neural or humoral feedback from the gastrointestinal tract can occur at any level of the CNS[2]. Indeed, sodium deprivation alters the responsiveness of some peripheral gustatory neurons to sapid sodium stimuli[3], raising the possiblity that some oral afferent activity relevant to ingestion might be modulated before it reaches the CNS. In a series of behavioural experiments, Gerard P. Smith, Harvey, J. Grill and this author have defined a preparation that limits each of these dimensions while preserving the essential features of behavioural control in question—gut-mediated termination of ingestion. In the following, the evidence needed for this definition is reviewed and the anatomical and electrophysiological studies that extend the inquiry to specific neural systems concerned with the sensory and motor control of ingestive behaviour are summarized.

ORAL STIMULI

Ingested food produces complex mixtures of olfactory, thermal, tactile and gustatory stimuli. In addition, the sensory neurophysiology of food constituents remains rudimentary. Although fats and oils are avidly consumed by many animals, the oral sensory activity that elicits this behaviour is poorly documented. At least when in short supply, protein intake is regulated. Some amino acids stimulate gustatory receptors, but probably only poorly when incorporated into proteins and polypeptides[4]. Sugars, acids, and alkaloids occur in most foodstuffs at concentrations that stimulate gustatory receptors. Carbohydrates are even more ubiquitous, and some species exhibit specific preferences for carbohydrates[5]. Again, the oral sensory apparatus that detects carbohydrates cannot be specified with certainty, but it appears not to involve the gustatory receptors that respond well to chemicals labelled 'sweet' by humans[6].

The sensory complexity of many foods, coupled with the inadequate characterization of the afferent sensory activity elicited by foods, complicates the neurophysiological analysis of feeding. It leaves unspecified the afferent activity needed to control ingestion, which is the terminal behaviour in any food-seeking sequence. This problem can be circumvented by using sucrose in solution (or some other sweet-tasting compound), particularly if the fluid is presented via an intraoral catheter, because this eliminates the added complexity of food-seeking behaviour[7]. When added to food, sucrose appears to provide little additional information for rats, but in the absence of other sensory cues, rats treat sucrose as food[8]. In the oral cavity, sucrose is detected by gustatory receptors and, as far as is known, primary gustatory sensory neurons terminate only in the nucleus of the solitary tract in the medulla[9]. Although some sensitivity to sucrose exists in each of the gustatory receptor subpopulations, in rats the taste buds in and near the nasoincisor ducts on the anterior hard palate are particularly sensitive to sugars and other compounds that taste sweet to humans[6,10]. Thus, sucrose can substitute for more complex foods, its peripheral receptors and primary afferent neurons are known, and the first central synapse of these neurons has been specified. In addition, this 'model food' has other pragmatic advantages. Sucrose solutions are easy to quantify and to deliver into the oral cavity. Water serves as an almost perfect control stimulus. Other sapid substances, such as quinine HCl, also elicit reliable behaviours that result in rejection of fluid from the oral cavity.

GASTROINTESTINAL STIMULI

If the oral sensory characteristics of food are complex, the sequence of events set off when food enters the GI tract is staggering (and well beyond the scope of this paper). The list of signals that might serve as feedback to terminate a meal includes activity in neurons that innervate the gut wall or the liver and hormonal responses to food or its circulating constituents and to the circulating consituents themselves. In fact, candidates in each of these categories have been shown to inhibit feeding behaviour. Stomach distension drives specific vagal afferent axons and, at least at large values, inhibits intake[11]. Both while in the gut and after entering the portal circulation, constituents of food such as carbohydrates, simple sugars, amino acids and fatty acids, activate vagal and other splanchnic afferent neurons[12]. When introduced into the stomach or directly into the duodenum, relatively small amounts of fat or carbohydrates reduce feeding behaviour[13]. The contribution of peripheral sensory neural signals in this inhibition cannot be stated accurately, but it is far from complete. Severing vagal or splanchnic nerves alters, but does not eliminate, the inhibiting effect that food in the gut has upon ingestive behaviour[14]. Similarly, the absorbed, circulating products of digestion, such as glucose or free fatty acids, have the potential for signalling satiety. Unless rapidly absorbed substances are used, however, these fluxes do not change significantly in the systemic circulation until after a normal meal has ended. Thus, if they provide information, it probably influences intermeal interval, rather than meal size.

The remaining candidate signals for terminating ingestion are the various peptide hormones and neurotransmitters that are known to be released during the early phases of digestion. Given exogenously, many of these peptides do inhibit food intake (Table 1)[15]. The three peptides most extensively investigated for their possible role in inducing satiety are cholecystokinin (CCK), bombesin and glucagon. All three apparently act on the periphery, because they do not cross the blood–brain barrier and are effective in producing satiety when given i.p.[16]. In addition, the satiating potency of each peptide can be blocked or attenuated by section of visceral nerves. The satiating influence of glucagon can be attenuated by section of just the hepatic branch of the vagus[17]. Blunting the CCK effect requires at least bilateral section of the gastric branches of the vagus[18]. Bombesin

Table 1 Gut peptides that inhibit food intake

Gut peptide	Inhibition of feeding	Inhibition of sham feeding	Toxic signs
Cholecystokinin	Yes	Yes	No
Bombesin	Yes	Yes	No
Gastrin	Yes	No	No
Secretin	Yes	No	No
Glucagon	Yes	No	No
Insulin	Yes	*	No
Somatostatin	Yes	*	No
Neurotensin	Yes	*	Yes
Substance P	Yes	*	Yes
Pancreatic polypeptide	Yes	*	No
Gastric inhibitory peptide	Yes	No	No

*Peptide has not been tested
(Reproduced with permission from Smith, ref. 15)

continues to exhibit its satiating potential until both subdiaphragmatic vagal trunks are cut and much of the sympathetic nervous system has been disconnected from the spinal cord[19].

Of the three, CCK is best suited as a probe for examining the central neural mechanisms that control ingestive behaviour. Although perhaps mediated by a single vagal branch, the satiation induced by glucagon can be modulated by an interaction between the diurnal cycle and the degree of food deprivation[20]. Bombesin not only has access to the CNS over a variety of visceral nerves, but also influences both meal size and intermeal interval, perhaps for as long as 24 h after a single exogenous dose[21]. Cholecystokinin, on the other hand, influences meal size alone and, at least at low doses, this influence is mediated by vagal neurons. In addition, we have demonstrated recently that the satiating potency of CCK is mediated by afferent fibres in the subdiaphragmatic vagus rather than by efferents alone or by a combination of visceral afferent and efferent fibres[22].

This demonstrationw as made possible by two distinct features of the rat vagus nerves (Figure 1). First, intracranially, the vagus separates into afferent

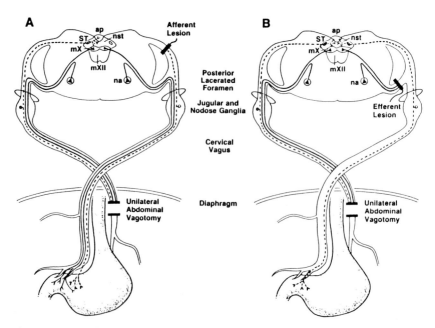

Figure 1 Schematic representation of the surgical preparations required for selective bilateral section of the **A** afferent or **B** efferent axons in the abdominal vagus nerves. The upper half of the diagrams shows the arrangement of the vagus nerves with respect to the medulla (coronal section); the lower half diagrams show the arrangement of the abdominal vagus nerves with respect to the lower oesophagus and the stomach. Dashed lines show the course of afferent axons, heavy solid lines show the course of efferent axons. Abbreviations: ap, area postrema; mX, dorsal motor nucleus of the vagus; mXII, hypoglossal nucleus; na, nucleus ambiguus; nst, nucleus of the solitary tract; ST, solitary tract (reproduced with permission from Smith *et al.*, ref. 22)

and efferent rootlets which segregate in two dimensions. The afferent fibres of the vagus and glossopharyngeal nerves reach the dorsolateral surface of the medulla as 2–4 rootlets at the level of the posterior lacerated or jugular foramen. The efferent axons collect into small rootlets which exit from the ventrolateral surface of the medulla further caudally and then run rostrally along the medial side of the accessory nerve to exit via the jugular foramen. Within the medulla, this separation is evident in the fact that vagal afferent axons penetrate the *dorsolateral* surface of the *rostral* medulla and form the descending solitary tract. The majority of vagal efferent fibres arise from cells in the dorsal motor nucleus of the vagus in the *caudal* medulla and exit from its *ventrolateral* surface[23]. Thus, within the cranium, vagal afferent axons are separated from most vagal efferent axons both dorsoventrally and anteroposteriorly. Given this anatomical separation, if the jugular foramen is expanded medially, it is possible to expose the ventral and lateral aspects of the medulla and to sever selectively either the afferent or efferent rootlets of the vagus under direct visual control (Norgren and Smith, in prep.).

The second important characteristic of the rat vagus is that, although the nerves rotate more than 90° around the oesophagus below the diaphragm, very few fibres actually switch from one trunk to the other[24]. Thus, if the afferent rootlets are cut intracranially on one side and the entire subdiaphragmatic trunk is severed before the vagus that reaches the contralateral medulla, then the subdiaphragmatic vagus is bilaterally de-afferented, but only unilaterally de-efferented. Conversely, if the efferents are cut intracranially, the subdiaphragmatic vagus is bilaterally de-efferented, but only unilaterally de-afferented.

In the paradigm used for our experiments, 6.0 μg/kg of synthetic CCK-8 results in an approximate 50% reduction in the spontaneous intake of a liquid diet. Given this dose of CCK, rats with their subdiaphragmatic vagus bilaterally de-afferented fail to exhibit premature satiety. Those with their subdiaphragmatic vagus bilaterally de-efferented are not different than control animals[22].

Cholecystokinin shares some of the advantages of sapid sucrose in that it is a quantifiable, chemically specific stimulus which is easy to deliver and whose sensory message reaches the CNS over defined afferent nerves that terminate in the nucleus of the solitary tract. It differs from the gustatory stimuli because relatively little is known about the nature of the critical sensory message. There are high-affinity CCK receptors concentrated in vagal axons[25] and on the circular muscle of the pylorus[26]. Exogenous CCK slows gastric emptying and induces gastric contractions[27]. Both these actions undoubtedly elicit indirect afferent activity in vagal nerves, but the receptors in vagal axons could also result in direct stimulation of afferent activity. Of the peptides that induce satiety, none is associated with identifiable visceral afferent activity. In fact, none of the suspected neural, hormonal or humoral factors has been established as contributing toward normal satiety under physiological conditions. Perhaps more discomfiting, none has been excluded either. This leaves us with CCK as a convenient probe for a model system, but without the reassurance offered by oral sucrose, that the experimental probe can serve as a minimal stimulus in the real world.

FEEDING BEHAVIOUR

For many species feeding behaviour is an elaborate process that requires considerable knowledge of the environment. An animal must not only find food, but do so in a manner that outwits possible competitors and avoids potential predators. Nature food sources are not uniformly distributed in time, density or quality. Successful foraging includes some notion of where and when a particular food will be available, as well as memory of the nutritional consequences of consuming it. Regardless of the diversity of behaviour and knowledge required for successful living in the wild, the final common behaviour in the process is ingestion or rejection. At least to an inexperienced animal, it is usually the oral and perhaps olfactory stimuli arising from food that determines whether it will be ingested and swallowed or rejected from the oral cavity.

Some years ago, Dr Harvey Grill and this author developed a procedure for examining this final decision in the sequence of feeding without any interference from the behaviours that normally precede it[7]. Rats are implanted with chronic intraoral cannulas that permit calibrated infusions of fluid stimuli. The animal's oral motor response to these stimuli is videotaped and subsequently scored by replaying the tape in slow motion or frame by frame. This procedure, subsequently dubbed the 'taste reactivity taste', elicits a lexicon of behavioural subunits that, depending upon the composition of the fluid stimuli, combine sequentially to produce a characteristic ingestive sequence, an equally distinct rejection sequence or graded composites of both sequences (Figure 2)[28]. The distinctiveness of these behaviours and their temporal relationship to swallowing have been ascertained using chronic EMG recording (Figure 3)[29]. The utility of the taste reactivity test as a model for more conventional measures of feeding behaviour has been documented

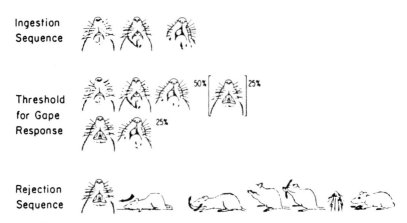

Figure 2 Behavioural units of the ingestion sequence (top), the rejection sequence (bottom) and a mixed sequence (middle). The ingestion sequence consists of mouth movements, tongue protrusions, and lateral tongue movements. The rejection sequence consists of gapes, chin rubs, head shakes, face washing, forelimb shaking, and paw wiping (reproduced with permission from Grill, ref. 28)

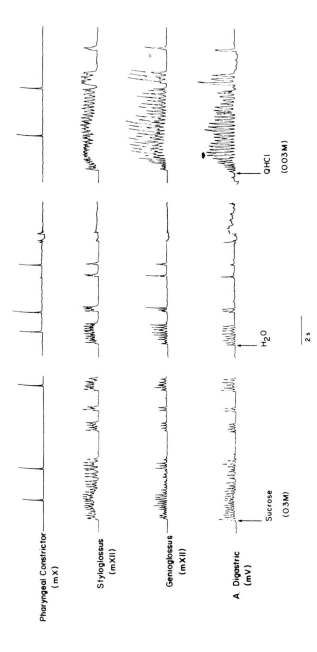

Figure 3 Integrated electromyographic activity from four muscles involved in oral motor activity after intraoral infusions of 0.3 M sucrose (left), distilled H_2O (centre), and 0.03 M quinine HCl (right). The low amplitude activity in the styloglossus, genioglossus and anterior digrastric muscles reflects mouth movements and tongue protrusions; the lower frequency, larger-amplitude activity (large arrowhead, lower right panel) reflects gaping. The isolated deflections in the pharyngeal constrictor channel indicate individual swallows (reproduced with permission from Travers and Norgren, ref. 29)

by using it with standard metabolic challenges that influence spontaneous food and fluid intake[28]. For present purposes, the most important of these challenges are food in the gut and injections of CCK. In most cases, a rat's orofacial response to a weak sucrose solution switches from one associated with ingestion to one associated with either active or passive rejection of the contents of the oral cavity[30]. Despite using simplified stimuli and abbreviated behaviour, this preparation preserves the essential elements of regulated feed behaviour, i.e. the response to the same oral signal can be changed as a function of signals from the gut that are normal consequences of ingested food. The same paradigm also contains the characteristics necessary for a model of motivated behaviour[31].

NEURAL CONTROL

For almost 40 years, the neural control of feeding behaviour was vested in the hypothalamus. The model was simple: after a meal, a ventromedial satiety centre inhibited a more lateral hypothalamic feeding centre. The heuristic value of a simple hypothesis, years of apparently confirmatory evidence and substantial scientific inertia maintained this conception as current for more than a decade as contradictory experiments accumulated. Indeed, some evidence for non-hypothalamic and even non-limbic system control was abroad by the early 1960s[32]. The critical events in undermining the hypothalamic theory of feeding behaviour have been reviewed elsewhere[33]. For the sake of brevity, these experiments can be grouped into three categories: (1) those demonstrating that the deficits attending hypothalamic lesions were not specific to feeding (and drinking) behaviour; (2) those implicating non-hypothalamic areas in the control of feeding behaviour; and (3) those documenting residual control of feeding behaviour in the absence of hypothalamic function.

In the present context, the experiments in the third category are most relevant because they establish the amount of CNS tissue necessary to support the rudiments of regulated ingestive behaviour. The original reason for developing the taste reactivity test was to develop a metric for examining ingestion and rejection in animals that fail to eat spontaneously. In our initial experiments, we tested two such preparations: the chronic thalamic rat and the chronic decerebrate rat[34]. The chronic thalamic preparation has all of its brain removed rostral to the thalamus and hypothalamus. Although the animals have what appear to be a histologically normal hypothalamus, they never again feed themselves. The chronic decerebrate preparation, in which the hypothalamus is neurally disconnected from the brainstem, also fails to feed itself, but in the taste reactivity tests it produces virtually normal oral motor responses to sapid stimuli, i.e. it ingests chemicals at the same concentrations that neurologically normal rats ingest them, and it rejects chemicals at the same concentrations that normal rats reject them. When food deprived, these chronic decerebrate preparations also reduce their intake of sucrose solution in the face of either a gastric preload of their normal milk diet or an injection of CCK (Figure 4)[30].

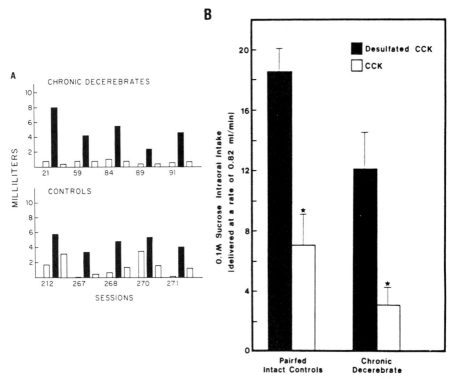

Figure 4 Intake of sucrose solutions by chronic decerebrate rats and pair-fed, intact controls with and without exogenous satiating stimuli. **A**: Intake of 0.03 M sucrose during three sequential daily tests in which the rats (numbers below abcissa) had been either tube-fed (12 ml milk diet; open bars) or 24 h food deprived (dark bars). **B**: Intake of 0.1 M sucrose after injections of either synthetic CCK octapeptide or its desulphated analogue (mean 5.8 μg/kg, i.p.) given 10 min prior to testing. In both experiments, the fluids were delivered via intraoral cannula, in A as discrete 50 μl trials and in B as a continuous infusion. **A** adapted with permission, from Grill, ref. 28 and Grill and Smith, ref. 38)

These experiments establish that at least simple forms of regulated ingestive behaviour can occur without the neural participation of the hypothalamus. The same evidence provides the final element in a minimal preparation for examining the basic neural mechanisms needed to organize meal taking in the rat.

BRAINSTEM SYSTEMS

Given a model that employs only a gustatory stimulus to elicit ingestion and a vagal visceral afferent stimulus to modulate it, within the brainstem, the neural systems capable of generating the behaviour might be quite restricted. As stated earlier, both the gustatory and vagal afferent axons first terminate in the nucleus of the solitary tract (NST), albeit at opposite ends[24,35]. Neurons in the rostral third of the NST respond to gustatory stimuli[9]; those in caudomedial NST respond to gut distension, peripheral CCK and other visceral stimuli[36]. In the rat, neurons from all levels of the

455

nucleus of the solitary tract project to the pontine parabrachial nuclei (PBN), with some evidence that the organization is at least partially maintained[37]. Neurons in the caudomedial parabrachial nuclei also respond to gustatory stimuli[38]. Although less well documented, various visceral afferent stimuli, such as changes in blood pressure, activate parabrachial neurons as well[39]. Of possible gastrointestinal related stimuli, apparently only intraportal sodium infusions have been used to test PBN neurons for visceral sensory responses[40]. Nevertheless, within the brainstem, two sets of nuclei contain sensory neurons that respond to the oral and abdominal stimuli, including those that serve in a reduced model for feeding behaviour.

Ingestion and rejection require the co-ordinated activity of neurons in the trigeminal motor nucleus, the facial nucleus and the hypoglossal nucleus. If swallowing is added, then neurons in and near the nucleus ambiguus must be included. Forebrain and cerebellar neurons do not project directly into the oral motor nuclei and, likewise, only a few cells in the midbrain appear to synapse in these nuclei. In rats, the interneurons that project to the oral motor nuclei are restricted to the midlateral parvicellular reticular formation extending from the level of the trigeminal motor nucleus caudally almost to the obex[41]. Within this distribution, modest concentrations of interneurons exist close to both the PBN and the NST but, otherwise, the cells are scattered among other neurons of similar morphology. Some of these other neurons make up the superior and inferior salivatory nuclei[42], and the same area is reputed to contain the pattern generator for rhythmic jaw movements[43]. In one recent experiment in anaesthetized rats, neurons ventral to NST that sent axons to either the facial or trigeminal motor nucleus were spontaneously silent and, for the most part, could not be excited by intraoral fluid stimuli or even by pinching the tongue[44].

The connections between the NST and the PBN and the reticular formation are not well characterized. Axons from all levels of NST pass through the parvicellular reticular formation on their way to the parabrachial nuclei, but synaptic connections en route have not been documented. By one estimate, however, only 25% of gustatory neurons in NST have axons that reach the pons[45]. In the rat at least, few if any gustatory neurons project rostral to the pons or into the spinal cord[38]. Thus, the axons of many second-order taste neurons must terminate within the NST itself or within the reticular formation. In some species, substantial anatomical and electrophysiological evidence exists for axonal connections between NST and specific respiratory and blood pressure regulatory zones within the reticular formation[46]. Although most PBN neurons apparently project to the forebrain, these nuclei also have local connections. If the adjacent Kolliker–Fuse nucleus is included, there are neurons that project through the reticular formation caudally to NST, as well as into the intermediolateral cell columns in the spinal cord[47]. All this anatomy provides a potential substrate for oral and visceral stimuli to influence the generation of ingestive behaviour in the brainstem, but no hints about specific mechanisms. The available electrophysiological experiments add only a little more.

INTERACTIONS

In the decerebrate preparation, the interaction of oral and visceral afferent neural activity that switches ingestion to rejection could occur at four different levels: on the periphery; in the nucleus of the solitary tract; in the parabrachial nuclei; and in the reticular formation systems that generate the behaviour. As mentioned in the introduction, salt deprivation altered the sensitivity of some peripheral gustatory neurons in the chorda tympani to sapid sodium[3]. Large doses of CCK (10–$15\,\mu$g/kg) apparently had little effect on the integrated chorda tympani response to gustatory stimuli[48]. The chorda tympani nerve, however, contains many axons that exhibit high sensitivity to NaCl, but very few that respond well to sucrose. Parallel effects have been reported for gustatory neurons in the NST: salt deprivation altered the sensitivity of second-order taste cells to sapid soium, but intravenous CCK had little effect[49]. The same research group has observed that intravenous infusions of glucose can reduce multi-unit responses in the NST to sapid sucrose[50]. Both stomach inflation and electrical stimulation of the cervical vagus influenced the responses of neurons in and near the NST which responded to real or surrogate gustatory stimulation[51]. A somewhat different paradigm failed to demonstrate any interaction between portal infusions of hypertonic saline or stimulation of the hepatic vagus and NST gustatory neurons[52]. On the periphery and in the first central relay, attempts to influence gustatory activity with humoral or visceral challenges have been equivocal. Each of these tests was carried out in anaesthetized rats. In unanaesthetized preparations (monkeys), the only direct test of the influence of satiation on gustatory responses in the NST was entirely negative[53].

Using the same paradigm, Rolls and his colleagues reported that presumed fifth-order gustatory neurons in orbitofrontal cortex reduced their responses to a particular sapid stimuli when that chemical was used to satiate the animal[54]. When a few neurons were tested in the anterior insula, an area known to receive projections from the thalamic gustatory relay[55], satiation had no influence on their responsiveness to sapid stimuli[56]. Aside from demonstrating that GI stimuli can influence the neural response to gustatory stimuli, the importance of these observations in behaving monkeys is difficult to assess. Although anencephalic humans exhibit differential responsiveness to sapid stimuli, the influence of satiation on these responses has not been reported[57]. If primates do have a primitive satiety system in the brainstem, it probably does not involve the nucleus of the solitary tract. It is possible, however, that such a system is not complete in the primate brainstem because, in Old World monkeys at least, the gustatory system appears to bypass the parabrachial nucleus, i.e. second-order gustatory neurons in the NST project monosynaptically to the thalamic gustatory relay[58].

In rodents, the parabrachial nuclei not only appear to be an obligatory synapse in the central gustatory projections, but also these nuclei are emerging as a crossroads for oral sensory, visceral afferent and other brainstem neural systems equal to that found in the nucleus of the solitary tract. In addition to receiving gustatory and visceral afferent projections from the NST, the parabrachial nuclei receive substantial projections from the spinal trigeminal nuclei, the spinal cord and the bulbar reticular formation[59]. For both the NST and the PBN, much of the evidence predicting complex interactions of sensory and other neural systems derives from anatomical data. Electrophysiological efforts at establishing convergene or interactions between the sensory systems that pass through the NST and PBN remain few and are scattered across disciplines[2]. A few relevant studies involving the NST were summarized above; even fewer relate to the PBN. Injections of hypertonic saline into the hepatic portal system excite some neurons in the PBN that also are driven by sapid sodium stimuli[52]. Similarly, a subset of PBN gustatory neurons also responded to electrical stimulation of either the cervical vagus nerve or the caudal, visceral afferent end of the NST[60]. In an ongoing study, we have yet to observe convincing evidence that stomach inflation influences parabrachial gustatory neurons (Evey and Norgren, unpublished observations, 1988). Although some interaction of gustatory and visceral sensory activity occurs both in the nucleus of the solitary tract and in the parabrachial nuclei, the relevance of the interactions to the onset and maintenance of satiety remains unclear.

The remaining level of possible interaction, the reticular formation systems that actually generate the oral motor ingestion and rejection behaviours, requires both anatomical and electrophysiological work before questions can be framed. As with many opposing functions, the muscles involved in both behaviours are much the same; only the pattern of activity changes[29]. The neuroanatomy of the system, therefore, seems unlikely to differentiate between the behaviours, because the motoneurons and most of the interneurons involved will be in common. Within the interneuronal network, it is necessary to identify cells with activity patterns that differ depending upon the behaviour being generated. It is this quality of a decision variable that distinguishes the analysis of ingestion and rejection from its subcomponent behaviours, such as rhythmic jaw movements or swallowing. Nevertheless, compared with ingestion, the neurophysiology of mandibular movement or swallowing is advanced[61] and provides a framework for examining the organization of rhythmic oral motor sequences.

Each of the components of ingestion or rejection behaviour consists of punctuated rhythmic movements that occur in various orders. This implies that an individual behavioural unit—a tongue protrusion or a swallow—may have separate, perhaps ballistic, generating circuits. The sequencing of these behavioural units is orderly and largely independent of sensory feedback or at least oral sensory feedback[62]. A change in visceral sensory feedback, however, can alter the sequence of behavioural units generated by the same oral stimulus. If oral and visceral afferent activity does not interact within the sensory relays of the NST and PBN, then the interaction probably involves the neurons that sequence the behavioural subunits. At minimum, these neurons must receive converging input from gustatory and visceral afferent areas and they must include or project to the interneurons that control the activity of the oral motor nuclei. Integrative areas with similar functional properties, such as the 'walking generator' in the midbrain[63] or the cardiovascular and respiratory areas of the ventral medulla[64], are distinct from the neurons which govern their behavioural subunits. Based on analogy with the interneurons involved in jaw movements and swallowing, however, the ingestion and rejection systems probably exist in close association with the oral sensory and motor nuclei.

Acknowledgement

Mrs Meredith Tulli's assistance with the bibliography was appreciated. The author's research reported here was supported by NIH (NS 20397) and the paper was written during a Research Scientist Development Award, Level II (MH 00653).

References

1. Young, R., Gibbs, J., Antin, J., Holt, J. and Smith, G. P. (1974). Absence of satiety during sham-feeding in the rat. *J. Comp. Physiol. Psych.*, **87**, 795–800
2. Norgren, R. (1983). Afferent interactions of cranial nerves involved in ingestion. *J. Autonom. Nerv. Syst.*, **9**, 67–77
3. Contreras, R. J., Frank, M. E. (1979). Sodium deprivation alters neural responses to gustatory stimuli. *J. Gen. Physiol.*, **73**, 569–94
4. Iwasaki, K., Kasahara, T. and Sato, M. (1985). Gustatory effectiveness of amino acids in mice: behavioral and neurophysiological studies. *Physiol. & Behav.*, **34**, 531–42
. Pritchard, T. C. and Scott, T. R. (1982). Amino acids as taste stimuli. II. Quality coding. *Brain Research*, **253**, 93–104
5. Sclafani, A. (1987). Carbohyrate taste, appetite, and obesity: An overview. *Neurosci. Biobehav. Rev.*, **11**, 131–53
6. Travers, S. P. and Norgren, R. (1987). Responses of neurons in the nucleus of the solitary tract to lingual and palatal stimulation with preferred chemicals. Proceedings of the Ninth International Symposium on Olfaction and Taste. *Ann. N Y Acad. Sci.*, **510**, 673–6
7. Grill, H. J. and Norgren, R. (1978). The taste reactivity test. I. Mimetic responses to gustatory stimuli in neurologically normal rats. *Brain Research*, **143**, 263–79
8. Mook, D. G. (1974). Saccharin preference in the rat: Some unpalatable findings. *Psych. Rev.*, **81**, 475–90
9. Norgren, R. (1984). Central neural mechanisms of taste. In Brookhart, J., Darien-Smith, I. and Mountcastle, V. (eds.) *Handbook of Physiology—The Nervous System III, Sensory Processes*, pp. 1087–28. (Washington DC: American Physiological Society)
10. Travers, S., Pfaffmann, P. and Norgren, R. (1986). Convergence of lingual and palatal gustatory neural activity in the nucleus of the solitary tract. *Brain Research*, **365**, 305–20
11. Paintal, A. S. (1973). Vagal Sensory Receptors and their reflex effects. *Physiol. Rev.*, **53**(1), 159–222
. Smith, M., Pool, R. and Weinberg, H. (1962). The role of bulk in the control of eating. *J. Comp. Phyiol. Psych.*, **55**, 115–20
12. Mei, N. (1986). Intestinal chemosensitivity. *Physiol. Rev.*, **65**, 211–37
13. Deutsch, J. A. and Gonzalez, M. F. (1981). Gastric fat content and satiety. *Physiol. & Behav.*, **26**, 673–6
. Liebling, D. S., Eisner, J. D., Gibbs, J. and Smith, G. (1975). Intestinal satiety in rats. *J. Comp. and Physiol. Psychol.*, **89**, 955–65
. Snowdon, C. T. (1975). Production of satiety with small intraduodenal infusions in the rat. *J. Comp. & Physiol. Psych.*, **88**, 231–8
. Tordoff, M. G. and Friedman, M. I. (1986). Hepatic portal glucose infusions decrease food intake and increase food preference. *Am. J. Physiol.*, **251**, R192–6
. Yin, T. H. and Tsai, C. T. (1973). Effects of glucose on feeding in relation to routes of entry in rats. *J. Comp. & Physiol. Psychol.*, **85**, 258–64
14. Kraly, F. S. and Gibbs, J. (1980). Vagotomy fails to block the satiating effect of food in the stomach. *Physiol. & Behav.*, **24**, 1007–10
. Louis-Sylvestre, J., Servant, J., Molimard, R. and Le Magnen, J. (1980). Effect of liver denervation on the feeding pattern of rats. *Am. J. Physiol.*, **239**, R66–70
15. Smith, G. P. (1983). The role of the gut in the control of food intake. *Viewpoints on Digestive Diseases*, **15**, 1–4

16. Oldendorf, W. H. (1981). Blood-brain barrier permeability to peptides: Pitfalls in measurement. *Peptides*, **2**(Suppl. 2), 109–11

17. Geary, N. and Smith, G. P. (1983). Selective hepatic vagotomy blocks pancreatic glucagon's satiety effect. *Physiol. & Behav.*, **31**, 391–4

18. Smith, G. P., Jerome, C., Cushin, B. J., Eterno, R. and Simansky, K. J. (1981). Abdominal vagotomy blocks the satiety effect of cholecystokinin in the rat. *Science*, **213**, 1036–7

19. Stuckey, J. A., Gibbs, J. and Smith, G. P. (1985). Neural disconnection of gut from brain blocks bombesin induced satiety. *Peptides*, **6**, 1249–52

20. Geary, N., Farhoody, M. and Gersony, A. (1987). Food deprivation dissociates pancreatic glucagon's effects on satiety and hepatic glucose production at dark onset. *Physiol. & Behav.*, **39**, 507–11

21. Mindell, S., DiPoala, J., Weiner, S., Gibbs, J. and Smith, G. P. (1985). Bombesin increases postprandial intermeal interval. *Soc. Neurosci. Abstr.*, **11**, 38

22. Smith, G. P., Jerome, C. and Norgren, R. (1985). Afferent axons in the abdominal vagus mediate the satiety effect of cholecystokinin in the rat. *Am. J. Physiol.*, **249**, R638–41

23. Contreras, R., Beckstead, R. and Norgren, R. (1982). An autoradiographic examination of the central distribution of the trigeminal, facial, glossopharyngeal and vagus nerves in the rat. *J. Auton. Nerv. Syst.*, **6**, 303–22

24. Norgren, R. and Smith, G. P. (1988). Central distributon of subdiaphragmatic vagal branches in the rat. *J. Comp. Neurol.*, **273**, 207–23

25. Moran, T. H., Smith, G. P., Hostetler, A. M. and McHugh, P. (1987). Transport of cholecystokinin (CCK) binding sites in subdiaphragmatic vagal branches. *Brain Res.*, **415**, 149–52

26. Smith, G. T., Moran, T. H., Coyle, J. T., Kuhar, M. J., O'Donohue, T. L. and McHugh, P. R. (1984). Anatomical localization of cholecystokinin receptors to the pyloric sphincter. *Am. J. Physiol.*, **246**, R127–30

27. Moran, T. J. and McHugh, P. R. (1982). Cholecystokinin suppresses food intake by inhibiting gastric emptying. *Am. J. Physiol.*, **242**, R491–7

28. Grill, H. (1980). Production and regulation of ingestive consummatory behavior in the chronic decerebrate rat. *Brain Res. Bull.*, **5**, 79–87

29. Travers, J. B. and Norgren, R. (1986). An electromyographic analysis of the ingestion and rejection of sapid stimuli in the rat. *Behav. Neurosci.*, **100**, 544–55

30. Grill, H. J. and Norgren, R. (1978). Chronic decerebrate rats demonstrate satiation but not baitshyness. *Science*, **201**, 267–9
Grill, H. J. and Smith, G. P. (1988). Cholecystokinin decreases sucrose intake in chronic decerebrate rats. *Am. J. Physiol.*, **254**, R853–6

31. Miller, N. E. (1957). Experiments on motivation: Studies combining psychological, physiological and pharmacological techniques. *Science*, **126**, 1271–8

32. Morgane, P. J. (1965). Alterations in feeding and drinking behavior of rats with lesions in globi pallidi. *Am. J. Physiol.*, **201**, 420–8

33. Norgren, R. and Grill, H. (1982). Brainstem control of ingestive behavior. In Pfaff, D. W. (ed.), *Physiological Mechanisms of Motivation*, pp. 99–131. (New York: Springer-Verlag)

34. Grill, H. J. and Norgren, R. (1978). The taste reactivity test. II. Mimetic responses to gustatory stimuli in chronic thalamic and chronic decerebrate rats. *Brain Res.*, **143**, 281–97

35. Hamilton, R. and Norgren, R. (1984). Central projections of gustatory nerves in the rat. *J. Comp. Neurol.*, **222**, 560–77

36. Raybould, H. E., Gayton, R. J. and Dockray, G. J. (1985). CNS effects of circulating CCK8: involvement of brainstem neurones responding to gastric distension. *Brain Res.*, **342**, 187–90
Kahrilas, P. J. and Rogers, R. C. (1984). Rat brainstem neurons responsive to changes in portal blood sodium concentration. *Am. J. Physiol.*, **247**, R792–9

37. Norgren, R. (1978). Projections from the nucleus of the solitary tract in the rat. *Neuroscience*, **3**, 207–18

38. Norgren, R. and Pfaffmann, C. (1975). The pontine taste area in the rat. *Brain Res.*, **91**, 99–117

39. Hamilton, R. B., Ellenberger, H., Liskowsky, D. and Schneiderman, N. (1981). Parabrachial areas as mediator of bradycardia in rabbits. *J. Auton. Nerv. Syst.*, **4**, 261–81

40. Rogers, R., Novin, D. and Butcher, L. (1979). Electrophysiological and neuroanatomical studies of hepatic portal osmo- and sodium receptive afferent projections within the brain. *J. Auton. Nerv. Syst.*, **1**, 183–202

41. Travers, J. B. and Norgren, R. (1983). Afferent projections to oral motor nuclei in the rat. *J. Comp. Neurol.*, **220**, 280–98
42. Contreras, R., Gomez, M. and Norgren, R. (1980). Central origins of cranial nerve parasympathetic neurons in the rat. *J. Comp. Neurol.*, **190**, 373–94
43. Chandler, S. H. and Tal, M. (1986). The effects of brain stem transections on the neuronal networks responsible for rhythmical jaw muscle activity in the guinea pig. *J. Neurosci.*, **6**, 1831–42
44. Evey, L., Travers, J. and Norgren, R. (1987). Characteristics of medullary neurons that project to the facial or trigeminal motor nuclei in the rat. *Soc. Neurosci. Abstr.*, **13**, 854
45. Ogawa, H., Imoto, T. and Hayama, T. (1984). Responsiveness of solitario-parabrachial relay neurons to taste and mechanical stimulation applied to the oral cavity in rats. *Exp. Brain Res.*, **54**, 349–58
46. Ross, C. A., Ruggiero, D. A. and Reis, D. J. (1985). Projections from the nucleus tractus solitarii to the rostral ventrolateral medulla. *J. Comp. Neurol.*, **242**, 511–34
47. Saper, C. B. and Loewy, A. D. (1980). Efferent connections of the parabrachial nucleus in the rat. *Brain Res.*, **197**, 291–317
48. Gosnell, B. A. and Hsiao, S. (1982). Lack of effect of cholecystokinin on the integrated chorda tympani response. *Soc. Neurosci.*, **8**, 201
49. Giza, B., Scott, T. and Antonucci, R. (1987). Cholecystokinin administration does not influence taste-evoked activity in rat NTS. *Soc. Neurosci. Abstr.*, **13**, 880
. Mark, G., Jacobs, K. and Scott, T. (1987). Taste responses in the NTS of Na-deprived rats. *Soc. Neurosci. Abstr.*, **13**, 333
50. Giza, B. and Scott, T. R. (1983). Blood glucose selectively affects taste-evoked activity in rat nucleus tractus solitarius. *Physiol. Behav.*, **31**, 643–50
51. Glenn, J. F. and Erickson, R. P. (1976). Gastric modulation of gustatory afferent activity. *Physiol. Behav.*, **16**, 561–8
. Bereiter, D. A., Berthoud, H. R. and Jeanreaud, B. (1981). Chorda tympani and vagus nerve convergence onto caudal brain stem neurons in the rat. *Brain Res. Bull.*, 7, 261–6
52. Hermann, G. E., Kohlerman, N. J. and Rogers, R. C. (1983). Hepatic-vagal and gustatory afferent interactions in the brainstem of the rat. *J. Auton. Nerv. Syst.*, **9**, 477–95
53. Yaxley, S., Rolls, E. T., Sienkiewicz, Z. J. and Scott, T. R. (1985). Satiety does not affect gustatory activity in the nucleus of the solitary tract of the alert monkey. *Brain Res.*, **347**, 85–93
54. Rolls, E. T., Yaxley, S., Sienkiewicz, Z. J. and Scott, T. R. (1985). Gustatory responses of single neurons in the orbitofrontal cortex of the macaque monkey. *Chem. Sens.*, **10**, 443
55. Pritchard, T. C., Hamilton, R., Morse, J. and Norgren, R. (1986). Projections from thalamic gustatory and lingual areas in the monkey. *Macaca Fascicularis. J. Comp. Neurol.*, **244**, 213–28
56. Yaxley, S., Rolls, E. T. and Sienkiewicz, Z. J. (1988). The responsiveness of neurons in the insular gustatory cortex of the macaque monkey is independent of hunger. *Physiol. & Behav.*, **42**, 223–9
57. Steiner, J. E. (1977). Facial expressions of the neonate infant indicating the hedonics of food-related chemical stimuli. In Weiffenbach, J. M. (ed.) *Taste and Development: The Genesis of Sweet Preferences.* Bethesda, MD: US Dept. of Health, Education, and Welfare, Public Health Service National Institutes of Health)
58. Beckstead, R., Morse, J. and Norgren, R. (1980). The nucleus of the solitary tract in the monkey: Projections to thalamus and other brainstem nuclei. *J. Comp. Neurol.*, **90**, 259–82
59. Cechetto, D., Standert, D. and Saper, C. (1985). Spinal and trigeminal dorsal horn projections to the parabrachial nucleus in the rat. *J. Comp. Neurol.*, **240**, 153–60
. King, G. W. (1980). Topology of ascending brainstem projections to nucleus parabrachialis in the cat. *J. Comp. Neurol.*, **191**, 615–38
60. Hermann, G. E. and Rogers, R. C. (1985). Convergence of vagal and gustatory afferent input within the parabrachial nucleus of the rat. *J. Auton. Nerv. Syst.*, **13**, 1–17
61. Amri, M. and Car, A. (1988). Projections from the medullary swallowing center to the hypoglossal motor nucleus: a neuroanatomical and electrophysiological study in sheep. *Brain Res.*, **441**, 119–26
. Chandler, S. and Tal, M. (1987). Brain-stem perturbations during cortically evoked rhythmical jaw movements: Effects of activation of brain-stem loci on jaw muscle cycle characteristics. *J. Neurosci.*, 7, 463–72

62. Berridge, K. C. and Fentress, J. C. (1987). Deafferentation does not disrupt natural rules of action syntax. *Behav. Brain Res.*, **23**, 69–76
    Berridge, K. C., Fentress, J. C. and Parr, H. (1987). Natural Syntax rules control acton sequence of rats. *Behav. Brain Res.*, **23**, 59–68
63. Garcia-Rill, E. and Skinner, R. D. (1987). The mesencephalic locomotor region. I. Activation of a medullary projection site. *Brain Res.*, **411**, 1–12
64. Caverson, M. M., Ciriello, J. and Calaresu, F. R. (1983). Direct pathway from cardiovascular neurons in the ventrolateral medulla to the region of the intermediolateral nucleus of the upper thoracic cord: an anatomical and electrophysiological investigation in the cat. *J. Auton. Nerv. Syst.*, **9**, 451–75
    Feldman, J. L., Loewy, A. D. and Speck, D. F. (1985). Projections from the ventral respiratory group to phrenic and intercostal motoneurons in cat: an autoradiographic study. *J. Neurosci.*, **5**, 1993–2000

Section V
Psychovisceral and behavioural aspects of gut function and dysfunction

36
Psychopathology in patients with irritable bowel syndrome

W. E. WHITEHEAD, P. ENCK, J. C. ANTHONY AND M. M. SCHUSTER

INTRODUCTION

Irritable bowel syndrome (IBS) is frequently thought to be a psychosomatic disorder because studies of medical clinic samples show a strong correlation between psychopathology and the diagnosis of IBS. In different studies 70–80% of patients are found to score in the abnormal range on various psychometric tests[1-11] and, when psychiatric interviews are used to assign psychiatric diagnoses, 72–100% of patients in medical clinic samples are found to have psychiatric disorders[2,12,13]. Moreover, more than half of patients with IBS report that their bowel symptoms are made worse by psychological stress[6,14,15].

Although these studies show a strong association between psychopathology and the diagnosis of IBS, they do not exhibit specificity. The types of psychological symptoms vary among patients with IBS: some IBS patients do not have clinically significant psychological symptoms, and the average symptom profile is similar to that seen in other chronic pain syndromes[9]. This lack of specificity is not compatible with a mechanistic interpretation in which psychological symptoms are seen as causes of IBS.

In the experiments which are summarized below, we sought to re-examine the relationship of psychopathology to IBS. To evaluate specificity, we added a control group of patients with lactose malabsorption (LMA), since lactose malabsorbers have chronic bowel symptoms which are indistinguishable from the symptoms of IBS but which are thought to be adequately explained by an absence of the enzyme lactase[16]. We have also compared medical clinic patients to people in the community who have the same bowel symptoms but who have not sought medical care for these symptoms. This enabled us to evaluate the hypothesis that psychological traits do not cause bowel symptoms but only influence which patients with bowel symptoms consult a doctor. Lastly, we have evaluated the contribution of a specific psychological mechanism, parental encouragement of the sick role during childhood, to the development of IBS.

PSYCHIATRIC DIAGNOSES IN IBS PATIENTS

Three studies[2,12,13] have been published in which the research diagnostic criteria of Feighner[17] or the operational criteria published in the third edition of the *Diagnostic and Statistical Manual of the American Psychiatric Association*[18] were used to assess the presence of psychiatric disorders in patients with IBS. These studies included 16 to 29 patients with IBS. The proportion of IBS patients found to have diagnosable psychiatric disorders was 72%[13] to 100%[2]. The spectrum of psychiatric disorders identified in these samples varied, but when the samples were pooled, the most common diagnoses were major depression (20%), generalized anxiety disorder (14%) and hysteria (20%). The diagnosis of hysteria was made on the basis of Feighner criteria[17], not on the basis of the current criteria for somatization disorder.

We used the Diagnostic Interview Schedule (DIS)[19] to detect psychiatric disorders in our study of 19 IBS patients, 19 LMA patients, and 10 normal controls. The DIS is a structured interview which was developed for the NIMH study of the epidemiology of mental illness in the United States. It is administered by lay interviewers and is scored by a computer program. Validation studies suggest that diagnostic decisions made on the basis of the DIS agree well with decisions made by psychiatrists using DSM III criteria, although the DIS appears to underestimate the prevalence of somatization disorder. In this study we employed interviewers who had participated in the East Baltimore component of the NIMH study; they were supervised by a psychologist who had also participated as a trainer/supervisor in the NIMH study.

Patients in our study were referred from the outpatient clinic of the Francis Scott Key Medical Center Division of Digestive Disease. Consecutive referrals who met the inclusion criteria were invited to participate in a psychological evaluation and in a study of colon motility and myoelectric activity. Patients were referred to the study if they complained of abdominal pain plus constipation or diarrhoea but had no evidence of a disease process based on their history and a physical examination by a gastroenterologist. All were tested for lactose intolerance by the hydrogen breath technique[20], and those who showed an increase in breath hydrogen concentration of $\geqslant 22$ ppm within three hours after ingesting 50 g of lactose were diagnosed LMA. The remainder were diagnosed IBS. Normal controls were recruited by advertisement and were paid to participate. Controls were also tested for lactose intolerance.

The results are shown in Figure 1. In contrast with previous studies[6,12,13], only 47% of IBS patients were found to have psychiatric diagnoses. This was significantly greater (significance of difference between proportions, $Z = 2.27$, $p < 0.05$) than the 20% of normal controls who had psychiatric diagnoses, but it was not different from the 42% of LMA patients with psychiatric diagnoses.

The most frequent diagnoses in both IBS patients and lactose malabsorbers were major depression, generalized anxiety disorder and phobias. Figure 1 gives the lifetime prevalence of these disorders in the Baltimore community[21]

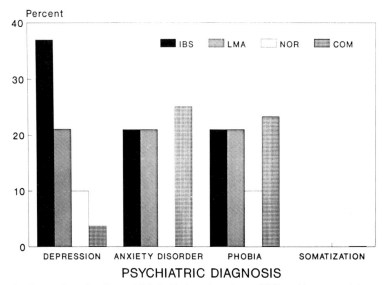

Figure 1 Proportion of patients with irritable bowel syndrome (IBS), and lactose malabsorption (LMA) who had psychiatric diagnoses when evaluated by the Diagnostic Interview Schedule[19]. Normal controls are abbreviated NOR. The lifetime prevalence of these diagnoses in the Baltimore community[21] is abbreviated COM

for comparison. It is apparent that the frequency of generalized anxiety disorders and phobias in IBS patients were consistent with the prevalence of these disorders in the community, but the prevalence of depression was greater in IBS patients than in the community. Based on psychometric tests completed by these same patients (see below) we also expected to see a high incidence of somatization disorder. No patient met criteria for this diagnosis, but this appears to be due to test insensitivity. The lietime prevalence of somatization disorder in the community made by the same criteria was also very low (0.17%).

PSYCHOMETRIC TESTING IN MEDICAL CLINIC PATIENTS WITH IBS

The subjects who participated in DIS interviews also completed the following psychometric tests: the Beck Depression Inventory[22], the trait scale of the Spielberger State–Trait Anxiety Inventory[23], the Pilowski Illness Behavior Questionnaire[24], and the Neuroticism–Extroversion–Openness Inventory[25]. For these comparisons, the IBS patients were subdivided into those who met restrictive diagnostic criteria for IBS given below[11] and those who satisfied more general criteria of abdominal pain plus altered bowel habits, which we refer to henceforth as functional bowel disorder (FBD). The restrictive diagnostic criteria were adapted from Manning *et al.*[26] and consisted of pain which is relieved by defaecation plus at least two of the following: looser stools with the onset of pain; more frequent stools with pain onset; abdominal distension; mucous by rectum; and a feeling of incomplete evacuation.

The psychometric data are given in Figures 2–4. IBS patients had significantly higher scores than normal controls on the Beck Depression Inventory (Figure 2), the Spielberger State–Trait Anxiety Scale (Figure 3) and on four subscales of the Illness Behaviour Questionnaire (Figure 4). They also tended to score higher than controls on the neuroticism scale of the NEO Inventory, but this difference was not statistically significant. These results are consistent with previously published reports[1–10] on IBS but, unfortunately, they are not specific to IBS; patients with other disorders (e.g. headaches) show similar psychological profiles[9]. Moreover, patients with LMA showed significant elevations on some of the same scales which distinguished IBS patients from normals.

SELF-SELECTION HYPOTHESIS

The finding that lactose malabsorbers, for whom there is an adequate organic explanation for bowel symptoms, had amounts and types of psychopathology similar to those seen in IBS patients raised doubts about whether psychological symptoms could be considered to be causally related to the development of bowel symptoms in IBS. One possible explanation for these findings was that psychological symptoms were unrelated to (i.e. independent of) bowel symptoms but influenced which of a spectrum of patients with IBS would decide to consult a physician.

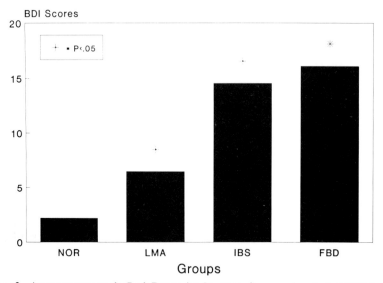

Figure 2 Average scores on the Beck Depression Inventory for normal controls (NOR), lactose malabsorbers (LMA), patients with irritable bowel syndrome (IBS) and patients with functional bowel disorder (FBD). Asterisks indicate that the group is significantly more depressed than the normal control group

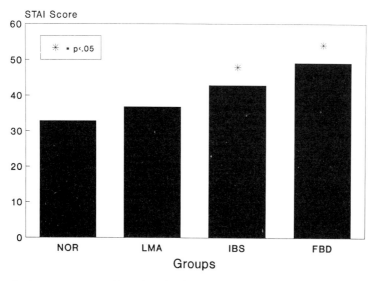

Figure 3 Average scores on the trait scale of the Spielberger State–Trait Anxiety Inventory. Abbreviations same as for Figure 2

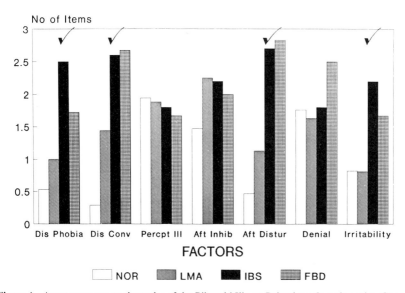

Figure 4 Average scores on the scales of the Pilowski Illness Behaviour Questionnaire. Groups are defined as in Figure 2. Scales are Disease Phobia (Dis Phobia), Disease Conviction (Dis Conv), Psychological vs. Somatic Perception of Illness (Percpt Ill), Affective Inhibition (Aft Inhibit), Affective Disturbance (Aft Distur), Denial, and Irritability. Check marks indicate that IBS patients were significantly different from normal controls

To test the self-selection hypothesis, we[11] compared women who had symptoms of IBS or LMA for which they had not consulted a doctor to a new sample of medical clinic patients with these disorders. The non-consulters were recruited by contacting the leaders of church women's societies and charities and asking them to participate in a study of bowel symptoms and psychological symptoms in exchange for a contribution to the organization's treasury. We were successful in recruiting 149 women who were demographically similar to our medical clinic population. These women were given a bowel symptom questionnaire to identify those who met diagnostic criteria for IBS or FBD, and a lactose breath test to identify lactose malabsorbers. A control group of women without bowel symptoms was also studied. After excluding women who had consulted a doctor for bowel symptoms (approximately 20% of each group), we were left with 16 IBS patients, 26 FBD patients and 28 LMA patients. These women were compared with 10 IBS patients, 12 FBD patients and 23 LMA patients who were evaluated in the medical clinic. Women in both samples completed the Hopkins Symptom Checklist[28].

The results, which are shown in Table 1, provided strong support for the self-selection hypothesis. For each diagnostic group, medical clinic patients showed more psychological symptoms than community non-consulters. Moreover, patients who satisfied restrictive diagnostic criteria for IBS, but had not consulted a doctor, had no more psychological symptoms than control subjects without bowel symptoms. This is shown for the standard scales of the MMPI in Table 2, for MMPI factor scores derived by Costa's group[29] in Table 3, for the NEO Inventory in Table 4, and for the Cornell Medical Index in Table 5. This suggests that psychological traits are unrelated to the development of IBS and that the correlation between psychological symptoms and IBS which is seen in medical clinic samples is an artifact of self-selection.

It is of some interest to note that non-consulting subjects who met criteria for FBD, but did not meet the more restrictive criteria for IBS, had significantly more psychological symptoms than asymptomatic controls on several psychometric inventories (Tables 1–5). Further analysis of this association showed that the global symptom index of the Hopkins Symptom Checklist and other measures of neuroticism were correlated significantly with the vague complaint of abdominal pain but not with reports of constipation or diarrhoea. Moreover, when subjects answered that their abdominal pain was relieved by defaecation and was associated with a change in bowel habits, there was no association with psychopathology. This suggests that a vague complaint of abdominal pain is not a reliable symptom of bowel dysfunction.

LEARNED ILLNESS BEHAVIOUR

The influence of psychological symptoms on self-selection for treatment is compatible with the psychiatric concept of somatization disorder or the older concept of hypochondriasis. However, this concept falls short of providing

Table 1 Medical clinic patients compared to community non-consulters on Hopkins symndrome checklist. Group means with standard deviations in parenthesis.

	Non-consulters				Medical clinic			Statistically significant effects
	NOR	FBD	IBS	LMA	FBD	IBS	LMA	
Somatization	0.43 (0.37)	0.73 (0.60)	0.34 (0.29)	0.55 (0.33)	1.27 (0.88)	1.34 (0.75)	1.22 (0.67)	S
Obsessive-compulsive	0.67 (0.53)	0.92 (0.71)	0.55 (0.55)	0.73 (0.51)	1.8 (0.94)	1.32 (1.07)	1.00 (0.73)	S
Interpersonal sensitivity	0.57 (0.49)	0.73 (0.66)	0.60 (0.64)	0.49 (0.35)	1.13 (0.99)	0.93 (0.85)	0.66 (0.57)	S
Depression	0.64 (0.49)	0.94 (0.91)	0.56 (0.63)	0.59 (0.50)	1.85 (1.88)	1.15 (0.76)	1.21 (0.89)	S/D
Anxiety	0.36 (0.33)	0.67 (0.81)	0.46 (0.80)	0.38 (0.31)	1.03 (0.84)	0.95 (1.22)	0.87 (0.64)	S
Hostility	0.31 (0.35)	0.71 (0.84)	0.30 (0.36)	0.36 (0.27)	1.25 (0.86)	1.05 (0.89)	0.65 (0.67)	S/D
Phobia	0.07 (0.14)	0.23 (0.39)	0.09 (0.17)	0.13 (0.19)	0.69 (0.94)	0.51 (0.87)	0.38 (0.42)	S
Paranoia	0.36 (0.43)	0.50 (0.39)	0.25 (0.44)	0.32 (0.36)	0.83 (0.79)	0.83 (0.98)	0.52 (0.56)	S
Psychoticism	0.25 (0.36)	0.35 (0.54)	0.17 (0.26)	0.13 (0.17)	0.78 (0.82)	0.32 (0.45)	0.27 (0.32)	S/D
Global symptoms index	0.45 (0.32)	0.69 (0.60)	0.41 (0.44)	0.46 (0.30)	1.08 (0.76)	1.01 (0.73)	0.87 (0.48)	S
Number of subjects	46	26	16	28	12	10	23	

S = Significant main effect for medical clinic sample vs. community non-consulters
D = Significant main effect for diagnosis: FBD vs. IBS vs. LMA.

471

Table 2 MMPI K-corrected scores in non-consulters. Group means with standard deviations in parentheses.

	FBD	IBS	LMA	NOR
HS	16.37 (4.66)^N	13.53 (2.67)^F	13.66 (3.05)^F	14.01 (3.45)
D	22.42 (6.72)	20.69 (5.34)	19.61 (3.87)	21.37 (4.85)
HY	24.58 (5.61)^N	20.94 (3.47)^F	21.04 (3.86)^F	22.02 (4.20)
PD	22.39 (4.94)	22.39 (3.68)	20.22 (4.01)	20.53 (4.10)
MF	39.81 (3.88)	38.69 (3.36)	39.61 (4.28)	39.04 (3.58)
PA	10.31 (3.54)	10.00 (2.97)	8.43 (2.90)^F	9.94 (3.62)
PT	29.88 (6.57)^N	27.56 (3.24)	26.14 (4.48)^F	27.18 (3.82)
SC	28.69 (6.92)	26.63 (2.83)	26.29 (3.79)	26.37 (5.15)
MA	18.37 (3.42)	17.91 (3.86)	18.58 (3.67)	18.16 (4.60)
SI	30.27 (10.44)	26.06 (12.33)	27.75 (6.98)	28.06 (8.10)
Number of subject	26	16	28	49

N indicates the group is significantly ($p < 0.05$) different from normal controls.
F indicates the group is significantly ($p < 0.05$) different from the FBD group.

Table 3 MMPI-GRC factor scores in non-consulters. Group means with standard deviations in parentheses.

	FBD	IBS	LMA	NOR
Neuroticism	24.77 (11.32)	20.56 (12.09)	18.00 (10.53)^F	20.53 (9.36)
Psychoticism	9.85 (7.36)	8.38 (6.78)	5.89 (3.53)^F	8.55 (7.02)
Religiosity	13.85 (4.44)	11.25 (3.57)^N	14.82 (5.25)^I	14.55 (4.66)
Extroversion	11.35 (4.19)	13.38 (5.52)	13.18 (2.87)	12.82 (4.20)
Cynicism	10.19 (5.24)	10.88 (5.39)	10.89 (5.20)	11.10 (5.58)
Somatic complaints	9.04 (6.35)^N	5.88 (4.50)	5.71 (5.20)^F	6.22 (5.58)
Inadequacy	11.62 (6.06)	10.13 (6.97)	11.29 (6.28)	11.49 (4.92)
Openness	7.58 (2.02)	7.75 (1.81)	8.21 (1.71)	7.22 (2.23)
Femininity	17.42 (3.56)	19.38 (3.05)^N	16.00 (3.13)^I	16.84 (4.14)
Number of subjects	26	16	28	49

N indicates the group is significantly ($p < 0.05$) different from normal controls.
F indicates the group is significantly ($p < 0.05$) different from the FBD group.
I indicates the group is significantly ($p < 0.05$) different from the IBS group.

Table 4 Neuroticism–extroversion–openness inventory scores in non-consulters. Group means with standard deviations in parentheses.

	FBD	IBS	LMA	NOR
Neuroticism	35.88 (6.60)^N	32.38 (9.13)	31.11 (5.27)^F	32.38 (7.62)
Extroversion	34.65 (4.83)	36.63 (7.81)	37.46 (3.77)^F	35.04 (7.11)
Openness	40.77 (4.85)	41.31 (9.39)	40.71 (4.65)	38.98 (7.44)
Agreeableness	38.19 (3.62)	38.44 (4.62)	39.86 (3.82)	39.38 (7.07)
Conscientiousness	29.69 (6.86)	29.25 (4.77)	31.89 (7.08)	30.26 (7.27)
Number of subjects	26	16	28	47

N indicates the group is significantly ($p < 0.05$) different from normal controls.
F indicates the group is significantly ($p < 0.05$) different from the FBD group.

472

Table 5 Cornell medical index scores in non-consulters group, means with standard deviations in parentheses.

	FBD	IBS	LMA	NOR
Sensory	1.46 (0.90)	2.31 (2.80)	1.29 (1.12)	1.43 (1.04)
Respiratory	1.27 (1.15)	1.25 (1.53)	1.25 (1.43)	1.04 (1.43)
Cardiovascular	2.31 (1.95)[N]	1.50 (1.55)	1.32 (1.42)[F]	1.20 (1.63)
Digestive	3.35 (2.95)[N]	2.63 (2.25)	2.43 (1.81)	2.12 (2.05)
Musculoskeletal	0.88 (1.37)	0.88 (1.36)	0.79 (1.07)	0.76 (1.27)
Skin	0.88 (1.18)	0.81 (1.22)	0.61 (1.26)	0.45 (1.00)
Neurological	1.88 (2.07)	1.44 (1.21)	1.21 (1.60)	1.14 (1.32)
Genitourinary	2.81 (1.98)	2.44 (2.50)	2.43 (1.57)	2.27 (1.92)
Fatigue	0.81 (1.50)	0.44 (0.89)	0.50 (1.00)	0.61 (1.08)
Illness frequency	0.31 (0.88)	0.00 (0.00)	0.00 (0.00)	0.08 (0.28)
Miscellaneous diseases	2.19 (1.70)[N]	2.38 (2.00)[N]	1.46 (1.29)	1.45 (1.39)
Activity	1.58 (1.06)[N]	1.00 (0.97)	0.79 (0.88)[F]	0.84 (1.14)
Anxiety	1.58 (2.32)	1.31 (1.89)	1.00 (1.70)	1.18 (1.75)
Depression	0.65 (1.41)[N]	0.31 (0.79)	0.07 (0.38)[F]	0.33 (0.72)
Nervousness	1.69 (1.49)	1.06 (1.53)	0.64 (1.13)[F]	0.96 (1.15)
Sensitivity	1.42 (1.63)	0.94 (1.18)	0.50 (0.75)[F]	0.96 (1.15)
Irritability	1.35 (1.67)[N]	0.63 (1.09)	0.36 (0.62)[F]	0.57 (0.87)
Fearfulness	1.38 (2.04)	1.38 (2.00)	0.71 (1.21)	0.73 (0.95)
All physical symptoms	19.73 (11.73)[N]	16.44 (11.56)	14.07 (8.64)[F]	13.39 (8.79)
All psychological symptoms	8.8 (8.47)[N]	5.63 (6.86)	3.29 (3.84)[F]	4.73 (4.69)
Number of subjects	26	16	28	49

N indicates the group is significantly ($p < 0.05$) different from normal controls.
F indicates the group is significantly ($p < 0.05$) different from the FBD group.

an explanation; it only names the phenomenon. We have been investigating whether childhood social learning of specific types of illness complaints may help to explain this phenomenon.

Our first study in this area[30], was a telephone interview of a random sample of 832 people in metropolitan Cincinnati. We asked a variety of questions to identify subjects with IBS, peptic ulcer disease and other presumed psychosomatic disorders. We also asked questions about the way subjects dealt with current health problems and about how their parents had responded to somatic complaints during the subject's childhood. Many of the questions dealt with how the subjects and their parents dealt with symptoms of a cold because we assumed this was a common illness experience which was objectively similar for most people.

In agreement with the suggestion made above, we found that subjects with IBS exhibited more illness behaviours suggestive of a somatization disorder than did subjects with peptic ulcer disease or asymptomatic controls. Subjects with IBS thought they had more colds than other people, felt their colds were worse than those of others, and were more likely to consult a doctor for treatment of a cold. These illness behaviours appeared not to be due simply to the presence of anxiety and depression since subjects with peptic ulcer disease reported comparable amounts of anxiety and depression, although they did not exhibit illness behaviour.

When we examined how parents had responded to cold symptoms during childhood, we found that subjects with IBS were more likely than peptic ulcer subjects or asymptomatic controls to report that their parents gave them gifts of treat foods when they had a cold as a child. We inferred that this reflected direct reinforcement of somatic complaints and supported the role of childhood social learning in the development of FBD. It is not clear from these findings, however, whether childhood social learning modified colon motility or only influenced the subject's tendency to notice and/or to report somatic complaints.

These data have not addressed the specificity of social learning about illness. In other research we[31] have found that parents respond differentially to the somatic complaints of their children and that young adult subjects tend to complain of, and to consult doctors for, the symptoms which their parents reinforced during their childhood. We are conducting additional reearch to see whether specific types of parental response to bowel complaints and modelling of bowel complaints by parents make a unique contribution to the development of FBD.

ROLE OF PSYCHOLOGICAL STRESS

Although the data now suggest that psychological symptoms are not inherently related to IBS, psychological stressors may nevertheless trigger exacerbations of bowel symptoms. Almy[32] and others[33,34] have shown that psychological stress or experimental pain can cause changes in colonic motility in both IBS patients and normal controls. Survey data collected by Drossman et al.[35] suggests that half of normals report that stress causes abdominal pain and two-thirds of normals report that stress causes a change in bowel habits. Data from laboratory stressor studies[10] and survey studies[35] suggest that IBS patients may exhibit a greater response to psychological stress than normal controls.

SUMMARY AND CONCLUSIONS

Medical clinic patients with IBS show an excess incidence of psychological symptoms, especially depression and somatization.

This association is an artifact of self-selection for treatment by neurotic indiviuals. Comparison of medical clinic IBS patients to people with the same symptoms who have not consulted a doctor shows that non-patients are psychologically normal.

Childhood social learning of specific patterns of illness behaviour provides a mechanism which may account for the association of somatization disorder with IBS.

Acknowledgements

Supported by grant DK31369 from the National Institute for Diabetes, Digestive and Kidney Diseases and by Research Scientist Award MH00133 from the National Institute of Mental Health.

References

1. Whitehead, W. E., Engel, B. T. and Schuster, M. M. (1980). Irritable bowel syndrome: Physiological and psychological differences between diarhea-predominant and constipation-predominant patients. *Dig. Dis. Sci.*, **25**, 404–13
2. Latimer, P., Sarna, S., Campbell, D., Latimer, M., Weaterfall, W. and Daniel, E. E. (1981). Colonic motor and myoelectric activity: A comparative study of normal subjects, psychoneurotic patients, and patients with irritable bowel syndrome. *Gastroenterology*, **80**, 893–901
3. West, K. L. (1970). MMPI correlates of ulcerative colitis. *J. Clin. Psychol.*, **26**, 214–29
4. Wise, T. M., Cooper, J. N. and Ahmed, S. (1982). The efficacy of group therapy for patients with irritable bowel syndrome. *Psychosomatics*, **23**, 465–9
5. Hill, O. W., Blendis, L. (1967). Physical and psychological evaluation of 'non-organic' abdominal pain. *Gut*, **8**, 221–9
6. Esler, M. D. and Goulston, K. J. (1973). Levels of anxiety in colonic disorders. *N. Engl. J.Med.*, **288**, 16–20
7. Palmer, R. L., Stonehill, E., Crisp, A. H., Waller, S. L. and Misiewicz, J. J. (1974). Psychological characteristics of patients with the irritable bowel syndrome. *Post. Grad. Med. J.*, **50**, 416–19
8. Cook, I. J., Van Eeden, A. and Collins, S. M. (1987). Patients with irritable bowel syndrome have greater pain tolerance than normal subjects. *Gastroenterology*, **93**, 727–33
9. Blanchard, E. B., Radnitz, C. L., Evans, E. D., Schwartz, S. P., Neff, D. F. and Gerardi, M. A. (1986). Psychological comparisons of irritable bowel syndrome to chronic tension and migraine headache and non-patient controls. *Biofeedback Self Regul.*, **11**, 221–54
10. Welgan, P., Meshkinpour, H. and Beeler, M. (1988). The effect of anger on colon motor and myoelectric activity in irritable bowel syndrome. *Gastroenterology*, **94**, 1150–6
11. Whitehead, W. E., Bosmajian, L., Zonderman, A. B., Costa, P. T. Jr. and Schuster, M. M. (1988). Symptoms of psychologic distress associated with irritable bowel syndrome: comparison of community and medical clinic samples. *Gastroenterology*. (In press)
12. Liss, J. L., Alpers, D. and Woodruff, R. A. Jr. (1973). The irritable colon syndrome and psychiatric illness. *Dis. Nerv. System.*, **34**, 151–7
13. Young, S. J., Alpers, D. H., Norland, C. C. and Woodruff, R. A. Jr. (1976). Psychiatric illness and the irritable bowel syndrome: Practical implications for the primary physician. *Gastroenterology*, **70**, 162–6
14. Chaudhary, N. A. and Truelove, S. C. (1962). The irritable colon syndrome: a study of the clinical features, predisposing causes, and prognosis in 130 cases. *Q. J. Med.*, **31**, 307–23
15. Hislop, I. G. (1971). Psychological significance of the irritable colon syndrome. *Gut*, **12**, 452–7
16. Paige, D. M. and Bayless, T. M. (1981). *Lactose Digestion: Clinical and Nutritional Implications.* (Baltimore: John Hopkins University Press)
17. Feighner, J., Robins, E., Guze, S., Woodruff, R., Winokur, G. and Munoz, R. (1972) Diagnostic criteria for use in psychiatric research. *Arch. Gen. Psychiatry*, **26**, 57–63
18. *American Psychiatric Association (APA): Diagnostic and Statistical Manual of Mental Disorders*, 3rd Edn. (1980). (Washington, DC: American Psychiatric Association)
19. Robins, L. N., Helzer, J. E., Croughan, J. and Ratcliff, K. S. (1981). National Institute of mental health diagnostic interview schedule: Its history, characteristics, and validity. *Arch. Gen. Psychiatry*, **38**, 381–9
20. Rosado, J. L. and Solomons, N. W. (1983). Sensitivity and specificity of the breath analysis test for detecting malabsorption of physiological doses of lactose. *Clin. Chem.*, **19**, 545–8
21. Robins, L. N., Helzer, J. E., Weissman, M. M., Orvaschel, H., Gruenberg, E., Burke, J. D. Jr. and Regier, D. A. (1984). Lifetime prevalence of specific psychiatric disorders in three sites. *Arch. Gen. Psychiatry*, **41**, 949–58
22. Beck, A. J., Ward, C. H., Mendelson, M., Mock, J. and Erbaugh, J. (1961). An inventory for measuring depression. *Arch. Gen. Psychiatry*, **4**, 561–71
23. Spielberger, C. D. (1983). *State–Trait Anxiety Inventory.* (Palo Alto: Consulting Psychologists)
24. Pilowski, S. (1983). *Manual for the Illness Behavior Questionnaire (IBQ)*, 2nd Edn. (Adelaide, Australia: University of Adelaide)

25. Costa, P. T. Jr. and McCrae, R. R. (1985). *The NEO Personality Inventory Manual.* (Odessa, Florida: Psychological Assessment Resources)
26. Manning, A. P., Thompson, W. G., Heaton, K. W. and Morris, A. F. (1978). Towards positive diagnosis of the irritable bowel. *Br. Med. J.*, **2**, 653–4
27. Whitehead, W. E. and Schuster, M. M. (1985). *Gastrointestinal Disorders: Behavioral and Physiological Basis for Treatment.* (New York: Academic Press)
28. Derogatis, L. R. (1983). *SCL-90-R: Administration, Scoring, and Procedures Manual II.* (Towson, Maryland: Clinical Psychometric Research)
29. Costa, P. T. Jr., Zonderman, A. B., McCrae, R. R. and Williams, R. B. Jr. (1985). Content and comprehensiveness in the MMPI: an item factor analysis in a normal adult sample. *Pers. Soc. Psychol.*, **48**, 925–33
30. Whitehead, W. E., Winget, C., Fedoravicius, A. S., Wooley, S. and Blackwell, B. (1982). Learned illness behavior in patients with irritable bowel syndrome and peptic ulcer. *Dig. Dis. Sci.*, **27**, 202–8
31. Whitehead, W. E., Busch, C. M., Heller, B. R. and Costa, P. T. Jr. (1986). Social learning influences on menstrual symptoms and illness behavior. *Health Psychol.*, **5**, 13–23
32. Almy, T. P. and Tulin, N. M. (1947). Alterations in colonic function in man under stress. I. Experimental production of changes simulating the 'irritable colon'. *Gastroenterology*, **8**, 616–26
33. Narducci, F., Snape, W. J. Jr., Battle, W. M., London, R. L. and Cohen, S. (1985). Increased colonic motility during exposure to a stressful situation. *Dig. Dis. Sci.*, **30**, 40–4
34. Welgan, P., Meshkinpour, H. and Hoehler, F. (1985). The effect of stress on colon motor and electrical activity in irritable bowel syndrome. *Psychosom. Med.*, **47**, 139–49
35. Drossman, D. A., Sandler, R. S., McKee, D. C. and Lovitz, A. J. (1982). Bowel patterns among subjects not seeking health care. *Gastroenterology*, **83**, 529–34

37
Neurobiological gut disorders

D. L. WINGATE

So far in this volume, emphasis has been laid upon the architecture and function of the innervation of the gut, and of the structural and functional relationships between the central (CNS) and enteric (ENS) nervous systems. The preceding sections lie within the domain of the neuroscientist; this section deals with psychophysical and behavioural aspects of human gut dysfunction, which is essentially the preverse of the clinician and psychologist. There is thus a gap to be bridged; not merely a gap between areas of scientific knowledge, but a gap between scientific disciplines. The title, 'Neurobiology of Gut Disorders', presupposes that gut disorders that are familiar to the clinician may be explained in terms that derive from the neurobiologist and, therefore, that the disjunction between neuroscience and clinical science can be remedied. Apparent dysfunction of the gut without an obvious cause that results in illness or in 'illness behaviour' is not a new phenomenon, nor is the idea that psychic (i.e. CNS) factors are implicated in such conditions. However, for the most part, such ideas have been derived from clinical observations that are essentially anecdotal rather than rigorously scientific.

The recent advance of enteric neuroscience offers the prospect that the pathophysiology of enteric neural dysfunction may become susceptible to systematic classification, as has become accepted for diseases of the CNS. Neuroscientists have defined the morphology and functional characteristics of the ENS and some of the complex linkages with CNS. Neuroendocrinologists have demonstrated homologies of specific peptide and amine neurotransmitters and neuromodulators between ENS and CNS. Neurophysiologists have demonstrated the importance of post-synaptic potential changes in the excitability of neurons within the nerve are important.

The information provided by neurobiology might be compared to the mapping of a metropolis. Just as a map may describe networks of streets and metro and bus routes, so does neurobiology describe both possible pathways and modes of transportation. However, our knowledge of cities teaches us that there are patterns of transport and communication that are not described by a map. Not all potential pathways are utilized all the time; the morning and afternoon rush hours from home to office and back again, and the evening migration to restaurants and theatres are not visible on the map. The analogy can be perused in terms of dysfunction: from our own experience we know that the narrowing of a main thoroughfare in a city can be much more disruptive than the total blockage of a side street. But even though a map is not of itself sufficient for survival in strange territory, it is an essential requisite. If, until now, physicians have seemed inept in the management of 'functional' disorders, it is because they have been travelling in uncharted territory. Must this continue? In scientific terms, it is now pertinent to ask whether the neurobiology of the gut has advanced to the point where it is possible to construct a rational taxonomy of enteric neural dysfunction that is comprehensible to scientist and clinician alike. Two avenues of recent research suggest an affirmative answer.

The first conceptual advance is that the vagus nerve is predominantly a sensory or afferent nerve. Far from being a motor nerve that conveys commands from the CNS to individual gastrointestinal effector units such as muscle or secretory cells, the vagi consist, for the most part, of afferent fibres conveying information from gastrointestinal sensory receptors to the CNS. At the simplest conceptual level, we should no longer think of the vagi as a command system from brain to gut but as an information (and perhaps also command) link from gut to brain. This raises an important question that also leads to the second major area of progress. The question is the identity of the motor neurons that control gastrointestinal effector units, if this function can no longer be attributed to the vagi. The answer is that it is now clear that the enteric nervous system provides not only the motor neurons to the muscular apparatus of the digestive tract, but also the motor programmes that govern its operation. The identification of periodic activity within the ENS, exemplified by the migrating motor complex (MMC) has, for the first time, enabled clinicians to monitor the integrity of the ENS, thereby providing an overlap between the interests of basic scientists and clinicians.

If, then, the vagus nerve can no longer be viewed as the efferent limb of a simple reflex arc, what then is the function of the 10–15% of fibres in the vagus that are clearly 'efferent'? These fibres synapse with enteric neurons — the ratio between the numbers of efferent vagal fibres and those of enteric neurons is in the order of 1:1000 to 1:10 000 — and appear to modulate the integrated output of the ENS. This has been shown directly in animal experiments by acute reversible vagal blockade, but this modulation has also been demonstrated in humans by studying the effects of waking and sleeping (CNS arousal) and the effects of somatosensory and psychological stress (CNS perturbation).

These new insights provide, for the first time, a rational biological framework into which familiar clinical phenomena may be inserted, making it indeed possible to construct a valid clinical schema of motor pathophysiology. The starting point is that motor dysfunction is, under all circumstances, a reflection of ENS dysfunction.

The simplest case is (Figure 1) neuropathy confined to the ENS: this might be considered as 'CNS-independent'. Enteric neuropathy is characterized by local deficits such as achalasia of the cardia and Hirschsprung's disease, and by rare general deficits such as visceral aganglionosis manifest as chronic

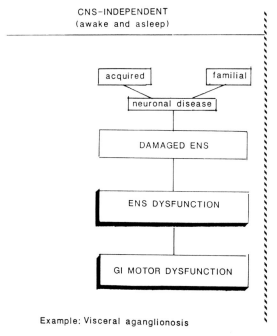

Figure 1   CNS-independent neuropathy

idiopathic intestinal pseudo-obstruction.

At the opposite end of the scale can be placed 'functional disorders' that appear to be totally 'CNS-dependent'. These are disorders that can be clearly attributed to mental stress often potentiated by psychiatric disorder. Characteristically, in such patients, symptoms subside with the withdrawal of stress and, unlike the enteric neuropathies, motor function is normal during sleep. Nevertheless, the expression of this category of disorders is (Figure 2) through enteric neural dysfunction, albeit intermittent and dependent upon CNS arousal.

The two preceding categories leave out a sizeable but unquantified fraction of the irritable bowel syndrome, where neither stress nor mental imbalance suffice to explain the abnormal modulation of gut motor activity. These are patients in whom there are suggestions of an organic aetiology. Such patients may date the onset of their illness as the sequel of an acute infective gastroenteritis, usually in the form of traveller's diarrhoea. Alternatively — or simultaneously — they may have identified dietary constituents that trigger their symptoms. In some such patients, stress may provide an additional provocation. A working supposition is that these patients suffer from irritability of enteric neurons, either due to minor damage by previous infection or due to antigenic challenge. It is possible that the sensitization may have occurred during an episode of bacterial or viral invasion. Such patients may be regarded as having dysfunction that is both CNS-dependent and CNS-independent (Figure 3) but, again, the final common pathway of

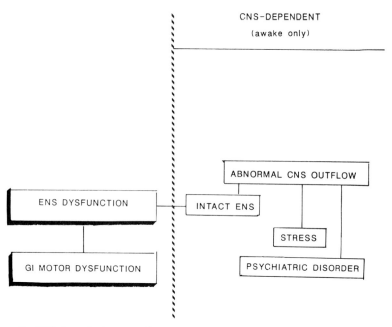

Figure 2   CNS-dependent neuropathy

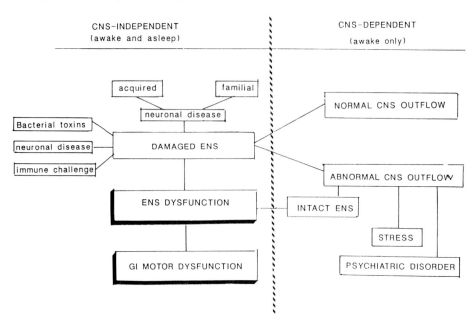

Figure 3   Both CNS-independent and CNS-dependent dysfunction (note that this figure includes Figure 2)

dysfunction is through the nerve networks of the ENS.

Fusion of these categories of disorders (Figure 4) provides a comprehensive scheme that is in accord with current knowledge and that unites both ends of the spectrum — neuropathic and psychophysiological — of enteric motor dysfunction, and that is comprehensible to basic scientist and clinician alike. It may not stand the test of time, but it may stimulate relevant research that could lead to its replacement by a better model.

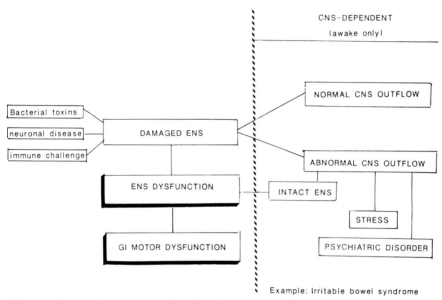

Figure 4   Neuropathic and psychophysiological enteric motor dysfunction (note that this figure includes Figures 1–3)

38
Epidemiology of the irritable bowel syndrome

W. G. THOMPSON

A functional gastrointestinal disorder may be defined as a variable combination of chronic or recurrent gastrointestinal symptoms not explained by structural or biochemical abnormalities[1]. The irritable bowel syndrome (IBS) is a functional gastrointestinal disorder attributed to the intestines with: abdominal pain, symptoms of disturbed defaecation (urgency, straining, feeling of incomplete evacuation, altered stool form (consistency) and altered bowel frequency/timing) and bloatedness or abdominal distension. Certain physiologic abnormalities have been associated with the IBS. They include a paradoxic increase in sigmoid motility in constipation, and the opposite in diarrhoea[2]; certain colon myoelectric abnormalities[3,4,5]; and increased small bowel motility in response to stress[6]. However, none of these explains how symptoms are generated or is sufficiently specific for the IBS to serve as a diagnostic marker. Even the observation that the abdominal pain of the IBS may be reproduced by intragut insufflation of balloons does not explain to what extent the IBS is a normal perception of altered physiology, or an altered perception of normal physiology[7,8].

The situation is further complicated by the likelihood that the IBS is a heterogeneous disorder. Can the diarrhoea-dominant IBS have the same pathogenesis of that of constipation, the gas–bloat syndrome or chronic abdominal pain? Will specific organic defects be found to explain the syndrome and its variants? Despite these unanswered questions, the IBS is an everyday reality in clinical practice. I will present evidence that it is very prevalent in western society, that it is chronic and that it is costly. On this basis it becomes a worthy subject of fundamental research.

PREVALENCE

In 1977 Dr Heaton and I administered a questionnaire to 301 healthy British adults (96% of those approached). There were roughly 100 young, middle-aged and elderly subjects[9]. Twenty-one per cent had experienced non-menstrual abdominal pain 6 times in the previous year, and 13.6% had their pain relieved by defaecation (Figure 1). This last group reported pain usually in the lower abdomen and were more likely than the remaining subjects to have constipation, diarrhoea and several symptoms previously shown to be associated with the irritable bowel. When defined as 'frequent loose stools' or 'frequent straining', diarrhoea and constipation occurred in 4 and 6% of these apparently healthy people. Thus functional bowel symptoms seemed to occur in 30% of the 301 subjects interviewed.

The above symptoms are indeed common in Western cultures (Table 1). Drossman and his colleagues using a modification of our questionnaire on 789 college students and hospital employees in North Carolina obtained results remarkably similar to ours[10,11]. Using random selection from the Cincinnati telephone directory Whitehead interviewed 832 people and identified the IBS in 8%[12]. Twenty-nine per cent of 1345 subjects had IBS in Michigan[13]. Using our criteria for the spastic colon type of IBS, studies in France and New Zealand report that 14% of apparently healthy subjects suffer the syndrome[14,15]. Among 202 citizens of Sydney, Australia, 32% had variable bowel habits, 8% had abdominal pain for 2 weeks or more in 6 months and 5% each had constipation and diarrhoea[16]. Less than half the respondents in these studies had reported their symptoms to a doctor (Table 1).

Functional abdominal symptoms are not confined to adults. Apley and Naish found that 11% of 1000 British schoolchildren suffered abdominal pain sufficiently severe to interfere with activities three times in 3 months[13]. There is some indication that such children are likely to have the IBS as adults.

In gastroenterology clinics in North America and Europe, 20–50% of referred patients had functional complaints, mainly the irritable bowel syndrome (Table 2)[18–24]. In contrast, the syndrome is said not to occur in

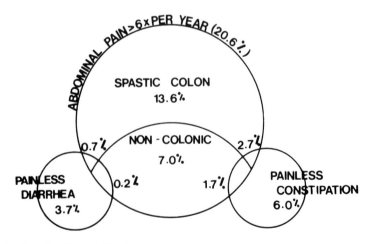

Figure 1   Functional bowel disorders in 91 (30.2%) of 301 apparently healthy individuals (non-patients) (from reference 59) see text.

Table 1 Prevalence of spastic colon type of IBS in apparently healthy individuals in several western countries

Author	Year	Study population	N	IBS (spastic colon type) %	Reported to MD (% of IBS)	Female %
Thompson and Heaton	1980[9]	UK	301	14	20	59
Drossman	1982[10]	USA	789	17	46	66
Sandler	1984[11]	USA	566	15	30	60
Whitehead	1982[12]	USA	832	8	36 (males) 49 (females)	63
Greenbaum	1984[13]	USA	1345	24	4 8	63
Welch	1985[14]	New Zealand	287	14	—	50
Bomelaer	1986[15]	France	1200	19	—	53

Table 2 Proportion of referrals to gastroenterology clinics that are functional

Author	Country	Year	Functional referrals (%)
Switz[18]	USA	1976	23
Ferguson[19]	Scotland	1977	31
Fielding[20]	Ireland	1977	52
Manning[21]	England	1977	29
Sullivan[22]	Canada	1983	17
Harvey[23]	England	1983	48
Kruis[24]	W. Germany	1984	23

Uganda[25,26]. It is rare among black South Africans living in rural areas, but the prevalence among those in urban centres is similar to that in western populations[27]. Although population studies are not available, the IBS appears to be prevalent in the Indian subcontinent and South America. One Japanese study determined that 7.1% of 356 university students and 6.1% of 400 company employees had IBS symptoms, and another found them in 20% of 2100 high school students[28,29].

The social implications of the IBS are interesting when we consider who, among the many sufferers, complain to doctors. The population studies mentioned above suggest that 50–65% of IBS sufferers are female (Table 1). In clinics, the female dominance seems to be greater (Table 3)[30-37]. In contrast, Indians and Sri Lankans who are referred to gastroenterologists for the IBS are only 20–30% female[38-41]. Thus, modern Western women with the IBS are more likely to become patients than men, whereas the opposite is the case among Indian sufferers.

Before World War II the IBS (or membranous colitis as it was then called) was said to be more common in the upper classes. A study from India indicates that the syndrome was more prevalent in private than public practice[38]. In most modern Western states where some form of health insurance is in place it is difficult to determine the importance of social class in IBS prevalence and reporting.

Table 3 Sex differences in IBS patients

Author	Year	Country	Female (%)	F/M ratio
Powel[30]	1818	England	100	1
White[31]	1905	England	85	6:1
Chaudhary and Truelove[32]	1962	England	65	2:1
Fielding[33]	1977	England	66	2:1
Ritchie and Truelove[34]	1980	England	74	3:1
Doteval[35]	1983	Sweden	70	2.5:1
Cann[36]	1983	England	80	4:1
Sullivan[22]	1983	Canada	74	3:1
Thompson[37]	1984	Canada	79	4:1
Mathur[38]	1966	New Delhi	28	1:3
Pimbarkar[39]	1970	Bombay	26	1:3
Bordie[40]	1972	Raipur	18	1:4
Mendis[41]	1982	Columbo	30	1:2

The IBS appears to be equally common in young, middle-aged and elderly healthy Western people, with the exception that constipation is more likely in the old[9]. The mean age of onset is about 29 years (range 1–63) and the interval between onset and reporting averages 4 years[20].

People with IBS symptoms who do not report them to doctors may have less severe symptoms. However, it seems likely that severity is a relatively unimportant determinant of health care seeking behaviour. As will be seen in subsequent chapters, Drossman and Whitehead established that IBS patients have more features of emotional disturbance than other patients, while IBS sufferers who do not see doctors have a psychologic make-up similar to controls[42,43]. These observations force us to consider the role of culture, sexual equality, idleness, wealth, fear of serious disease, emotion and other factors in the patient's decision to seek help.

PROGNOSIS

There is evidence that IBS sufferers have symptoms over long periods of their lives (Table 4). Chaudhary and Truelove[32] reported that 63% of their 126 patients continued to have symptoms 1–12 years later. Waller and Misciewicz[44] found little improvement in their 50 patients over 1 year. Holmes and Salter[45] found that 57 out of their 77 patients continued to suffer from the syndrome for 6 years: in only 4 was the diagnosis changed — all had benign disease. Sullivan[22] and Svendsen[46] in two further studies reported that less than 3% of their patients diagnosed as having the IBS were found to have organic disease 2 years later. Harvey[47] noted that of 97 IBS patients seen in clinic 74% remained symptomatic at 5–8 years, 26% severely so, and none had organic disease. The IBS is therefore a chronic disease and the diagnosis, once made, seldom needs revision. Data are available to support the notion that a positive diagnosis may be made with a high degree of confidence from the history[21,24]. Thus, repeated consultations or tests are inappropriate without new symptoms.

COST AND CONSEQUENCES

Irritable gut symptoms are very common amongst ordinary individuals. Although they are chronic, there is evidence neither that functional symptoms

Table 4 Prognosis in IBS

Author	Year	Patients	Follow-up (years)	Results
Chaudhary[32]	1962	126	1–10	63% still symptomatic
Waller[45]	1969	50	1	no change
Holmes[46]	1982	77	6	5% symptomatic (4 alternate benign diagnosis)
Sullivan[22]	1983	184	2	6 organic disease
Svendson[46]	1985	112	2	3 organic diseases
Harvey[47]	1987	97	5–8	74% symptomatic (26% severe), no organic disease

cause any physical harm themselves nor that they presage more serious illness. Nevertheless, many sufferers seek medical attention and become patients. Such health care seeking may trigger tests and treatments which are costly and may be more harmful to the patient's well-being than the disorder itself.

In the United States, functional gut complaints account for more physician visits that inflammatory bowel disease, and the days in hospital are similar for the two disorders[48]. The use of drugs in such a benign, non-life-threatening, non-crippling disorder staggers the imagination. Six per cent of Britons use laxatives at least weekly[9]. In the United States there are more than 120 over-the-counter medications for constipation for which $368 million was spent in 1982[49]. The cost of anticholinergics, tranquilizers, antidepressants and the countless other drugs used for functional disorders must be enormous, yet in few instances is efficacy proven.

Because of the fear of organic disease and the absence of a test that identifies the irritable gut, those sufferers of functional disorders who see doctors undergo much investigation. Of 527 outpatients in a general practice, 24% had altered bowel habit, abdominal pain or rectal bleeding[50]. Although these symptoms are said by some to be features of serious colonic disease, only one polyp was found in this group. In the remaining 76%, two cases and cancer and three polyps were found. The authors of this report concluded that a self-completed questionnaire that sought information about symptoms was 'of little value in the early detection of colorectal carcinoma'. Dent found the above symptoms so frequently among a random sample of people in Sydney that he came to the same conclusion[16]. Of 97 Ottawa outpatients referred for barium enema, in whom IBS symptoms were very common, only 18 had organic disease including 11 polyps but no cancer[51]. The complaints of IBS patients (i.e. abdominal pain, altered bowel habit, gas discomfort and even bright red blood from haemorrhoids or fissures) cause physicians to order investigations to exclude serious abdominal disease. The yield seems no greater than if asymptomatic persons were similarly tested.

Consultation, upper- and lower-gut barium contrast examinations, upper and lower endoscopy, ultrasonography and intravenous pyelography are frequently and fruitlessly performed for functional symptoms. Twenty-one of 22 patients with recurrent upper abdominal pain had their pain reproduced by balloon insufflation in the upper gut[52]. This group had 76 consultations, 72 procedures directed at the biliary tree, 53 barium studies, 25 endoscopies and 36 laparotomies, all negative. The average per patient bill for this was $1,528 in equivalent Canadian funds. Such a broadside of investigation is not only costly but dangerous. To be sure, one must be cautious of a missed colon cancer in the over-40 patient, but one should exercise some judgement.

An even more sinister consequence of the irritable gut is unnecessary surgery, a disturbing fact observed by Ryle 50 years ago[53]. Of 119 patients undergoing appendectomy, the organ was inflamed in only 60[54]. Those whose appendix was normal were far more likely than those with inflamed appendices to be female, to have had a severe emotional experience in the 6 months prior to the surgery and to continue to have bowel symptoms a year later. IBS patients were found to have undergone four times more appendectomies and in women three times more hysterectomies than a similar group with ulcerative colitis[55]. Fielding[56] found that 50 IBS patients, compared to age and sex-matched controls were very much more at risk of surgery, repeated surgery and abdominal surgery. Enquiry often reveals that the surgery resulted in the removal of a normal appendix, uterus or gall bladder and, in the case of multiple surgery, lysis of adhesions. Perhaps it should not surprise us that 16% of IBS patients in one clinic turned to alternative medicine.

CONCLUSIONS

Is the IBS a qualitative, or merely quantitative departure from the psychophysiological reactions of normal people[57]?

The IBS occurs in up to one-third of adults in Western countries, yet most do not report the symptoms. It is apparent that severity of symptoms is not the only motive a patient may have for consulting a doctor. Discovery of the cultural, fearful and emotional factors underlying the patient's visit may provide vital clues as to how that patient may best be helped. Whatever the cause of the complaints, care of such patients is costly. Clinical and basic research into the nerve–gut relationships in persons with and without symptoms should lead to a better understanding of how these symptoms are generated and/or perceived. This in turn may identify pathophysiological markers which would allow inexpensive and reliable diagnosis of the irritable bowel, reduce morbidity and save resources for the detection and cure of more serious disease. Although the symptoms of the irritable bowel are not those of cancer or IBD, these diseases may occur coincidently[37,58]. Thus, there will always be a need to be alert for the signs and symptoms of organic disease. Nonetheless, these common functional gut conditions demand a positive, confident diagnosis if the physician is to be believed by the patient and if costly, unnecessary and harmful tests are to be avoided. Improved understanding through basic and psychological research should also permit more effective treatment and halt the use of expensive and ineffective drugs, none of which are without hazard.

References

1. Thompson, W. G., Dotevall, G., Drossman, D., Heaton, K. W. and Kruis, W. (1988). Irritable Bowel syndrome: Guidelines for the Diagnosis. Working Team Report, International Congress of Gastroenterology, Rome
2. Connell, A. M. (1962). The motility of the pelvic colon. II. Paradoxical motility in diarrhoea and constipation. *Gut*, **3**, 342–8
3. Snape, W. J., Carlson, G. M. and Cohen, S. (1976). Colonic myoelectric activity in the irritable bowel syndrome. *Gastroenterology*, **70**, 326–30
4. Taylor, I., Darby, C. and Hammond, P. (1978). Comparison of recto-sigmoid myoelectrical activity in the irritable colon syndrome during relapses and remissions. *Gut*, **19**, 923–9
5. Bueno, L., Fioramonti, J., Rukebusch, Y., Frexinos, J. and Coulom, P. (1980). Evaluation of colonic myoelectrical activity in health and functional disorders. *Gut*, **21**, 480–5
6. Kumar, D. and Wingate, D. L. (1985). The irritable bowel syndrome: a paroxysmal motor

disorder. *Lancet*, **2**, 973–7

7. Swarbrick, E. T., Hegarty, J. E., Bat, L., Williams, C. B. and Dawson, A. M. (1980). Site of pain from the irritable bowel. *Lancet*, **1**, 443–6

8. Moriarty, K. J. and Dawson, A. M. (1982). Functional abdominal pain: further evidence that whole gut is affected. *Br. Med. J.*, **1**, 1670–2

9. Thompson, W. G. and Heaton, K. W. (1980). Functional bowel disorders in apparently healthy people. *Gastroenterology*, **79**, 283–8

10. Drossman, D. A., Sandler, R. S., McKee, D. C. *et al.* (1982). Bowel dysfunction among subjects not seeking health care. *Gastroenterology*, **83**, 529–34

11. Sandler, R. S., Drossman, D. A., Nathan, A. P. *et al.* (1984). Symptom complaints and health care seeking behaviour in subjects with bowel dysfunction. *Gastroenterology*, **87**, 314–18

12. Whitehead, W. E., Winget, C., Fedaravicius, A. S. *et al.* (1982). Learned illness behavior in patients with irritable bowel syndrome and peptic ulcer. *Dig. Dis. Sci.*, **27**, 202–8

13. Greenbaum, D., Abitz, L., Van Ergeren, L. *et al.* (1984). Irritable bowel syndrome prevalence, rectosigmoid motility and psychometrics in symptomatic subjects not seeing physicians [abstr.] *Gastroenterology*, **86**, 1097

14. Welch, G. W., Hillman, L. C. and Pomare, E. W. (1985). Psychoneurotic symptomatology in the irritable bowel syndrome: a study of reporters and non-reporters. *Br. Med. J.*, **291**, 1382–4

15. Bommelaer, G., Rouch, M., Dapoigny, M. *et al.* (1986). Epidemiologie des troubles fonctionnels dans une population apparement saine. *Gastro. Clin. Bio.*, **10**, 7–12

16. Dent, O. F., Goulston, K. J., Zubrzycki, J. and Chapuis, P. H. (1986). Bowel symptoms in an apparently well population. *Dis. Col. Rect.*, **29**, 243–7

17. Apley, J. and Naish, N. (1958). Recurrent abdominal pain: a field study of 1000 school children. *Arch. Dis. Child.*, **33**, 165–70

18. Switz, D. M. (1976). What the gastroenterologist does all day. *Gastroenterology*, **70**, 1048–50

19. Ferguson, A., Sircus, W. and Eastwood, M. A. (1977). Frequency of 'functional' gastrointestinal disorders. *Lancet*, **2**, 613–4

20. Fielding, J. F. (1977). A year in outpatients with the irritable bowel syndrome. *J. Ir. Med. Sci.*, **146**, 162–5

21. Manning, A. P., Thompson, W. G., Heaton, K. W. *et al.* (1978). Towards positive diagnosis of the irritable bowel. *Br. Med. J.*, **2**, 653–4

22. Sullivan, S. N. (1983). Management of the IBS: a personal view. *J. Clin. Gastrointestinol.*, **5**, 499–502

23. Harvey, R. F., Salih, S. Y., Read, A. E. (1983). Organic and functional disorders among 2000 outpatients. *Lancet*, **1**, 632–4

24. Kruis, W., Thieme, C. H., Weinzierl, M. *et al.* (1984). A diagnostic score for the irritable bowel syndrome. *Gastroenterology*, **87**, 1–7

25. Painter, N. S. (1972). Irritable or irritated bowel. *Br. Med. J.*, **2**, 46

26. Burkitt, D. P., Walker, A. R. P. and Painter, N. S. (1972). Effect of dietary fibre on stools and transit times, and its role in the causation of disease. *Lancet*, **2**, 1408–12

27. Segal, I. and Walker, A. R. P. (1984). The irritable bowel syndrome in the black community. *J. South Afr. Med.*, **64**, 885–6

28. Inoue, M. (1983). Irritable colon syndrome. *J. Clin. Med.*, **41**, 495–504

29. Kaji, I., Namiki, M. (1985). IBS. *J. Gastroenter.*, **80**, 1671–2

30. Powell, R. (1818). On certain painful affections of the intestinal canal. *Med. Trans. RCP.*, **6**, 106–17

31. White, W. M. (1905). A study of 60 cases of membranous colitis. *Lancet*, **2**, 1229–35

32. Chaudhary, N. A. and Truelove, S. C. (1962). The irritable colon syndrome. *Q. Med. J.*, **31**, 307–22

33. Fielding, J. F. (1977). A year in out-patients with the irritable bowel syndrome. *J. Ir. Med. Sci.*, **146**, 162–5

34. Ritchie, J. A. and Truelove, S. C. (1980). Comparison of various treatments for irritable bowel syndrome. *Br. Med. J.*, **281**, 1317–19

35. Dotevall, G., Svedlund, J. and Sjodin, I. (1982). Symptoms in irritable bowel syndrome. *Scand. Gastroenterol. J.*, **79** (Suppl.), 124–7

36. Cann, P. A., Read, N. W., Brown, C. *et al.* (1983). Irritable bowel syndrome relation of disorders in the transit of a single meal to symptom patterns. *Gut*, **24**, 405–11

37. Thompson, W. G. (1984). Gastrointestinal symptoms in the irritable bowel compared to peptic ulcer and inflammatory bowel disease. *Gut*, **25**, 1089–92
38. Mathur, A. K., Tandon, B. N. and Prakash, O. M. (1966). Irritable bowel syndrome. *J. Indian Med. Assoc.*, **46**, 651–6
39. Pimbarker, B. D. (1971). Irritable colon syndrome. *Indian Pract.*, **24**, 65–71
40. Bordie, A. K. (1972). Functional disorders of the colon. *J. Indian Med. Assoc.*, **58**, 451–5
41. Mendis, B. L. J., Wijesiriwardena, B. C., Sheriff, M. H. R. *et al.* (1982). Irritable bowel syndrome. *J. Ceylon Med.*, **27**, 171–81
42. Drossman, D. A., McKee, D. C., Sandler, R. S. *et al.* (1988). Psychosocial factors in the irritable bowel syndrome: a multivariate study of patients and non-patients with IBS. *Gastroent.*, **95**. (In press)
43. Whitehead, W. E., Bosmajian, L., Zonderman, A. *et al.* (1988). Psychological distress associated with irritable bowel syndrome: comparison of community and medical clinic samples. *Gastroent.*, **95**. (In press)
44. Waller, S. L., Misciewicz, J. J. (1969). Prognosis in the irritable bowel syndrome. *Lancet*, **2**, 753–6
45. Holmes, K. M. and Salter, R. H. (1982). Irritable bowel syndrome — a safe diagnosis? *Br. Med. J.*, **285**, 1533–4
46. Svendsen, J. H., Munck, L. K. and Andersen, J. R. (1985). Irritable bowel syndrome — prognosis and diagnostic safety. *Scand. J. Gastroenterol.*, **20**, 415–18
47. Harvey, R. F., Mauad, A. C. and Brown, A. M. (1987). Prognosis in the irritable bowel syndrome: a 5-year prospective study. *Lancet*, **1**, 963–5
48. *Report to the Congress of the United States of the National Commission on Digestive Diseases*, Vol. 1 (DHEW PUBL NO [NIH] 79–1878), US Dept of Health, Education and Welfare, Bethesda, Md., 1979, 10
49. Glaser, M. and Chi, J. (July 1983). Thirty-fifth annual report on consumer spending. *Drug Top*, **4**, 18–20
50. Farrands, P. A. and Hardcastle, J. D. (1984). Colorectal screening by self-completion questionnaire. *Gut*, **25**, 445–7
51. Thompson, W. G., Patel, D. G., Tao, H., *et al.* (1982). Does uncomplicated diverticular disease cause symptoms? *Dig. Dis. Sci.*, **27**, 605–8
52. Kingham, J. G. C. and Dawson, A. M. (1985). Origin of chronic right upper quadrant pain. *Gut*, **26**, 783–8
53. Ryle, J. A. (1928). Chronic spasmodic afflictions of the colon and the diseases which they simulate. *Lancet*, **2**, 1115–19
54. Creed, F. (1981). Life events and appendectomy. *Lancet*, **1**, 1381–5
55. Burns, D. G. (1986). The risk of abdominal surgery in irritable bowel syndrome. *J. South Afr. Med.*, **7**, 91
56. Fielding, J. F. (1983). Surgery and the irritable bowel syndrome: the singer as well as the song. *J. Ir. Med.*, **76**, 33–4
57. Almy, T. P. (1980). The irritable bowel syndrome: back to square one? *Dig. Dis. Sci.*, **25**, 401–3
58. Isgar, B., Harmon, M., Keye, A. D. *et al.* (1983). Symptoms of irritable bowel in ulcerative colitis in remission. *Gut*, **24**, 190–2
59. *Gastroenterology*, (1980). **79**, 283–8

39
Why does the patient with functional GI complaints go to the doctor?

D. A. DROSSMAN

INTRODUCTION

In this chapter, I will try to respond to the question posed by the title, in the light of eights year of research of the clinical, epidemiologic and psychological aspects of the irritable bowel s yndrome. The answer has clinical relevance, for bowel disturbances are common, yet only a subset of these people ever seek medical attention, and the reason they come is not fully explained by the degree of bowel dysfunction.

Also, our findings[1], recently supported by the research of Drs Whitehead and Schuster at John Hopkins University[2] and Drs Talley and Phillips from the Mayo Clinic[3], allow us to develop a new conceptualization that conveys how psychologic processes interact with the altered bowel physiology to explain the patient's experience of illness and his/her resultant behaviours. This information should allow us to put aside timeworn dualistic efforts to try to determine whether IBS is organic *or* psychiatric. Both are operative, and more will be accomplished by combining research efforts to understand both the mechanisms and the clinical consequences of the functional bowel disorders.

THE BACKGROUND

The irritable bowel syndrome is the most prevalent of the functional gastrointestinal disorders, and is characterized by chronic or recurrent bowel dysfunction, usually associated with abdominal pain. Since there is no biological marker, a diagnosis is made by clinical assessment of characteristic symptoms (pain, constipation, diarrhoea) and the absence of other medical aetiologies to explain the symptoms. In Rome, in 1988, based on the report of an international working team, Dr Thompson presented guidelines for diagnosis of irritable bowel which can be used for clinical practice and research[4].

Given our broad definition, the IBS is the most common chronic bowel disorder, and it produces a considerable health care burden. Seen primarily in young people, it is reported in 12% of primary care patients and may lead to frequent hospitalizations[5]. From a survey of the American Gastroenterological Association, we found that the IBS comprises the largest diagnostic group in a gastroenterologist's practice[6]. Despite its high prevalence, a full understanding of the mechanisms underlying the disorder eludes us, and many seek, or at least hope, to find the one aetiology that will explain the illness.

There is good evidence that physiologic disturbances underlie patient complaints. Numerous studies indicate that IBS patients have increased motor reactivity and possibly decreased pain thresholds in response to various stimuli (e.g. food, hormones, psychologic stress, rectal distension). The disorder is exhibited throughout the gastrointestinal tract and is probably mediated by a variety of biological mechanisms now under study[7]. I believe that the IBS is biologically multi-determined; it is unlikely that a single cause or treatment will be found to explain this diverse symptom complex. Furthermore, the physiologic findings are not sufficient to explain the behavioural observations seen in these patients.

Psychologically, IBS patients are abnormal. They report higher stress and neuroticism scores, and have a higher prevalence of psychiatric diagnoses. The extent of these findings cannot be attributed merely to having chronic bowel symptoms, since patients with other chronic GI diseases do not score as high. And since IBS patients *do* have physiological disturbances, we cannot say that IBS is a psychiatric disorder[7]. So trying to understand the IBS as *either* biologically *or* psychiatrically determined is insufficient.

THE QUESTION

These data seem to reflect a selection bias related to the patient subset that is selected for evaluation. Since the behavioural characteristics of non-patients with IBS had not been known, perhaps the psychologic findings characterize only those with IBS who go to the doctor. Our research group therefore decided to test the question: '*Do the psychosocial observations in IBS relate to all with bowel disturbance...or mainly to those who see physicians?*' Our hypothesis was that the previously reported abnormal psychological scores would be seen more in patients than IBS non-patients, and IBS non-patients psychologically would be similar to normals.

PRELIMINARY INFORMATION

We addressed this question in a preliminary fashion through surveys we administered in the early 1980s. Using a questionnaire[8] similar to that of Thompson's[9], we found that among our university and hospital population

15% have symptoms consistent with a diagnosis of IBS and, of this group, only 38% (6% of the survey population) have seen physicians for bowel complaints[10]. We therefore had three convenient samples to study: those with IBS symptoms who had (patients) and those who had not (non-patients) been to physicians, and subjects without bowel problems (normals).

Given that IBS patients seem to report many other symptoms, we first surveyed this population to determine whether patients were different from non-patients in the frequency of non-gastrointestinal symptoms or in their health care seeking tendencies. Indeed, we found that people with IBS symptoms who saw physicians reported 3.1 ($\pm$ 0.5) non-gastrointestinal complaints compared to 2.2 ($\pm$ 0.3) for IBS non-patients and 1.3 ($\pm$ 0.1) for normals. Then, when we controlled for the number of symptoms, we found that IBS patients were significantly more likely than the other two groups to see physicians for these other non-gastrointestinal complaints[10]. These findings indicate that bowel symptoms do not appear sufficient to explain why IBS patients go to doctors. They suggest that IBS patients are behaviourally different from IBS non-patients in the way they experience and act upon symptoms *in general*. The next step was to study whether psychologic factors influence these behaviours.

TESTING THE QUESTION

Beginning in 1983, with the collaboration of Drs Bob Sandler, Daphne McKee, Elliot Cramer, Betsy Lowman, Amy Burger and Ms Madeline Mitchell, our project co-ordinator, we undertook a more comprehensive multi-disciplinary case-control medical and psychologic evaluation of our three subject groups. IBS patients were referred from internal medicine and family medicine practices at North Carolina Memorial Hospital and the UNC Student health services. If they fulfilled our IBS criteria[8] and had a negative complete medical evaluation by us, then their data were included in the analysis. IBS non-patients were selected by survey if they fulfilled our IBS symptom criteria, had never been to a doctor for these symptoms, and also had a negative medical exaination. Normal subjects were selected if they had no bowel symptoms.

Subjects were given a battery of questionnaires including a demographic and health history questionnaire, diary cards to determine prospectively pain frequency and severity (McGill Pain Questionnaire[11]) and stool frequency, and standardized psychological tests to assess personality (Minnesota Multiphasic Personality Inventory), stressful life events (Life Experiences Survey[12]), mood (Profile of Mood States), illness behaviour (Illness Behavior Questionnaire[13]) and social support.

The data were analysed by multivariate analyses of covariance to assess differences in symptoms and psychological scores between our three groups. Because pain symptoms and stool frequency might independently lead to doctor visits and may also affect the psychosocial scores, we covaried for these symptoms in the psychosocial data analysis.

The results obtained on 238 subjects (72 patients, 82 non-patients and 84 normals)[1] were as follows. The groups consisted primarily of young white females. Seven patients (8.8%) were excluded because we found other diagnoses to explain their bowel symptoms. These included inflammatory bowel disease (2 patients), pancreatic insufficiency, dumping syndrome, lactose intolerance, persistent occult GI bleeding, infectious diarrhoea. Also, 2 non-patients were excluded when *Giardia l amblia* infections were diagnosed.

In terms of GI symptoms, patients reported more stools per week (9.8 ± 0.98) than non-patients (6.7 ± 1.0; $p < 0.001$) and normals (7.3 ± 1.0; $p < 0.004$); more days of pain (8.2 ± 0.53) than the other two groups (5.6 ± 0.54 for non-patients, 1.1 ± 0.54 for normals; $p < 0.001$) and greater pain intensity scores (McGill Pain Rating Index 9.05 ± 0.89) than the other two groups (5.64 ± 0.92 for non-patients, 3.20 ± 0.92 for normals). Patients also reported more other gastrointestinal and non-gastrointestinal symptoms but, after performing a logistic regression analysis co-varying for pain score and stool frequency, these other symptoms did not differentiate patients from IBS non-patients. In other words, abdominal pain and diarrhoea were the primary symptom predictors of patient status.

When controlling for demographic factors, pain scores and stool frequency in the multivariate analysis, we found that the psychosocial scores still discriminated the groups: patients scored significantly higher than non-patients ($p < 0.001$) and normals ($p < 0.001$), but the non-patients were not different from normals ($p = 0.207$). These findings can be demonstrated by describing some of the univariate results.

Figure 1 shows the mean values of the MMPI scales for the three groups. IBS patients had significantly higher scores than normals on scales 1 (hypochondriasis), 2 (depression), 3 (hysteria) and 7 (psychasthenia) an a lower score on Ego Strength. Also, patients had higher scores than IBS non-patients on scales L (Lie), 1 and 2 and again a lower score on Ego Strength.

Furthermore, when we look at the prevalence of clinically abnormal MMPI subscale scores (T score > 70) in each group, for most of the clinical scales (1,2,3,7,8), 20–33% of patients had pathologic scores when compared to non-patients ($< 10\%$) and normals ($\leqslant 5\%$).

These data are interpreted to mean that IBS patients have a greater tendency to report pain and other somatic complaints when under stress, to display concern about health and bodily functions, to require reassurances about their health, to have less coping ability and to deny or misrepresent psychological information so as to be seen in a favourable light. *These findings are not found to the same degree in IBS non-patients who are psychologically not different from normals.*

What about stress? When we look at the reporting of stressful life events, we get some insight not only into differences in the frequency of these events, but also the way in which stressful experiences are perceived. With the Life Experiences Survey, subjects depict meaningful life events occurring during the preceding 6 months, denote them as positive or negative, and rate them on an intensity scale 0–3. Figure 2 compares the mean positive and negative life event scores and number of life events for this test. The hatched score equals the sum of each life event multiplied by the perceived intensity or impact of that event rated 0–3.

MMPI SCALES BY GROUP
(adjusted means)

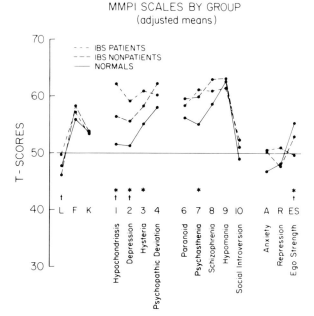

Figure 1 Minnesota Multiphasic Pain Inventory (MMPI). Adjusted mean T-scale scores for IBS patients. IBS non-patients and normal subjects. T-scale scores are derived from a normally distributed reference population. A score of 50 is the mean and 70 (2 S.D. from the mean) is considered clinically abnormal. Significant differences between groups are indicated as follows: * = patients vs. normals; + = patients vs. non-patients. $p < 0.001$ for scales 1,2,3,7; $p < 0.01$ for scale L, $p < 0.04$ for scale ES (reprinted with permission from reference 1)

As seen on the left-hand graph, patients reported lower scores for positive life events than did non-patients ($p < 0.007$) and normals ($p < 0.006$), indicating that as a group patients report fewer good experiences occurring in their lives. As shown on the right, IBS non-patients reported higher negative life event scores than normals ($p < 0.018$), but contrary to our predictions, IBS patients reported *lower* scores than non-patients and even tended to score lower than normals. However, we can also look at how a negative event was perceived and rated. Note that the ratio of the average negative score (hatched bars) to the average number of items (open bars) is less for Patients (1.1) than for the other two groups (1.9 non-patients, 1.8 normals). This suggests that IBS patients minimize the impact of negative events on their lives by rating them lower, and this is supported by the L scale differences on the MMPI. These data fit clinical observations. For example, when at a social gathering, some people, when learning of my area of research, may comment about their bowel difficulties and how it must be due to stress from work, the children, etc. However, the patient sitting in my office will not only discount these possibilities, but will defend against them (It's *definitely* not stress... everything is fine!').

Illness behaviour is another psychological dimension describing how

497

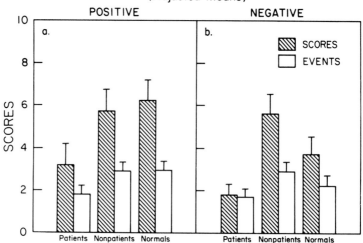

Figure 2 Life Experiences Survey (LES). **a**: positive stress; **b**: negative stress. Adjusted mean scores (hatched bars) and mean number of events chosen ($\pm$ SD of mean) for 0–6 months preceding study visit (reprinted with permission from reference 1)

symptoms are experienced and acted upon. In using the Illness Behavior Questionnaire, we found that patients reported that symptoms were more disruptive to their lives (Illness Disruption Subscale) when compared to non-patients ($p < 0.001$) and normals ($p < 0.001$). Also, patients were more concerned about health issues in general (Health Worry Subscale; $p < 0.001$) and believed illness caused more emotional distress (Affective Disturbance Subscale $p < 0.012$) than normals.

To summarize, when controlling for age and symptom differences, IBS patients are characterized by: (1) a higher frequency of pathological MMPI scores; (2) more illness behaviours; (3) fewer positive life events; and (4) a tendency to deny or minimize negative psychological states and experiences. In contrast, IBS non-patients psychologically were not different from normals and are distinguished from IBS patients by: (1) greater positive life events (LES); (2) higher ego strength; (3) fewer somatic concerns and health worries (IBQ); and (4) less denial/minimization of negative psychological states. These observations of non-patients may be adaptive psychological traits, helping to explain why they choose *not* to see physicians.

A final point to consider is: 'What is the basis for the psychologic findings among IBS patients?' The answer to this question is obviously very complex and is poorly studied (Dr Whitehead in Chapter 36 has more to say about this topic). My belief is that, in part, IBS patients may be conditioned from childhood to communicate certain feelings through bodily symptoms. For example, consider the young child who, in anticipation of beginning school, develops an anxiety attack. If rather than attending to the child's feelings about school, the parent keeps the child home because of concomitant symptoms of abdominal pain or diarrhoea, the child may deal with future episodes of anxiety through bodily complaints. As part of our research, we interviewed our study subjects to determine the possible role for early childhood events on group status[14]. We found that patients were different from normals by reporting a childhood history with more bowel complaints and reinforcement of illness behaviours as evidenced by greater parental attention when ill and more frequent school absences and doctor visits. Patients were also distinguished by reporting a higher prevalence of family illness, death and divorce, and a greater tendency toward conflicted or dependent relationships with the mother. We also found that IBS patients were distinguished from non-patients by reporting more doctor visits as a child when ill. These data suggest the possibility that, for certain families, stresses are handled through attention to illness and reinforcement of illness behaviours.

CONCUSION

We conclude that, in the IBS, the bowel disturbance is not sufficient to explain patient status. Rather our data has shown that psychological factors interact with the altered bowel physiology to determine why patients come to the doctor. These findings may serve as a model for other functional bowel disorders and possibly for chronic illness in general. Illness exists on a continuum from the experience of a physical sensation (nociception) to the recognition of it as a departure from normal (illness), to behavioural effects such as buying medication or seeing the doctor (health care utilization) and finally, to exaggerated or abnormal illness behaviours. We believe that it is the interaction of physiological and psychosocial processes that determines the person's threshold for going to a physician. So, for a given IBS patient, there may be a great deal of psychological disturbance with little physiologic findings, causing him/her to seek help or, conceivably, more physiologic effect with less psychologic disturbance. The result is that, to obtain an optimal clinical iresponse, it is important for the physician to address both the physiological and psychological determinants of the patients illness and subsequent behaviours.

Acknowledgements

Supported by Grant AM29934 from the National Institutes of Health (NIADDK) and by the Core Center in Diarrheal Diseases, University of North Carolina School of Medicine.

References

1. Drossman, D. A., McKee, D. C., Sandler, R. S., Mitchell, C. M., Cramer, E. M., Lowman, B. C. and Burger, A. L. (1988). Psychosocial factors in the irritable bowel syndrome: A multivariate study of patients and nonpatients with IBS. *Gastroenterology*, **95**, 701–8

2. Whitehead, W. E., Bosmajian, L., Zonderman, A., Costa, P. and Schuster, M. M. (1988). Role of psychological symptoms in irritable bowel syndrome: Comparison of community and clinic samples. *Gastroenterology*, **95**, 709–14

3. Talley, N. J., Phillips, S. F., Melton, L. J., Bruce, B., Hench, A. R. and Zinsmeister, A. R. (1988). A controlled study of psychosocial factors in presenters and nonpresenters with functional bowel disease (FBD). *Gastroenterology* (*Abstract*), **94**, A454

4. Thompson, W. G., Drossman, D. A., Dotevall, G., Heaton, K. W. and Kruis, W. (1988). Irritable bowel syndrome: guidelines for the diagnosis. Presented at *ROMA* 88: *XIII International Congress of Gastroenterology*, September 4–10, Rome

5. Mendeloff, A. I. (1983). Epidemiology of irritable bowel syndrome. In Chey, W. Y. (ed.) *Functional Disorders of the Digestive Tract*, pp. 13–19. (New York: Raven Press)

6. Mitchell, C. M. and Drossman, D. A. (1987). Survey of the AGA membership relating to patients with functional GI disorders. *Gastroenterology*, **92**, 1282–4

7. Mitchell, C. M. and Drossman, D. A. (1987). The irritable bowel syndrome: understanding and treating a biopsychosocial illness disorder. *Ann. Behav. Med.*, **9**, 13–19

8. Drossman, D. A., Sandler, R. S., McKee, D. C. and Lovitz, A. J. (1982). Bowel patterns among subjects not seeking health care. Use of a questionnaire to identify a population with bowel dysfunction. *Gastroenterology*, **83**, 529–34

9. Thompson, W. G. and Heaton, K. W. (1980). Functional bowel disorders in apparently healthy people. *Gastroenterology*, **79**, 283–8

10. Sandler, R. S. and Drossman, D. A. (1984). Symptom complaints and health care seeking behavior in subjects with bowel dysfunction. *Gastroenterology*, **87**, 314–18

11. Melzack, R. (1975). The McGill Pain Questionnaire: Major properties and scoring methods. *Pain*, **1**, 277–99

12. Sarason, I. G., Johnson, J. H. and Siegel, J. M. (1978). Assessing the impact of life changes: development of the life experiences survey. *J. Consult. Clin. Psychol.*, **46**, 932–46

13. Pilowsky, I. and Spence, (1983). *Manual for the Illness Behavior Questionnaire* (*IBQ*), 2nd Edn. (Adelaide: University of Adelaide Press)

14. Lowman, B. C., Drossman, D. A., Cramer, E. M. and McKee, D. C. (1987). Recollection of childhood events in adults with irritable bowel syndrome. *J. Clin. Gastroent.*, **9**, 324–30

40
Life events and the onset of functional abdominal pain

F. CREED, T. CRAIG AND R. FARMER

INTRODUCTION

Gastroenterologists have long considered that psychological factors play a major part in causing the Irritable Bowel Syndrome (IBS)[1]. But when we reviewed the literature recently we found that the evidence for this was, scientifically speaking, poor[2]. Most of the research has used questionnaires upon which IBS patients have indicated that they feel more anxious than controls. Palmer *et al.*[3] found that a group of IBS patients has a mean anxiety score higher than that of a group of normal controls; Esler and Goulston found that this was only so for those with diarrhoea as a predominant symptom[4].

There are two problems with such research. First, IBS patients seem to say 'Yes' to every symptom about which they are asked. The second is that, as Figure 1 demonstrates, many of the IBS subjects recorded their anxiety as within normal limits. Is it fair, therefore, to claim that their bowel symptoms are caused by anxiety?

Since these studies were performed there have been a number of studies which have used standardized clinical interviews, not self-rated questionnaires, and there is now good evidence[5-9] that psychiatric disorder is two to three times more common among patients with functional abdominal pain than it is in patients with organic gastrointestinal disease (Table 1). But such psychiatric disorder recorded among clinic patients might be a *consequence* of the pain, rather than its cause; unless it can be demonstrated that the psychiatric disorder *preceded* the onset of abdominal pain. Only two studies have distinguished patients with such disorder (Table 1).

In order to investigate more clearly the role of psychological factors in functional abdominal pain, we have studied the onset of bowel symptoms in relation to stressful life events (environmental changes, the paradigm of which is bereavement) and the onset of psychiatric disorder, placing great emphasis on the exact dating of each of these. In order to do this we needed groups of patients with a clear onset of abdominal pain, which could be accurately

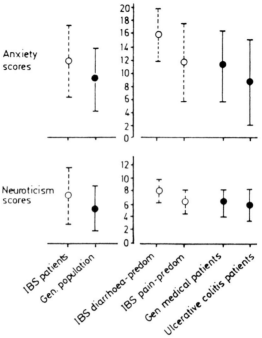

Figure 1 Anxiety scores in IBS patients compared to general population and ulcerative colitis controls according to Palmer *et al.*[3] (left) and Esler and Goulston[4] (right)

Table 1 Prevalence of psychiatric disorder, assessed using standardized interviews, among patients attending gastroenterology clinics (a) with functional abdominal pain and (b) with organic gastro-intestinal disease

	No.		Functional abdominal pain (%)	Organic disease
McDonald and Bouchier[5]	32	CIS	53	20
Colgan *et al.*[9]	37	CIS	57	6
Kingham and Dawson[6]	22	HRS	64	—
Craig and Brown[7]	79	PSE	42 (34)	18 (16)
Ford *et al.*[8]	48	PSE	42 (31)	6 (0)

CIS = Clinical Interview Schedule.
HRS = Hamilton Depression Rating Scale.
PSE = Present State Examination.
Figures in parentheses refer to psychiatric disorder that was present *before* the onset of the abdominal pain.

dated. We also needed reliable instruments that could accurately date and quantify (a) the life events and (b) any resulting psychiatric disorder.

We have applied this research method to those patients seeking treatment for abdominal pain, in order to see whether severe life events were more common before the onset of functional abdominal pain than before the onset of organic abdominal illness. By using this model, the assessment of life events can be made before it is known whether the patient will receive an organic diagnosis (such as appendicitis or peptic ulcer) or a 'functional' one (most commonly IBS), so that both patient and experimenter are 'blind' to the eventual diagnosis at the time that environmental stress is measured.

METHOD

The first study[10] chose patients aged 17–30 years undergoing appendicectomy, over one-third of whom had an appendix that was classified as not acutely inflamed. The second study[7] included patients aged 18–60 years attending a gastroenterology clinic who had a clear onset or recurrence of abdominal pain within one year of the clinic attendance. The third study[11] involved patients aged 17–35 years who were admitted to hospital having taken an overdose. These patients are well-known to have undergone recent crises and they are included in the present report to illustrate the similarity between the life changes preceding the onset of functional bowel disturbance and those preceding self-poisoning. Each of the abdominal pain groups had a community comparison group.

Measures

In order to measure psychiatric symptoms accurately we used the Present State Examination[12]. A trained interviewer establishes the presence or absence of 40 psychiatric symptoms over the preceding month. Each symptom is rated as absent, present in mild or marked form. Thus difficulty getting off to sleep during at least ten nights over the last month is scored mild if it is one hour or more, marked if it is two hours or more. To be classified as a case of psychiatric disorder a patient must have experienced 11 or more symptoms, and for the disorder to be classified as depression, for example, these 11 symptoms must include marked depressed mood together with one or more of the following: autonomic symptoms of anxiety, psychomotor slowness, pathological guilt. Such an exact definition of psychiatric disorder leads to over 90% agreement between trained psychiatrists.

The measurement of life events is more complicated. Some researchers have tried to use self-administered questionnaires, but one such questionnaire includes the item: 'Over the last six months, have you experienced concern over the health or behaviour of a family member (major illness, accidents, etc.)?' This leaves the patient to decide who is a family member, which illnesses should be considered major and the result is only dated to the nearest six months. The depressed patient with chronic abdominal pain might be so preoccupied with health problems that he or she ticks the above item on the grounds that a distant aunt has chronic heart disease, whereas a healthy control subject might ignore such illness. In this way, those with functional abdominal pain would appear to have experienced more life events than the healthy comparison group because of reporting error. In addition, the lack of exact dating means that the patient might include events ocurring *after* the onset of abdominal pain.

To ensure a truly objective and reliable measure of environmental stress the Life Events and Difficulties Schedule (LEDS)[13] defines at the outset those people to be included (usually first-degree relatives and household members only) and the exact nature of life events. For example, 'being off work' through illness is included only if the patient is off for at least four weeks; if the breadwinner in the family is off for a minimum of eight weeks; or if there is objective evidence of marked financial hardship.

When an event is recorded it is accurately dated; any events occurring after the onset of abdominal pain are excluded from subsequent analysis. The objective threat of the event is then rated by a group of experienced raters to whom the circumstances of the event are presented. Each event is rated on two four-point scales. The first scale refers to the immediate (short-term) threat; the second scale refers to the long-term threat — that which remains after one week. A house move is regarded as low threat in both the long and short-term. Accidents and examinations can score high (1 or 2) on short-term threat, but often drop to a lower rating by the end of a week. Bereavement, marital separation and the break-up of a close heterosexual relationship, on the other hand, generally carry a high threat rating on both scales (these are referred to as severe events).

Life event results are expressed as the proportion of subjects who have experienced an event of a particular type in a given period. Thirty-eight weeks is the period commonly used because this time is important in the aetiology of depression. This period is long enough to include those severe events, such as bereavement, which may affect the individual for some months afterwards, but not so long that distorted data might result from poor recall.

Statistical significance of differences between groups has been assessed using the χ^2 test.

RESULTS

The demographic details of the samples indicate that, in both studies, those with functional abdominal pain included more females whereas in the organic illness groups there was a slight predominance of males. The subjects in the gastroenterology clinic were older than those undergoing appendioectomy and a greater proportion were married. There were no significant differences between the demographic characteristics of the subjects in the self-poisoning group and those of the community comparison group for the appendicectomy study.

The commonest diagnoses in the gastroenterology clinic sample were peptic ulcer (41%) for the organic group; irritable bowel syndrome (35%), dyspepsia (18%) and abdominal pain (44%) for the functional group. For convenience, hereafter 'organic' refers to organic gastroenterology clinic patients and acute appendicitis patients; 'functional' refers to the remaining clinic patients and those with a not acutely inflamed appendix.

All the groups considered were similar in the proportion who had experienced any kind of life event over the previous 38 weeks. This result is important because it demonstrates that all groups were interviewed with similar intensity.

However, when we considered only those events rated as severely threatening in the long term (severe events) a distinct pattern emerged: the functional abdominal pain groups had experienced these severe events in a proportion similar to the self-poisoning group and significantly greater than either the organic ($p < 0.01$) or healty comparison ($p < 0.0001$) groups (Figure 2). Analysis by sex did not affect these findings. The high rate of severe events is very similar to that found in depressed patients[13].

The most frequent type of severe event in the case of the functional abdominal pain group involved a major disruption of close relationships; a marital separation, a family member leaving home or break-up of a serious girl–boyfriend relationship (Table 2). Since these events almost always

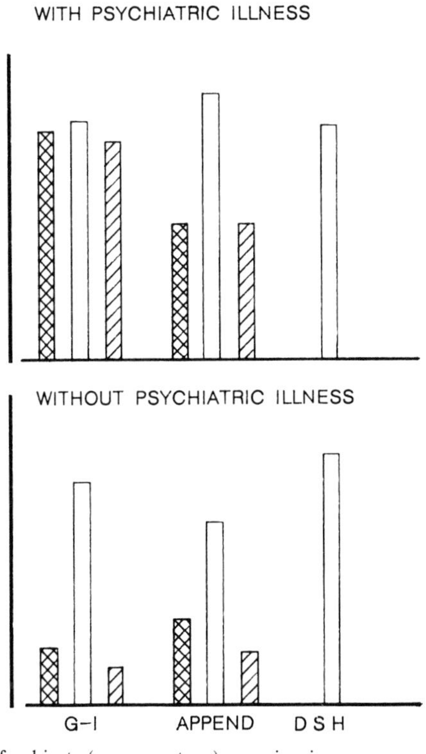

Figure 2 Proportion of subjects (as percentage) experiencing a severe event during 38 weeks before onset of abdominal pain, or interview in case of comparison subjects. (G–I = patients attending gastroenterology clinic, Append = patients undergoing appendicectomy, DSH = patients admitted following deliberate self harm).
Above: subjects with psychiatric illness; **below**: subjects without psychiatric illness. Cross hatching = organic abdominal disease (appendicitis or peptic ulcer, etc.); open bars = functional abdominal disorder (including appendix not acutely inflamed/deliberate self-harm subjects); diagonal hatching = community comparison subjects

Table 2 Proportion of subjects with a severe event categorized as a 'row'

Gastro-clinic		Appendicectomy	Percentage	DSH
Organic	5%	Acutely inflamed	6	
(n = 56)		(n = 63)		
Functional	28%*†	Not acutely inflamed	27	33%
(n = 79)		(n = 56)		(n = 80)
Comparison	7%	Comparison	2	
(n = 135)		(n = 62)		

*$p < 0.0001$ compared to community comparison group
†$p < 0.001$ compared to organic/acutely inflamed groups

included arguments we have called them 'row' events, which occurred in the functional abdominal pain groups approximately five times as often as the organic illness and healthy comparison groups, and nearly as often as those in the overdose group.

I indicated earlier that approximately one-third of the functional abdominal pain group had symptoms of depression sufficiently severe to be classified as a 'case' of psychiatric illness that had developed prior to the onset of the abdominal pain. It is therefore appropriate to consider whether the excess of severe life events found in the functional pain group is attributable to those with depression. Such events are known to be associated with the onset of depression.

To our surprise this was not the case. The lower part of Figure 2 includes only those subjects who did not have depression and, once again, the functional pain group has a clear excess of severe life events compared to the organic and community comparison groups. They are similar to those patients who take an overdose but do not have severe depression.

DISCUSSION

It has been emphasized that accurate measurement is important if we are to obtain reliable results relating environmental stress to the onset of functional bowel symptoms. This limited the present studies to those patients who have a clear onset of pain. However, many patients with chronic pain are able to describe an early acute onset (between a third and a half of clinic IBS patients have had a normal appendix removed previously[6,14–16]) and similar stress factors may have antedated their abdominal symptoms.

Our work is not entirely unique. Ford et al.[8] also used the LEDS, although they ignored depression and limited their study to anxiety. They found that the weighted life event scores for the functional pain group were twice that of the events experienced by the organic group. Canton et al.[17] used a similar method and found that patients having a normal appendix removed had experienced life events very similar to a group of depressed patients attending a psychiatrist.

The ways in which severe events may lead to patients presenting with functional abdominal pain are somewhat speculative at present. However, there is experimental evidence that emotional stress can alter colonic motility[18-20], so the experience of a severe life event may lead to painful contractions of the colon in those who are constitutionally predisposed to develop them. In addition, where psychiatric symptoms are present, depression or anxiety may lead to a lowered pain threshold and this may contribute to the experience of abdominal pain.

Since environmental stress leads to the onset of functional symptoms, reflief of the psychological problems should relieve the pain. We are working on this at present. The exact ways in which stress affect colonic function are complex and will require the combined skills of gastroenterologists, physiologists and psychiatrists.

Acknowledgements

These studies were performed while Francis Creed held a Leverhulme Mental Health Research Fellowship and Tom Craig held a Medical Research Council Grant.

References

1. Thompson, W. G. (1984). The irritable bowel. *Gut*, **25**, 305–20
2. Creed, F. H. and Guthrie, E. (1987). Psychological factors and the irritable bowel syndrome. *Gut*, **28**, 1307–18
3. Palmer, R. L., Stonehill, E., Crisp, A. H., Waller, S. L. and Misiewicz, J. J. (1974). Psychological characteristics of patients with the irritable bowel syndrome. *Postgrad. Med. J.*, **50**, 416–19
4. Esler, M. D. and Goulston, K. J. (1973). Levels of anxiety in colonic disorders. *N. Engl. J. Med.*, **288**, 16–20
5. Macdonald, A. J. and Bouchier, P. A. D. (1980). Non-organic gastrointestinal illness: a medical and psychiatric study. *Brit. J. Psych.*, **136**, 276–83
6. Kingham, J. G. C. and Dawson, A. M. (1985). Origin of chronic right upper quadrant pain. *Gut*, **26**, 783–8
7. Craig, T. K. and Brown, G. W. (1984). Goal frustrating aspects of life event stress in the aetiology of gastrointestinal disorder. *J.Psychosom. Res.*, **28**, 411–21
8. Ford, M. J., Miller, R. McC., Eastwood, J. and Eastwood, E. A. (1987). Life events, psychiatric illness and the irritable syndrome. *Gut*, **28**, 160–5
9. Colgan, S., Creed, F. H. and Klass, H. (1988). Psychiatric disorder and abnormal illness behaviour in patients with upper abdominal pain. *Psychological Medicine*. (In press)
10. Creed, F. H. (1981). Life events and appendicectomy. *Lancet*, **1**, 1381–5
11. Farmer, R. and Creed, F. H. (1988). Life events, hostility and self-poisoning. *Brit. J. Psychiat.* (In press)
12. Wing, J. K., Cooper, J. E. and Sartorius, N. (1974). *The Measurement and Classification of Psychiatric Symptoms: an Instruction Manual for the Present State Examination and CATEGO Programme*. (London: Cambridge University Press)
13. Brown, G. W., Harris, T. (1978). *Social Origins of Depression*. (London: Tavistock)
14. Chaudhury, N. A. and Truelove, S. C. (1962). The irritable colon syndrome. *Quart. J. Med.*, **31**, 307–22
15. Lane, D. (1973). The irritable colon and right iliac fossa pain. *Med. J. Austr.*, **1**, 66–7
16. Keeling, P. W. N. and Fielding, J. F. (1975). The irritable bowel syndrome: a review of 50 consecutive cases. *J. Ir. Coll. Phys. Surg.*, **4**, 91–4
17. Canton, G., Santonastaso, P. and Fraccon, I. G. (1984). Life events, abnormal illness behaviour and appendectomy. *Gen. Hosp. Psych.*, **6**, 191–5
18. Almy, T. P. (1951). Experimental studies on the irritable colon. *Am. J. Med.*, **10**, 60–7
19. Chaudhury, N. A. and Truelove, S. C. (1961). Human colonic motility: a comparative study

of normal subjects, patients with ulcerative colitis, and patients with irritable colon syndrome. *Gastroenterology*, **40**, 27–36

20. Wangel, A. E. and Deller, D. J. (1964). Intestinal motility in man. III. Mechanism of constipation and diarrhoea with particular reference to irritable colon syndrome. *Gastroenterology*, **48**, 69–84

41
Differential effects of mental and physical stress on perception of gastrointestinal distension

J. F. ERCKENBRECHT, C. HOEREN, G. SKODA AND P. ENCK

Stress alters GI functions probably by interfering with efferent neural pathways from the CNS to the gut. In the present study we investigated the effects of physical and mental stress on the perception of GI distension, which mainly involves afferent neural pathways.

Physical and mental stress was applied to 10 and 11 healthy male volunteers (age 18–30 years). Mental stress was exerted by three different tests. The Dichotomous Listening Test is an acoustical test for investigating the ability of concentration and prompt replies to special audible signals. The visual Colour Word Conflict Test is mainly to differentiate between the optical impression and the correct reading of coloured numerals in a quick sequence. The Mental Arithmetic Test is performed by summing up figures of the decimal system within limited time.

Physical stress was produced by the Ice Water Test. The volunteers were asked to put their non-dominant hand into 4°C cold water — continuously at first and, after a short break, in intervals. The mental stress situation covered a period of 35 min whereas the physical stress lasted about 10 min. The single tests were interrupted by short breaks of 5–15 min.

Heart rate, systolic and diastolic blood pressure served as variables indicating stress effects in the cardiovascular system.

Perception of GI distension was determined by introducing a balloon 30 cm into the rectosigmoid and repetitively inflating this intrarectal balloon from 10–250 ml of air until the volunteers perceived an urge to defaecate and lower abdominal pain, respectively.

The results ($\bar{x}$) were compared to a control situation without stress.

Mental and physical stress increased heart rate and blood pressure (Figure 1). However, volumes to induce an urge to defaecate were significantly increased during physical stress, but were unaffected by mental stress. In contrast, the intrarectal volumes causing lower abdominal pain were significantly decreased by mental stress, but were unaffected by physical

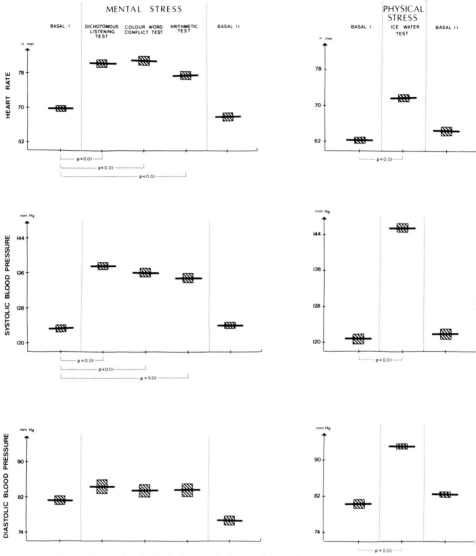

Figure 1 Effects of mental and physical stress in the cardiovascular system

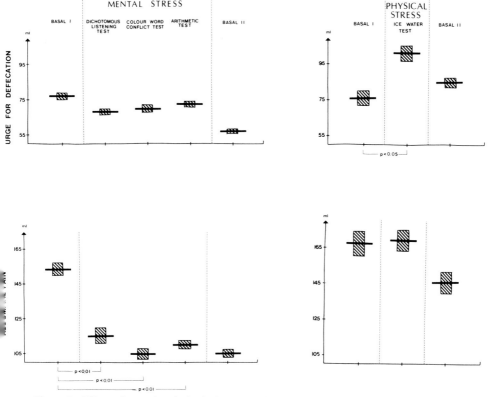

Figure 2 Effects of mental and physical stress on intrarectal volumes to induce an urge for defaecation and lower abdominal pain, respectively.

stress (Figure 2). No significant correlations were found between stress-induced changes in the GI tract and the cardiovascular system.

We conclude that perception of GI distension is differentially affected by mental and physical stress. These effects are unrelated to stress-induced changes in the cardiovascular system.

42
Effects of psychological stress on oesophageal pressures in chronic oesophageal chest pain patients and healthy volunteers

J. E. RICHTER, K. O. ANDERSON, C. B. DALTON
AND L. A. BRADLEY

Clinical experience and experimental evidence indicates that oesophageal motility can be altered by psychologic stress. Non-propulsive oesophageal contractions have been observed in normal subjects and patients during stressful interviews[1,2]. Stacher et al.[3,4] demonstrated that unpredictable noise bursts induce simultaneous oesophageal contractions of increasing amplitude in healthy volunteers. In a more recent investigation from our laboratory, psychological stressors produced significant increases in contraction amplitudes and velocities of peristaltic contractions generated by wet swallows among normal subjects[5].

The documented effects of stress on oesophageal motility suggests that psychological factors may play an important role in oesophageal motility disorders. This possibility is further supported by the observation from several laboratories that patients with such disorders frequently have psychiatric diagnoses and personality profiles charaterized by anxiety about somatic functioning and the tendency to develop gastrointestinal symptoms in response to stress[6,7]. We therefore undertook to examine the effects of acute psychological stress on patients with oesophageal motility disorders and compare their stress reaction to those of healthy volunteers.

MATERIALS AND METHODS

Study populations

Patients with non-cardiac chest pain
Nineteen patients, 11 men, 8 women, mean age 48 years (range 31–65 y), with non-cardiac chest pain (CP) participated in this study. All patients had

suffered recurrent substernal chest pain for a mean of 28 months (range 4 w to 12 y). Coronary arteriography showed normal coronary arteries in ten patients and non-obstructive disease in nine patients. Musculoskeletal examinations revealed no trigger points on the anterior or posterior chest wall associated with the reproduction of their chest pain. All patients had either normal upper gastrointestinal X-rays or endoscopy to exclude oesophagitis. Baseline oesophageal manometry was normal in nine patients and revealed the nutcracker oesophagus in ten patients[8]. Mean distal contraction amplitude for the patients with normal manometry was 92 ± 30 mmHg ($\pm$ SD) and 218 ± 10 mmHg for the patients with the nutcracker oesophagus compared to 99 ± 40 mmHg for our laboratory control group of 95 healthy volunteers. All patients underwent a Bernstein test[9], edrophonium test[10] and balloon distension test[11], in an attempt to reproduce their suspected oesophageal chest pain. All patients with normal baseline manometry had their chest pain reproduced by at least one of the three oesophageal provocative tests. Eight of the ten patients with the nutcracker oesophagus had similar reproduction of their chest pain by provocative testing.

Healthy control subjects

Twenty healthy paid volunteers, 11 men, 9 women, mean age 31 years (range 22–55 y), served as control groups. Potential subjects were excluded if they presented any history of oesophageal symptoms or any disorder known to alter oesophageal function.

Recording apparatus

Oesophageal manometry was performed using a round 8 lumen standard polyvinyl catheter (diameter 4.5 mm), Arndorfer Specialties, Inc, Greendale, Wisconsin, USA). The catheter amd manometric recording equipment were the same as those used in our previous studies of oesophageal motility[10,12]. Systolic and diastolic blood pressures were obtained manually from subjects' left arms using a standard occluding cuff. Heart rate was determined by palpating the left radial artery pulse, counting the beats over 30 s and multiplying by two.

Stressors

Intermittent noise

The noise stressor consisted of 10 min of 100 dB white noise (i.e. tones with a wide range of frequencies) with random, unpredictable bursts and pauses delivered via headphones.

Cognitive problems[13]

Two letters were printed together on ten cards and displayed sequentially to subjects. Each letter varied as to four variables: type of letter (A or T); letter colour (red or green); letter size (large or small); and border surrounding the letter (circle or square). One of the eight variable values (e.g. red) was chosen as the correct answer to each ten-card problem. On every trial the subject pointed to one letter on the card and the experimenter told the subject if the letter contained the correct answer. Although the subjects initially had to guess which letter contained the correct value, they could use the experimental feedback to determine the correct answer. In order to increase the amount of stress experienced, several unsolvable problems were included in the series.

Behavioural and self-report measures

Subjective anxiety was assessed by an abbreviated version of the State Anxiety Scale (SAS) of the State–Trait Anxiety Inventory[14]. The SAS is a reliable measure of situational anxiety, i.e. a transitory emotional state that is characterized by subjective feelings of tension and apprehension. The abbreviated SAS consisted of four items with a four-point response scale. A total SAS score (range 4–16) was determined by summing the responses. The higher the score, the more situational anxiety there was.

In order to assess the multi-dimensional nature of anxiety[15], a behavioural measure of situational anxiety was included. Behavioural measures may provide a more objective assessment of anxiety than self-report measures that are influenced by factors such as cultural values and social desirability. One or two trained observers independently rated on five-point scales the extent to which the subject (a) followed instructions; (b) exhibited signs of anxiety (e.g. crying, groaning, shaking); (c) moved around unnecessarily; and (d) adjusted to the procedure. The ratings were made at the end of each baseline and stressor period. The four ratings from each period were summed to form a total anxiety behaviour score with higher scores indicating more anxiety. The mean percentage agreement for the total anxiety behaviour scores between observers was 83.5%.

Experimental studies

Subjects were studied in the supine position after an overnight fast. The manometry catheter was positioned permitting measurements of oesophageal contractions from 3 and 8 cm above the lower oesophageal sphincter. After a 10 min rest period for adaptation, participants were exposed to four 10 min experimental periods. These consisted of two pairs of baseline followed by stressor periods separated by a 5 min rest period. During the baseline periods, subjects were asked to lie quietly. Subjects were then exposed to each stressor continuously for the entire 10 min period. The order of the stressors was randomized. Measures of anxiety, heart rate and supine blood pressure were recorded during the last minute of each of the four study periods.

Each experimental period was divided into 5 min segments. Initially participants were allowed to swallow on an *ad lib.* basis. This interval was used to determine whether an increased number of spontaneous or simultaneous contractions occurred during stressful stimulation. Next participants were given ten 5 ml wet swallows every 30 s. This latter interval permitted an assessment of the effects of stressful stimuli on the parameters of oesophageal peristalsis.

All motility tracings were coded and read by an investigator blinded to the experimental conditions. The pressure values at 3 and 8 cm above the lower oesophageal sphincter were combined and are described subsequently as distal oesophageal contractions. For each contraction parameter, the mean value for ten wet swallows was determined for each study. Contraction amplitude, duration and velocity were measured by traditional methods[12]. The *ad lib.* swallow interval was evaluated for the combined frequency of spontaneous and/or simultaneous contractions. To compensate for the irregular oesophageal baseline secondary to respiration (normal for our laboratory: 5.0 ± 2.1 mmHg), these waves were required to have an amplitude greater than 10 mmHg.

Statistical analysis

The first set of analyses were performed to evaluate changes in stressor responses among the CP patients. Each of eight dependent variables was entered in separate 2 x 2 x 2 analyses of variance (ANOVA) with the between-subject factor of sequence and the within-subject factors of period (baseline vs. stressor) and stressor (noise vs. cognitive problems). Sequence refers to whether the cognitive problems or noise were presented as the first stressor. Given the large number of ANOVAs, the Bonferroni equation was used to adjust the α-level. The α-level for three oesophageal motility variables was set at 0.017 (0.05 divided by the number of variables); the α-level for the two anxiety measures was set at 0.025; and the α-level for the three heart rate and blood pressure variables was set at 0.017. When ANOVA indicated a significant F-ratio for a dependent variable, analysis of covariance (ANCOVA) was used to compare the stressor responses of CP patients with nutcracker oesophagus to those of CP patients with normal baseline manometry. The second set of analyses used ANCOVA to compare the changes in stressor response of CP patients to those of control subjects. The baseline values of each dependent variable served as the covariates in each ANCOVA in order to control for the initial differences between groups.

RESULTS

The CP patients were found to be significantly older ($\bar{x}$ 48 years) than the healthy volunteers ($\bar{x}$ 31 years, $p < 0.01$). Given this age difference, a preliminary set of ANOVAS was performed to determine if the stressor responses of a subset of 6 older control subjects (mean age, 43 years) were significantly different from those of the 14 younger control subjects (mean age, 25 years). No significant differences were found between these two groups of control subjects on any of the eight dependent variables. Thus, the age differences between the CP patients and control subjects does not appear to be of confounding variable affecting oesophageal or behavioural responses to the stressors.

Oesophageal contraction amplitude

Exposure to both noise and cognitive problems produced significant increases in distal mean contraction amplitude of CP patients with the nutcracker oesophagus, CP patients with normal baseline manometry, and healthy control subjects. Both groups of CP patients demonstrated greater increases during cognitive problems than during the noise stressor ($p = 0.01$). Control subjects, in contrast, responded similarly to both stressors. The ANCOVA revealed significant differences among group responses to the stressors ($p = 0.01$). As shown in Figure 1, patients with the nutcracker oesophagus had a greater increase in contraction amplitude during the cognitive problems than control subjects ($p = 0.004$). The CP patients with normal baseline manometry tended to show a smaller increase in contraction amplitude during cognitive problems than the nutcracker patients ($p = 0.03$) but did not differ from control subjects ($p = 0.10$). During the noise stressor, patients with the nutcracker oesophagus tended to have a greater increase in contraction amplitude than the other two groups ($p = 0.05$).

None of the control subjects produced oesophageal contractions during the stressors that met the criteria for the nutcracker oesophagus. However, four CP patients with normal baseline manometry increased their contraction amplitudes into the nutcracker range ($> 180 \, \text{mmHg}$) during the cognitive problems. A similar change was not observed during the noise stressor.

Oesophageal contraction duration, velocity and abnormal wave forms

Neither of the two CP patient groups nor the controls showed significant increases in contraction duration during the stressor relative to the baseline periods. However, two CP patients developed abnormal durations ($> 6 \, \text{s}$) during the cognitive problems. The velocity of oesophageal contractions was not significantly affected by the stressors. Likewise, there was no significant change in the frequency of abnormal contractions (spontaneous and/or simultaneous waves) during stressor as compared to baseline periods in any of the three groups.

Subjective anxiety and anxiety-related behaviours

The CP patients reported significantly greater subjective anxiety during the cognitive problems relative to the preceding baseline period ($p = 0.01$). The

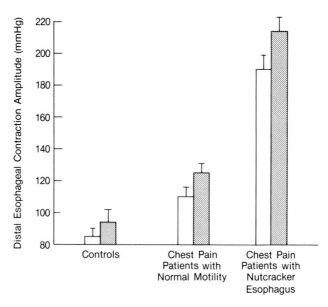

Figure 1 Effects of psychological stress (difficult cognitive problems) on distal oesophageal peristaltic contraction amplitude in healthy control subjects ($n = 20$), chest pain patients with normal oesophageal motility ($n = 9$), and chest pain patients with nutcracker oesophagus ($n = 10$). Open bars = baseline study; shaded bars = stress study. Data presented as $\bar{x} \pm$ SE. Exposure to cognitive problems produced significant increases in distal oesophageal contraction amplitude among all three groups. After controlling for baseline differences, patients with the nutcracker oesophagus demonstrated significantly greater ($p = 0.004$) increases in contraction amplitude than control subjects. The chest-pain patients with normal oesophageal motility tended to show a smaller increase than the nutcracker patients ($p = 0.03$) but did not differ from control subjects ($p = 0.10$)

control subjects' report of anxiety were greater during stressor than during baseline periods ($p = 0.002$) and for the noise relative to the cognitive problems ($p = 0.01$). However, the CP patients' anxiety ratings during the stressors were not significantly different from those of the control subjects.

Figure 2 demonstrates that CP patients and control subjects produced greater anxiety-related behaviour during stressor than during baseline periods ($p = 0.001$). The anxiety related behaviour of the nutcracker patients did not differ from that of CP patients with normal baseline manometry. Both patients and control subjects produce greater anxiety behaviour during the cognitive problems as compared to noise ($p = 0.001$). However, the CP patients demonstrated greater increases in anxiety related behaviour during both stressors than the control subject ($p = 0.01$).

Heart rate and blood pressure

The CP patients' and control subjects' heart rates, systolic and diastolic blood pressures were not significantly affected by the stressors. The ANCOVA

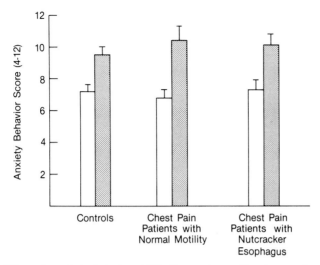

Figure 2 Effects of psychological stress (difficult cognitive problems) on anxiety behaviour scores in healthy control subjects, chest-pain patients with normal manometry, and chest-pain patients with the nutcracker oesophagus. Exposure to cognitive problems produced significant increases ($p = 0.001$) in anxiety scores as assessed by two independent observers among all three groups. The chest pain patients demonstrated greater increases in anxiety behaviour scores than the control subjects ($p = 0.01$)

revealed that the mean systolic blood pressures of patients during baseline and stressor periods tend to be greater than those of control subjects ($p = 0.05$).

Chest pain

One patient experienced chest pain during the stressor studies. This 61-year-old gentleman had a normal baseline oesophageal manometry. The noise replicated his chest pain in association with minimal increases in oesophageal pressures, i.e. contraction amplitude increased from 127 to 144 mmHg and contraction duration increased from 4.1 to 4.3 s. Measures of situational anxiety, however, markedly changed with increases of 160% in the SAS score and 140% in the total anxiety behavioural score.

DISCUSSION

Kronecker and Meltzer[16] observed in 1883 that 'psychic upset' could induce oesophageal contractions. Subsequent studies reported evidence of an association between psychological stress and spontaneous oesophageal contractions[1-4,17,18]. The present study, however, is the first to evaluate critically with modern manometric technology the effects of acute laboratory stressors on various parameters of oesophageal motility in patients with non-cardiac chest pain and oesophageal motility disorders. Unpredictable loud noises and difficult cognitive problems produced significant increases in mean distal peristaltic oesophageal contraction amplitudes among chest pain patients and healthy control subjects. Thus, an increase in contraction amplitude appears to be the primary oesophageal response to stress. Unlike previous studies[1-4], we did not find an increased frequency of simultaneous or spontaneous contractions in response to stressful stimuli. These earlier studies must be reviewed with caution because their equipment frequently was not optimal[1,2] and the amplitude criterion used for simultaneous contractions could be easily confused with normal respiratory variation[3,4].

The magnitude of oesophageal responses to stress varied as a function of the subject group and laboratory stressor. Among control subjects, both stressors elicited comparable increases in contraction amplitudes. However, among the CP patients, the cognitive problems induced greater increases in contraction amplitude than the noise stressor. During these problems, patients with the nutcracker oesophagus demonstrated a significantly greater increase in contraction amplitude than control subjects, even after compensating for baseline differences in oesophageal pressures. The amplitude change in CP patients with normal baseline manometry tended to be less than that of the nutcracker patients but greater than that of control subjects. Four of the CP patients developed high amplitude contractions during the cognitive problem stressor; this response was not observed among the control subjects. Paralleling the changes in oesophageal contraction amplitude, the CP patients also demonstrated greater subjective and behavioural anxiety during the cognitive problems as compared to noise. Our results therefore suggest a possible spectrum of oesophageal responsiveness to various psychological stressors with the greatest response in patients with the nutcracker oesophagus.

Although both stressors significantly affected behavioural and self-report measures of anxiety, these increases were of a relatively low magnitude. Furthermore, the stressors did not significantly change heart rate or blood pressure. However, reliable mean increases in contraction amplitude across subject groups were still found. The stressors chosen for this study were intended to be analogous to those experienced in the individual's home and work environment, without risking subject injury as might occur with the cold pressor test. Thus, it is not surprising that mean increases in contraction amplitude ranged only from 10 to 17% of the baseline values. However, four highly responsive patients experienced increases in individual contraction amplitude ranging from 24 to 74%. These amplitude changes are comparable to those produced by pharmacologic provocative agents such as edrophonium[10]. We plan to investigate the effects of more intense stressors of longer duration on oesophageal pressures.

In summary, this study demonstrates that patients with non-cardiac chest pain react to psychological stress with increases in oesophageal contraction amplitude. These increases were greatest for patients with the nutcracker oesophagus. As with previous studies, a low correlation was found between the presence of abnormal contraction pressures and chest pain[10,19,20]. These observations lead us to hypothesize that conventionally measured oesophageal contraction abnormalities, particularly the nutcracker oesophagus, may simply be manometric markers of a clinical pain syndrome rather than being directly responsible for chest pain. Additional investigations are needed to fully understand the interplay of oesophageal contraction abnormalities, non-cardiac chest pain and psychological stress. If a consistent temporal relationship is found among these three variables, it may be possible to teach individuals effectively to use coping techniques (e.g. relaxation training, stress management training) in order to reduce the negative effects of stress and pain.

References

1. Wolf, S. and Almy, T. P. (1949). Experimental observations on cardiospasm in man. *Gastroenterology*, **13**, 401–21
2. Rubin, J., Nagler, S., Spiro, H. M. and Pilot, M. L. (1962). Measuring the effect of emotions on esophageal motility. *Psychosom. Med.*, **24**, 170–6
3. Stacher, G., Schmeierer, C. and Landgraf, M. (1979). Tertiary esophageal contractions evoked by acoustic stimuli. *Gastroenterology*, **44**, 49–54
4. Stacher, G., Steinringer, H., Blau, A. and Landgraf, M. (1979). Acoustically evoked esophageal contractions and defense reaction. *Psychophysiology*, **16**, 234–41
5. Young, L. D., Richter, J. E., Anderson, K. O., Bradley, L. A., Katz, P. O., McElveen, L., Obrecht, W. F., Dalton, C. and Snyder, R. M. (1987). The effects of psychological and environmental stressors on peristaltic esophageal contractions in healthy volunteers. *Psychophysiology*, **24**, 132–41
6. Clouse, R. E. and Lustman, P. J. (1982). Psychiatric illnesses and contraction abnormalities of the esophagus. *New Engl. J. Med.*, **309**, 1337–42
7. Richter, J. E., Obrecht, W. F., Bradley, L. A., Young, L. D. and Anderson, K. O. (1986). Psychological similarities between patients with the nutcracker esophagus and irritable bowel syndrome. *Dig. Dis. Sci.*, **31**, 131–8
8. Benjamin, S. B., Gerhardt, D. C. and Castell, D. O. (1979). High amplitude, peristaltic esophageal contractions associated with chestpain and/or dysphagia. *Gastroenterology*, **77**, 478–83
9. Bernstein, L. M. and Baker, L. A. (1958). A clinical test for esophagitis. *Gastroenterology*, **34**, 760–81
10. Richter, J. E., Hackshaw, B. T., Wu, W. C. and Castell, D. O. (1985). Edrophonium: a useful provocative test for esophageal chest pain. *Ann. Intern. Med.*, **103**, 14–21
11. Richter, J. E., Barish, C. F. and Castell, D. O. (1986). Abnormal sensory perception in patients with esophageal chest pain. *Gastroenterology*, **91**, 845–52
12. Richter, J. E., Wu, W. C., Johns, D. N., Blackwell, J. N., Nelson, J. L., Castell, J. A. and Castell, D. O. (1987). Esophageal manometry in 95 healthy adult volunteers: variability of pressures with age and frequency of 'abnormal' contractions. *Dig. Dis. Sci.*, **32**, 583–92
13. Klein, D. C., Fencil-Morse, E. and Seligman, M. E. P. (1976). Learned helplessness, depression, and the attribution of failure. *J. Pers. Soc. Psych.*, **33**, 508–16
14. Spielberger, C. D., Gorsuch, R. L. and Lushene, R. E. (1970). *Manual for the State–Trait Anxiety Inventory*. (Palo Alto: Consulting Psychologists Press)
15. Bernstein, D. A., Borkovec, T. D. and Coles, M. G. H. (1986). Assessment of anxiety. In Ciminero, A. R., Calhoun, K. S. and Adams, H. E. (eds.) *Handbook of Behavioral Assessment*, 2nd Edn., pp. 353–403. (New York: Wiley)
16. Kronecker, H., Meltzer, S. J., (1883). Der Schluck-mechanismus, seine erregung und seine Hemmung. *Arch. Anat. Physiol.* (Suppl.), **7**, 328–62
17. Jacobson, E. (1927). Spastic esophagus and mucous colitis: etiology and treatment of progressive relaxation. *Arch. Int. Med.*, **39**, 433–45
18. Faulkner, W. B. Jr. (1940). Severe esophageal spasm: an evaluation of suggestion-therapy as determined by means of the esophagoscope. *Psychosom. Med.*, **2**, 139–40
19. Clouse, R. E., Staiano, A., Landau, D. W. and Schlacter, J. L. (1983). Manometric findings

during spontaneous chest pain with presumed esophageal 'spasm'. *Gastroenterology*, **85**, 395–402

20. Peters, L. J., Maas, L. C., Petty, D. A., Dalton, C. B., Penner, D., Wu, W. C., Castell, D. O. and Richter, J. E. (1988). Spontaneous noncardiac chest pain; evaluation by 24 hour ambulatory motility and pH monitoring. *Gastroenterology*, **94**, 878–86

43
Acute mental stress and the function of the stomach, the pancreas and the gastroduodenal motility: a short review

G. HOLTMANN, R. KRIEBEL AND M. V. SINGER

This short review deals with the findings and concepts of psychophysiological research with respect to the function of the stomach and the exocrine pancreas, as well as to the gastroduodenal motility in humans. With the exception of naturally occurring stressful events, different acute stressors such as noise, mental arithmetic, cold pressure have been used in human research. Only results of studies or case reports on effects of acute mental stress will be considered. However, two case reports on the effects of real-life stress which might be classified as chronic stress are considered, since in these studies there is only a limited period of stress.

There is a long history of research on the relationship between the psyche and the function of the upper gastrointestinal tract. In the classical studies of William Beaumont[1] in 1833, influences of different emotional states on the secretion and motility of the stomach have been documented. Beaumont described a person named Alexis St. Martin who, as a result of an injury, had a permanent gastric apertura. Beaumont was therefore able to observe changes of gastric secretion and changes of the colour of gastric mucosa in response to different psychic conditions. The mucosa of the stomach became red and the flow of gastric juice increased when Alexis St. Martin felt angry or fearful. Almost 100 years later, Wolf and Wolff[2] reported similar observations in their fistulated patient Tom. In addition, these authors observed changes of gastric emptying in response to emotions such as fearfulness.

ACUTE MENTAL STRESS AND GASTRIC ACID SECRETION

In this century several studies in subjects with gastric fistulas or in healthy humans have confirmed and extended Beaumont's observations. However,

523

the results are partly inconclusive. In the studies of Bennet and Venable[3] and Wolf and Wolff[2] anxiety was induced and revealed different results. Whereas Wolf and Wolff described a pailor of the mucosa and a diminished acid secretion in response to anxiety, Bennet and Venable observed an increased acid secretion. Similar contradictory results have been reported in a number of different studies (see Table 1 and Refs 4–19). These studies indicate that neither the quality of the stressor nor the secretory state (interdigestive, post-prandial or exogenously stimulated) of the stomach, is probably the determinant factor for gastric acid response to stress.

As stated by Eichhorn and Tracktir[16] as early as 1955, the contradictory results might be due to a lack of standardized methods in investigations on the effects of emotions on the gastrointestinal tract. They suggested using highly standardized instructions and evoking specific emotions by means of hypnosis. However, studies[2,3] in which specific emotional patterns were induced by means of hypnosis also yielded contradictory results.

The different gastric acid responses to acute standardized stressors might be attributed partly to different hypnotical instructions and/or different experimental settings. However, under standardized experimental conditions, Wittkower[4] found in several healthy subjects different responses of gastric acid output to the same hypnotically induced emotions. Wittkower stated that one person always reacted in the same way to a given stressor (e.g. with an increase or decrease of gastric acid output in response to anxiety), but different persons reacted differently to the same stimulus. This finding indicates that not only the quality of a stressor but different individual factors determine individual gastric acid responses to stress.

One important factor determining individual stress responses might be the individual experience with stressful events. In subjects habituated to special kinds of stressors, there might be different responses compared with subjects who are not habituated. However, volunteers participating in psychophysiological studies on the gastrointestinal tract should be habituated to the experimental setting (not to the stressor) in order to minimize the discomfort from the nasogastric tubes used to collect gastric juice which might superimpose the effects of the experimental stressor.

Another important modulator of individual stress responses has to be mentioned: the ability to cope with stress varies from person to person. This might depend on personal experience on the one hand and differences of personality traits on the other hand. Studies by Eichhorn and Tracktir[9] and our group[19] showed, that the gastric acid response to acute mental stress depend on specific personality traits. Whereas Eichhorn and Tracktir found that changes of gastric acid output during an anxiety inducing stress situation (induced by hypnosis) were correlated with the personality trait anxiety we found a significant correlation between the personality trait impulsivity and changes of gastric acid output during a stress period of performing mental arithmetic and solving anagrams against a financial reward[19]. Therefore, not only the quality of a stressor but the individual's reagibility has to be considered. In addition the relationship between the investigator and the subject might have some influence on gastric acid output; it is a matter of fact that this is difficult to control.

Most studies have been performed without an adequate control experiment and the design of most studies does not exclude experimenters effects. For example, if the experimenter induces specific emotional patterns and is aware of gastric acid responses, there might be conscious or unconscious influences on behaviour. In our opinion it is necessary that the experimenters are unaware of gastric acid responses if valuable conclusions are to be reached.

On the other hand the state of gastric acid secretion has to be known, i.e. whether it is interdigestive, meal-stimulated or stimulated by exogenous hormones such as gastrin (see Table 1). Different methods to measure gastric

Table 1 Effects of various kinds of psychological stressors on gastric acid responses in humans

Authors	Stressors	Response of gastric acid output	Sample size	Subjects
Wittkower[4]	Different emotional stressors (e.g. anxiety, fear)	Standardized stressors evoked divergent responses in different persons	7	Healthy volunteers
Hoelzel[5]	Real life-threatening situation	Biphasic, initially decrease followed by an increase (i)	1	Author
Floyer and Jenning[6]	Real-life examination	No significant effect (m)	16	Students
Mahl[7]	Real life	Increase	8	Healthy volunteers
Heller et al.[8]	Real life	Increase	10	Patients peptic ulcer
Eichhorn and Tracktir[9]	Hypnotically	(i)	24	Healthy volunteers
	fear,	Decrease		
	anger,	Decrease		
	contentment	Increase		
Shay[10]	Psychologic interview	Increase (i)	1	Peptic ulcer
Seymour and Weinberg[11]	Stressful interview	Increase (i)	24	Peptic ulcer
Badgley et al.[12]	Mental arithmetics	Decrease (i)	12	Healthy volunteers
Norman[13]	Response contingent stressor	Biphasic, initially decrease followed by an increase	18	Healthy volunteers
Stacher et al.[14]	Hypnotically induced anxiety	Biphasic, initially decrease followed by an increase (i)	4	Healthy volunteers
Thompson et al.[15]	Cold stress	Biphasic, initially decrease followed by an increase (m)	4	Healthy volunteers
Peters and Richardson[16]	Real life	Increase (uncontrolled) (i, p)	2	Prisoners
Sonneberg et al.[17]	Noise	No effect (p)	12	Healthy volunteers
Oktendalen et al.[18]	5-day physical/mental stress	Increase of BAO and MAO (i, p)	12	Military cadets
Holtmann et al.[19]	Mental arithmetics, solving anagrams	Individual resp. dependent on personality traits (m)	12	Healthy volunteers

i = interdigestive (basal) secretion, p = pentagastrin stimulated
m = meal stimulated secretion, ni = no information given
o = other

acid output (aspiration, pH-meter with a radiocapsule, intragastric titration) have been used and might influence the results.

Because of the large number of confounding variables it is difficult to compare different studies and to draw a firm conclusion on the action of acute psychological stress on gastric acid secretion. There is just one consistent finding: In all studies on subjects with peptic ulcer disease an increase of gastric acid output was observed independent from the stressor used. This might indicate a specific stress response in peptic ulcer patients.

ACUTE MENTAL STRESS AND PANCREATIC EXOCRINE SECRETION

In animals (dogs and cats) there is a long tradition of studies on the brain–gut axis. However, with respect to the effects of acute mental stress on pancreatic exocrine secretion in humans, there is a lack of knowledge. In 1928, Wittkower[20] demonstrated in a single case study that anger decreased duodenal flow rate (without measurement of pancreatic enzymes), whereas anxiety and contentment increased duodenal flow rate. Studies by Thompson et al.[21] showed a biphasic response of post-prandial pancreatic enzyme output, with an initial increase followed by a decrease induced by a cold labyrithine stimulation. Recently we have shown[22], that acute psychological stress (solving angrams and doing mental arithmetics against a financial reward) initially increased pancreatic enzyme output, followed by a significant decrease of enzyme output after the end of a 60 min stress period. However, pancreatic enzyme output per interdigestive motility cycle was not changed.

Table 2 Effects of various kinds of stressors on gastroduodenal motility

Authors	Stressor	Response of gastroduodenal motility (method)	Sample size	Subjects
Cann et al.[27]	Dichotomous listening	No significant effect on gastric emptying (gc)	8	Healthy volunteers
McRae et al.[24]	Dichotomous listening	Decrease of MMC frequency (rt)	11	Healthy volunteers
Stanghellini et al.[29]	Vertigo, cold pain	Antral phasic pressure response to a meal decreased (lp)		
Thompson et al.[28]	Vertigo	Decreased gastric emptying of a meal (mr)	4	Healthy volunteers
Valori et al.[25]	Video game, driving, delayed auditory feedback, sleep interruption	Decrease of MMC frequency (rt)	37	Healthy volunteers
Holtmann et al.[26]	Mental arithmetic, solving anagrams	Duration of IMC increased (lp)	14	Healthy volunteers

gc = gamma camera, mr = markers recovery, rt = radio-telemetric, lp = low-compliance perfusion, MMC = migrating motor complexes

Mental stress induced a reduction of duodenal flow rate and a significant increase of pancreatic enzyme concentration. Chronic mental stress might cause recurring increases in pancreatic enzyme concentration and, thus, play some role in the pathogenesis of chronic pancreatitis, as already hypothesized by Kaplan[23], but this merely speculative assumption has not been proved clinically. Studies on the effects of acute mental stress on exogenously stimulated pancreatic exocrine secretion are missing; the effects of chronic stress on the pancreatic exocrine function are completely unknown.

ACUTE MENTAL STRESS AND GASTRODUODENAL MOTILITY

In healthy humans acute mental stress (induced by noise, mental arithmetic or cold pressure test) seems to increase the duration of the interdigestive migrating complex (IMC) and to decrease the frequency of recurrence of duodenal phase III complexes of the interdigestive motility cycle and to decrease post-prandial motility[24-26]. However, in healthy volunteers, the gastric emptying pattern was not changed by dichotomous listening[27] but significantly inhibited by vertigo induced by labyrinthine stimulation[28]. Cold pain and labyrinthine stimulation decreased the antral phasic pressure response to a meal[29].

Up to now motility studies have suffered from methodological problems. Tubes used to perfuse the intestinuum may induce discomfort, which might superimpose the experimental stressor; telemetric measurement of motility is of limited value as it is only just possible to identify phase III complexes of the IMC, but not to perform a more detailed analysis of motility patterns. Gastric emptying studies using a gamma camera are easy to perform, but they do not give information about contractility patterns. The future of these studies might be seen in very small pressure transducers which allow ambulatory motility recordings. To perform studies with these instruments highly sophisticated hardware and software are required.

POSSIBLE MEDIATORS OF THE STRESS RESPONSES OF THE GASTROINTESTINAL TRACT

Several mechanisms have been proposed to explain the stress-induced changes of motility and secretion of the stomach and the pancreas. Previous studies have shown that adrenergic and/or opioid pathways have to be taken into account. Stanghellini and co-workers[29] demonstrated that stress responses of the human gastrointestinal tract were changed or even abolished by an α-receptor-blocking agent or a morphine antagonist. On the other hand, the gastric acid responses might be mediated by changes of gastrointestinal hormones such as gastrin or pancreatic polypeptide. Stadil and Reheld[30] showed that epinephrine given intravenously increases plasma gastrin levels and therefore induces changes of acid gastric secretion. Nevertheless, in a more recent study[31] noradrenaline, given intravenously in a dose to maintain plasma levels which are observed during mental stress did not significantly change gastric acid output.

Another possible mediator of changes of gastric acid secretion is the cholinergic (vagal) activity. In humans, vagal activity cannot be measured directly. However, it is widely assumed, that plasma levels of pancreatic polypeptide (PP) reflect vagal tonus[32]. In the study of Oktendalen et al.[18] the increases of pancreatic polypeptide levels induced by sham feeding were significantly stronger after a four-day period of physical and psychological stress than before the stress period. Therefore, these data give evidence for the role of the N. vagus in the stress-induced changes of the upper gastrointestinal motility and secretion of the stomach and pancreas.

It has been shown that the administration of single peptides into the brain or into peripheral veins mimics stress responses[33] and the use of peptide antagonist (e.g. naloxone) might change or abolish stress responses[29]. These findings might not lead to the conclusion that these hormones or receptors are responsible for stress responses. Stress responses of the intact organism are characterized by an interaction of different hormonal and nervous systems[34], therefore, a lack of knowledge about mechanisms mediating stress-induced changes of gastric and pancreatic secretion as well as of gastroduodenal motility has to be noted.

CONCLUSIONS

As shown in this short review, historical case reports, as well as uncontrolled and controlled studies, indicate that acute mental stress induced by different methods has some influence on the secretion of the stomach, the exocrine pancreas and the motility of the upper gastrointestinal tract. The patterns of response, however, have only been incompletely investigated so far. Much basic research under well-controlled conditions has still to be made in order to quantify the influence of acute mental stress on the gastrointestinal tract.

Acknowledgements

The preparation of the manuscript and studies of our group cited in this paper were supported by grants from the Deutsche Forschungsgemeinschaft (Si 228/7-1,2).

References

1. Beaumont, W. (1833). *Experiments and Observations on the Gastric Juice and the Physiology of Digestion*. (Platsburg: F.P. Allen)
2. Wolf, S. and Wolff, H.G. (1947). *An Experimental Study of a Man and his Stomach*. (New York: Oxford University Press)
3. Bennet, T.I. and Venables, J.F. (1920). The effect of emotions on gastric secretion and motility in the human being. *Br. Med. J.*, **2**, 662–3
4. Wittkower, E. (1931). Zur affektiven Beeinflussbarkeit der Magensekretion. *Klin. Wochenschr.*, **10**, 1811–13
5. Hoelzel, F. (1942). Fear and gastric acidity. *Am. Dig. Dis.*, **9**, 188

6. Floyer, M. and Jennings, D. (1946). Fractional test-meals on students awaiting examination results. *Lancet*, , 356–7
7. Mahl, G. F. (1950). Anxiety, HCl secretion and peptic ulcer etiology. *Psychosom. Med.*, **12**, 158–64
8. Heller, M. H., Levine, J. and Sohler, Th. P. (1953). Gastric acid and normally produced anxiety. *Psychosom. Med.*, **15**, 509–12
9. Eichhorn, R. and Tracktir, J. (1955). The relationship between anxiety, hypnotically induced emotions and gastric secretion. *Am. J. of Dig. Dis.*, **29**, 422–33
10. Shay Sun, D. C. H., Dlin, B. and Weiss, E. (1958). Gastric secretory response to emotional stress in a case of duodenal ulcer: A consideration of possible mechanisms involved. *J. Appl. Physiol.*, **12**, 461–7
11. Seymour, C. T. and Weinberg, J. A. (1959). Emotions and gastric acid activity. *J.A.M.A.*, **171**, 1193–7
12. Badgley, L. E., Spiro, H. M. and Senay, E. (1969). Effect of mental arithmetic on gastric secretion. *Psychophysiology*, **5**, 633–7
13. Norman, A. (1969). Response contingency and human gastric acidity. *Psychophysiology*, **5**, 673–82
14. Stacher, G., Berner, D. and Naske, R. (1976). Effect of hypnotically suggestion on basal and betazol-stimulated gastric acid secretion. *Gastroenterology*, **69**, 656–61
15. Thompson, D. G., Richelson, E. and Malagelada, J. R. (1983). Pertubation of upper gastrointestinal function by cold stress. *Gut*, **24**, 277–83
16. Peters, M. N. and Richardson, C. T. (1983). Stressful life events, acid hypersecretion, and ulcer disease. *Gastroenterology*, **84**, 114–19
17. Sonnenberg, A., Donga, M., Erkenbrecht, J. F. and Wienbeck, M. (1984). The effect of mental stress induced by noise on gastric acid secretion and mucosal blood flow. *Scand. J. Gastroenterology*, **19**(Suppl. 89), 45–8
18. Oktendalen, O., Guldvog, I., Opstad, P. K., Berstad, A., Gedde-Dahl, D. and Jorde, R. (1984). The effect of physical stress on gastric secretion and pancreatic polypeptide levels in man. *Scand. J. Gastroenterol.*, **19**, 770–8
19. Holtmann, G., Kriebel, R., Singer, M. V., Goebell, H. and Stäcker, K. H. (1987). Do personality traits modify gastric acid secretion in a stressful situation? *Gastroenterology*, **92**, 1439
20. Wittkower, E. (1928). Über den Einfluß der Affekte auf den Gallefluß. *Klin. Wochenschr.*, **7**, 2193–3194
21. Thompson, D. G., Richelson, E. and Malagelada, J. R. (1983). Pertubation of upper gastrointestinal function by cold stress, *Gut*, **24**, 277–83
22. Holtmann, G., Singer, M. V., Kriebel, R., Layer, P., Stäcker, K. H., Goebell, H. (1988). Effects of mental stress on interdigestive gastric acid output, pancreatic enzyme output and gastroduodenal motility. *Gastroenterology*, **94**, A191
23. Kaplan, M. H. (1986). Pathogenesis of pancreatitis: a unified concept. *Int. J. Pancr.*, **1**, 5–8
24. McRae, S., Younger, K. and Thompson, D. L. (1982). Sustained mental stress alters human jejunal motor activity. *Gut*, **23**, 404–9
25. Valori, R. M., Kumar, D. and Wingate, D. L. (1986). Effects of different types of stress and the 'prokinetic drugs' on the control of the fasting motor complex in humans. *Gastroenterology*, **90**, 1890–1900
26. Holtmann, G., Singer, M. V., Kriebel, R., Stäcker, K. H. and Goebell, H. (1988). Mentaler Stress verlängert die Zykluslänge der interdigestiven gastro-duodenalen Motiltät. *Klin. Wochenschr.*, **66**, 206–7
27. Cann, P. A., Read, N. W., Cammack, N. W., Childs, H., Holden, S., Kashman, R., Longmore, I., Nix, S., Simms, N., Swallow, K. and Weller, J. (1983). Physiological stress and the passage of a standard test meal through the stomach and small intestine in man. *Gut*, **24**, 236–42
28. Thompson, D. G., Richelson, E. and Malagelada, J. R. (1982). Pertubation of gastric emptying and duodenal motility through central nervous system. *Gastroenterology*, **83**, 1200–6
29. Stanghellini, V., Malagelada, J.-R., Zinsmeister, A. R., Go, V. L. W. and Kao, P. C. (1984). Stress-induced gastroduodenal motor disturbances in humans: possible humoral mechanisms. *Gastroenterology*, **85**, 83–91
30. Stadil and Rehfeld (1973). Release of gastrin by epinephrine in man. *Gastroenterology*, **65**, 210–15
31. Graeffner, H., Bloom, S. R., Farnebo, L. O. and Järhult, J. (1987). Effects of physiological

increases of plasma noradrenaline on gastric acid secretion and gastrointestinal hormones. *Dig. Dis. Sci.*, **3**, 715–19

32. Schwartz, T. W., Stenquist, B., Olbe, L. and Stadil, F. (1979). Synchronous oscillation in the basal secretion of pancreatic polypeptide and gastric acid. Depression by cholinergic blockade of pancreatic polypeptide concentrations in plasma. *Gastroenterology*, **76**, 14–19

33. Roze, C., Dubrasquet, C. J. and Vaille, C. (1980). Central inhibition of basal pancreatic and gastric secretions by icv administered β-endorphin in rats. *Gastroenterology*, **78**, 659–64

34. Axelrod, J. and Reisine, T. D. (1984). Stress hormones: their interactions and regulation. *Science*, **224**, 452–9

44
The irritable bowel syndrome: biological and non-biological links

N. E. DIAMANT AND S. M. MCHUGH

INTRODUCTION

A universally acceptable definition of the irritable bowel syndrome (IBS) is presently lacking. As a result, research aimed at understanding the basic nature of the 'disorder' has lacked direction, and management strategies have been of limited success[1]. Much of the difficulty can be related to the absence of a satisfactory model capable of integrating the multiple facets of this disorder. In the first part of this chapter, we discuss aspects of IBS that have confounded research efforts intended to delineate the essential nature of IBS. In the latter part, we present an illness behaviour model as a better conceptual model for both understanding the disorder and for orienting future research.

It is clear that a model sufficiently comprehensive to provide a sensible approach to the IBS must take into consideration a number of factors. First, the definition of the IBS must incorporate both biological processes and illness behaviour and experience. Secondly, the designation of the IBS is a generic one, that is, IBS must be viewed as being heterogeneous with respect to aetiology and pathogenesis, the mechanisms whereby symptoms are experienced, and how and why individuals come to seek medical care. Thirdly, the approach to IBS must be dimensional as opposed to categorical[2,3]. In other words, normative and pathological processes are viewed as a continuum, whether looking at physiological, psychological or behavioural responses, and these responses are probably interrelated. Fourthly, the intimate relationship between the central nervous system (CNS) and the enteric nervous system (ENS) should not be isolated from the cognitive processes.

The models for IBS employed in the past, have directed attention to one or more aspects such as disordered physiology of portions of the digestive tract, psychiatric disorders, psychophysiological interactions between brain and gut, and patient behaviour. The biological model, the psychiatric disease model and the psychophysiological model have been unsatisfactory, since no specific disease process, psychiatric disorder, psychophysiological response, pathophysiological marker, or symptoms complex has been found that characterizes the IBS. The biopsychosocial model proposed by Engel[4] includes a consideration of biological, psychological and social dimensions, but fails adequately to articulate the interactions between these dimensions. In a later paper, Engel[5] details the systemic approach permitting application of the biopsychosocial model. Latimer has proposed a behavioural model of IBS where physical motor activity and behaviour, verbal responses, and physiological functioning are considered in trying to understand a given individual's clinical picture[2]. However, this model suffers mostly from its inadequacies as a more general approach, not refuting its usefulness on an individual basis.

Physical symptoms have been the usual criteria employed to define IBS and this approach underscores the limitations of the biomedical model. These symptoms commonly include disordered bowel activity, with or without the presence of abdominal pain or discomfort, along with other symptoms usually taken to infer disordered colonic function. Thompson has suggested five different symptom complexes: spastic colon, constipation (spastic or atonic), painless diarrhoea, burbulence (gas) and the chronic abdomen[6]. Manning et al.[7] have also pointed out that certain symptoms such as pain relief with defaecation, frequent and loose stools with painful onset, abdominal distension, mucous in the stool and a sense of incomplete evacuation, tend to be discriminatory symptoms. However, at most, approximately 75% of patients with the diagnosis of IBS have one particular symptom on presentation[7,8], and symptoms such as constipation and diarrhoea may be present in less than 30% of the patients[8]. This lack of symptom consistency has forced clinicians and researchers to consider additional discriminating characteristics of the IBS.

The search in other realms has been similarly unsatisfactory in providing a basis for defining the IBS for a number of reasons. First, physiological dysfunction or pathology has been demonstrated in some patients to involve various regions of the gut outside the intestines (e.g. stomach[9], oesophagus[10]) gut functions other than motility (e.g. acid secretion[10]) and other organ systems than the gut (e.g. urinary[11], cardiovascular[10,12] and respiratory tracts[13]). Symptoms are similarly ubiquitous[14]. Secondly, regardless of the physiological, pathological or psychiatric abnormality felt to be more common in the IBS group, there is always a large group of patients that falls within the range of normality for the particular parameter under study[10-22]. Thirdly, there has almost uniformly been a poor or inconsistent correlation between demonstrable abnormalities and symptoms[15,16,18,23]. Fourthly, many of the demonstrable physiological abnormalities and symptoms are not unique to patients with IBS but may be found in other physiological or pathophysiological states (inflammatory bowel disease[24,25], carbohydrate intolerance[26], stress in normal individuals[27], physiological states such as eating, awake, sleeping, etc.).

The multiple clinical pictures, the marked overlap with normal states, and the variable organ and system involvement, does not give one much confidence that a single physiological or psychological defect exists to explain the IBS. Furthermore, it is well documented that many, if not a majority of, individuals in the general population with the physical symptoms of IBS do not seek medical attention[28,29]. The feature common to those subjects diagnosed as IBS is therefore not a specific group of physical symptoms or the presence of any specific demonstrable abnormality, but the *seeking of medical attention.*

THE ILLNESS BEHAVIOUR MODEL FOR IBS

We would argue that IBS can best be understood within the framework of an illness behaviour model[30]. Illness behaviour has been defined by Mechanic[31] as the manner in which persons monitor their bodies, define and interpret their symptoms, take remedial action, and use the health care system and various other sources of help. The illness behaviour model as elaborated by McHugh and Vallis makes the distinction between disease and the illness experience while integrating both (Figure 1)[30].

According to an illness behaviour model, biological processes are but one of several factors determining help-seeking. In fact, psychological processes and sociocultural factors are given a major role, since these factors determine an individual's subjective experience of distress, their affective state and the nature of help-seeking. The model is portrayed in a somewhat linear fashion rather than considering cause and effect issues in more circular fashion[5]. This does not mean that the interactions between factors are unidirectional but that the net result or output is an adaptational response by the individual. According to the illness behaviour model, the initiation of the process occurs in the interaction between physiological events, including autonomic arousal

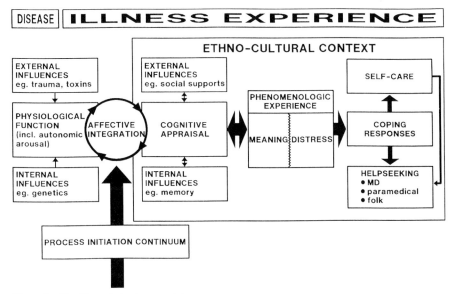

Figure 1 The illness-behaviour model
Psychovisceral and behavioural aspects of gut function and dysfunction

and the cognitive appraisal processes, whereby the interaction is integrated by the affective state, all occurring in a sociocultural context. Viewed in linear fashion, meaning is attached to the individual's experience and is associated with some form of subjective distress, which in turn leads to adaptational behaviour which may or may not include medical help-seeking.

Since medical help-seeking is a central focus of the illness behaviour model, the model in turn can be seen as particularly suited to the study of IBS. Recent studies provide evidence to support the usage and application of an illness behaviour model to the IBS[32,33].

McHugh and Vallis have discussed the illness behaviour model in detail, and illustrated its potential to deal with disease and the illness experience[30]. The general principles outlined by these authors are readily applicable to the irritable bowel synrome. The interactions among physiological function, pathological processes, genetic make-up, social and cultural supports and experiences, memory, affect and cognitive appraisal become of importance.

Physiological functions

Physiological dysfunction could result from: disease process (motor, hormonal or secretory disorders) the extremes of variation in normal functioning (motor, hormonal or secretory) a state of altered autonomic arousal or physiologial stimulation; specific behaviours, e.g. dietary and eating habits; a combination of these factors.

The illness behaviour approach dictates that biological processes involved in the production of symptoms should not be restricted to disease processes. That is, non-disease physiological processes such as autonomic arousal, the fed state, the state of wakefulness or sleep, as well as response system variability and genetic endowment can contribute to eliciting troublesome symptoms. In some subjects, psychological abnormalities and/or physiological disturbances may only become apparent under conditions of stimulation. This stimulation may be normal and physiological (eating) or unusual (periods of variable stress). In other subjects no such relationship to stimuli may be found. In addition, affect and cognitive processes help determine how individuals respond to their environment and internal cues to attach meaning to symptoms and to decide whether they should seek help. In this perspective, it is apparent how a large group of patients with irritable bowel syndrome can have normal values for any physiological or psychological parameter that is studied.

The variability in physiological findings in so-called IBS patients has raised many questions. Are IBS patients normal or abnormal? Do the observed findings represent more of a quantitative than a qualitative difference from the general population? Are there permanent physiological or pathological changes in patients with the IBS? Zegans[34] has reviewed the various ways in which stress responses may come to be associated with organ pathology. In IBS patients there is no data on whether in some individuals continuous autonomic stimulation produces permanent physiological or pathological change, or whether in others behavioural conditioning sets up powerful conditioned reflexes which help maintain ongoing physiological variation and symptoms. There are experimental paradigms, for example, taste aversion conditioning[35,36] or the nausea and vomiting associated with cancer chemotherapy[37,38] which provide evidence to support the latter hypothesis of behavioural conditioning. These aspects require serious academic consideration and testing in patients with IBS.

Cognitive appraisal

Individuals are not passive recipients of information from their environment but, instead, actively and selectively process information which has a marked impact on their behaviour. This selective processing is determined by a number of factors including attentional demands, the influence of past memory, and the cognitive schemata held (the ways in which individuals organize information). Within the cognitive appraisal process, there are concepts such as self-efficacy[39] whereby personal judgements depend on how capable an individual feels about implementing patterns of coping behaviour in new, unpredictable or stressful situations. These judgements are good predictors of behaviour in many situations, such as coping with acute pain and subsequent avoiding behaviour. The concept of self-efficacy has been shown to be relevant in IBS[40]. Negative cognitions or catastrophizing where certain thoughts and images are related to increased distress and decreased ability to cope can have an adverse effect on behaviour and subjective distress[41].

It is easy to see what impact a cognitive scheme relating to a vicious circle of constipation, abdominal pain and laxative intake, or the distress of an episode of faecal incontinence associated with a bout of diarrhoea, might have on the behaviour of a patient with the irritable bowel syndrome. Furthermore, there is evidence for a learned basis for much illness behaviour in general[31] and specifically for patients with gastrointestinal disease[42].

Affective integration

The illness behaviour model incorporates the undeniable role for affect or emotion in the illness experience. Emotion is viewed as an integrative experience interacting with physiological, behavioural and cognitive phenomena[43]. More precisely, these co-variables comprise the emotional reaction whereby charged emotional states can be associated with increased physiological activity and, in turn, symptom perceptions can be studied through physiological reactivity. In the context of the IBS where negative affective states are common[21,22], individuals' affective state may amplify or make chronic both the experience of symptoms and the behavioural responses of the individual. Depending on the nature of psychological disturbance, the role played by affect may vary considerably between individuals.

Previous emphasis has been on psychiatric disorders as opposed to psychological functioning and represents the persistence of the biomedical approach to IBS in contrast to the exploration of psychological factors associated with an illness behaviour model approach[40]. Since only approximately 50% of IBS patients can reliably be labelled with a diagnosis of psychiatric illness, subtypes are diverse[21,21] and it is appropriate to explore further the illness behaviour approach. This approach should also provide insight into the relationships between genetic factors and learned illness behaviours in determining the development of the IBS.

Social support and sociocultural influences

Social support variables such as marital relationships and social contacts, along with the quality of those relationships, can reduce illness directly by influencing the perception of control and of available coping responses or indirectly by reducing stress levels and one's ability to cope with stress. This is not unique to the IBS. On the other hand, specific sociocultural factors are quite apparent in influencing help-seeking associated with IBS symptoms. In India, males are much more likely to seek medical help for the IBS, while in North America and Europe, females predominate[44]. Sociocultural influences include, in a broader context, such things as political processes, acessibility to health care, and family and religious backgrounds. These influences play a role in determining not only who may seek attention, but why certain types of help are sought.

Meaning and experience of distress

Distress is the subjective experience of an individual attaching meaning to symptoms and attempting to make sense out of the illness[45]. This combination of distress and meaning determines the individual's adaptational response. Some people concentrate on somatic symptoms and ignore psychological and social factors; for others, the distress may be primarily psychological. Environmental stressors themselves may cause focusing on somatic symptoms and lead to help-seeking in IBS[21]. This type of variability is readily apparent in the irritable bowel population.

Coping

In adapting to distress, an individual may seek some form of help, look after him/herself, or do nothing. Each individual has a different repertoire of coping skills and their coping response is subject to many variables, including past learning experience and the severity and type of distress. The amount of physiological dysfunction, the affective integration and the cognitive appraisal which have finally led to the meaning and the experience of the distress, are of particular importance in directing the coping response. That only a minority of individuals with irritable bowel symptomatology apparently seek medical help[28,29] brings the potential importance of the illness behaviour model into focus.

CONCLUSIONS

The illness-behaviour model proposes that a more comprehensive definition of the IBS is required (Table 1). This definition would group IBS under the category of 'functional gastrointestinal disorders'. Irritable bowel syndrome would be defined as a functional gastrointestinal disorder attributable to dysfunction of one or more levels of the gut, i.e. stomach, small bowel or colon, and which is associated with medical help-seeking. Characteristic features would include: (a) somatic symptoms and (b) illness behaviour factors. Specifically this diagnosis labels only those who seek medical attention as 'patients'. This definition provides for research into multiple factors which lead to a common outcome, that is, a patient labelled as having IBS. Each one of the many factors, biological and non-biological, must be separately considered and then placed in an interactive framework with all the other potential factors. The model gives impetus to comparisons among individuals who identify no gastrointestinal symptoms, those who experience typical IBS-like somatic symptoms but who do not seek medical attention, and those symptomatic individuals who become 'patients' by seeking medical attention. This dissection and understanding of the multiple interactions should provide more effective management strategies directed and individualized to consider the important factors in each particular patient or patient group.

Table 1 Definition of Irritable bowel syndrome

A functional gastrointestinal disorder attributable to dysfunction of one or more levels of the gut and which is associated with medical help-seeking.
Characteristic features
(a) Somatic symptoms:
    abdominal pain
    disturbed defaecation
    bloating or feeling of abdominal distension
(b) Illness behaviour factors (i.e. affective, cognitive appraisal, sociocultural, individual coping styles, sense of distress) that distinguish individuals seeking medical attention (i.e. patients) from individuals with similar symptoms who do not seek medical attention

References

1. Klein, K. B. (1988). Controlled treatment trials in the irritable bowel syndrome: a critique. *Gastroenterology*, **95**, 232–41
2. Latimer, P. R. (1981). The irritable bowel syndrome. A Behavioural model. *Behav. Res. & Ther.*, **19**, 475–83
3. Latimer, P. (1983). *Functional Gastrointestinal Disorders*: A behavioural Medicine Approach. (New York: Springer Publishing)
4. Engel, G. (1977). The need for a new medical model: A challenge for biomedicine. *Science*, **196**, 129–36
5. Engle, G. (1984). Clinical application of the biopsychosocial model. In Reiser, D. E. and Rosen, D. H. (eds.) *Medicine as a Human Experience*. (Baltimore: University Park Press)
6. Thompson, W. G. (1984). The irritable bowel. *Gut*, **25**, 305–20
7. Manning, A. P., Thompson, W. G., Heaton, K. W. and Morris, A. F. (1978). Towards positive diagnosis of the irritable bowel. *Br. Med. J.*, **2**, 653–4

8. Fielding, J. F. (1983). Detailed history and examination assist positive clinical diagnosis of the irritable bowel syndrome. *J. Clin. Gastroenterol.*, **5**, 495–7

9. Fielding, J. F. and Doyl, G. D. (1982). The prevalence and significance of gastritis in patients with lower intestinal irritable bowel (irritable colon) syndrome. *J. Clin. Gastroenterol.*, **4**, 507–10

10. Smart, H. L. and Atkinson, M. (1987). Abnormal vagal functions in irritable bowel syndrome. *Lancet*, **2**, 475–8

11. Whorwell, P. J., Lupton, E. W., Erduran, D. and Wilson, K. (1986). Bladder smooth muscle dysfunction in patients with irritable bowel syndrome. *Gut*, **27**, 1014–17

12. McAllister, C. and Fielding, J. F. (1988). Patients with pulse rate changes in irritable bowel syndrome. Further evidence of altered autonomic function. *J. Clin. Gastroenterol.*, **10**, 273–74

13. Collins, S. M. (1988). Is irritable bowel syndrome the asthma of the gut? *Gastroenterology*, **94**, A494

14. Whorwell, P. J., McCallum, M., Creed, F. H. and Roberts, C. T. (1986). Non-colonic features of irritable bowel syndrome. *Gut*, **27**, 37–40

15. Kellow, J. E. and Phillips, S. F. (1987). Altered small bowel motility in irritable bowel syndrome is correlated with symptoms. *Gastroenterology*, **92**, 1885–93

16. Trotman, I. F. and Price, C. C. (1986). Bloated irritable bowel syndrome defined by dynamic 99mTc bran scan. *Lancet*, **2**, 364–6

17. Cook, I. J., van Eccden, A. and Collins, S. M. (1987). Patients with irritable bowel syndrome have greater pain tolerance than normal subjects. *Gastroenterology*, **93**, 727–33

18. Cann, P. A., Read, N. W., Brown, C., Hobson, N. and Holdsworth, C. D. (1983). Irritable bowel syndrome: relationship of disorders in the transit of a single solid meal to symptom patterns. *Gut*, **24**, 405–11

19. Lasser, R. B., Bond, J. H. and Levitt, M. D. (1975). The role of intestinal gas in functional abdominal pain. *N. Engl. J. of Med.*, **70**, 524–26

20. Snape, W. J. Jr., Carlson, G. M. and Cohen, S. (1976). Colonic myoelectric activity in the irritable bowel syndrome. *Gastroenterology*, **70**, 326–30

21. Creed, F., Guthrie, F. (1987). Psychological factors in the irritable bowel syndrome. *Gut*, **28**, 1307–18

22. Sammons, M. T. and Karoly, P. (1987). Psychosocial variables in irritable bowel syndrome: a review and proposal. *Clin. Psychol. Rev.*, **7**, 187–204

23. Oettle, G. J. and Heaton, K. W. (1987). Is there a relationship between symptoms of the irritable bowel syndrome and objective measurements of large bowel function? A longitudinal study. *Gut*, **28**, 146–9

24. Isgar, B., Hurman, M., Kaye, M. D. and Whorwell, P. J. (1983). Symptoms of irritable bowel syndrome in ulcerative colitis in remission. *Gut*, **24**, 190–2

25. Bazzocchi, G., Ellis, J., Meyer, J., Mena, I., Reddy, S. N., Moreno-Ossett, E. and Snape, W. J. Jr. (1988). Colonic scintigraphy and manometry in constipation, diarrhea and inflammatory bowel disease. (Abstract). *Gastroenterology*, **94**, A29

26. Rumessen, J. J. and Gudonard and Hyer, G. (1988). Functional bowel disease: Malabsorption and abdominal distress after ingestion of fructose, sorbitol and fructose-sorbitol mixtures. *Gastroenterology*, **95**, 695–700

27. Valori, R. M., Kumar, D., Wingate, D. L. (1986). Effects of different types of stress and of 'prokinetic' drug on the control of the fasting motor complex in humans. *Gastroenterology*, **90**, 1890–1900

28. Thompson, W. G. and Heaton, K. W. (1980). Functional bowel disorders in apparently healthy people. *Gastroenterology*, **79**, 283–8

29. Sandler, R. S., Drossman, D. A., Nathan, H. P. and McKee, D. C. (1984). Symptom complaints and health care seeking behaviour in subjects with bowel dysfunction. *Gastroenterology*, **28**, 314–18

30. McHugh, S. and Vallis, M. (1986). Illness behaviour: Operationalization of the biopsychosocial model. In McHugh, S. and Vallis, T. M. (eds.) *Illness Behaviour: A multidisciplinary model.* (New York: Plenum Press)

31. Mechanic, D. (1986). Illness behaviour: an overview. In McHugh, S. and Vallis, T. M. (eds.) *Illness Behaviour: A Multi-disciplinary Model.* (New York: Plenum Press)

32. Drossman, D. A., McKee, D. C., Sandler, R. S., Mitchell, M., Cramer, E. M., Lowman, B. C. and Burger, A. C. (1988). Psychosocial factors in the irritable bowel syndrome. A multivariate

study of patients and non-patients with irritable bowel syndrome. *Gastroenterology*, **95**, 701–8

33. Whitehead, W. A., Bosmajian, L., Zonderman, A. B., Costa, P. T. Jr. and Schuster, M. M. (1988). Symptoms of psychological distress associated with irritable bowel syndrome. Comparison of community and medical clinic samples. *Gastroenterology*, **95**, 709–14
34. Zegans, L. (1982). Stress and the development of somatic disorders. In Goldberger, L. and Breznitz, S. (eds.) *Handbook of Stress: Theoretical and Clinical Aspects*. (New York: Free Press)
35. Garb, J. L. and Stunkard, A. J. (1974). Taste aversions in man. *Am. J. Psychiatry*, **131**, 1204–7
36. Logue, A. W. (1985). Conditioned food aversion learning in humans. *Ann. NY. Acad. Sci.*, **443**, 316–29
37. Morrow, G. R. and Morrell, C. (1982). Behavioral treatment for the anticipatory nausea and vomiting induced by cancer chemotherapy. *N. Engl. J. Med.*, **307**, 1476–80
38. Andrykowski, M. A., Redd, W. H. and Hatfield, A. K. (1985). Development of anticipatory nausea: A prospective analysis. *J. Cons. Clin. Psychol.*, **53**, 447–54
39. Turk, D. and Rudy, T. (1986). Living with chronic disease: The importance of cognitive appraisal. In McHugh, S. and Vallis, T. M. (eds.) *Illness Behaviour: A Multidisciplinary Mode*. (New York: Plenum Press)
40. McHugh, S., Segal, Z., Lico, S. and Diamant, N. E. (1987). Confidence over bowel control. (Abstract). *Gastroenterology*, **92**, 1527
41. Beck, A. T., Rush, A. J., Shaw, B. F. and Emery, G. (1979). *Cognitive Therapy of Depression*. (New York: Guilford Press)
42. Whitehead, W. E., Winget, C., Fedoravicius, A. S., Wooley, S. and Blackwell, B. (1982). Learned illness behaviour in patients with irritable bowel syndrome and peptic ulcer. *Dig. Dis. Sci.*, **27**, 202–7
43. Lang, P., Cuthbert, B. and Melamud, B. (1986). Cognition, emotion and illness. In McHugh, S. and Vallis, T. M. (eds.) *Illness Behaviour: A Multi-disciplinary Model*. (New York: Plenum Press)
44. Pimbarker, B. D. (1971). Irritable colon syndrome. *Indian Pract.*, **24**, 65–71
45. Kleinman, A. (1986). Illness meanings and illness behaviour. In McHugh, S. and Vallis, T. M. (eds.) *Illness Behaviour: A Multi-disciplinary Model*. (New York: Plenum Press)

Sumary of section V

W. G. THOMPSON

Dr Schuster opened the four-hour discussion by contrasting the traditional paradigm of the irritable bowel as a psychosomatic disease with the evidence of gut disorder as a cause of symptoms. These two views might be considered the two solitudes of functional gut disease. Although the solitudes surfaced throughout the afternoon, it should be clear that they are not mutually exclusive and that both psychologic and physical factors are involved. Dr Wingate discussed his work on the migrating motor complex as a marker of enteric neural activity or the 'gut brain'. He pointed out that, in his work and in several other studies, IBS subjects appear to be more sensitive to psychologic and physical stimuli. I pointed out that functional gut disease was very prevalent in western societies and that the irritable bowel alone likely constitutes 10–20% of sufferers. This condition tends to affect people for long periods of their lives. Most sufferers do not see a physician but those who do generate considerable cost.

Dr Drossmann then addressed the question as to why IBS patients see a physician. It has long been noticed that psychological, personality and psychosocial problems are more prevalent in IBS than other groups. Dr Drossman's studies, however, point out that, although this is true for patients with the IBS those IBS sufferers who do not see doctors have a similar psychosocial profile to controls. He raised the notion of illness behaviour. Dr Whitehead picked up this theme by citing evidence from his own work that individuals with the IBS who see physicians have problems such as somatization, anxiety, depression, etc., to a greater extent than non-patients with the IBS and controls. His earlier work suggested that illness behaviour is learned in childhood and that those IBS subjects with illness behaviour characteristics select themselves for a visit to the doctor. Dr McHugh in his poster and in the discussion, presented evidence for the concept that cognitive, affective and social factors may determine illness behaviour.

Dr Schuster then reviewed what is known about the relationship of IBS symptoms to motility phenomena. He cited the pioneer work of Drs Almy and Connell. Many observers have noted that IBS patients are more sensitive to stresses and drugs. He advanced the notion that it is not the stimulus but the response that is important. Dr Creed then presented his work on one such stimulus. Stressful, threatening life events, such as bereavement, marital break-up or loss of job, may precipitate the onset of IBS symptoms. Dr Erckenbrecht demonstrated that mental and physical stress have similar effects on the cardiovascular system, but paradoxical effects on the gut. Dr Richter, using the term 'the irritable oesophagus', demonstrated that the subjects with non-cardiac chest pain had different contractile and anxiety reactions to stress. Like the irritable bowel syndrome, the irritable oesophagus syndrome is multi-factorial (see Dr Holzl's poster on the irritable bowel syndrome). Dr Holtmann noted similar stressors have different effects on different parts of the gut. It seems clear that stressors affect gut function in curious ways. We are not, however, in a position to predict the manner in which the gut will respond to a certain stress.

Dr Diamant presented a multi-dimensional schema. He said that there are no symptomatic or physiologic absolutes in functional gut disease and proposed an 'illness-behaviour model'. Since illness behaviour is one factor that IBS patients have in common, it is the one we should be testing. Time does not permit a discussion of the remaining interesting posters which were presented at the meeting.

All participants thanked Dr Falk for the opportunity of dialogue between fundamental scientists and clinical scientists. It is clear that there are now better lines of communication between the two solitudes. There remains, however, a challenge to basic scientists to study patients rather than animals. Equally, there is a challenge to physicians to define which patients are studied, remembering Dr Almy's question 'is the irritable bowel a quantitative or qualitative departure from the psychophysiologic reactions of normal people?'

Poster abstracts and short communications

Part I
The Enteric Nervous System:
Circuits and Development

1
Electrophysiological analysis of synaptic inputs to chemically identified intestinal secretomotor neurons

J. C. BORNSTEIN, J. B. FURNESS AND M. COSTA

It is now clear that water and electrolyte transport across the intestinal mucosa is under neuronal control[1]. Both cholinergic and non-cholinergic secretomotor neurons with cell bodies in the submucous ganglia have been identified in the guinea-pig small intestine. However, there are four neurochemically distinct groups of submucous neurons in this organ. Almost half the neurons are immunoreactive for vasoactive intestinal peptide (VIP), dynorphin (DYN) and galanin (GAL). The other three groups of neurons are all immunoreactive for choline acetyltransferase (ChAT) and can be distinguished from each other by their immunoreactivity for different neuropeptides. ChAT neurons of one group are immunoreactive for neuropeptide Y (NPY), cholecystokinin (CK), calcitonin gene-related peptide (CGRP), somatostatin (SOM) and, in many cases, GAL. There are also neurons immunoreactive for both ChAT and substance P (SP) and neurons reactive only for ChAT.

There is considerable evidence that the DYN/GAL/VIP neurons are the non-cholinergic secretomotor neurons[1]. Both the ChAT/CCK/CGRP/ (GAL)/NPY/SOM neurons and the ChAT/SP neurons project from the submucosa to the mucosa and so may be secretomotor neurons. To understand the control of water and electrolyte transport, it is necessary to know the physiological characteristics of the chemically defined neurons. By using combined intracellular recording and immunohistochemical methods, we have shown that the DYN/GAL/VIP and the ChAT/CCK/CGRP/ (GAL)/NPY/SOM neurons have distinctive patterns of synaptic inputs[2]. Submucous neurons were impaled with microelectrodes filled with 0.5% Lucifer yellow (a fluorescent dye) in 0.5 M KCl solution. Each impaled neuron was injected with dye after its synaptic inputs and other cell properties had been determined. The injected dye was used to relocate the impaled neuron after the preparation had been processed for immunohistochemical localization of VIP or NPY.

We have now extended these studies to the SP-immunoreactive submucous neurons and have also used lesioned preparations to establish the sources of the fibres responsible for different synaptic potentials. The ChAT/CCK/CGRP/(GAL)/NPY/SOM neurons receive excitatory input from cholinergic neurons via nicotinic receptors to produce fast excitatory synaptic potentials (fast e.s.p.'s). Some of these cholinergic inputs arise from myenteric neurons and others from submucous neurons. The DYN/GAL/VIP neurons receive excitatory input from cholinergic neurons in both the myenteric and submucous plexuses, inhibitory input from noradrenergic sympathetic neurons and non-noradrenergic myenteric neurons and slow excitatory input from non-cholinergic neurons. In contrast, the ChAT/SP neurons do not exhibit fast e.s.p.'s or inhibitory synaptic potentials. The ChAT/SP neurons are unlikely to be cholinergic secretomotor neurons as it would be expected that such neurons would receive a substantial excitatory synaptic input; it is thus probable that the ChAT/CCK/CGRP/(GAL)/NPY/SOM neurons are the cholinergic secretomotor neurons (see also ref. 1).

As a result of this work we are able to propose anatomically, neurochemically and physiologically defined neuronal circuits which control water and electrolyte transport.

References

1. Keast, J. R. (1987). *Rev. Physiol. Biochem. Pharmacol.*, **109**, 1–59
2. Bornstein, J. C., Costa, M. and Furness, J. B. (1986). *J. Physiol.*, **381**, 465–82

2
Characterization of opiate binding to nerve membranes of myenteric plexus (MP), deep muscular plexus (DMP), submucous plexus (SMP) and muscle layers (CM, LM and MM) of canine small intestine

H.-D. ALLESCHER, S. AHMAD, P. KOSTKA, C. Y. KWAN
AND E. E. DANIEL

The objective of these studies was to obtain relatively purified and well-characterized membranes from the various components (nerve and muscle) of the small intestine and to determine the presence and nature of opioid receptors in these membranes. Previous studies[1] revealed atropine and tetrodotoxin (TTx) sensitive as well as insensitive excitation of small intestine by agonists with μ- and δ-selectivity. Agonists with κ-selectivity had only TTx-sensitive inhibitory effects. The various muscle layers were separated by dissection; the myenteric plexus accompanied longitudinal muscle (LM), the deep muscular plexus was contained within the circular muscle. The mucosa was removed from the tissue remaining after removal of the muscularis externa, leaving the muscular mucosa (MM) and submucous plexus. Separated layers were characterized morphologically. Nerve membranes were separated from muscle membranes after homogenization of the tissues using differential centrifugation and various sucrose density gradients. The purified synaptosomal nerve membranes were characterized by the ^{3}H-saxitoxin binding, by the content of VIP and substance P measured by radioimmunoassay and by their morphological appearance as well as low levels of 5'-nucleotidase. Smooth muscle plasma membrane fractions had high 5'-nucelotidase activity, negligible saxitoxin binding and were clear vesicles in electronmicroscopy. Opiate binding was studied using a non-selective antagonist ^{3}H-diprenorphine and a non-selective agonist, ^{3}H-ethorphine (10^{-6} M). Opioid receptor subtypes in the various fractions were

Table 1 Percentage of x Enrichment over PNS*

	Kd (nM)	Bmax (fmol/mg)	μ	δ	κ	3H-DPN	3H-STXC	5-NT
MP	0.12	400	40	40	10–20	24x	20x	1.7x
DMP	0.18	500	40	40	10–20	47x	50x	3x
SMP	0.2	500	65	35	0–5?	14x	16x	0.9x
LM	—	—	—	—	—	4.5x	4x	12x
CM	—	—	—	—	—	0.7x	0.3x	20x

*pns = post-nuclear supernatant

studied using various highly selective agonists (D-pen2-dpen5-enkephalin for δ-receptors, PL017-morphiceptin for μ-receptors and U-50488-H and dynorphin 1-13 for κ receptors). Saturation data, kinetic data and displacement curves were calculated using computer analysis (EBDA/LIGAND). [^{3}H]-ethylketocycloacosine in the presence and absence of blocking ligands for μ and δ receptors was used to confirm the existence of κ receptors. No evidence of specific opiate receptor binding was obtained in purified membranes from muscle layers. On the other hand, a high density of opiate-binding sites was found in all nerve membranes (see Table 1).

We conclude that membranes from nerve plexuses with neuronal cell bodies (MP) as well as from those without (DMP) contain three types of opiate-receptors, a minority (10–20%) of κ-receptors and nearly equal numbers (40%) of μ- and δ-receptors. No evidence of specific opiate binding on muscle membranes was obtained. The submucous plexus seems to contain more μ- than δ-receptors and probably no, or only a small number, of κ-receptors. The mechanism of TTx and atropine-resistant contractile effects in canine small intestine is probably mediated through actions on neuronal μ- and δ-membranes. Opioid control of mucosal function is also likely to be mediated through μ- and δ-receptors.

Acknowledgements

Supported by MRC of Canada and DFG Al 245/1-1.

References

1. Fox and Daniel (1987). *Am. J. Physiol.*, **253**, G179–88

3
Ultrastructure and localization of different neuropeptide-containing nerve elements in the small intestine

E. FEHÉR

The localization and the function of different neuropeptides in the enteric nervous system has been intensively examined in view of their possible role as transmitters or modulator[1,2,3]. A large number of peptide-containing nerve cell bodies and fibres were demonstrated immunohistochemically in the different parts of the alimentary tract of the mammals[4,5,6]. However, only a few papers described neuropeptide-containing fibres in the gut at electronmicroscopic level[7,8,9].

Electronmicroscopic analysis was required to decide whether the immunoreactive nerve terminals form synapses with each other or with neuronal perikarya, or whether they are closely situated to the supposed effector cells. The aim of the present study was to examine the ultrastructural features of different immunoreactive nerve elements (substance P, vasoactive intestinal polypeptide, somatostatin, neuropeptide Y, calcitonin-gene-related peptide and galanin), as well as their relationships to the supposed effector cells and their synaptology in the wall of the small intestine (in rats, cats and guinea-pig) using immunoelectron microscopic (peroxidase-antiperoxidase, PAP) technique.

The immunoreactive nerve cell bodies were found in both myenteric and submucous plexuses. They were medium to large in size (20–40 μm), with round or multipolar cell bodies having eccentrically located nucleus, containing mitochrondria, rough surface endoplasmic reticulum, a well-developed Golgi apparatus and some dense-cored vesicles. The peroxidase products were diffusely arranged in the cytoplasm, the cytoplasmic organelles were generally devoid of immunoreactivity, while a strong reaction was found on the outer surface of their membrane. Additionally, labelled small (10 μm) cells were also observed within the intramural ganglia, especially in the submucous ganglia.

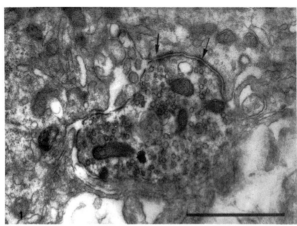

Figure 1 Somatostatin immunoreactive nerve terminal making synapse (arrows) on the surface of the unlabelled nerve cell body. Note, that this terminal contains a large number of small clear vesicles. Bar scale = 1 μm ($\times$ 54 000)

The immunoreactive nerve terminals established a dense network around the unlabelled nerve cell bodies and could be found in all layers of the small intestine. They had an average diameter of 0.2 μm and contained high numbers of synaptic vesicles. About 30% of the observed immunoreactive profiles were of small diameter without any synaptic vesicles. In the varicosity, the peroxidase reaction linked to the outer surface of vesicular and mitochondrial membranes and aggregates at the synaptic sites. Most of the immunoreactive nerve terminals contained a large number of small clear vesicles and some large dense-cored vesicles of 80–120 nm in diameter.

Most of the immunoreactive nerve terminals were surrounded by other neuronal elements without any synaptic contact. However, real synaptic contacts were sometimes found within the ganglia, between the labelled nerve terminals and unlabelled nerve cell body (Figure 1). Both symmetrical and asymmetrical synapses could be observed where the post-synaptic sites were denser. In the muscle layer the immunoreactive nerve fibres were observed running parallel to the long axis of the smooth muscle cells. The gaps between the neuronal profiles and the adjacent smooth muscle cell membrane was 20–2000 nm (Figure 2), sometimes less than 20 nm. These immunoreactive nerve fibres were also widespread in association with the blood vessels, especially arterioles. They have an intimate topographical connection with the basement membranes of the capillary walls. A large number of immunoreactive nerve fibres were found in the tunica mucosa, being very close to the epithelial cells of the Lieberkühn crypts and villi.

These findings provide a morphological basis for the possibility that these neuropeptide-containing nerve fibres may influence the blood flow of the small intestine and may participate in the regulation of the epithelial cell function and the activity of the smooth muscle cells. Some of these neuropeptides may act as neurotransmitters as well as having a neuromodulatory effect on the other intrinsic nerve elements.

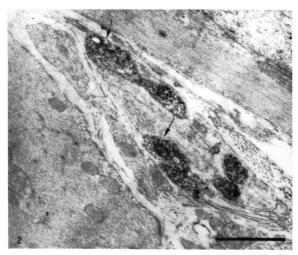

Figure 2 Vasoactive intestinal polypeptide immunoreactive nerve terminals (arrows) in a very close situation to the smooth muscle cells. Bar scale = 1 μm (x 38 000)

References

1. North, R. A. (1982). Electrophysiology of the enteric nervous system. *Neuroscience*, **7**, 315–25
2. Barthó, L. and Holzer, P. (1985). Search for a physiological role of substance P in gastrointestinal motility. Commentary. *Neuroscience*, **16**, 1–32
3. Furness, J. B., Costa, M., Morris, J. L. and Gibbins, I. L. (1987). Novel neurotransmitters and the chemical coding of neurones. *Advances in Physiological Research*, pp. 143–165. (New York: Plenum Press)
4. Sundler, F., Hakanson, R., Larsson, J. L., Brodin, E. and Nilsson, G. (1977). Substance P in the gut: an immunochemical and immunohistochemical study of its distribution and development. *Substance P: Nobel Symposium*, **37**, pp. 59–65. (New York: Raven Press)
5. Schultzberg, M., Dreyfus, C. F., Gershon, M. D., Hökfelt, T., Elde, R. P., Nilsson, G., Said, S. I. and Goldstein, M. (1978). VIP-enkephalin-substance P and somatostatin-like immunoreactivity in neurons intrinsic to the intestine: Immunohistochemical evidence from organotypic tissue cultures. *Brain Res.*, **155**, 239–48
6. Furness, J. B. and Costa, M. (1987). *The Enteric Nervous System*. (Edinburgh: Churchill Livingstone)
7. Probert, L., De Mey, J. and Polak, J. M. (1981). Distinct subpopulations of enteric-type neurones containing substance P and vasoactive intestinal polypeptide. *Nature*, **294**, 470–1
8. Fehér, E. and Léránth, C. (1983). Light and electron microscopic immunocytochemical localization of VIP-like activity in the rat small intestine. *Neuroscience*, **10**, 97–106
9. Fehér, E. and Burnstock, G. (1986). Ultrastructural localization of substance P, vasoactive intestinal polypeptide, somatostatin and neuropeptide Y immunoreactivity in perivascular nerve plexuses of the gut. *Blood Vessels*, **23**, 125–36

4
Mechanisms of release of conventional neurotransmitters and neuropeptides from enteric nerves in normal and diabetic rat intestine

A. BELAI AND G. BURNSTOCK

The release of endogenous vasoactive intestinal polypeptide (VIP), calcitonin gene-related peptide (CGRP) and substance P from enteric nerves of isolated rat ileum and the role of extracellular calcium in the release mechanism have been investigated. Evaluation of simultaneous release of acetylcholine (ACh) and adenosine 5′-triphosphate (ATP) from enteric nerves was used for comparison. Segments of mucosa-free ileum were superfused with Bülbring-modified Krebs solution and the concentration of the peptides in the superfusate was quantitated using enzyme-linked immunosorbent assay (ELISA) and ACh and ATP with luminometric methods. Electrical stimulation and high potassium (76 mM and 110 mM) were used as depolarizing stimuli. A summary of the results is shown in Table 1.

The electrical stimulation-induced release of ACh, ATP, substance P and CGRP was shown to be dependent on extracellular calcium, as omission of Ca^{2+} or addition of the Ca^{2+}-channel blocker, cadmium, inhibited the release of the neurotransmitters from enteric nerves. K^+-depolarization increased the release of ACh, ATP and substance P. Endogenous release of

Table 1

Transmitters	Ca^{2+}-dependent release during electrical stimulation	Release during K^+ depolarization
Ach	√	√
ATP	√	√
Substance P	√	√
CGRP	√	×
VIP	×	×

VIP, however, was not inhibited in Ca^{2+}-free media or in the presence of cadmium, and K^+-depolarization failed to induce the endogenous release of both VIP and CGRP from enteric nerves. The results will be discussed in relation to the role of voltage-sensitive and receptor-operated calcium channels in the mechanism of enteric neurotransmitter release.

The effect of streptozotocin-diabetes on the endogenous release of these neurotransmitters from enteric nerves was investigated. The concentrations of ACh, ATP and substance P released during electrical stimulation from enteric nerves of diabetic rat ileum was similar in magnitude to that of controls. However, despite the increased VIP-like immunoreactivity in the enteric nerves of diabetic rat ileum, electrical stimulation did not cause increase in release of VIP. The lack of increase in electrical stimulation-induced release of CGRP from diabetic rat ileum was consistent with the decreased CGRP-like immunoreactivity in enteric nerves. This defective release of VIP and CGRP in the diabetic ileum was restored after acute short-term application of insulin *in vitro*. The significance of the effect of diabetes on VIP and CGRP and the reversal of the defective release by acute insulin application *in vitro* is discussed in relation to the possible involvement of inositol phosphatides.

5
Neuroendocrine complex (NEC) and interstitial cell of Cajal (ICC) in the region of Meissner's plexus (MP) in the human GI tract

H. G. SCHMIDT AND A. SCHMID

So far, the NEC has been investigated in detail only in the appendix[1]. The NEC is postulated to be the starting-point of carcinoids[2]. The ICC has so far been investigated in MP only in the small bowel[3]. We carried out an ultrastructural study of the presence of NECs and ICC in MP of the upper and lower gastrointestinal tract. We also investigated ultrastructurally the significance of the NEC in microcarcinoidosis of the stomach in pernicious anaemia and in gastrointestinal carcinoids.

METHOD

Patient group A

NEC and ICC were studied in endoscopic biopsies from 240 patients (P): oesophagus, 50 P (normal oesophagus, oesophagitis, Barrett's oesophagus, heterotopic gastric mucosa in proximal oesophagus); stomach, 75 P (normal stomach, gastric ulcer, carcinoma, diabetes mellitus, amyloidosis); duodenum, 25 P (normal duodenum, duodenal ulcer); colon, 90 P (normal colon, ulcerative colitis, Crohn's disease, diabetes mellitus, amyloidosis, spastic colon, AIDS).

Patient group B

In each of 23 patients with pernicious anaemia 6 step biopsies from the stomach were investigated.

Patient group C

In 24 patients with carcinoids, endoscopic or surgical biopsies taken from the centre and the margin of the tumour were investigated: 5 P had gastric, 3 P duodenal, 5 P ileal, 1 P caecal, and 9 P rectal carcinoids.

RESULTS

Patient group A

15/240 P had NECs: 2 P in heterotopic gastric mucosa in proximal oesophagus; 1 P in Barrett's oesophagus; 10 P in the stomach; 2 P in the rectum. Per NEC, usually 1–2, maximally 5, endocrine cells were found. On the basis of the morphology of the endocrine granules, at least three different types of endocrine cells were distinguishable. Endocrine cells and the nerve fibres surrounding them were enclosed within a basement membrane. 19/240 P showed ICC: 3 P in the oesophagus; 13 P in the stomach and 3 P in the colon. The ICC were characterized by pronounced rough endoplasmic reticulum and usually possessed a number of cytoplasmic processes. Contact between ICC and nerve fibres was of two basic types: (1) cytoplasmic processes of ICC penetrated the basement membrane of the Schwann cells and entered into direct, synapse-like contact with the cell membrane of the Schwann cells or axolemma, (2) nerve fibres were located in 'recesses' of the ICC, no basement membrane being found in the region of the contact zone between the ICC and the nerve fibre. A basement membrane was to be seen on the circumference of the nerve fibre opposite the contact zone, and extended partially over the adjacent portions of the ICC.

Patient group B

18/23 P showed, as a rule, in several of the step biopsies removed from each P, and in particular in corpus biopsies, NECs that were mostly multiple per biopsy. The number of endocrine cells per NEC varied from 1 to about 30. At least five different types of endocrine cells were differentiable. The nerve fibres belonging to the NECs were usually located in the periphery of the NECs. Approximately 30% of the extraepithelial endocrine cell nests revealed no nerve fibres. In 6 P, ICC were found to be in direct contact with NECs.

Patient group C

13/24 P were NEC-positive: 4 gastric, 2 duodenal, 4 ileal, 1 caecal, and 2 rectal carcinoids. Most of the NECs were located in the margin of the tumours. The number of endocrine cells per NEC was a minimum of 1, and could not be accurately determined in large NECs.

CONCLUSIONS

NECs and ICC can occur in MP in the upper and lower human gastrointestinal tract. The majority of the extraepithelial endocrine cell nests in microcarcinoidosis of the stomach in pernicious anaemia represent NECs. NECs are possibly starting-points of at least some of the gastrointestinal carcinoids.

Acknowledgements

Supported by the J. and F. Marohn Foundation.

References

1. (1983). *Gastroenterol.*, **84**, 490
2. (1983). *Virch. Arch.*, **401**, 17
3. (1965). *Okajimas. Fol. Anat. Jap.*, **40**, 409

POSTER ABSTRACT

6

Disposition and morphology of myenteric neurons immunoreactive for dynorphin A(1-8) in guinea-pig and rat small intestine

G. T. PEARSON, D. J. LEISHMAN, M. J. GRAY AND G. M. LEES

Corbett et al.[1] suggested that dynorphin A(1-8) may be an endogenous neurotransmitter or neuromodulator, actions mediated via κ-opioid receptors. Although this neuropeptide has been demonstrated immunohistochemically in submucous plexus neurons[2] and dynorphin A and A(1-13) have been found in guinea-pig and rat enteric nerve cell bodies and fibres[3,4], the occurrence of dynorphin A(1-8) (Dyn) in myenteric plexus neurons of the small intestine has not previously been reported.

Antibodies (Peninsula RAS-8697N and 61022) with a high selectivity for Dyn revealed, in both guinea-pig and rat small intestine, immunoreactive fibres in myenteric ganglia and their interconnecting strands, in the tertiary plexus and the deep muscular plexus of the circular muscle. In the guinea-pig, numerous immunoreactive somata were observed in myenteric ganglia and, as reported[2], in those of the submucous plexus. In contrast, there were no immunoreactive cell bodies in either plexus of the rat small intestine, though many immunoreactive fibres were seen in the myenteric plexus. It should be noted that no colchicine pre-treatment was used in any of the present studies.

Useful correlations between peptide-immunoreactivity and cell type have already been described[2,5]. Since, however, immunohistochemical reactions may not reveal adequate detail for morphological classification[5] intracellular staining with Lucifer yellow has been employed. Random impalement of 296 neurons in four preparations resulted in staining of approximately equal numbers of Dogiel type I and II neurons. Immunoreactivity was confined to Dogiel type I cells (88/144). Thus, the proportion of Dyn-immunoreactive neurons was 61% of Dogiel type I cells; therefore, constituting about 30% of *all* myenteric plexus neurons. In a parallel study using a monoclonal antibody to [Leu]enkephalin (NOC1), we found that only 43% (50/116) of

Dogiel type I neurons were immunoreactive; as expected[3,5], no Enk-immunoreactivity was present in other morphological categories. In these and other preparations, the myenteric plexus consistently contained greater numbers of Dyn-immunoreactive neurons than of Enk-containing neurons. For both neuropeptides, the principal locus was the Type Ia rather than the Type Ib subclass[2], a higher proportion of which was immunoreactive for Dyn (52%) than for Enk (18%).

These data strongly suggest that dynorphin A(1-8) is an important neuropeptide in the enteric nervous system and provide supportive evidence for the proposal[3] that there is a population of Dyn-containing neurons that is distinct from Enk-containing neurons in the myenteric plexus.

References

1. Corbett, A. D., Paterson, S. J., McKnight, A. T., Magnan, J. and Kosterlitz, H. W. (1982). *Nature*, **299**, 79–81
2. Pearson, G. T., Gray, M. J. and Lees, G. M. (1988). *J. Neurosci.* (In press)
3. Costa, M., Furness, J. B. and Cuello, A. C. (1985). *Neuropeptides*, **5**,445–8
4. Vincent, S. R., Dalsgaard, C.-D., Schultzberg, M., Hokfelt, T., Christensson, I. and Terenius, L. (1984). *Neuroscience*, **11**, 973–87
5. Bornstein, J. C., Costa, M., Furness, J. B. and Lees, G. M. (1984). *J. Physiol.*, **351**, 313–25

7
Synaptophysin: a marker for enterochromaffin and intestinal neuromuscular junctions

B. WIEDENMANN, B. KOMMERELL AND W. W. FRANKE

Synaptophysin is a major integral membrane glycoprotein of a certain class of small (30–80 nm diam.) neurosecretory vesicles, including presynaptic vesicles, but also vesicles of various neuroendocrine cells of both neuronal and epithelial phenotype. Using synaptophysin-specific antibodies, we have isolated cDNA clones from rat nervous tissue libraries which identify a 2.5 kb mRNA in rat and human cells, including neuroendocrine tumours, that contains a reading frame for a polypeptide of 307 amino acids with a total molecular weight of 33 312. The deduced amino acid sequence reveals four hydrophobic domains and a carboxy-terminal tail of 89 amino acids, which is located on the vesicle outside. Using immunofluorescence microscopy we show that this polypeptide is also expressed in normal human enterochromaffin cells, in the myenteric and submucous plexus of Auerbach and Meissner, and neuromuscular junctions. Furthermore, our studies show, using immunoblotting and immunohistochemical techniques, that synaptophysin is expressed in almost all intestinal carcinoids, including metastases.

In summary, our data show that synaptophysin is a broad marker for neuroendocrine normal and neoplastic cells of the intestinal tract. Our studies suggest that synaptophysin could also be used as tool for the investigation of gastrointestinal motility and secretion disorders.

8
Neuropathology of congenital intestinal motility disorders

**J. MEBIS, F. PENINCKZ, K. GEBOES, E. EGGERMONT
AND V. DESMET**

INTRODUCTION

Congenital abnormalities of the enteric nervous system in the hindgut cause significant disturbances of normal intestinal motility. This may result in variable symptoms, including diarrhoea, chronic constipation and acute bowel obstruction. Differential diagnosis, and hence appropriate treatment, may be obtained by combining findings of clinical, radiological, manometrical and morphological investigations. The application of histochemistry to intestinal biopsies appears to be an especially valuable tool for separating cases of true Hirschsprung's disease showing aganlionosis coli from cases that mimic Hirschsprung's disease through other neural abnormalities, and cases that resemble Hirschsprung's disease but do not show obvious innervational abnormalities[1].

This report summarizes the findings we obtain by enzyme- and immuno-histochemistry, performed on biospy material from paediatric patients with intestinal motility disturbances. Not only classical, perpendicular cryostat sections of superficial biopsies, but miorodissected tissular sheets of intestinal segments are used to study the innervation.

MATERIALS AND METHODS

Biopsy material from 171 patients presenting with intestinal motility disorders, is used for this study. It comprises 342 (160 cases) superficial rectal forceps biopsies, taken above the normal hypoganglionic zone[2], and 58 intestinal resection specimens from cases diagnosed as Hirschsprung's disease on forceps biopsies. In addition, intestinal segments from eight human fetuses (19–24 weeks of gestational age), and six newborns are obtained at autopsy and used as controls.

For mucosal biopsies perpendicular cryostat sections are stained with a double enzymehistochemical technique[3], revealing neuronal cell bodies by NADH-diaphorase histochemistry, and nerve fibres by acetylcholinesterase histochemistry.

Specimens obtained after surgical intervention or at autopsy are processed as a whole, without sectioning. They are properly stretched and fixed in Pearson's fixative. By microdissection under stereomicroscopical control, the different tissular sheets of the intestinal wall are separated. These tissular sheets are stained by acetylcholinesterase histochemistry or immunohisto-chemistry for S-100 protein[4].

RESULTS

Superficial rectal biopsies

The double enzymehistochemical staining on superficial rectal biopsies allows the identification of four different staining patterns. Accordingly the biopsy material is divided into: cases showing submucosal ganglia, containing at least one nerve cell with a large cytoplasm, and rare mucosal nerve fibres (normal innervation pattern, $n = 34$); cases showing an aganglionic submucosa with hypertrophic nerve fascicles, and a mucosal neural hyperpla-sia of variable degree (Hirschsprung's disease pattern, $n = 79$); cases (all newborns) showing submucosal ganglia, containing nerve cells with only a small cytoplasmic rim, and practically no mucosal nerve fibres (immature innervation pattern, $n = 5$); and cases showing submucosal ganglia, and a clearly increased number of nerve fibres, limited to the muscularis mucosae ($n = 42$).

Intestinal segments obtained in the control group

Auerbach's plexus is distinctly present from the most distal border of the internal anal sphincter, and extends uninterrupted orally. In the anal canal the plexus is composed of ganglia and nerve fascicles. The latter form a widely meshed neural network, composed of irregular polygons. At many corners of the latter, clusters of nerve cells are found forming rounded, well-delineated ganglia. Many extrinsic nerve fascicles merge with Auerbach's plexus of the anal canal. At the transition of the anal canal to the rectal ampulla, the plexus arrangement suddenly changes. In the rectal ampulla, ganglia are irregular and interconnected by short nerve fascicles, creating a narrowly meshed neural network. Unlike in the anal canal, all intersections of nerve fascicles now contain nerve cells.

Intestinal segments obtained in cases of Hirschsprung's disease

Cases of Hirschsprung's disease are subdivided according to neuroanatomical criteria related to the length of the aganglionic segment.

One case is recognized as an *ultrashort form of Hirschsprung's disease*, with abnormalities restricted to the anal canal. Anganglionosis associated with neural hyperplasia is found in a superficial biopsy taken at 3 cm above the dentate line. Similar abnormalities are seen in the full-thickness biopsy taken at the distal end of the rectosigmoidectomy specimen. The remaining part of the resection specimen shows a myenteric and submucosal ganglionated plexus, similar to the one found in the control group. It is estimated that only the most distal 4 cm of the anorectum is aganglionic for this case.

In cases of *classical Hirschsprung's disease* ($n = 53$), abnormalities are found in the anorectum and may extend all the way or not in the sigmoid or descending colon. Several extrinsic nerve fascicles enter the aganglionic rectum via its retroperitoneal wall. They pierce the outer muscle layer, reach the connective tissue septum, separating the outer and inner layer of the musculosa, and follow a fairly straight, ascending course throughout the more oral aganglionic rectum and colon. They finally merge with Auerbach's plexus of the normal, ganglionic oral colon via a transition segment. The length of this segment varies, as well as the arrangement of its ganglionated neural plexuses. In some cases ganglia occur more distally at the antimesenteric border than at the mesenteric border; in other cases the neural network shows paucicellular ganglia and solitary nerve cells. In yet other cases an occasional hypertrophic, extrinsic nerve fascicle is found among normal looking ganglia. Numerous nerve fascicles branch off from the ascending, extrinsic fascicles and proliferate into all layers of the intestine. They are responsible for the neural hyperplasia characteristic for Hirschsprung's disease.

In cases of *ultralong Hirschsprung's disease* abnormalities are found in the anorectum, and extend into the transverse colon ($n = 3$), throughout the entire colon ($n = 6$), or even into the distal ileum ($n = 2$). The anorectum, sigmoid and descending colon show similar neural abnormalities as in classical forms. Since the intramurally ascending nerve fascicles nowhere meet a normal ganglionated plexus, they end as tapering nerves. Consequently, the musculosa of the aganglionic colon proximal to the splenic flexure only shows occasional small nerve fascicles. The latter enter the colonic wall accompanying the mesenteric vascular truncs, and run at right angles to the intestinal axis.

In one case the anorectum, colon, appendix and distal part of the ileum is aganglionic, except for a limited segment of the transverse colon, and appendix, showing myenteric and submucosal ganglia.

DISCUSSION

Application of double enzymehistochemical staining to superficial rectal biopsies offers a reliable method for recognizing the neural abnormalities of the aganglionic colon and diagnosing true Hirschsprung's disease. By analysing intestinal specimens with a microdissection technique, we collect additional information on the neuroanatomy of the hindgut in normal and pathological conditions.

Our findings inthe control material demonstrate the present of Auerbach's plexus in the anal canal of the normal human intestine. Despite the fact that ganglia are less numerous in the anal canal than in the rectal ampulla, such terms as 'hypoganglionosis of the anal canal' and 'anganglionosis of the anal sphincter' are misleading or incorrect.

Compared with the normal innervation pattern found in the control group, the neural abnormalities we found in biopsies obtained from patients with motility disturbances can be interpreted as the morphological expression of neuronal agenesis, neuronal hypogenesis or neuronal immaturity.

In *neuronal agenesis* the ganglionated plexuses are absent in the anal canal and in a variable part of the more oral intestine. Extrinsic nerves still enter the aganglionic intestinal wall. They occur as intramurally ascending nerve fascicles, which give rise to a neural hyperplasia in the anorectum and distal colon. True Hirschsprung's disease is the result of such neuronal agenesis. Depending on clinical criteria[1], and on the extent of the neuroanatomical abnormalities, one can recognize: an ultrashort form of Hirschsprung's disease, limited to the anal canal; a classical form of Hirschsprung's disease, extending from the anorectum into the sigmoid or descending colon; and an ultralong form of Hirschsprung's disease, extending beyond the splenic flexure of the colon or occasionally up to the terminal ileum.

Aganglionosis of the intestine has been explained by a failure of normal neuroblast migration[5] or by a disturbance of the microenvironment[6] in the developing gut. The latter hypothesis is supported by the finding of an intermediate, ganglionic segment in a case of so-called double segmental aganglionosis with a skipped ganglionic area.

In *neuronal hypogenesis* the myenteric plexus shows paucicellular ganglia and solitary nerve cells. Hypogenesis may be seen in association with true Hirschsprung's disease in the transition zone betwen ganglionic and aganglionic bowel segments. This transition zone has to be resected together with the aganglionic segment. Neuronal hypogenesis is also found as an isolated congenital defect[7]. Thus, a normal migration of neuroblasts has to occur in these conditions, since nerve cells are present. Innervational disturbances in hypogenesis should therefore result from a local disturbance in the microenvironment, which has to be less pronounced or which occurs later than the one responsible for agenesis.

The cytologic characteristics of submucosal nerve cells in the rectum of newborns suggest the existence of *neuronal immaturity*. It has been demonstrated that during fetal development there is a progressive maturation of nerve elements, which continues in the first years of life[8]. At birth, one can expect rectal, submucosal ganglia showing at least one nerve cell with a well-developed cytoplasm among smaller immature ones. If these ganglia only contain immature nerves cells in children born at term, a neuronal maturation retardation[9] has to be diagnosed.

Finally, there are cases characterized by the presence of submucosal ganglia associated with nerve fibre hyperplasia limited to the muscularis mucosae. These previously reported[10,11] abnormalities cannot be classified as one of the subcategories described here. Since surgical intervention was not indicated in these cases, the myenteric plexus could not be evaluated.

To unravel the pathogenesis of these neuronal abnormalities other investigations will be necessary.

References

1. Kaiser, G. and Bettex, M. (1982). Chapter IV. Clinical generalities. In Holschneider, M. (ed). *Hirschsprung's Disease*, pp. 43–53. (Stuttgart: Hippokrates Verlag Gmbh)
2. Aldridge, R. T. and Campbell, P. E. (1968). Ganglion cell distribution in the normal rectum and anal canal. A basis for the diagnosis of Hirschsprung's disease by anorectal biopsy. *J. Pediat. Surg.*, **3**, 475–90
3. Mebis, J., Penninckx, F., Geboes, K. and Desmet, V. (1985). Histochemistry on rectal biopsies in the diagnosis of Hirschsprung's disease. *Acta Gastroenterol. Belg.*, **48**, 29–38
4. Mebis, J., Geboes, K. and Desmet, V. (1988). A microdissection technique for the en face visualisation of enteric component neural plexuses throughout the human gut. *VIII International Symposium on Morphological Sciences*, Rome, 10–15 July
5. Okamoto, E. and Ueda, T. (1967). Embryogenesis of intramural ganglia of the gut and its relation to Hirschsprung's disease. *J. Pediat. Surg.*, **2**, 437–43
6. Gershon, M. D., Epstein, M. C. and Hegstrand, L. (1980). Colonization of the chick gut by progenitors of enteric serotonergic neurons: distribution, differentiation and maturation within the gut. *Dev. Biol.*, **77**, 41–51
7. Meier-Ruge, W. (1969). New aspects in the pathology of the hypoganglionic megacolon. *Verh. Dtsch. Ges. Pathol.*, **53**, 237
8. Bughaighis, A. G. and Emery, J. L. (1971). Functional obstruction of the intestine due to neurological immaturity. *Progr. Pediat. Surg.*, **3**, 37–52
9. Erdohazi, M. (1974). Retarded development of the enteric nerve cells. *Dev. Med. Child. Neurol.*, **16**, 365
10. Toorman, J., Bots, G. Th. A. M. and Vio, P. M. A. (1977). Acetylcholinesterase-activity in rectal mucosa of children with obstipation. *Virchows Arch. Pathol. Anat.*, **376**, 159–64
11. Chow, C. W. and Campbell, P. E. (1983). Short segment Hirschsprung's disease as a cause of discrepancy between histologic, histochemical and clinical features. *J. Pediat. Surg.*, **18**, 167–71

9
Identification of the intrinsic innervation of human colonic smooth muscle

F. ANGEL AND T. L. PEETERS

INTRODUCTION

Human studies are essential for a good understanding of colonic motility and its nervous control, in health and disease. However, it is extremely difficult to make precise observations because of the multiple complex factors simultaneously involved in the control of motility. Furthermore, colonic electrical activities recorded *in vivo* show a high degree of variability. These activities are also modified by excitatory or inhibitory nervous inputs. Experiments on isolated segments of colonic muscle may eliminate a number of variables observed during experiments *in vivo* and help to provide a better understanding of colonic motility. More particularly, it seems essential to determine the nature of the neurons which modulate and control directly the activity of colonic smooth muscle cells.

A number of studies have been done concerning the pharmacological effects of exogenously applied non-peptide substances on human colonic smooth muscle layers[1-3]. Circular[4] and longitudinal[3,5] strips of human colonic smooth muscle responded to acetylcholine by a contraction and to noradrenaline by a relaxation. Serotonin induced either relaxant or contractile responses[6]; bradykinin relaxed taenia coli preparations[7,8]. Peptides have seldom been tested. One study undertaken by Couture *et al.*[9] in 1981 showed that longitudinal and circular strips of human colon contract in the presence of various peptides such as bradykinin, substance P, neurotensin and bombesin, and relax in the presence of vasoactive intestinal polypeptide. Only a few studies have been made on human colonic muscle *in vitro* which give information about the nature of the motor nerves to colonic muscle. Crema *et al.* in 1968[10] showed the existence of a non-adrenergic, non-cholinergic nerve-mediated relaxation[9].

In an attempt to determine the nature of motor nerves which synapse on human colonic smooth muscle, this present work was initiated to establish

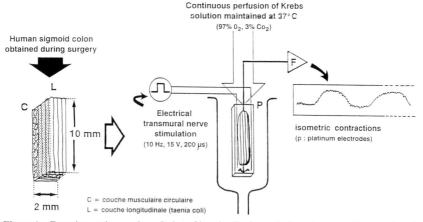

Figure 1 Experimental procedure. Strips of longitudinal muscle from human colon are placed in a superfusion apparatus, continuously perfused with warmed Krebs solution. Intramural nerves are electrically stimulated by means of two platinum electrode wires. The superfusate can be collected for RIA techniques

spontaneous mechanical activities developed by human taenia coli and its responses to transmural nerve stimulation. Furthermore, a pharmacological study was undertaken simultaneously to determine the nature of the neurotransmitters involved in the responses to electrical, transmural nerve stimulation.

MATERIAL AND METHODS

Strips of taenia coli (longitudinal muscle layer) from the human sigmoid colon were obtained from patients undergoing partial colectomy for carcinoma. Longitudinally oriented strips were dissected from the taenia coli after dissecting off the mucosa and the submucosa. Strips of muscle were then 'strung-up' in a glass-chambered superfusion apparatus. To record isometric tension, one end of the strip was securely anchored to a steel hook; the other end was attached to an isometric force transducer (10 Hz, 20 μs, 12 V). Intramural nerves were electrically stimulated by two platinum wire electrodes placed parallel to the strip. Modified Krebs solution[11] warmed to 37°C passed continuously over the muscle. In one set of experiments, the solution was collected in chilled test tubes for radioimmunoassay of gut peptides and more particularly of vasoactive intestinal polypeptide (VIP). The experimental set-up is illustrated diagrammatically in Figure 1.

RESULTS

Longitudinal muscle of human colon exhibited resting tone and spontaneous phasic mechanical activity (Figure 2) which consisted of small contractions (frequency ranging from 22 to 34 cycles per min) superimposed on larger

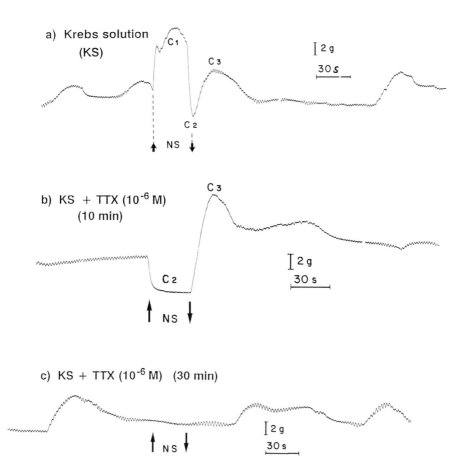

Figure 2 Responses to electrical, transmural nerve stimulation (frequency, 10 Hz; pulse duration, 200 μs; tension, 12 V) in normal Krebs solution (2a); in a solution containing TTX (10^{-6} M), after 10 min (2b) and after 30 min (2c). Note that spontaneous mechanical activities are not altered in the presence of TTX (2c)

contractions in amplitude and duration (frequency ranging from 1 contraction per min to 1 contraction every 2–4 min). Transmural nerve stimulation (square pulses: 10 Hz frequency, 200 μ duration, 12 V tension) for 30 s periods induced a triphasic response which consisted of three components (Figure 2a): the first one (C_1) occurred at the beginning of the stimulation. C_1 faded rapidly and was replaced by a transient relaxation (C_2). It was followed by a powerful contraction (C_3) at the end of the stimulation. The contractile components C_1 and C_3 of the response to nerve stimulation were blocked in the presence of tetrodotoxin (10^{-6} M) perfused during 10 min, leaving a deep relaxation (Figure 2b). However, after a 30 min perfusion of TTX

$(10^{-6}M)$, the entire response to nerve stimulation was abolished (Figure 2c) showing that it was a nerve-mediated response. Furthermore, the response to nerve stimulation was unaltered by adrenergic antagonists (phentolamine, propranolol; 10^{-6} M). Atropine $(10^{-6}$ M) induced a decrease of C_1, but left C_3 unaltered. These pharmacological experiments suggest that the existence of excitatory cholinergic nerves, excitatory and inhibitory NANC nerves in the longitudinal muscle of the human colon.

A preliminary study was then undertaken to test the hypothesis that the putative neurotransmitters VIP and substance P (SP) could be involved in the response to intramural nerve stimulation.

The exogenous application of the two peptides was first tested. SP induced a dose-dependent $(10^{-7}, 10^{-6}, 10^{-5}$ M) contraction which faded with time during SP perfusion. Since the excitatory response C_1 faded during nerve stimulation, the effect of prolonged application of SP was examined. We reasoned that, if SP or a SP-like peptide was the neurotransmitter involved in the contractile response to intramural nerve stimulation, desensitization by prolonged application of SP should abolish the excitatory response to nerve stimulation. Accordingly, the following experiments were undertaken.

The muscle strip was exposed to SP $(10^{-5}$ M) until the response to SP faded. Nerves were then electrically stimulated. In all experiments, the excitatory component C_1 of the response to nerve stimulation was decreased. An example is shown in Figure 3. After desensitization to SP $(10^{-6}$ M) the contraction C_1 was significantly $(p<0.05)$ decreased from 6.11 ± 0.99 g (control experiment) to 2.49 ± 0.56 g.

As far as VIP is concerned, the exogenous application of the peptide $(10^{-6}$ M) induced in some experiments a decrease in muscle tone and in all experiments an inhibition of spontaneous activity. No desensitization to VIP could be achieved. We therefore tried to determine whether VIP was released during intramural nerve stimulation.

As shown in Table 1, nerve stimulation did not produce any significant increase of VIP release in the superfusate in normal Krebs solution. However, the presence of TTX $(10^{-6}$ M) in the superfused Krebs solution produced a slight increase of VIP release in control experiments (133.75 ± 2.76 pg/ml) and a very significant $(p<0.05)$ increase of VIP release during nerve stimulation (168.5 ± 18.1 pg/ml), when the relaxation induced by nerve stimulation was the most pronounced (Figure 2).

DISCUSSION

The present work provides evidence for the existence of three kinds of motor nerves synapsing on the colonic smooth muscle cells: excitatory nerves that are cholinergic; and non-cholinergic, non-adrenergic inhibitory and excitatory nerves. Adrenergic nerves have also been described morphologically in the colon[12]. However, our preparations did not respond to adrenaline or noradrenaline (unpublished data). The non-cholinergic and non-adrenergic nerves in the human colon have not been specifically identified morphologically. So their existence can be generally inferred from physiological or

TACHYPHYLAXIS TO SUBSTANCE P (SP)

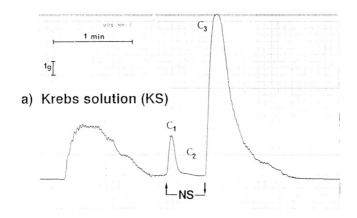

a) Krebs solution (KS)

b) KS + SP (10^{-6} M)

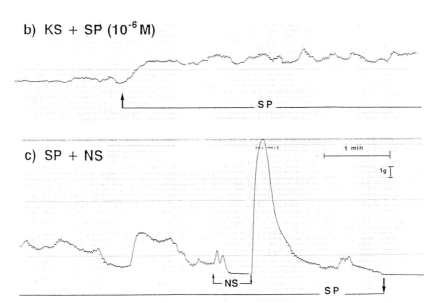

c) SP + NS

Figure 3 Tachyphylaxis to substance P. Intramural nerves were electrically (10 Hz, 200 μs, 12 V) stimulated in normal Krebs solution (3a). Substance P perfusion (10^{-6} M) was then undertaken until the baseline returned to control values. Then, intramural nerves were stimulated (3c). The component C_1 was significantly reduced

pharmacological evidence. To start with the identification of the neur-otransmitters involved in the response to nerve stimulation, the effects of exogenously applied substance P were tested on spontaneous contractile activity. It was shown that substance P had powerful excitatory effects and that it acted directly on colonic smooth muscle cells. The existence of non-cholinergic excitatory fibres has been suggested by the fact that some

Table 1 Release of VIP, expressed in pg/ml in the superfusate in control conditions and during transmural nerve stimulation when the muscle strips are perfused by normal Krebs solution or a solution containing tetrodotoxin (TTX, 10^{-6} M). It is important to note that the release of VIP is highly significant ($p < 0.05$) during TTX perfusion and is correlated to an increase of C_2 amplitude

	KS Before NS (10 Hz 15 U 200 μs)	KS + NS	KS + TTX(10^{-6} M)	KS + TTX(10^{-6} M) + NS (10 min. perf.)	TTX(10^{-6} M) + NS (30 min. perf.)
VIP pg/ml	106.12 ± 5.31	102.94 ± 5.42	133.75 ± 2.76*	178.50 ± 18.60*	104.30 ± 6.51

n = 16; m ± SEM; *$p < 0.05$; KS = Krebs solutions; NS = Nerve stimulation (10 Hz, 200 μs, 12 V)

contractions, induced in human colonic smooth muscle *in vitro* by electrical field stimulation, persisted in the presence of anticholinergic substances but were tetrodotoxin-sensitive[4,10]. Substance P has already been shown to exert its stimulant action through the activation of specific receptors since its effects were not influenced by a variety of classical inhibitors[13]. Furthermore, several lines of evidence in the literature suggest that substance P might be involved in the non-cholinergic excitatory response to electrical transmural nerve stimulation[4,11].

Finally, the fact that desensitization to substance P decreased the excitatory component of the response to nerve stimulation in our experiments provides evidence that substance P or a related substance might be an excitatory transmitter in human colonic smooth muscle.

Some of the present data, with others, support the hypothesis that VIP or a closely related peptide mediated the inhibitory component of the response to electrical, transmural nerve stimulation[11]. However, the release of VIP during nerve stimulation is significant when the excitatory nerve inputs are blocked in the presence of tetrodotoxin and when the relaxation induced by nerve stimulation is particularly deep. After 30 min perfusion of tetrodotoxin, whereas the entire response to nerve stimulation is blocked by tetrodotoxin, there was no more release of VIP. The exact mechanisms by which VIP released seems to be emphasized are still undetermined. Further experiments are needed to potentiate these data.

Acknowledgements

The authors thank the surgery departments of Professors Adloff and Grenier for providing human colon. They also express their appreciation to Christine Scheer for secretarial work and to Bernard Lafleuriel for illustrations.

References

1. Bennett, A. and Whitney, B. (1966). A pharmacological study of the motility of the human gastrointestinal tract. *Gut*, **7**, 307–16
2. Bennett, A. (1975). Pharmacology of colonic muscle. *Gut*, **16**, 307–11
3. Bucknell, A. and Whitney, B. (1964). A preliminary investigation of the pharmacology of the human isolated taenia coli preparation. *Br. J. Pharmacol.*, **23**, 164–75
4. Huizinga, J. D., Stern, H. S., Chow, E., Diamant, N. E. and El-Sharkawy, T. Y. (1985). Electrophysiologic control of motility in the human colon. *Gastroenterology*, **88**, 500–11
5. Fishlock, D. J. and Gunn, A. (1970). The action of angiotensin on the human colon in vitro. *Br. J. Pharmacol.*, **39**, 34–9
6. Burleigh, D. E. and Trout, S. J. (1986). Morphine attenuates cholinergic nerve activity in human isolated colonic muscle. *Br. J. Pharmacol.*, **88**, 307–13
7. Fishlock, D. J. and Parks, A. G. (1963). A study of human colonic muscle in vitro. *Br. Med. J.*, **14**, 666–7
8. Fishlock, D. J. (1966). Effect of bradykinin on the human isolated small and large intestine. *Nature*, **5070**, 1533–5
9. Couture, R., Mizrahi, J., Regoli, D. and Devroede, G. (1981). Peptides and the human colon: an in vitro pharmacological study. *Can. J. Physiol. Pharmacol.*, **59**, 957–64
10. Crema, A., Del Tacca, M., Frigo, G. M. and Lecchini, S. (1968). Presence of a non-adrenergic inhibitory system in the human colon. *Gut*, **9**, 633–7

11. Angel, F., Go, V. I.. W. and Szurszewski, J. H. (1984). Innervation of the muscularis mucosae of canine proximal colon. *J. Physiol.*, **357**, 93–108

12. Capurso, C., Friedmann, C. A. and Parks, A. G. (1968). Adrenergic fibres in the human intestine. *Gut*, **9**, 678–82

13. Couture, R. and Regoli, D. (1982). Mini review: smooth muscle pharmacology of substance P. *Pharmacology*, **24**, 1–25

10
Neural regulation of the *in vitro* release of colonic peptide YY

T. R. KOCH, K. H. SOERGEL, J. A. CARNEY AND V. L. W. GO

INTRODUCTION

Peptide YY (PYY) is a 36 amino acid peptide with amino-terminal tyrosine (Y) and carboxyl-terminal tyrosine (Y) amide that has been localized within 'open type' enteric endocrine cells[1]. A proportion of enteric PYY appears to be co-localized with enteroglucagon[2,3].

In humans, PYY is present in the ileum and colon with highest concentrations in the distal colon[4]. The majority of circulating PYY in humans appears to be released from the colorectal region[5]. In human subjects, its potential physiological endocrine effects include inhibition of gastric secretion[6], delay of gastric emptying[7] and increase in mouth-to-caecum transit time[8].

Possible regulation of gut endocrine cell secretion by enteric neural input is poorly understood. Previous morphological studies have shown that enteric extraepithelial endocrine cells are present in close proximity to non-myelinated nerve fibres[9]. In our present study, to examine possible neural regulation of PYY release, we used a specific radioimmunoassay to measure *in vitro* release of PYY from human colonic mucosa in the basal state, during activation of intramural nerves and during neural blockade.

METHODS

Tissue samples

Histologically and grossly normal human colon was obtained at surgery from patients who had a carcinoma, polyps or diverticulosis, and was transported to the laboratory in ice-cold oxygenated Krebs solution. The mucosal–submucosal layer was removed by microdissection; PYY was extracted into boiling 0.1 N HCl and was neutralized with assay buffer prior to determination by specific radioimmunoassay[4].

High performance liquid chromatography (HPLC)

Separation of immunoreactive PYY by our HPLC system has been previously described[4]. A Beckman model 332 liquid chromatograph was employed and included a Rainin Short One Column (C18) with a gradient of 25–45% CH_3CN in 0.1% trifluoroacetic acid buffer. Immunoreactive PYY was separated from solution collected during *in vitro* superfusion of human colonic mucosa. The system was independently calibrated with porcine PYY and human neuropeptide Y.

Release of PYY

By microdissection, strips (8 x 8 mm) of colonic mucosal–submucosal layer were prepared that were free of submucosal connective tissue but contained underlying muscularis mucosae and submucosal plexus. Each strip was bisected: one half was frozen prior to PYY extraction; the other half was pinned mucosal side upward in a 1 ml organ bath for superfusion with oxygenated Krebs solution at $37°C$[10]. After 1 h of equilibration, 1 min samples of solution were collected with a polyethylene pipette and added to chilled polypropylene tubes containing aprotinin (500 IU) and 50 μl of 1% bovine serum albumin. Intramural nerves were then field-stimulated for 1 min by current (400 μs square wave pulses at varying frequencies) passing across platinum electrodes with 10 mm separation. Cholinergic and then adrenergic receptor antagonists were superfused, followed by the neural toxin, tetrodotoxin. After the completion of each experiment, each strip was removed and frozen prior to PYY extraction and determination.

Immunocytochemical localization of PYY

Each colonic specimen was incubated for 20 h in 4% neutral buffered formalin. An indirect immunoperoxidase technique[11] was used to localize PYY-containing cells. Sections (3 μm) were prepared from paraffin blocks for immunostaining using rabbit Ab 80 raised against porcine PYY[4]. In previous work, we have shown that rabbit Ab 80 recognizes human PYY[4]. Controls included peptide absorption experiments, substitution of non-immune rabbit serum for the primary antibody, and substitution of non-immune goat serum for the secondary antibody. Peptide YY immunoreactivity was extinguished by pre-adsorption with porcine PYY (10 μg/ml anti-serum), but not by pre-adsorption with human neuropeptide Y (100 μg/ml) or human pancreatic polypeptide (100 μg/ml). The numbers of PYY-containing cells in the lower and upper halves of colonic crypts ($n = 7$ specimens) were estimated by counting PYY cells within 6 random fields per section (using sections cut parallel to the mucosal surface epithelium) and then averaged. The area of the field was determined from micrometer measurements.

RESULTS

HPLC

As shown in Figure 1, one immunoreactive peak which appeared to coelute with porcine PYY was separated from the superfusion solution. Using this elution gradient, human neuropeptide Y would have eluted 8 min later.

Mucosal–submucosal concentrations of PYY

At the beginning of each superfusion experiment ($n = 10$), the mean [SE] concentration of PYY was 4147 [851] ng/g wet tissue, while at the completion of these experiments, the mean [SE] concentration of PYY was unchanged at 4463 [931] ng/g (paired Student's t-test: $p > 0.05$).

Release of PYY

Basal release of PYY (Figure 2) was measured by radioimmunoassay in superfusion solution ($n = 10$ specimens). In our preliminary studies, release of PYY during electrical field stimulation at different frequencies was examined. During electrical field stimulation at 1 Hz, there was a trend toward increased PYY release from normal colonic mucosa (Figure 2). This increase in release of PYY was blocked by atropine (Figure 2). By contrast, stimulation at higher frequency (8 Hz) did not increase the release of PYY, most likely by further activating intramural inhibitory nerves (Figure 2). The latter result was not altered by addition of α- and β-adrenergic receptor antagonists (Figure 2). As shown in Figure 3, basal PYY release was not altered by addition of cholinergic and α- and β-adrenergic receptor

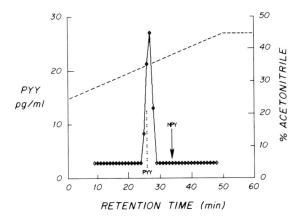

Figure 1 High-performance liquid chromatographic separation of immunoreactive PYY from superfusion solution. Elution of porcine PYY is indicated by the dotted line; human neuropeptide (NPY) would have eluted 8 min later

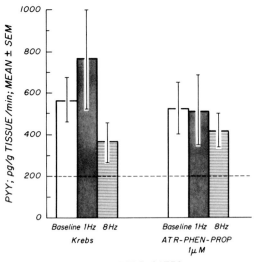

Figure 2 Basal release and field-stimulated release of PYY ($n = 10$ specimens). There was a trend toward increased release of PYY during low-frequency field stimulation (1 Hz); this effect was blocked by atropine sulphate (ATR). Release of PYY during high-frequency field stimulation (8 Hz) was not altered by phentolamine mesylate (PHEN) and propranolol · HCl (PROP). The dotted horizontal line indicates the lower detection limit of the radioimmunoassay

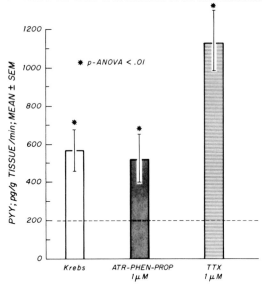

Figure 3 Release of PYY from human colonic mucosa ($n = 10$ specimens). Basal release of PYY was not altered by atropine sulphate (ATR), phentolamine mesylate (PHEN) and propranolol · HCl (PROP). Release of PYY was significantly increased ($p < 0.01$) by the neural toxin, tetrodotoxin (TTX). The dotted horizontal line indicates the lower detection limit of the radioimmunoassay

antagonists, but was significantly increased ($p < 0.01$) by neural blockade with tetrodotoxin.

Distribution of PYY-containing cells

In the lower half of the colonic crypts, immunoreactive PYY was identified within 'open-type' endocrine cells (Figure 4). In the upper half of the colonic crypts, immunoreactive PYY was present within rare, partially stained, thin cells (Figure 5). The average number of PYY cells in the lower half of crypts

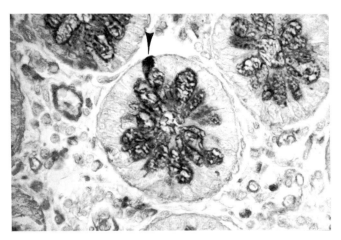

Figure 4 Immunostaining for PYY in human colonic mucosa ($n = 7$ specimens). In the lower half of colonic crypts, PYY was localized (arrowhead) to 'open type' endocrine cells (counterstained with alcian blue–periodic acid–Schiff stain; original magnification x 640)

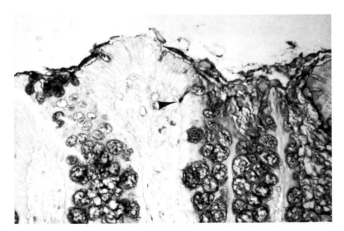

Figure 5 Immunostaining for PYY in human colonic mucosa ($n = 7$ specimens). In the upper half of colonic crypts, PYY was localized (arrowhead) to rare, partially stained, thin cells (counterstained with alcian blue–periodic acid–Schiff stain; original magnification x 640)

(mean $\pm$ SE: 8.0 ± 1 cells/mm^2) was greater than in the upper half of crypts (mean $\pm$ SE: 3.5 ± 0.3 cells/mm^2) (paired Student's t-test: $p < 0.05$). No immunoreactive PYY was present within nerve fibres.

DISCUSSION

Neural regulation of gut endocrine peptide release is supported by at least two previous observations. First, extraepithelial gut endocrine cells have been shown morphologically to be in close proximity to non-myelinated nerve fibres[9]. Secondly, the density of both gastric gastrin and somatostatin cell populations has been found to increase after vagotomy in animal models[12,13].

In our present study, radioimmunoassay of superfusion solutions was used to measure *in vitro* release of PYY from human colonic mucosa. The results suggest that release of PYY from human colonic mucosa was increased by activation of intramural excitatory (cholinergic) nerves and by blockade of intramural inhibitory (non-adrenergic, non-cholinergic) nerves.

Using the basal release of PYY and the concentration of PYY in human colonic mucosa, our study suggests that depletion of PYY stored in PYY-containing cells would require 5 days. This could explain the significantly lower density of PYY-containing cells in the upper half, compared with the lower half of colonic crypts, and the appearance of rare, partially stained, thin PYY cells near the mucosal surface. Further studies should be helpful in determining whether increased plasma concentrations of PYY in specific human colonic disorders[5] might be related to alteration of the neural regulation of PYY release.

SUMMARY

Peptide YY was measured in solutions obtained by *in vitro* superfusion of human colonic mucosa. Release of PYY was increased by activation of muscarinic-cholinergic intramural nerves and by blockade of non-adrenergic, non-cholinergic inhibitory intramural nerves. Peptide YY-containing cells were more commonly present in the lower half of the colonic crypts. In the upper half of the colonic crypts, partial staining of PYY cells suggested a lower PYY content. Active inhibitory neural input may be important in regulating the basal release of PYY, and PYY cells may become depleted during their migration from the base of the colonic crypt to the surface epithelium.

Acknowledgements

The authors extend their sincere gratitude to Lisa Go and Diane Roddy for technical assistance, to Cindy Stanislav for editorial assistance and to Dr Joseph Szurszewski for scientific input. This work was partially supported by grant DK34988-D from National Institutes of Health and by Merit Review grant 5020-09P from the Veterans Administration.

References

1. El-Salhy, M., Grimelius, L., Wilander, E., Ryberg, B., Terenius, L., Lundberg, J. and Tatemoto, K. (1983). Immunocytochemical identification of polypeptide YY (PYY) cells in the human gastrointestinal tract. *Histochemistry*, **77**, 15–23
2. Ali-Rachedi, A., Varndell, I., Adrian, T., Gapp, O., Van Noorden, S., Bloom, S. and Polak, J. (1984). Peptide YY (PYY) immunoreactivity is co-stored with glucagon-related immunoreactants in endocrine cells of the gut and pancreas. *Histochemistry*, **80**, 487–91
3. Bottcher, G., Alumets, J., Håkanson, R. and Sundler, F. (1986). Co-existence of glicentin and peptide YY in colorectal L-cells in cat and man. An electron microscopic study. *Regul. Peptides*, **13**, 283–91
4. Roddy, D. R., Koch, T. R., Reilly, W. M., Carney, J. A. and Go, V. L. W. (1987). Identification and distribution of immunoreactive peptide YY in the human, canine and murine gastrointestinal tracts: species-related antibody recognition differences. *Regul. Peptides*, **18**, 201–12
5. Koch, T. R., Roddy, D. R. and Go, V. L. W. (1987). Abnormalities of fasting serum concentrations of peptide YY in the idiopathic inflammatory bowel diseases. *Am. J. Gastroenterol.*, **82**, 321–6
6. Adrian, T., Savage, A., Sagor, G., Allen, J., Bacarese-Hamilton, A., Tatemoto, K., Polak, J. and Bloom, S. (1985). Effect of peptide YY on gastric, pancreatic, and biliary function in humans. *Gastroenterology*, **89**, 494–9
7. Allen, J., Fitzpatrick, M., Yeats, J., Darcy, K., Adrian, T. and Bloom, S. (1984). Effects of peptide YY and neuropeptide Y on gastric emptying in man. *Digestion*, **30**, 255–62
8. Savage, A., Adrian, T., Carolan, G., Chatterjee, V. and Bloom, SD. (1987). Effects of peptide YY (PYY) on mouth to caecum intestinal transit time and on the rate of gastric emptying in healthy volunteers. *Gut*, **28**, 166–70
9. Aubock, L. and Hofler, H. (1983). Extraepithelial intraneural endocrine cells as starting points for gastrointestinal carcinoids. *Virch. Archiv. A.*, **401**, 17–33
10. Koch, T. R., Carney, J. A., Go, V. L. W. and Szurszewski, J. H. (1988). Spontaneous contractions and some electrophysiologic properties of circular muscle from normal sigmoid colon and ulcerative colitis. *Gastroenterology*. (In press)
11. Nakane, P. K. and Pierce, G. M. Jr. (1966). Enzyme-labelled antibodies: preparation and application for the localization of antigens. *J. Histochem. Cytochem.*, **14**, 929–31
12. Delince, P., Willems, G. and de Graef, J. (1978). Antral gastrin cell proliferation after vagotomy in rats. *Digestion*, **18**, 27–34
13. Mulholland, M., Bonsack, M. and Delaney, J. (1985). Proliferation of gastric endocrine cells after vagotomy in the rat. *Endocrinology*, **117**, 1578–84

11
Intrinsic nerves of the pancreas after cutting the extrinsic pancreatic nerves in dogs

H. J. HÜCHTEBROCK, W. NIEBEL, M. V. SINGER, H. GOEBELL AND W. G. FORSSMANN

Little is known about the influence of cutting the extrinsic pancreatic nerves on the morphology and function of the intrapancreatic nerves in dogs. For this reason, intrapancreatic nerves of mongrel dogs were studied, using electronmicroscopy and immunocytochemistry, after truncal vagotomy (TV; $n = 5$), after coeliac and superior mesenteric ganglionectomy (G; $n = 6$) and after a combination of both operations (TVG; $n = 8$), i.e. removing all extrinsic nerves of the pancreas. Four dogs with intact extrinsic and intrinsic pancreatic nerves were used as controls. Studies were performed 1–2 weeks and up to 5 months after one or both denervation procedures. For immunohistochemical and electronmicroscopic studies, the animals were perfused with glutaraldehyde–formaldehyde/picric acid solution and the tissue was embedded in epon or paraffin.

RESULTS

Both immunohistochemical and electronmicroscopic studies revealed that only in the early phase (up to 30 days) after operation degeneration signs of intrapancreatic nerves occurred. After 60 days, hypertrophy of pancreatic nerve fibres was observed. The most striking finding was that the integrity of the intrapancreatic ganglia and nerves was almost preserved after complete extrinsic denervation (TVG). In controls, there was a strong intrapancreatic innervation with vasoactive intestinal polypeptide (VIP) and peptide histidine isoleucine (PHI), substance P and neuropeptide Y (NPY) nerves. NPY-nerves significantly decreased after the different denervation procedures but the other peptidergic nerves were not altered by TV, G or TVG.

CONCLUSIONS

We conclude that the dog pancreas contains extensive intrinsic peptidergic nerves which, with the exception of NPY nerves, are greatly independent of the integrity of the extrinsic nerves. This morphological finding is supported by physiological studies which suggest that the pancreatic secretory response to exogenous hormones mainly depends on an intact intrinsic innervation of the gland.

References

(1986). *Gastoenterology*, **90**, 355–61

12
Innervation of the pancreas before and after vagotomy

R. RADKE

INTRODUCTION

The neural status of the pancreas seems to be particularly interesting: two differentiated morphological and functional parts are unified in one organ. Moreover, the closer the exocrine cells are situated to the islets of Langerhans, the more intense is the innervation of these peri-insular cells[1,2]. Apart from the acinar–insular nervous relationships there is some evidence that a nervous connection between pancreas and the small intestine does exist. It has been shown that a dog's pancreas *in situ* responds much more strongly than the transplanted denervated Proc. uncinatus after giving Trypthophane intraluminally. This and other results support the existence of an enteropancreatic reflex[3]. What is the significance of the vagus nerves in this respect? Our study aimed to ascertain whether bilateral truncal vagotomy leads to any qualitative ultrastructural changes in the pancreatic nervous system of the dog.

MATERIALS AND METHODS

Light microscopy

The pancreas of pigs, cats and rats was stained with acetylcholinesterase[4].

Electron microscopy

Pancreatic tissue of dogs and rats were fixed in glutaraldehyde or potassium permanganate[5]. The material from bilaterally truncular vagotomized dogs was removed at post-operative intervals of 7, 14 days and 5 months.

RESULTS AND CONCLUSIONS

The main sources of the pancreatic nervous system are the ganglia (Figure 1). A large number of nerve cells are situated in these structures, forming interneuronal contact zones. The transmitter of the varicosities is, for example, VIP (Figure 1b). The intrapancreatic ganglia act among other things as a pacemaker in hormone liberation[6].

The exocrine pancreas contains a dense nervus plexus stemming from the ganglion. Every acinus is surrounded by nerve fibres. Considerably more nervous tissue was found in the islets of Langerhans (Figure 2). The finding was confirmed by ultrastructural investigations. A neuroinsular complex originates in the islets of Langerhans. Almost every B-cell of the canine's pancreas seemed to be innervated (Figure 3). In addition, the other cell types (A-, D- and PP-cells) have numerous neurocellular contact zones (Figure 4).

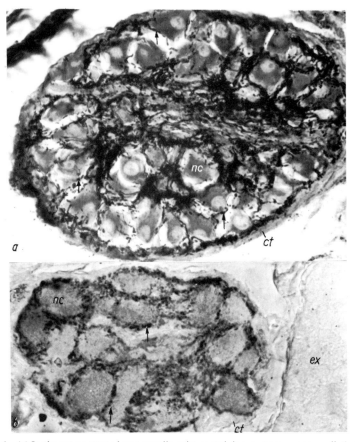

Figure 1 (a) In the cat pancreas large ganglia exist containing numerous nerve cells (*nc*) which are surrounded by synapses (arrow). A relatively thick layer of connective tissue (*ct*) encloses every ganglion. (b) A large number of VIP-varicosities surround every nerve cell (*nc*) of these cats ganglia. Osmic acid method (a); PAP-method (anti-VIP: 1:250). (a) x300; (b) x480

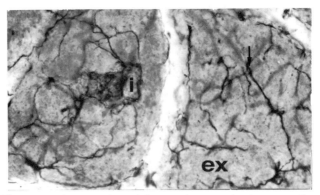

Figure 2 The pancreatic nerves (arrow) form a dense net in the organ. Every acinus is surrounded by nerve fibres. The islets of Langerhans (i) can be clearly differentiated by the much more concentrated insular plexus. Cat. Acetylcholinesterase. (x150)

The islets of Langerhans have been described in their entirety 'as the neuroparaneuronal control centre of the exocrine pancreas'. In this case, the intra-insular nerves should therefore not make contact with the endocrine cells but with the capillaries, in order to secrete into the insulo-acinar portal system[7]. This, together with the islet cell hormones, controls the exocrine pancreas. We have commented on this elsewhere[8].

Electron microscopic (Figure 3)[1] and immunohistochemical studies[9] show that external denervation (truncular vagotoma) obviously has no structural implications for the pancreatic nervous system. The majority of the nerve endings in both the exocrine and endocrine pancreas do not stem from external nerves as has been described[10] but are the terminals of the nervous system of the organ itself.

What is the functional interpretation of the fact that B-cell and acinar cell are linked by the same terminal nerve ending (Figure 3a[5])? It seems feasible that insulin secretion and the ecbolic pancreas function are related because both cell populations can be innervated by the same nerve. A linear correlation can be established between the B-cell reserve and the function of the exocrine pancreas in patients with chronic pancreatic disease[11].

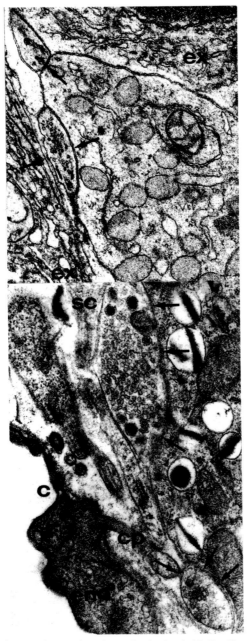

Figure 3 (a) Simultaneous innervation of an endocrine (probably B-cell) and exocrine pancreatic cell (ex) by one and the same axon (arrow). (b) Note the endothelial cell process (cp) of the fenestrated capillary (c) penetrating the basal membrane to establish contact with an axon; end = endothelial cell; sc = Schwann cell. Potassium permanganate (a) and glutaraldehyde perfusion (b)k. (a) x26 000, (b) x35 000

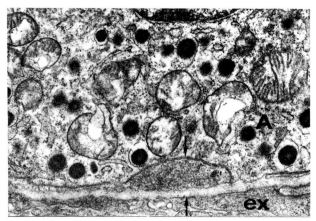

Figure 4 Simultaneous innervation (arrow) of an A-cell and acinus cell (ex) of dog pancreas after vagotomy (5 months). Glutaraldehyde. (x30 000)

References

1. Radke, R., Radke, M. and Radke, C. (1985). Licht- und elektronenmikroskopische Untersuchungen zur Innervation des exokrinen Pankreas. *Z. mikrosk-anat. Forsch.*, **99**, 1–17
2. Radke, R. and Štach, W. (1986). Do B-cell and peri-insular acinar cells have nerves in common? *Acta Anat.*, **127**, 65–8
3. Singer, M. V. (1981). *Neurohormonale Kontrolle der Pankreassekretion.* Nachweis eines enteropankreatischen Reflexes. (Stuttgart, New York: Georg Thieme Verlag)
4. Gomori, G. (1952). *Microscopic Histochemistry, Ptinciples and Practice.* (Chicago: University of Chicago Press)
5. Hökfelt, T. and Jonsson, G. (1968). Studies on reaction and binding of monoamines after fixation and processing for electron microscopy with special reference to fixation with potassium permanganate. *Histochemie*, **16**, 45–67
6. Stanger, J. I. and Samols, E. (1985). Role of intrapancreatic ganglia in regulation of periodic insular secretions. *Am. J. Physiol.*, **248**, E522–30
7. Fujita, T. and Kobayashi, S. (1979). Proposal of a neurosecretory system in the pancreas. An electron microscope study in the dog. *Arch. Histol. Jap.*, **42**, 277–95
8. Radke, R. and Stach, W. (1986). Are the islets of Langerhans neuro-paraneuronal control centers of the exocrine pancreas? *Arch. Histol. Jap.*, **49**, 411–20
9. Forssmann, W. G. and Greenberg, J. (1978). Organspecific innervation by autonomic nerve fibres as revealed by electron microscopy. *Front. Horm. Res.*, **12**, 5–73
10. Smith, P. H. and Madson, K. L. (1981). Interactions between autonomic nerves and endocrine cells of the gastroenteropancreatic system. *Diabetologia*, **20**, 314–24
11. Stock, K.-P., Domschke, S., Pichel, J., Schneider, M. and Domschke, W. (1985). Einschränkung von Insulinnerven und exokriner Pankreassekretion bei chronischer Pankreatitis. *Dt. med. Woschenschr.*, **110**, 134–6

SHORT COMMUNICATION

13
Immunohistochemistry of efferent and afferent pathways in components neural plexuses of the human pharyngo-oesophagus

J. MEBIS, K. GEBOES, J. JANSSENS, G. VANTRAPPEN, P. MOERMAN AND V. DESMET

INTRODUCTION

On deglutition a stripping wave of contraction created in the oropharynx passes the relaxed cricopharyngeus and descends uninterrupted into the oesophageal body. This behaviour is well documented by radiological, manometrical and electromyographical investigations in both animals and humans[1]. Yet, detailed morphological descriptions of the neuromuscular apparatus mediating this action are rare, especially for humans. The purpose of this study was: (a) to reinvestigate the anatomy of the musculature in the human pharyngo-oesophagus by a microdissection technique; and (b) to stain the dissected tissular sheets of the wall immunohistochemically in order to reveal the intramural ganglionated plexuses and the innervation of striated muscle cells.

MATERIALS AND METHODS

Pharyngo-oesophageal specimens, including the whole larynx, trachea and retrotracheal part of the oesophagus, were obtained by autopsy on three human fetuses, two newborns and two adults. The tubular gut was clamped at both ends and the lumen distended with Pearson's fixative. After 2 h of immersion fixation the clamped ends were removed, the specimen was opened lengthwise and pinned flat to paraffin filled dishes. All tissue handling is performed in 0.1 M phosphate pH 7.2, 0.1% Triton X-100 under a dissecting microscope (magnifications up to x40). During dissection the fixed specimens were opened at the dorsal or ventral midline, the trachea removed, the laryngeal cartilages carefully dissected free from the surrounding tissues and the different tissular layers of the gut wall separated. The sheets thus obtained were stained immunohistochemically for S-100 protein to visualize Schwann cells of the neural plexuses, neurofilament protein to visualize nerve cell perikarya, nerve fibres and motor endplates, and myelin basic protein to visualize myelinated nerves. Stained sheets were investigated by stereomicroscopy. Neuromuscular structures of special interest were selected and studied by conventional lightmicroscopy.

RESULTS

Anatomy of the musculature

The major band of cricopharyngeal muscle fibres both arises and inserts on the posterolateral aspects of the cricoid cartilage. It forms a continuous string of striated muscles around the sides and back of the pharyngo-oesophageal junction, crossing the dorsal midline without the formation of a raphé. The anatomy of the musculature in the proximal oesophagus is complex. In the inner layer, the course of the muscle fibres is elliptical and the inclination varies according to the level of the segment. For the outer layer, a stout tendinous band, attached to the dorsal aspect of the cricoid cartilage, gives origin to two separate muscle bands whose fibres, gathered by smaller accessory muscle slips, form thick anterolateral longitudinal muscle masses descending in parallel with and on either site of the trachea. At the 'most cervical segment' (corresponding to the first three tracheal cartilage rings) the inner muscle layer is incompletely covered by the outer layer, leaving a 'bare' area at the ventral and a 'V-shaped area of Laimer' at the dorsal aspect (Figure 1).

Ganglionated plexuses

From the proximal margin of the inner layer of the oesophageal musculosa Auerbach's plexus extends uninterrupted distally. It is present as an irregular

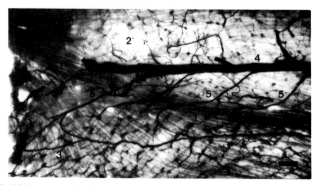

Figure 1 S-100-immunostained outer muscle sheet of the retrotracheal human oesophagus: (1) main longitudinal muscle mass; (2) bare areas; (3) V-shaped area of Laimer; (4) right recurrent laryngeal nerve; (5) oesophageal branches (Fetus 24 w, ▬▬▬ = 1 mm)

polygonal neural network composed of ganglia and branching interganglionic connections (Figure 2), corresponding to nerve fibre bundles that can be divided into primary (interganglionic), smaller secondary (interfascicular) and tertiary fascicles. The latter course into the connective tissue of both layers of the musculosa. Clusters of nerve cells are located within the confines of intersections of primary and secondary fascicles (intrafascicular ganglia) or may be found outside the confines of these fascicles (parafascicular ganglia). Many intersections do not contain nerve cells. Neurofilament stains reveal in detail the cellular composition of the ganglia: multipolar Dogiel type I nerve cells are present, showing many fine dendrites and a single coarse axon.

The submucosal neural network consists of a deep submucosal ganglionated (Henle's) plexus connected with an aganglionic, branching neural network extending through the more luminal submucosa towards the mucosa. In the 'most cervical segment' submucosal nerve cells are not found. However, in the more aboral submucosa Henle's plexus consists of paucicellular ganglia within a very wide meshed neural network facing the inner layer of the musculosa (Figure 3). A ganglionated plexus of Meissner is absent throughout the retrotracheal oesophagus.

Innervation of striated muscles

Myelin-basic-protein stains reveal three separate pathways for the motor innervation of striated muscle cells in the cricopharyngeus, and in both layers of the oesophageal musculosa.

(1) Fascicles of myelinated nerves enter the cricopharyngeus muscle at the far, left and right, posterior margin of the flattened sphincter. They fall apart into smaller nerve fibre bundles and, finally, in separate nerve fibres. The latter terminate in typical motor endplates on striated muscle cells of the cricopharyngeus.

(2) Nerve fascicles directed to the outer layer of the oesophageal musculosa

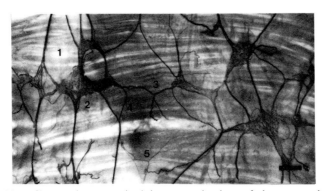

Figure 2 Neurofilament immunostained inner muscle sheet of the retrotracheal human oesophagus: (1) inner muscle layer; (2) intrafascicular ganglia of Auerbach's plexus; (3) primary; (4) secondary; (5) tertiary fascicles (Adult, ▬▬▬ = 1 mm)

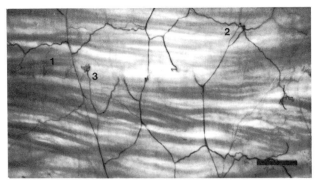

Figure 3 Neurofilament-immunostained inner muscle sheet of the retrotracheal human oesophagus: (1) inner muscle layer; (2) ganglia of Henle's plexus; (3) complex encapsulated neural ending. (Adult, ▬▬▬ = 1 mm)

merge with a wide-meshed neural network, located in the adventitia and perimuscular connective tissue. At several places, smaller nerve fibre bundles separate from this network. They fall apart into different nerve fibres, each one terminating in typical motor endplates (NF stains) on striated muscle cells (Figure 4).

(3) Nerve fascicles directed to the inner layer of the oesophageal musculosa pierce the external layer to merge with Auerbach's plexus. They traverse the ganglia (primary and secondary fascicles) without interruption and leave the plexus (tertiary fascicle) for the internal muscle layer. As in the outer layer, these nerve fibre bundles fall apart in separate nerve fibres terminating in typical motor endplates on striated muscle cells (Figure 5).

Terminal sensory innervation

Some large-sized myelin basic protein positive nerve fibres leave major nerve fascicles of the myenteric neural network and course into the inner muscle

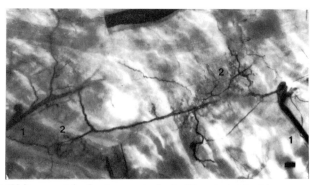

Figure 4 S-100-immunostained outer muscle sheet of the retrotracheal human oesophagus: (1) oesophageal branch of the recurrent laryngeal nerve; (2) cluster of motor endplates (Fetus 24 w, ▬▬▬ = 0.1 mm)

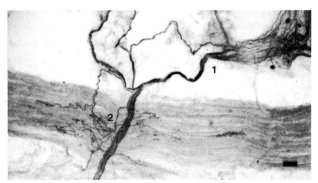

Figure 5 Neurofilament-immunostain of the motor innervation for striated muscle cells in the inner sheet of the oesophageal musculosa: (1) nerve fascicles and ganglion of Auerbach's plexus; (2) branching pattern of motor nerves to striated muscle cells (Adult, ▬▬▬ = 0.1 mm)

layer. They terminate in a spiral, wrapped-around striated muscle cells. When stained for neurofilaments these neuromuscular structures showed small-sized nerve fibres raising a spray of endings on the striated muscle cells in addition to the large spiralling nerve endings; they correspond to neuromuscular spindles.

Other complex nerve endings were found in the connective tissue which accommodates Auerbach's plexus, or in the deep submucosal connective tissue facing the musculosa. They are attached to Auerbach's or Henle's plexus via a single, large-sized nerve fibre. At their distal end these fibres bifurcate and raise twisting and tapering endings, forming complex globular neural structures (Figure 6).

DISCUSSION

Our observations on the anatomy of the musculature of the cricopharyngeus and retrotracheal part of the oesophagus in man correspond largely to

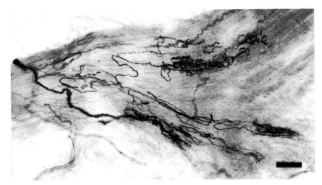

Figure 6 Neurofilament-immunostained submucosal sheet. A cluster of complex encapsulated neural structures is present in the deep submucosal connective tissue of the retrotracheal human oesophagus (Adult, ▬▬▬ = -.1 mm)

original descriptions given by Birmingham and Able and to pictorial illustrations made by Netter[2].

Our observations confirm previously reported findings[3] that, in the oesophageal musculosa, only the 'most cervical segment' is exclusively striated and that the transition zone corresponds to the remainder of the retrotracheal oesophagus. Consequently, in the 'most cervical segment' a significant part of the neural network must reflect the presence of motor pathways for striated muscle cells; while in the more aboral transition zone there must be a gradient changing this microanatomical organization of the neural network towards an arrangement as is seen in the smooth muscle oesophagus[4].

Two intramural ganglionated plexus are present in the retrotracheal part of the human oesophagus: Henle's plexus and Auerbach's plexus. In the submucosa, ganglia are seen only in the deep submucosa (Henle's plexus) and not in the superficial submucosa: Meissner's plexus, normally facing the muscularis mucosae, is absent. Yet, since in the 'most cervical segment' of the oesophagus, ganglia of Henle's plexus are also absent, the first submucosal ganglia appear more or less simultaneously with the development of muscularis mucosae. Hence, it is tempting to speculate that Henle's plexus is responsible for the innervation of the muscularis mucosae. The presence of numerous branching nerve fascicles, connecting Henle's plexus with the neural network of the muscularis mucosae supports this hypothesis.

In the musculosa, Auerbach's plexus is distinctly present in the fully striated 'most cervical segment': 50 ganglia/cm^2 in the newborn[5]. The density of ganglia increases over 100 ganglia/cm^2 throughout the remainder of the retrotracheal oesophagus[5], while transition to smooth muscle takes place.

Staining for myelin basic protein reveals the immediate extramural origin of myelinated nerve fascicles and their intramural course within the confines of the myenteric neural network. It proves that the recurrent laryngeal nerve provides motor innervation to the retrotracheal part of the oesophagus, and that the course of these motor fibres is different for both layers of the musculosa. Some fascicles run direct to striated muscle cells in the outer layer, other fascicles pierce the outer layer and traverse Auerbach's plexus through the ganglia to terminate on striated muscle cells of the inner layer. This explains the occurrence of a striking number of ramifying myelinated nerve fascicles in Auerbach's plexus at the 'most cervical segment' of the oesophagus. In the more aboral neural network, a reduction in number and size of myelinated nerve fascicles gradually occurs. The findings do not provide evidence for the role of nerve cells in ganglia of Auerbach's plexus at the fully striated 'most cervical segment' of the human oesophagus.

A few myelinated nerve fibres do not simply terminate on striated muscle cells, but show a more elaborated configuration of their endings forming neuromuscular spindles and complex globular neural structures. Richly innervated muscle spindles are found in the inner layer of the retrotracheal oesophageal musculosa. In analogy with the muscle spindles of skeletal muscle, we can speculate that they represent the mechanoreceptors in the striated part of the human oesophagus. Complex encapsulated neural endings, attached to Auerbach's and Henle's plexus, resemble specialized neural endings of the human skin[6]. These endings may represent proprioceptive elements of the human striated oesophagus.

References

1. Vantrappen, G. and Hellemans, J. (1974). *Diseases of the Esophagus*. (Berlin: Springer-Verlag)
2. Fransen, G. and Valembois, P. (1974). Anatomy and Embryology. In Vantrappen, G. and Hellemans, J. (eds.) *Diseases of the Esophagus*, pp. 1–16. (Berlin: Springer-Verlag)
3. Meyer, G. W., Austin, R. M., Brady, C. E. and Castell, D. O. (1986). Muscle anatomy of the human esophagus. *J. Clin. Gastroenterol.*, **8**, 131–4
4. Mebis, J., Geboes, K., Janssens, J., Desmet, V. and Vantrappen, G. (1987). Immunohistochemistry of ganglionated plexuses and of motor and sensory pathways in the human oesophagus. *Dig. Dis. Sci.*, **32**, 921
5. Mebis, J., Geboes, K., Janssens, J., Desmet, V. and Vantrappen, G. (1986). Micro-anatomy of the human oesophageal myenteric plexus and of its relations with the extrinsic nerves. In *Third European Symposium of Gastrointestinal Motility*, p. 37. (Bruges)
6. Miller, M. R., Ralston, H. J. and Kasamara, M. (1958). The pattern of innervation of the human hand. *Am. J. Anat.*, **102**, 183–218

14
Modulation of cholinergic neurons in canine antrum is not mediated by serotoninergic or adrenergic interneurons

E. A. MAYER, C. B. M. KOELBEL, G. VAN DEVENTER, W. J. SNAPE, JR. AND H. M. ENNES

INTRODUCTION

The neurokinins substance P, neurokinin A and neurokinin B have been identified in mammalian nerves, including the enteric nervous system[1,2]. The respective receptors, the NK-1, NK-2 and NK-3, mediate primarily excitatory responses to these peptides[3-10]. Based on immunohistochemical[1] and electrophysiological[11] studies, substance P has been identified as major excitatory neurotransmitter in the basic peristaltic circuitry within the mammalian ENS[1,12]. However, *in vivo*, substance P has been shown to inhibit small intestinal motility by stimulating inhibitory, cholinergic interneurons[13].

We have previously shown that neurokinin A is the most potent agonist for longitudinal muscle contraction and net acetylcholine release from cholinergic motor neurons in canine antral muscle, suggesting that both of these responses are mediated by a NK-2 receptor[14]. In the current study, by using a tritiated acetylcholine release assay, we sought to determine if, in addition to their stimulatory effect, neurokinins can also inhibit cholinergic motorneurons. We also wanted to determine if stimulatory and inhibitory effects are mediated by specific neurokinin receptors on the cholinergic motorneuron, or mediated by different interneurons. To determine if respective neurokinin effects are mediated by receptors on neurons within the myenteric plexus or on nerve terminals located within the longitudinal muscle, we compared the response in muscle strips with and without attached myenteric plexus.

METHODS

Tissue preparation

Thirty mongrel dogs, 15–30 kg, male and female, were anaesthetized with phenobarbital sodium. The stomach was removed and placed in modified Krebs solution at room temperature (137.4 Na$^+$, 5.9 K$^+$, 2.5 Ca^{2+}, 1.2 Mg^{2+}, 134.0 Cl$^-$, 15.5 HCO$_3^-$, 1.2 PO$_4^{2-}$, and 11.5 glucose, all mM). Sections of muscle coat from the anterior wall of the midantrum were prepared as described previously[15]. Longitudinally cut muscle strips, with or without attached myenteric plexus, were used. The lower end of a strip was attached to a stationary metal hook and the upper end to a Grass Instrument isometric strain gauge mounted on a Harvard Apparatus isometric stand. Tension was recorded on a Beckman model R-711 polygraph.

Measurement of ^{3}H acetylcholine release

Muscle strips were incubated in Krebs solution containing ^{3}H-choline (0.2 μM; 80 Ci/mmol) and eserine (50 mM) for one hour as described previously[15]. Incubation was followed by a continuous superfusion of Krebs-containing albumin (300 mg/l). After a washout period of 1 h the superfusate was collected and the tissue was exposed to peptides and/or EFS. Results of spontaneous and stimulated release of radioactivity were expressed as distintegrations per min (dpm) per gram tissue. Under these experimental conditions, the validity of assuming total tritium released during stimulation as a measure of ^{3}H-acetylcholine released has been demonstrated previously and validated for our system[16-18]. The release of ^{3}H-acetylcholine during the second stimulation was expressed as fraction of the release during the first stimulation.

RESULTS

Inhibition of cholinergic neurons

To determine if neurokinins can inhibit cholinergic motorneurons in addition to their stimulatory effect, we studied the effect of neurokinin A (NKA), a NK-2 agonist, and substance P methylester (SPME), a specific NK-1 agonist, on spontaneous and stimulated ^{3}H-acetylcholine release from longitudinal muscle strips with and without attached myenteric plexus.

No inhibitory effect on either peptide on spontaneous release was seen. In contrast, SPME, showed a dose-dependent inhibitory effect on ^{3}H-Ach release stimulated by electrical field stimulation (EFS; stimulation frequency: 10 Hz, pulse duration: 0.5 ms, stimulus duration: 1 min, stimulus strength: 25 V). The maximal inhibition (59 $\pm$ 11%; $n = 6$; $p < 0.05$) was observed in response to SPME 10^{-7} M. No inhibitory effect of NKA (10^{-11} M to 10^{-6} M) on EFS-stimulated ^{3}H-Ach release was seen in either preparation.

To determine if the inhibitory effect of SPME on stimulated ^{3}H-Ach release from strips with attached myenteric plexus was mediated by interneurons containing neuropeptides or neuromodulators with inhibitory effects on cholinergic motorneurons, we first evaluated the effect of adrenergic blockers, of the opioid receptor antagonist naloxone and of the prostaglandin synthesis inhibitory indomethacin on SPME-induced inhibition. As shown in Figure 1, pretreatment of tissues with phentolamine and propranolol (both 10^{-6} M) or naloxone (10^{-6} M) did not prevent the inhibition of EFS-stimulated ^{3}H-Ach release by SPME. In contrast, pretreatment with indomethacin (10^{-5} M for 10 min) abolished the inhibitory effect.

To determine if the inhibition seen with SPME could be reproduced by exogenous inhibitory modulators, we studied the effect of enkephalin, dynorphin and prostaglandin E_2 (PGE_2) on ^{3}H-Ach release, stimulated by EFS. Only PGE_2 (10^{-5} M) significantly reduced stimulated ^{3}H-Ach release by $32 \pm 8\%$ ($n = 6$; $p < 0.05$), whereas the two opioids were without effect.

Stimulation of cholinergic neurons

To determine if the stimulatory effect of NKA on spontaneous ^{3}H-Ach release is a direct effect on the cholinergic motorneuron or if it is mediated

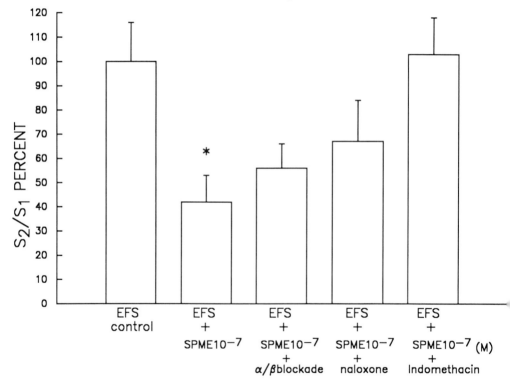

Figure 1 Release of ^{3}H-acetylcholine induced by electrical field stimulation (EFS). Shown are means $\pm$ SE after different treatments as indicated. Results are expressed as percentage of release induced by EFS alone;* indicates significant difference from control and indomethacin group ($p < 0.05$; $n = 5$–6 for each group)

by interneurons containing excitatory neuromodulators, we measured NKA-stimulated ^{3}H-Ach release in the absence and presence of hexamethonium $(10^{-4}\,M)$, and the serotonin receptor antagonist methysergide $(10^{-6}\,M)$. Neither blocker had a significant effect on NKA-stimulated ^{3}H-Ach release.

DISCUSSION

Neurokinins released from myenteric neurons or from collaterals of spinal afferents within the myenteric plexus may be the major excitatory non-cholinergic neuromodulators of gastrointestinal muscle[19]. In the current study we have shown that exogenous neurokinins can both stimulate and inhibit the release of acetylcholine from neurons in the myenteric plexus of canine antral muscle. These effects appear to be mediated by different neurokinin receptors.

We had previously shown that neurokinin A is the most potent member of the neurokinin family to stimulate net acetylcholine release from antral myenteric plexus[14]. Substance P has been shown to stimulate cholinergic interneurons[20], and the release of other neuroregulators[21-24]. In the current study we found that, in the canine antrum, the stimulation of acetylcholine release by neurokinin A is unaffected by hexamethonium and by the serotonin receptor antagonist methysergide. Therefore, neither cholinergic nor serotoninergic interneurons are mediating the stimulatory effect on cholinergic motorneurons. Since specific antagonists for gastrin-releasing peptide receptors are currently not available, and since desensitization to this peptide in our assay is not possible without depleting [^{3}H]-acetylcholine stores, we cannot rule out the possibility that neurokinin-induced release of gastrin-releasing peptide contributes to the stimulatory effect.

Even though no inhibitory effect of neurokinins was observed on spontaneous acetylcholine release and on basal contractile activity, substance P methylester, a specific agonist of the NK-1 receptor, inhibited the increase in acetylcholine release secondary to electrical depolarization of myenteric neurons by electrical stimulation. This inhibition was not seen with neurokinin A or neurokinin B. We have previously shown that the contractile response to electrical field stimulation with the parameters used in the current study is completely blocked by tetrodotoxin and atropine[14]. Thus the current results are consistent with the hypothesis that a NK-1 receptor located either on cholinergic motorneurons or on interneurons mediates the inhibitory neurokinin effect. The presence of inhibitory neurokinin receptors on cholinergic neurons in the guinea pig ileum has been suggested previously[7]. Substance P has also been shown to stimulate the release of opioids[21] which, in turn, can modulate acetylcholine release. Our results indicate that prostaglandins play a significant role in the inhibitory effect of substance P methylester on acetylcholine release, since indomethacin prevented the inhibition, and exogenous prostaglandin E_2 mimicked the inhibition. We have previously shown that prostaglandin E_2 is involved in the inhibitory effect of somatostatin on stimulated acetylcholine release[15]. The generation of arachionic acid metabolites, including prostaglandins from membrane phospholipids in response to neuropeptides has been reported[25]. Thus it is conceivable that prostaglandins are liberated from muscle and/or neurons in response to NK-1 receptor activation. Even though catecholamines and opioids do not seem to play a role in inhibitory effect of substance P methylester, the current results do not rule out that other inhibitory neuropeptides, such as somatostatin or VIP mediate the effect and that prostaglandin release is associated with the action of these inhibitory peptides.

References

1. Furness, J. B. and Costa, M. (1982). Identification of gastrointestinal neurotransmitters. In Bertaccini, G. (ed.) *Handbook of Experimental Pharmacology*, pp. 383–460. (Berlin: Springer)
2. Harmar, A. J. (1984). Three tachykinins in mammalian brain. *Trends Neurosci.*, **7**, 57–60
3. Buck, S. H., Burcher, E., Shults, C. W., Lovenberg, W. and O'Donohue, T. L. (1984). Novel pharmacology of substance K-binding sites: a third type of tachykinin receptor. *Science*, **226**, 987–9
4. Burcher, E. and Buck, S. H. (1986). Multiple tachykinin binding sites in hamster, rat and guinea-pig urinary bladder. *Eur. J. Pharmacol.*, **128**, 165–77
5. Burcher, E., Buck, S. H., Lovenberg, W. and O'Donohue, T. L. (1986). Characterization and autoradiographic localization of multiple tachykinin binding sites in gastrointestinal tract and bladder. *J. Pharmacol. Exp. Therap.*, **236**, 819–31
6. Fosbray, P., Featherstone, R. L. and Morton, I. K. M. (1984). Comparison of potency of substance P and related peptides on [^{3}H]acetylcholine release, and contractile actions, in the guinea-pig ileum. *Naunyn-Schmiedeberg's Arch. Pharmac.*, **326**, 11–115
7. Kilbinger, H., Stauss, P., Erlhof, I. and Holz, P. (1986). Antagonist discrimination between substypes of tachykinin receptors in guinea-pig ileum. *Naunyn-Schmiedeberg's Arch. Pharmacol.*, **334**, 181–7
8. Lee, C. M., Iversen, L. L., Hanley, M. R. and Sandberg, B. E. B. (1982). The possible existence of multiple receptors for substance P. *Naunyn-Schmiedeberg's Arch. Pharmacol.*, **318**, 281–7
9. Lee, C. M., Campbell, J., Williams, B. J. and Iversen, L. L. (1986). Multiple tachykinin binding sites in peripheral tissues and in brain. *Eur. J. Pharmacol.*, **130**, 209–17
10. Regoli, D., Drapeau, G., Dion, S. and D'Orleans-Juste, P. (1987). Minireview: Pharmacological receptors for substance P and neurokinins. *Life Sci.*, **40**, 109–117
11. Wood, J. D. (1987). Physiology of the enteric nervous system. In Johnson, L. R. (ed.) *Physiology of the Gastrointestinal Tract*, Vol. 1, p. 77. (New York: Raven Press)
12. Wood, J. D. (1987). Neurophysiological theory of intestinal motility. *Japan J. Smooth Muscle Res.*, **23**, 143–86
13. Daniel, E. E., Gonda, T., Domoto, T., Oki, M. and Yainahara, N. (1982). The effect of substance P and Met[5]-enkephalin in dog ileum. *Can. J. Physiol. Pharmacol.*, **60**, 830–40
14. Koelbel, C. B., Van Deventer, G., Snape, W. J. Jr. and Mayer, E. A. (1987). Differences in the stimulation of antral and colonic smooth muscle by mammalian tachykinins. *Gastroenterology*, **92**, 1475
15. Koelbel, C. B., Van Deventer, G., Khawaja, S., Mogard, M., Walsh, J. H. and Mayer, E. A. (1988). Somatostatin modulates cholinergic neurotransmission in canine antral muscle. *Am. J. Physiol.*, **254** (*Gastrointest. Liver Physiol.* **17**), G201–9
16. Szerb, J. C. (1976). Storage and release of labelled acetylcholine in the myenteric plexus of the guinea-pig ileum. *Can. J. Pharmacol.*, **54**, 12–22
17. Wu, Z. A. C., Kisslinger, S. C. and Gaglinella, T. S. (1982). Functional evidence of cholinergic nerve endings in the colonic mucosa of the rat. *J. Pharmacol. Exp. Ther.*, **221**, 664–9
18. Yau, W. M. and Youther, M. L. (1982). Direct evidence for a release of acetylcholine from myenteric plexus of guinea pig small intestine by substance p. *Eur. J. Pharmacol.*, **81**, 665–8
19. Bartho, L. and Holzer, P. (1985). Search for a physiological role of substance P in gastrointestinal motility. *Neuroscience*, **16**, 1–32

20. Fox, J. E. T. and Daniel, E. E. (1986). Substance P: a potent inhibitor of the canine small intestine in vivo. *Am. J. Physiol. (Gastrointest. Liver Physiol.*, **13**), G21–7

21. Garzon, J., Hoellt, V., Sanchez-Blazquez, P. and Herz, A. (1989). Neural activation of opioid mechanisms in guinea pig ileum by excitatory peptides. *J. Pharmacol. Exp. Ther.*, **240**, 642–9

22. Hermansen, K. (1980). Effects of substance P and other peptides on the release of somatostatin, insulin, an glucagon in vitro. *Endocrinology*, **107**, 256–61

23. Olpe, H. R., Heid, J., Bittiger, H. and Steinmann, M. W. (1987). Substance P depresses neuronal activity in the olfactory bulb in vitro and in vivo: possible mediation via gamma-aminobutyric acid release. *Brain Res.*, **412**, 269–74

24. Regal, J. F. and Johnson, D. E. (1983). Indomethacin alters the effects of substance P and VIP on isolated airway smooth muscle. *Peptides*, **4**, 581–84

25. Axelrod, J., Burch, R. M. and Jelsema, C. L. (1988). Receptor-mediated activation of phospholipase A_2 via GTP-binding proteins: arachidonic acid and its metabolites as second messengers. *Trends Neurosci.*, **11**, 117–23

· Costa, M., Furness, J. B. and Llewellyn-Smith, I. J. (1987). Histochemistry of the enteric nervous system. In Johnson, L. R. (ed.) *Physiology of the Gastrointestinal Tract.* Vol. 1, pp. 1–41. (New York: Raven Press)

· Domoto, T., Berezin, J. I., Fox, J. E. T. and Daniel, E. E. (1983). Does substance P comediate with acetylcholine in nerves of opposum esophageal muscularis mucosa? *Am. J. Physiol.*, **245** (*Gastrointest. Liver Physiol.*), G19–28

· Wormser, U., Laufer, R., Hart, Y., Chorev, M., Gilon, C. and Selinger, Z. (1986). Highly selective agonists for substance P subtypes. *EMBO J.*, **5**, 2805–8

SHORT COMMUNICATION

15
Gastrointestinal aspects of autonomic neuropathy

P. KEMPLER, A. VÁRADI, F. SZALAY, E. KÁDÁR, E. REGŐS AND B. VESZTER

Autonomic neuropathy (AN) is a well recognized but poorly understood syndrome, in which cardiovascular and gastrointestinal symptoms usually dominate the clinical picture. Resting tachycardia, orthostatic hypotension [1-3] and decreased left ventricular performance[4] may be present. AN is associated with a high mortality[5,6] secondary to silent myocardial infarction[7], major arrhythmias, cardiorespiratory arrest[8] and other causes not yet explained. Gastrointestinal symptoms might make miserable the patients' everyday life. Motor abnormalities of oesophagus, stomach and bowels are consequences of parasympathetic (PS) damage[9], with drug metabolism also being altered in these patients. Reflux oesophagitis is a common clinical sign[9]. A definite gastroparesis is, however, rare; although, in some cases, vomiting may be intractable and need surgical treatment[10]. Impaired gallbladder contractility due to PS damage is an important risk factor in the pathogenesis of cholelithiasis[11]. A catastrophic watery diarrhoea with several nocturnal exacerbations and faecal incontinence may occur, but its mechanism is not well understood[12]. Post-prandial hypotension is supposed to be due to sympathetic (S) neuropathy. Autonomic abnormalities have been reported in patients with irritable bowel syndrome[9].

Diabetes mellitus[1,3,12,14] and chronic alcoholism[13,15] are well known aetiologic factors of AN. However, no data are available on the occurrence of AN in patients with chronic liver diseases.

The aim of our present study was to evaluate autonomic function in patients with liver diseases of alcoholic and non-alcoholic origin and to compare their results with those of diabetic patients.

PATIENTS

Examined groups were:

(1)   126 patients with Type 1 (insulin-dependent) diabetes mellitus (DM)

(age: 14–57, mean: 34·4 years; mean duration of diabetes: 11·6 years);
(2) 99 patients with chronic alcoholism were divided on the basis of clinical, laboratory and histological data into three groups:
    (a) group A/I: 33 patients without liver disease (age: 25–55, mean: 42·6 years),
    (b) group A/II: 33 patients with liver disease but without cirrhosis (age: 29–55, mean: 42 years),
    (c) group A/III: 33 patients with alcoholic cirrhosis (age: 29–56, mean: 45 years);
(3) 10 patients with primary biliary cirrhosis (PBC, age: 34–69, mean: 52 years)
(4) 12 patients with cirrhosis of other origin (COO) (3 patients were HBsAg-positive; 'cryptogenic' cirrhosis was present in 9 patients, age: 31–64, mean: 52 years)
(5) 40 controls (K) (healthy subjects, age: 20–55, mean, 36·5 years).

METHODS

The quantitative determination of cardiovascular reflex disturbances as a simple non-invasive method was chosen for the evaluation of AN. Cardiovascular reflex tests were performed by Ewing's criteria[1,2]. Parasympathetic integrity was evaluated by beat-to-beat variation, by Valsalva ratio and standing ratio, and by sympathetic function by blood pressure response to standing and to sustained handgrip test[1,2,14,15]. Methods, as well as normal, borderline and abnormal values are summarized in Table 1[1].

RESULTS AND DISCUSSION

Table 2 shows mean values of cardiovascular reflex parameters in the various patient groups and in controls. All parameters in the five patient groups

Table 1

| | Beats/min. | | 30/15 | | Valsalva | | Handgrip | |
	Au	C/E	Au	C/E	Au	C/E	Au	C/E
K	—	—	—	—	—	—	—	—
A/I	+ <0.05	+ 0.05	+ + 0.01	+ 0.01	—	—	—	—
A/II	+ + + <0.001	+ + 0.001	+ + + 0.001	+ + 0.001	+ + + 0.001	+ + 0.001	+ + 0.01	+ 0.01
A/III	+ + + <0.001	+ + 0.001	+ + + 0.001	+ + 0.001	+ + + 0.001	+ + 0.001	+ + + 0.001	+ + 0.001
PBC	+ + + <0.001	+ + 0.001	+ + + 0.001	+ + 0.001	+ + + 0.001	+ + 0.001	+ + + 0.001	+ + 0.001
COO	+ + 0.01	+ 0.05	+ + 0.01	+ + 0.001	+ + 0.01	+ + 0.001	+ + + 0.001	+ + 0.001
DM	+ + + <0.001	+ + 0.001	+ + + 0.001	+ + 0.001	+ + 0.01	+ 0.01	+ + + 0.001	+ + 0.001

+ p < 0.05   + p < 0.05
+ + p < 0.01   + + p < 0.001
+ + + p < 0.001   + + + p < 0.01

Table 2 Mean values of cardiovascular reflex parameters in the various patient groups and in controls ($\bar{x} \pm SD$)

Groups	Beat-to-beat variation (beats/min)	30/15 ratio	Valsalva ratio	Sustained handgrip test (mmHg)
K	23.2 ± 7.3	1.14 ± 0.07	1.68 ± 0.28	24.0 ± 5.5
A/I	17.4 ± 7.2[+]	1.09 ± 0.06[++]	1.58 ± 0.49	18.9 ± 7.1
A/II	10.5 ± 5.4[+++]	1.01 ± 0.05[+++]	1.37 ± 0.28[+++]	15.6 ± 0.9[++]
A/III	7.9 ± 3.9[+++]	1.00 ± 0.03[+++]	1.15 ± 0.28[+++]	13.1 ± 6.8[+++]
PBC	11.0 ± 6.9[+++]	1.03 ± 0.04[+++]	1.12 ± 0.13[+++]	13.9 ± 7.4[+++]
COO	12.3 ± 6.6[++]	1.03 ± 0.06[++]	1.33 ± 0.22[++]	15.0 ± 7.4[+++]
DM	15.2 ± 9.8[+++]	1.05 ± 0.09[+++]	1.49 ± 0.32[++]	17.1 ± 9.6[+++]

Significance of differences compared to controls (Student's unpaired t-test):
[+]$p < 0.05$; [++]$p < 0.001$; [+++]$p < 0.01$.

showed a significant reduction compared to controls, except Valsalva-ratio and sustained handgrip test in group A/I.

Severity of PS neuropathy was defined by Ewing[1,2] as follows. Early PS damage: one of the three heart rate tests is abnormal. Definite PS involvement: two or three of the heart rate tests are abnormal. Number of patients with abnormal parameters by various reflex texts as well as with early PS, definite PS and PS + S neuropathy is summarized in Table 3. Incidence of abnormal parameters by four reflex tests, as well as incidence of PS and S damage, was found to be significantly higher in groups A/II and A/III compared to group A/I. Between groups A/II and A/III a significant difference was found only in respect of definite PS damage ($p<0.05$). Thus the major difference was found between groups A/I and A/II, i.e. between alcoholics with and without hepatic damage.

Abnormal blood pressure test to standing occurred in two diabetics only, therefore this method is not shown on Tables 2 and 3. All results in controls were normal. A severe gastroparesis was found in two diabetics.

Our data revealed AN with a prevalence not negligible in all groups examined, even in chronic liver diseases of non-alcoholic origin. AN in chronic alcoholism is related not only to chronic alcohol intoxication but to parenchymal hepatic damage. Autonomic failure has to be considered as a possible cause of gastrointestinal symptoms in liver diseases. The poor prognosis of AN further deteriorates the chances of survival of liver patients.

Table 3 Incidence of patients with abnormal reflex parameters and with early PS, definite PS, PS, PS + S neuropathy in the various patient groups

Groups	No. of patients total	Beat-to-beat variation (beats/min)	30/15 ratio	Valsalva ratio	Sustained handgrip test (mmHg)	PS neuropathy (definite)	PS neuropathy (all)	PS + S neuropathy
K	40	0	0	0	0	0	0	0
A/I	33	7	7	0	4	1	13	4
A/II	33	20^+	19^+	6^+	15^+	11^+	30^+	15^+
A/III	33	28^{++}	27^{++}	12^{++}	18^{++}	26^{++}	31^+	18^+
PBC	10	5	5	6^{+++}	5	6^{++}	8	5
NANPBC	12	5	5	2^+	4	3	8	4
DM	126	54^+	58^+	14^+	49^{++}	36^{++}	85^{++}	49^+

Significance of differences compared to group A/I (χ^2 test, Fischer's exact test):
$^+ p < 0.05$; $^{++} p < 0.01$; $^{++} p < 0.001$

References

1. Ewing, D. J. and Clarke, B. F. (1982). Diagnosis and management of diabetic autonomic neuropathy. *Br. Med. J.*, **285**, 916–18
2. Ewing, D. J., Martyn, Ch. N., Young, R. J. and Clarke, B. F. (1985). The value of cardiovascular autonomic function tests: 10 years experience in diabetes. *Diabetes Care*, **8**, 491–7
3. Runge, M. and Kühnau, J. (1983). Die autonome kardiale Neuropathie. *Dtsch. med. Wschr.*, **108**, 190–213
4. Zola, B., Kahn, J. K., Juni, J. E. and Vinik, A. I. (1986). Abnormal cardiac function in diabetics with autonomic neuropathy in the absence of ischemic heart disease. *J. Clin. Endocrinol. Metab.*, **63**, 208–14
5. Ewing, D. J., Cambell, B. F. and Clarke, B. F. (1976). Mortality in diabetic autonomic neuropathy. *Lancet*, **1**, 601–3
6. Hasslacher, Ch. and Bächler, G. (1983). Prognose der kardialen autonomen Neuropathie bei Diabetikern. *Münch. Med. Wschr.*, **125**, 375–7
7. Faerman, I., Faccio, E., Milei, J., Nunez, R., Jadzinsky, M., Fox, Dora and Rapaport, M. (1977). Autonomic neuropathy and painless myocardial infarction in diabetic patients. *Diabetes*, **26**, 1147–58
8. Kahn, J. K., Sisson, J. C. and Vinik, A. I. (1987). QT interval prolongation and sudden cardiac death in diabetic autonomic neuropathy. *J. Clin. Endocrinol. Metab.*, **64**, 751–4
9. Guy, R. I. C., Sharma, A. K., Thomas, P. K. and Watkins, P. J. (1983). Gastroparesis diabeticorum: the role of surgery and the histological abnormalities of the vagus nerve. *Diabetologia*, **25**, 160
10. Smart, H. L. and Atkinson, M. (1987). Abnormal vagal function in irritable bowel syndrome. *Lancet*, **1**, 475–8
11. Vogelberg, K. H., Kübler, H. G. W., Cicmir, J. and Rathman, W. (1984). Gallenblasenkontraktilität, Cholelithiasis und autonome Neuropathie bei Diabetes mellitus. *Dtsch. med. Wschr.*, **109**, 1712–15
12. Watkins, P. J. (1982). Diabetic neuropathy II. *Br. Med. J.*, **285**, 557–8
13. Duncan, G., Johnson, R. H., Lambie, D. G. and Whiteside, E. A. (1980). Evidence of vagal neuropathy in chronic alcoholics. *Lancet*, **2**, 1053–7
14. Kempler, P., Váradi, A., Regös, E., Veszter, B., Oravetz, L. and Kiss, È. (1987). Cardiovascular autonomic neuropathy in diabetes mellitus. *J. Mol. Cell. Cardiol.*, **19**, 43
15. Kempler, P., Váradi, A., Regös, È., Veszter, B., Oravetz, L. and Kiss, È. (1987). Cardiovacular autonomic neuropathy in diabetes mellitus, in chronic alcoholism and in patients suffering from diabetes and alcoholism simultaneously. *Diabetologia*, **30**, 538A

POSTER ABSTRACT

16
Structural alterations of the enteric nervous system in Crohn's disease

A. VON HERBAY, G. SCHÜRMANN, T. MATTFELDT,
M. BETZLER AND P. MÖLLER

Operative specimens from 11 patients with Crohn's Disease were studied in multiple transmural biopsies (up to 20) taken along each specimen. The enteric nervous system (ENS) was marked by means of immunohistochemistry for protein S-100, and was studied with light microscopy. Morphological findings in the ENS were quantified by morphometry, and correlated to the extent of inflammatory or fibrous alterations in its respective localization (bowel section, tissue layer).

Compared to normal controls, several alterations in the ENS were found:

(1) degenerative alterations of submucosal ganglion cells and nerve fibres;
(2) proliferation of submucosal nerve fibres, in part representing neuromas;
(3) degenerative alterations in ganglion cells of Auerbach's plexus;
(4) augmented nerve fibres in the lamina propria mucosae.

The extent of lesions in the ENS correlated approximately with the extent of inflammatory or fibrous lesions in the specimen. Moreover, similar lesions were sometimes, but not always, found in grossly normal resection margins.

These findings are interpreted as degenerative and reactive, e.g. proliferative alterations of the enteric nervous system in Crohn's Disease. Their pathophysiologic relation and their functional implications are discussed.

POSTER ABSTRACT

17
Ultrastructural studies of the intestinal nervous system in diabetes mellitus, amyloidosis, AIDS and Whipple's disease

H. G. SCHMIDT AND A. SCHMID

In diabetes mellitus (DM) and amyloidosis, gastrointestinal motility disorders may occur in consequence of an autonomic neuropathy. Recently, autonomic neuropathy has also been described in AIDS. Whipple's disease may also be associated with an involvement of the central nervous system. We examined ultrastructurally Meissner's plexus in endoscopic biopsies from the gastrointestinal tract in DM, amyloidosis, AIDS and Whipple's disease and, additionally, the vagus nerve in surgical biopsies in DM.

METHOD

Gastric biopsies were obtained from 30 diabetics (D) – 13 D had no diabetic late complications; 11 D had late complications with no gastrointestinal motility disorders and 6 D had diabetic gastroparesis. Rectal biopsies were available from 34 D – 10 D had no diabetic late complications; 14 D had late complications with no gastrointestinal motility disorders and 10 D had late complications associated with motility disorders such as diarrhoea, constipation or megacolon. Surgical biopsies of the vagus nerve (surgery for ulcer, carcinoma, etc.) of 16 D were investigated – 6 D with no diabetic late complications; 8 D with late complications but no gastrointestinal motility disorders and 2 D with gastroparesis diabetica (surgery for extreme gastroparesis).

Amyloidosis

Rectal biopsies of 10 patients with amyloidosis associated with amyloid deposits in the rectal mucosa were studied. Of these patients 4 had gastrointestinal motility disorders.

AIDS

Rectal biopsies were taken from 4 patients with full-blown AIDS; 4 with AIDS-related complex and 4 HIV-positive patients were studied.

Whipple's disease

Duodenal biopsies from 7 patients with Whipple's disease were examined. Controls for the abovementioned patient groups were gastric biopsies from 10, and rectal biopsies from a further 10 non-diabetics with no gastrointestinal disease, and also surgical vagal biopsies obtained in 6 non-diabetics.

RESULTS

Diabetes mellitus

Half of the D with gastrointestinal motility disorders, and one-third of D with late complications but no motility disorders, had, in the stomach or rectum, nerval changes such as axon-ballooning, axonal cytolysosomes, an increase in lipofuscin and lysosomes in Schwann cell cytoplasm, and multilayered thickening of Schwann cell basement membrane. In the stomach of 2 D, a few Schwann cells with no axons were seen. Several of these changes were sometimes found in one and the same nerve fibre. A maximum of 10% of the nerve fibres per biopsy revealed changes. In the vagus nerve 2/2 D with gastroparesis, and 4/8 D with late complications but no motility disorders, showed changes in a maximum of 5% of the nerve fibres per biopsy, such changes including axon ballooning, accumulation of glycogen, paracrystalline substances, lysosomes and lipofuscin in Schwann cell cytoplasm, Schwann cells with no axons, collagen pockets and multilayered thickening of Schwann cell basement membrane.

Amyloidosis

In 2 patients with and 2 without motility disorders, a maximum of 3% of the nerve fibres per biopsy revealed an intra-axonal increase of mitochondria, and an intra-axonal accumulation of osmiophilic homogeneous or layered structures.

AIDS

Two out of four patients with full-blown AIDS revealed a few scattered tubuloreticular structures (TRS) in Schwann cell cytoplasm, and axon-cytolysosomes.

Whipple's disease

One out of seven patients who also revealed CNS manifestation of the disease, had Whipple's bacteria in various stages of degradation up to and including phagolysosomes in Schwann cell cytoplasm in more than 30% of the nerve fibres per biopsy.

CONCLUSIONS

Ultrastructural studies of Meissner's plexus and vagus nerve in diabetes mellitus, and of Meissner's plexus in amyloidosis, AIDS and Whipple's disease reveal in some of the patients characteristic and uncharacteristic, nerval changes for each of the diseases.

18
Hirschsprung's disease: recent advances in the understanding of its pathophysiology

M. HANANI, O. Z. LERNAU, O. ZAMIR AND S. NISSAN

INTRODUCTION

Hirschsprung's disease (HD) is characterized by the total absence of the intrinsic ganglion cells of the myenteric and submucous plexuses in varying lengths of the distal bowel[1]. Another typical finding in the aganglionic bowel is the proliferation of cholinergic and adrenergic nerve fibres[2,3]. The functional obstruction that is observed in HD is usually explained by the absence of normal peristalsis and the constriction in the diseased segment. These findings fail to account for all the aspects of the disease; for example, the great variability in the clinical presentation and the lack of correlation between the severity of the symptoms and the length of the aganglionic segment[2]. This suggests that factors other than the absence of the neurons are also involved. Recent immunhistochemical findings indicate that aganglionosis is associated with a complex alteration of many types of nerve fibres. The emerging view is that HD may not simply represent a denervation effect, but rather a complex alteration of neuromuscular function. The aim of this paper is to discuss the current research on HD and to present some recent data on the role of the proliferating fibres in HD.

CHARACTERISTICS OF THE NERVE FIBRES IN THE AGANGLIONIC BOWEL

Morphology and histochemistry

An increase in the size and number of adrenergic and cholinergic fibres has been demonstrated by histochemical methods[2,3], yet their structure is poorly understood. Ultrastructural studies on these fibres[4] showed that the intramuscular layer and the circular muscle are more richly innervated than in the normal bowel, in accord with light microscopic observations. However, the nerve fibres looked normal, in contrast to their hypertrophic appearance under the light microscope. Recent work utilizing electron microscopy of ACh-ase-stained fibres also demonstrated the innervation of muscle by these fibres[5]. Interestingly, Garrett et al.[2] found that patients with severe neonatal obstruction had dense ACh-ase positive innervation of the circular muscle in the aganglionic segment. Patients with mild symptoms had the fewest nerves. This suggests that cholinergic nerves are functional in the aganglionic bowel and may have abnormally high activity leading to an increased release of ACh, which causes muscle spasm. Similar observations have not been reported by other authors but they are supported by in vitro studies on isolated aganglionic segments showing that the cholinergic nerves in HD are functional and may release excessive amounts of ACh[6,7].

Immunohistochemistry

Immunostaining of nerves has demonstrated that in HD the number of peptidergic nerves is reduced, but a considerable number of fibres containing VIP, substance P and other peptides do exist[8,9,10]. An exception to this rule was the increase in the number of fibres containing neuropeptide Y (NPY)[11]. This peptide is known to coexist with noradrenaline (NA) and may be contained in the numerous noradrenergic fibres found in HD. There is very little information on the physiology of the peptidergic fibres in the aganglionic bowel. We have shown that non-adrenergic, non-cholinergic nerves are functional in the aganglionic bowel[7].

Several nerve-specific antibodies have been used to investigate the nature of the innervation of the aganglionic bowel. These include antibodies for the proteins neuron-specific enolase and S-100 (which is found in glial cells)[12]. It is noteworthy that, unlike the ACh-ase method, immunostaining did not reveal nerve fibres as hypertrophic[12]. This is in accord with the electronmicroscopic findings[4] and suggests that the hypertrophic appearance may simply reflect a high enzymatic activity. Further insight was obtained by the use of the antibody, D_7, which recognizes a subset of bowel neurons. No D_7 immunoreactive fibres were found in the aganglionic segment[13]. Clearly, the use of antibodies holds promise for the diagnosis as well as the study of the physiology and pathogenesis of HD[14].

Origin of the nerve fibres

The origin of the proliferating fibres is not clear. Several authors assume that these are extrinsic cholinergic and noradrenergic fibres[3,15]. This is probably correct regarding the noradrenergic fibres, but the cholinergic fibres may originate in proximal, ganglionic regions. Likewise, the source of the peptidergic fibres is obscure, most of them (e.g. those containing VIP, substance P and enkephalin) are probably enteric in origin, whereas others may be extrinsic[11]. Some nerve types may have both extrinsic and enteric origins (e.g. VIP and NPY nerves[11]).

Physiology and pharmacology of nerve fibres in the anganglionic segments

Since the available techniques do not allow direct electrical recordings from these nerves, indirect methods have been employed for studying their physiology and pharmacology. Isolated muscle strips were used and nerve activity was assessed by measuring muscle contractions in response to various nerve-specific stimuli. Nerve activation by electrical field stimulation (EFS) produced relaxation followed by contractions in control preparations, whereas aganglionic segments responded with strong contraction only. This contraction was blocked by atropine[7,15,17,18]. We have found that after blockade with atropine the aganglionic segment also showed relaxation during EFS[7]. This response was also not diminished by adrenergic blockers (Figure 1). This indicates that, first, the cholinergic fibres in the diseased area are functional and apparently release excessive amounts of ACh. This conclusion is based on the findings that the muscle response to muscarinic agonists is normal (see p. 615). The results are in accord with the increased amounts of ACh found in HD[19]. Secondly, functional non-adrenergic non-cholinergic nerve fibres are present in the aganglionic bowel. The identity of the inhibitory transmitter is still unknown, but it may be one of the peptides that can be found in the affected segment.

Noradrenergic fibres can be effectively stimulated with nicotinic agonists such as dimethyl phenyl piperazinium iodide (DMPP). DMPP evokes relaxation in the normal intestine due to NA release[7,20]. Reports on its effect on the aganglionic segment are conflicting[21,22]. Our own work[7] however,

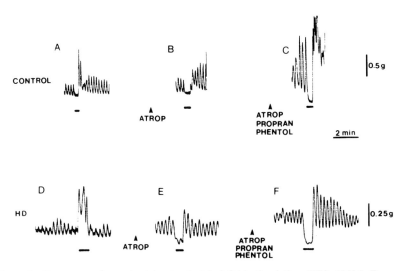

Figure 1 Responses of muscle strips to electrical field stimulation (EFS; 10 Hz). Top row, normal bowel; bottom row, aganglionic bowel. **A**: control response to EFS. **B**: the response in the presence of atropine (10^{-6} M). **C**: in the presence of atropine and the adrenergic blockers phentolamine and propranolol (both 10^{-5} M). **D**: control response. **E**: in the presence of atropine (10^{-6} M). **F**: in the presence of adrenergic blockers (both 10^{-5} M)

has clearly demonstrated that DMPP is less effective in relaxing the muscle in aganglionic compared to normal segments. Since it has been shown that muscle response to NA in HD is similar to normal controls[23], it follows that the noradrenergic fibres in HD secrete less transmitter in spite of their proliferation[2,3] and the greater amounts of NA that they contain[17].

The combination of: (1) increased release of ACh; (2) decreased release of NA; and (3) diminished amounts of non-adrenergic, non-cholinergic inhibitory transmitter, will tend to produce muscle contractions in the aganglionic bowel. Variations in one or more of these factors have been observed among different patients and may explain the great variability in the clinical presentation in HD.

WHAT CAUSES MUSCLE SPASM IN THE AGANGLIONIC SEGMENT?

According to Ehrenpreis[24], clear mechanical obstruction exists in the aganglionic bowel which he described to be in 'a state of spastic contraction'. This view is supported by most of the workers in the field (although Nixon[24a] claimed that affected segment is not always narrowed). *In vitro* work[16] showed that the electrical properties of the muscle cells from the aganglionic segment are similar to those obtained in control samples. It should be noted, however, that these controls were taken from the ganglionic part of the colon, which shows some deviations from colon of normal patients[2]. It can be concluded that, in general, the aganglionic segment is contracted, although exceptions may occur.

Physiological experiments support the above conclusion. Blockade of nerve activity of intestinal segments *in vitro* greatly enhanced muscle contractions[25] and Wood[26] has proposed that there is a tonic activity of myenteric neurons causing the release of an inhibitory neurotransmitter that opposes the spontaneous tendency of the circular muscle to contract. When the intrinsic nervous activity is missing, as in HD or during nerve blockade, muscle activity will be expected to increase. This hypothesis is very useful when attempting to understand the normal function of the enteric nervous system and the pathophysiology of HD[26], but it is probably not complete and should be modified to account for the following points: (1) in Chagas' disease the enteric ganglia are missing or damaged but the affected segment appears to be dilated[27]; (2) if the only difference between normal and aganglionic bowel is the absence of ganglion cells, the severity of the symptoms should be clearly correlated with the extent of aganglionosis. As noted above, such correlation does not always exist. It therefore appears that, in addition to absence of ganglion cells, other factors (possibly nerve fibre activity) contribute to the disease.

The tonically active myenteric neurons proposed by Wood[26] apparently play a key role in the function of the intestine, but there is little evidence for such cells from intracellular recordings. We have observed rhythmic firing of action potentials from a very small fraction ($< 1\%$) of myenteric neurons

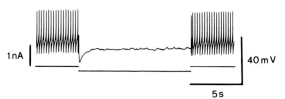

Figure 2 Spontaneous activity recorded from a myenteric neuron of the guinea-pig duodenum. The bottom record is the current trace. The current was injected in order to suppress the action potentials. No synpatic activity can be observed during current injection, suggesting that the activity is intrinsic to the neuron

from the guinea-pig, both in tissue culture[28] and in the freshly dissected preparation (Figure 2).

IS THERE AN ALTERATION IN THE PROPERTIES OF THE SMOOTH MUSCLE IN HD?

One of the hypotheses for explaining the apparent constriction of the aganglionic segment was that the sensitivity of the intestinal muscles increased due to the absence of the normal innervation (denervation hypersensitivity). It was assumed that ACh released from the nerves would evoke stronger contractions in the hypersensitivie muscle[24]. However, there is no clear support for this idea. In different studies, the sensitivity of the aganglionic bowel to ACh was found to be higher[21] than normal, lower[28,29] or normal[6,23]. Part of the disagreements may be due to the use of ACh as the cholinergic agonist. The presence of high ACh-ase activity in the aganglionic samples may have affected the results. Several authors report normal responses to ACh in HD[23,30]. We also studied this question, using the muscarinic agonist carbachol (which is ACh-ase resistant) and found that there is no significant difference between muscle responses to this agent in normal and diseased specimens. Likewise, the sensitivity of the muscle in HD to NA appears to be normal[23]. These findings are in accord with the view that the motility dysfunction in HD is mainly neurogenic rather than myogenic.

CONCLUSIONS

Despite many years of study, the pathophysiology of HD is still obscure, but it seems that this disease involves more than simple denervation. The data from recent work presented above strongly suggest that many types of nerve are present in the aganglionic bowel. These nerves may be functional and may affect the motility by releasing various neurotransmitters. It is likely that these nerves will be the subject of further study in the coming years.

References

1. Whitehouse, F. R. and Kernohan, J. W. (1948). Myenteric plexus in congenital megacolon. *Arch. Int. Med.*, **82**, 75–111

2. Garrett, J. R., Howard, E. R. and Nixon, H. H. (1969). Autonomic nerves in rectum and colon in Hirschsprung's disease. *Arch. Dis. Childh.*, **44**, 406–17

3. Gannon, B. J., Noblett, H. R. and Burnstock, G. (1969). Adrenergic innervation of bowel in Hirschsprung's disease. *Br. Med. J.*, **3**, 338–40

4. Howard, E. R. and Garrett, J. R. (1970). Electron microscopy of myenteric nerves in Hirschsprung's disease and in normal bowel. *Gut*, **11**, 1007–14

5. Ito, Y., Tatekawa, I., Nishiyama, F. and Hirano, H. (1987). Ultrastructural localization of acetylcholinesterase activity in Hirschsprung's disease. *Arch. Pathol. Lab. Med.*, **111**, 161–5

6. Frigo, G. M., Del Tacca, M., Lecchini, S. and Crema, A. (1973). Some observations on the intrinsic nervous mechanism in Hirschsprung's disease. *Gut*, **14**, 35–40

7. Hanani, M., Lernau, O. Z., Zamir, O. and Nissan, S. (1986). Nerve mediated responses to drugs and electrical stimulation in aganglionic muscle segments in Hirschsprung's disease. *J. Pediatr. Surg.*, **21**, 848–51

8. Bishop, A. E., Polak, J. M., Lake, D. B., Bryant, M. G. and Bloom, S. R. (1981). Abnormalities of the colonic regulatory peptides in Hirschsprung's disease. *Histopathology*, **5**, 679–88

9. Larsson, L. T., Malmfors, G. and Sundler, F. (1983). Peptidergic innervation in Hirschsprung's disease. *Z. Kinderchir.*, **38**, 301–4

10. Tsuto, T., Okamura, H., Fukui, K., Obata-Tsuto, H. L., Terubayashi, H., Tanagihara, J., Iwai, N., Majioma, S., Yanaihara, N. and Ibata, Y. (1985). Immunohistochemical investigation of gut hormones in the colon of patients with Hirschsprung's disease. *J. Pediatr. Surg.*, **20**, 266–70

11. Hamada, Y., Bishop, A. E., Federici, G., Rivosecchi, M., Talbot, I. C. and Polak, J. M. (1987). Increased neuropeptide Y-immunoreactive innervation of aganglionic bowel in Hirschsprung's disease. *Virch. Arch. A.*, **411**, 369–77

12. Hall, C. L. and Lampert, P. W. (1985). Immunohistochemistry as an aid in the diagnosis of Hirschsprung's disease. *Am. J. Clin. Pathol.*, **83**, 177–81

13. Fujimoto, T., Reen, D. J. and Puri, P. (1987). Immunohistochemical characterization of abnormal innervation of colon in Hirschsprung's disease using D_7 monoclonal antibody. *J. Pediatr. Surg.*, **22**, 246–51

14. Tam, P. K. H. (1986). An immunochemial study with neuron-specific-enolase and substance P of human enteric innervation – the normal developmental pattern and abnormal deviations in Hirschsprung's disease and pyloric stenosis. *J. Pediatr. Surg.*, **21**, 227–32

15. Okamoto, E. and Okasora, T. (1987). Cause of constriction in the aganglionic segment in Hirschsprung's disease. In Kasuya, H., Nagao, M. and Matsuo, Y. (eds.) *Gastrointestinal Function*, Vol. 5, pp. 53–65. (Amsterdam: Excerpta Medica)

16. Kubota, M., Ito, Y. and Ikeda, K. (1983). Membrane properties and innervation of smooth muscle cells in Hirschsprung's disease. *Am. J. Physiol.*, **244**, G406–15

17. Nirasawa, Y., Yokoyama, J., Ikawa, H., Morikawa, Y. and Katsumata, K. (1986). Hirschsprung's disease: catecholamine content, Alpha-adrenoceptors, and the effect of electrical stimulation in aganglionic colon. *J. Pediatr. Surg.*, **21**, 136–42

18. Larsson, L. T., Malmfors, G., Wahlestedt, C., Leander, S. and Hakanson, R. (1987). Hirschsprung's disease: a comparison of the nervous control of ganglionic and aganglionic smooth muscle in vitro. *J. Pediatr. Surg.*, **22**, 431–5

19. Ikawa, I., Yokoyama, Y., Morikawa, Y., Hayashi, A. and Katsumata, K. (1980). Quantitative study of acetylcholine in Hirschsprung's disease. *J. Pediatr. Surg.*, **15**, 48–52

20. Bennett, A. and Stockley, H. R. (1975). The intrinsic innervation of the human alimentary tract and its relation to function. *Gut*, **16**, 443–53

21. Wright, P. G. and Shepherd, J. J. (1965). Response to drugs of isolated human colonic muscle from a case of Hirschsprung's disease. *Lancet*, **2**, 1161–4

22. Beleslin, D. B., Bumbic, S. and Terzic, B. (1980). Action of drugs on the human colonic preparations of Hirschsprung's disease. *Neuropharmacology*, **19**, 1125–30

23. Penninckx, F. and Kerremans, R. (1975). Pharmacological characteristics of the ganglionic and aganglionic colon in Hirschsprung's disease. *Life Sci.*, **17**, 1387–94

24. Ehrenpreis, (1970). *Hirschsprung's Disease*. (Chicago: Year Book Medical Publishers)

24a. Nixon, H. H. (1977). Hirschsprung's disease: a commentary. *Ann. Chir. Infant.*, **18**, 219–29

25. Wood, J. D. (1972). Excitation of intestinal muscle by atropine, tetrodotoxin and xylocain. *Am. J. Physiol.*, **222**, 118–25

26. Wood, J. D. (1987). Physiology of the enteric nervous system. In Johnson, L. R. (ed.)

Physiology of the Gastrointestinal Tract, 2nd edn., pp. 67–109. (New York: Raven Press)

27. Smith, B. (1972). *The Neuropathology of the Alimentary Tract*. (London: Edward Arnold)
28. Hanani and Burnstock, G. (1985). Synaptic activity of myenteric neurons in tissue culture. *J. Auton. Nerv. Syst.*, **5**, 155–64
29. Hiramoto, Y. and Kiesewetter, W. B. (1974). The response of colonic muscle to drugs: an in vitro study of Hirschsprung's disease. *J. Pediatr. Surg.*, **9**, 13–20
30. Kamijo, K., Hiatt, R. B. and Koelle, G. (1953). Congenital megacolon. A comparison of the spastic and hypertrophied segments with respect to cholinesterase activities and sensitivities to acetylcholine, DPF and the barium ion. *Gastroenterology*, **24**, 173–85

Part II
Nerves and the Upper Gastrointestinal Tract

19
Calcitonin gene-related peptides I and II: distinct effects on gastric acid secretion in humans

C. BEGLINGER, W. BORN, P. HILDEBRAND, J. FISCHER AND K. GYR

The human calcitonin (CT) gene-related peptides (CGRP I AND CGRP II) are protein products of two closely related CT/CGRP genes. The two neuropeptides have been recognized throughout the gut including the stomach. In animals, CGRP I inhibits gastric acid secretion. Here, we compared in healthy volunteers effects of i.v. infusions of CGRP I and CGRP II to those on gastric acid secretion

METHODS

Twelve healthy subjects were studied on different days. Gastric acid secretion was measured continuously by aspiration using a marker perfusion technique (PEG 4000 as a non-absorbable marker). Step-doses of CGRP I and CGRP II (79–320 pmol/kg/h) were given on continuous pentagastrin (PG) stimulation (100 ng/kg/h) and compared to CT (88–352 pmol/kg/h) and saline (control). Furthermore, the effects of continuous i.v. infusions of CGRP I and CGRP II (79 pmol/kg/h), CT (88 pmol/kg/h) or saline (control) were determined on graded PG (50–800 ng/kg/h) stimulation.

RESULTS

The results are shown in Table 1.

SUMMARY

CGRP I did not inhibit PG-stimulated acid secretion. However, CGRP II and CT inhibited summated acid responses to graded PG by 20% and 28%

Table 1 Summated incremental gastric secretory responses to step-doses of pentagastrin (mean ± SEM)

	0 (control)	CGRP I (79 pmol/kg/h)	CGRP II (79 pmol/kg/h)	CT (88 pmol/kg/h)
Acid, mmol	9.9 ± 70.7	9.8 ± 0.8	8.0 ± 1.0*	7.1 ± 0.9**
Volume, ml	72 ± 7	68 ± 11	63 ± 14	48 ± 6**

* $p < 0.05$, ** $p < 0.01$

respectively ($p < 0.05$ and $p < 0.01$). These effects were recognized with low and absent with high doses of PG suggesting competitive inhibition. Step-doses of CGRP II and CT also induced a dose-dependent decrease of acid output ($p < 0.05$), whereas CGRP I was ineffective (acid output in mmol/15 min: control 6.4; CGRP I 6.7; CGRP II 5.2; CT 4.8).

CONCLUSION

CGRP II, unlike CGRP I, inhibits gastric acid secretion in humans. The results imply that CGRP I and CGRP II at the level of the stomach have distinct biological properties in humans. As CGRP II is a neuropeptide, a regulatory function in the control of acid secretion can be envisaged.

Acknowledgements

Supported by the Swiss National Science Foundation, grant No. 3.866-0.85.

20
Corticotropin-releasing hormone (CRH): lack of effect on gastric acid secretion in humans

C. BEGLINGER, C. SIEBER, J. BELTINGER, K. GYR, J. GIRARD AND G. A. STALDER

CRH is a hypothalamic peptide which has been shown to co-ordinate endocrine behavioural and autonomic responses to stress. Recent immuno-histochemical and radioimmunoassay studies have revealed the presence of CRH-like immunoreactivity not only in the brain but in peripheral tissues, among them the gut, of various species, including humans. These findings support a peripheral source and role for CRH. Systemic administration of CRH on human gastric acid secretion has not been determined yet. The purpose of the present study was to compare the effects of i.v. infusion of CRH at two different doses (0.6 and 1.8 μg/kg/h) to normal saline (control) on pentagastrin (PG)-stimulated acid secretion (100–1600 ng/kg/h) in healthy volunteers.

METHODS

Six healthy volunteers were studied on three different days. Gastric acid secretion was measured continuously by aspiration using a marker perfusion technique (PEG 4000 as a non-absorbable marker). Saline or one dose of the peptide was given throughout the study. Blood was drawn in regular intervals for plasma ACTH and cortisol levels by RIA.

RESULTS

The results are shown in Tables 1 and 2. CRH induced a dose-dependent increase in plasma cortisol and ACTH concentrations ($p < 0.05$).

Table 1 Acid output (mmol/min)

| | PG (ng/kg/h) | | |
	100	400	1600
Saline (control)	0.14 ± 0.02	0.30 ± 0.05	0.41 ± 0.05
CRH (0.6 µg/kg/h)	0.16 ± 0.03	0.36 ± 0.04	0.46 ± 0.06
CRH (1.8 µg/kg/h)	0.13 ± 0.02	0.33 ± 0.03	0.44 ± 0.02

Table 2 Plasma hormone data

| | Saline | | CRH (0.6 µg/kg/h) | |
	Basal	90 min	Basal	90 min
ACTH (ng/l)	50 ± 13	57 ± 13	50 ± 16	112 ± 24*
Cortisol (nmol/l)	246 ± 41	228 ± 42	238 ± 73	486 ± 40*

Data are mean ± SEM, *$p < 0.05$

SUMMARY

i.v. CRH does not inhibit PG-stimulated gastric acid secretion in humans.

The biological potency of the peptide is demonstrated by its effects on ACTH and cortisol secretion. We conclude that CRH is not a regulator of gastric acid secretion under these conditions.

Acknowledgements

Supported by the Swiss National Science Foundation, grant No. 3.866-0.85.

21
Pathways of inhibition of gastric acid secretion by injection of neuropeptide Y into the paraventricular nucleus of the hypothalamus of rats

G. A. HUMPHREYS, J. S. DAVISON AND W. L. VEALE

INTRODUCTION

The hypothalamus and autonomic regions of the medulla and spinal cord play important roles in the regulation of the cephalic phase of gastric acid secretion[1]. The paraventricular nucleus of the hypothalamus (PVN) is of particular interest because it maintains direct neural connections with autonomic preganglionic cell groups in the medulla and spinal cord. For example, the PVN gives rise to descending projections which end in the dorsal motor nucleus of the vagus[2,3], an area containing preganglionic parasympathetic cell bodies which contribute vagal motor fibres to the stomach[4]. Discrete populations of PVN cells also innervate the spinal intermediolateral cell column at the thoracic level[5-8] where sympathetic preganglionic neurons of the splanchnic nerves reside[9,10]. A small population of PVN neurons send axon collaterals to both the spinal cord and the medulla[8,11]. The PVN may, therefore, be in a position to alter, synchronously, the activity of sympathetic and parasympathetic fibres innervating the abdominal viscera[12,16].

The PVN has also been shown to modulate the transmission of visceral sensory information as it enters the central nervous system. For example, vagal sensory and PVN afferents converge in the nucleus tractus solitarius (NTS)[5,8,13]. Electrical stimulation and lesion of the PVN has been shown to alter the sensitivity of gastric vagal reflexes relayed in the NTS[14,15].

The PVN receives neural input from medullary areas which, collectively, function to process, gate and relay primary visceral sensory information to various other areas of the brain[11,16]. The noradrenergic (A2) cell group in the dorsal vagal complex receives visceral sensory information from vagal and glossopharyngeal afferents[16,17]. A moderate proportion of the A2 noradrenergic cells of the NTS then project directly to the PVN[17]. A significant output of non-noradrenergic NTS neurons ends in the A1 cell group of the ventro-lateral medulla[17,18], an area thought to function in the maintenance of blood presure[20]. The A1 area then heavily innervates the PVN[16,17].

Neuropeptide Y (NPY) is present in many of these medullary catecholaminergic cells and the A1 cell group is thought to be a major source of NPY in the PVN[18,19]. NPY is found widely distributed in the central nervous system but is in particularly high density within fibres and terminals of the PVN[20]. In addition to the catecholaminergic cells of the medulla, a significant proportion of NPY in the PVN originates within the arcuate nucleus of the hypothalamus[21], which functions to regulate release of adenohypophyseal hormones.

Injection of NPY into the PVN of rats stimulates feeding behaviour[22] and has been shown to reduce gastric acid output in fasted and anaesthetized rats[23].

In view of the anatomical and electrophysiological evidence supporting a role for the PVN in autonomic regulation of gastric activity, this paper examines the peripheral autonomic pathways involved in mediating the inhibition of gastric acid secretion following injection of NPY into the PVN.

METHODS

Male Sprague–Dawley rats weighing 300–400 g were fasted for 20–22 h and anaesthetized with a mixture of ketamine (90 mg/kg), xylazine (18 mg/kg) and pentobarbital (6.5 mg). The stomach of each rat was prepared for perfusion with warm saline (1.2 ml/min) by passing an inflow tube into the stomach through the oesophagus. The perfusate was collected and titrated automatically (Radiometer) through a duodenal outflow tube inserted into the stomach.

Subdiaphragmatic vagotomies were performed acutely on some rats by cutting the gastric vagal branches at a distance 1 cm cranial to the cardiac sphincter. Splanchnotomies were performed 1-2 weeks before experimentation by surgically removing the coeliac ganglia and surrounding plexi of nerves. Pentagastrin (0.05 μg/min) and atropine (1.0 μg/min) were infused continuously (5 μl/min) through a jugular cannula. Surgery was followed by a 40 min stabilization period, then 5, 50 or 200 pmol of NPY in 100 nl saline or saline alone was injected into the PVN using stereotaxic techniques. Gastric acid output was measured for 180 min following injection. At the end of each experiment, the injection site was marked with India ink for later histological determination of its location. Mucosal blood flow was measured in the acid secreting portion of the fundus using the hydrogen clearance technique[24].

RESULTS

Injection of NPY into the PVN caused a dose-dependent inhibition of interdigestive gastric acid output in the anaesthetized rat[23]. Gastric acid output was suppressed by $7.1 \pm 1.4\,\mu$eq/10 min, 20 min after injection of 200 pmol of NPY into the PVN and was sustained throughout the 180 min measurement period. This inhibition was abolished by atropine, subdiaphragmatic vagotomy and splanchnotomy (see Figure 1).

Continuous intravenous infusion of pentagastrin resulted in baseline levels of acid output ($32.1 \pm 2.8\,\mu$eq/10 min) which were significantly higher ($p < 0.001$) than baseline levels in unstimulated rats ($8.7 \pm 0.6\,\mu$eq/10 min). Injection of 200 pmol of NPY into the PVN was followed by a decrease in rate of gastric acid output which was statistically different from saline injected controls from 30–110 min after injection. The inhibitory effect of PVN injections of 200 pmol of NPY in gastrin-stimulated rats was absent in atropine treated and splanchnotomized rats (see Figure 2).

Mucosal blood flow in unstimulated rats was not altered by injection of NPY into the PVN (data not shown).

DISCUSSION

Injection of NPY into the PVN of anaesthetized rats has been shown previously to inhibit interdigestive gastric acid output in a dose-dependent manner[23]. This effect was limited to the PVN, since injections made into other hypothalamic areas were followed either by no change or by an elevation of acid output[23].

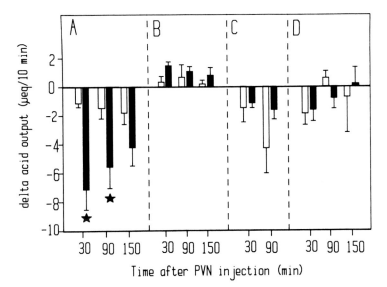

Figure 1 Time course of change of gastric acid output relative to baseline 30, 90 and 150 min after injection of 200 pmol NPY (solid bars) or 100 nl saline (open bars) into the PN of unstimulated rats. **A**, untreated; **B**, subdiaphragmatic vagotomy; **C**, atropine treated; **D**, splanchnotomized; **Star**, - group means which are statistically different from saline injected controls ($p < 0.05$, Student t-test)

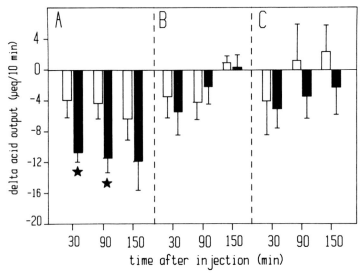

Figure 2 Time course of change of gastric acid output relative to baseline 30, 90 and 150 min after injection of 200 pmol NPY (solid bars) or 100 nl saline (open bars) into the PVN of pentagastrin stimulated rats. **A**, untreated; **B**, atropine treated; **C**, splanchnectomized; **Star**, group means which are statistically different from saline injected controls ($p < 0.05$, Student t-test)

The inhibition was absent in vagotomized, splanchnotomized and in atropine-treated rats. This suggests that both the vagal cholinergic and splanchnic autonomic pathways are involved in mediating the inhibition.

Pentagastrin was used to stimulate acid output and increase baseline measurements, in order to determine if the magnitude of the inhibition was limited by low baseline levels of acid output. This was especially important in the atropinized and vagotomized groups where the baseline acid outputs were decreased.

These results show that pentagastrin-stimulated acid output was also inhibited by PVN injection of NPY. The magnitude of the inhibitory response in gastrin-stimulated rats was slightly, but not significantly, greater than in the unstimulated state. The inhibition was sustained throughout the 180 min post-injection measurement period and an estimate of duration of effect will require experimentation on conscious rats.

The NPY induced inhibition of pentagastrin-stimulated acid output was abolished by atropine and splanchnotomy. This effect could be explained if NPY simultaneously suppressed vagal cholinergic output and increased splanchnic nerve activity to the gut. However, this is unlikely to be the only mechanism operating since blocking transmission in one or other of the autonomic nerves would only attenuate but not abolish the response. The most likely explanation is that the inhibitory mechanism is dependent on an interaction between sympathetic and cholinergic parasympathetic motor neurons or their released products at the gut level. In this case, blocking transmission proximal to the level of interaction in either nerve would abolish the response. Examples of this type of interaction are known to occur in the gut. For example, acetylcholine and vagus nerve activity impairs, presynaptically, the release of norepinephrine from sympathetic neurons and vice versa[25]. The mechanism in this case is unknown.

Also, the inhibitory effect of NPY in the PVN was probably not secondary to a sympathetically induced decrease of mucosal blood flow as indicated by the hydrogen clearance technique and by the failure of NPY to produce inhibition in the atropinized, gastrin-treated animals.

In summary, injection of NPY into the PVN of anaesthetized rats resulted in a prolonged inhibition of gastric acid output in both unstimulated and pentagastrin-stimulated states. The effect was dependent on cholinergic vagal and splanchnic nerve integrity and is not caused by a decrease in mucosal blood flow.

References

1. Taché, Y. (1988). CNS peptides and regulation of gastric acid secretion. *Annu. Rev. Physiol.*, **50**, 19–39
2. Willett, C. J., Rutherford, J. G., Gwyn, D. G. and Leslie, R. A. (1987). Projections between the hypothalamus and the dorsal vagal complex in the cat: an HRP and autoradiographic study. *Brain Res. Bull.*, **18**, 63–71
3. Rogers, R. C., Kita, H., Butcher, L. L. and Novin, D. (1980). Afferent projections to the dorsal motor nucleus of the vagus. *Brain Res. Bull.*, **5**, 365–73
4. Laughton, W. B. and Powley, T. L. (1987). Localization of efferent function in the dorsal motor nucleus of the vagus. *Am. J. Physiol.*, **R13-25**
5. Saper, C. B., Loewy, A. D., Swanson, L. W. and Cowan, W. M. (1976). Direct hypothalamo-autonomic connections. *Brain Res.*, **117**, 305–12
6. Ono, T., Nishino, H., Sasaka, K., Muramoto, K., Yano, I. and Simpson, A. (1978). Paraventricular nucleus connections to spinal cord and pituitary. *Neurosci. Letts.*, **10**, 141–6
7. Gilbey, M. P., Coote, J. H., Fleetwood-Walker, S. and Peterson, D. F. (1982). The influence of the paraventriculo-spinal pathway, and oxytocin and vasopressin on sympathetic preganglionic neurons. *Brain Res.*, **251**, 283–90
8. Swanson, L. W. and Kuypers, H. G. J. M. (1980). The paraventricular nucleus of the hypothalamus: cytoarchitectonic subdivisions and organization of projections to the pituitary, dorsal vagal complex, and spinal cord as demonstrated by retrograde fluoresence double-labeling methods. *J. Comp. Neurol.*, **194**, 555–70
9. Porter, J. P. and Brody, M. J. (1985). Neural projections from paraventricular nucleus that subserve vasomotor functions. *Am. J. Physiol.*, **R271-81**
10. Smith, O. A. and DeVito, J. L. (1984). Central neural integration for the control of autonomic responses associated with emotion. *Annu. Rev. Neurosci.*, **7**, 43–65
11. Swanson, L. W. and Sawchenko, P. E. (1983). Hypothalamic integration: organization of the paraventricular and supraoptic nuclei. *Annu. Rev. Neurosci.*, **6**, 269–324
12. Powley, T. L. and Laughton, W. (1981). Neural pathways involved in the hypothalamic integration of autonomic responses. *Diabetologia*, **20**, 378–87
13. Rogers, R. C. and Nelson, D. O. (1984). Neurons of the vagal division of the solitary nucleus activated by the paraventricular nucleus of the hypothalamus. *J. Auton. Nerv. Syst.*, **10**, 193–7
14. Rogers, R. C. and Hermann, G. E. (1985). Vagal afferent stimulation-evoked gastric secretion suppressed by paraventricular nucleus lesion. *J. Auton. Nerv. Syst.*, **13**, 191–9
15. Rogers, R. C. and Hermann, G. E. (1985). Gastric-vagal solitary neurons excited by paraventricular nucleus microstimulation. *J. Auton. Nerv. Syst.*, **14**, 352–62
16. Sawchenko, P. E. and Swanson, (1982). The organization of noradrenergic pathways from the brainstem to the paraventricular and supraoptic nuclei in the rat. *Brain Res. Rev.*, **4**,

275–325

17. Sawchenko, P. E. (1982). Anatomic relationships between the paraventricular nucleus of the hypothalamus and visceral regulatory mechanisms: implications for the control of feeding behavior. In Hoebel, B. G. and Novin, D. (eds.) *Neural Basis of Feeding and Reward*, pp. 259–74. (Brunswick, ME: Haer Inst.)

18. Everitt, B. J., Hokfelt, T., Terenius, L., Tatemoto, K., Mutt, V. and Goldstein, M. (1984). Differential coexistence of neuropeptide Y (NPY)-like immunoreactivity with catecholamines in the central nervous system of the rat. *Neuroscience*, **11**, 443–52

19. Sawchenko, P. E., Swanson, L. W., Grzanna, R., Howe, P. R. C., Bloom, S. R. and Polak, J. M. (1985). Colocalization of neuropeptide Y immunoreactivity in brainstem catecholamine neurons that project to the paraventricular nucleus of the hypothalamus. *J. Comp. Neurol.*, **241**, 138–53

20. Chronwall, B. M., Dimaggia, D. A., Massari, V. J., Pickel, V. M., Ruggerio, D. A. and O'Donohue, T. L. (1985). The anatomy of neuropeptide Y-containing neurons in rat brain. *Neuroscience*, **15**, 1159–81

21. Bai, F. L., Yamano, M., Shiotani, Y., Emson, P. C., Smith, A. D., Powell, J. F. and Tohyama, M. (1985). An arcuato-paraventricular and -dorsomedial hypothalamic neuropeptide Y-containing system which lacks noradrenalin in the rat. *Brain Res.*, **331**, 172–5

22. Stanley, B. G. and Leibowitz, S. F. (1985). Neuropeptide Y injected in the paraventricular hypothalamus: A powerful stimulant of feeding behavior. *Proc. Natl. Acad. Sci. USA*, **82**, 3940–3

23. Humphreys, G. A., Davison, J. S. and Veale, W. L. (1988). Injection of neuropeptide Y into the paraventricular nucleus of the hypothalamus inhibits gastric acid secretion in the rat. *Brain Res.* (In press)

24. Motonobu, M., Motoyuki, M., Miyake, T. and Uchino, H. (1982). Contact electrode method in hydrogen gas clearance technique: a new method for determination of regional gastric mucosal blood flow in animals and humans. *Gastroenterology*, **82**, 457–67

25. Gershon, M. D. (1981). The enteric nervous system. *Annu. Rev. Neurosci.*, 227–72

22
Nerves, neurohumours and gastric acid secretion

D. F. MAGEE

We have studied gastric acid and pepsin secretion in conscious dogs with vagally innervated and denervated secreting mucosa for years. Our conclusions and results are often at variance with those derived from the currently popular *in vitro* studies and are hard to explain as simple binding between stimulus and receptor.

We find that cholinergic agents are good stimulants of acid and pepsin secretion from both innervated and denervated mucosa and that the dose response curves and maximal doses are the same in both preparations[1]. From denervated mucosa pentagastrin has a much lower secretory maximum for acid than from the innervated mucosa, and pepsin is not stimulated at all from the former as it is with methacholine. The maximal secretory dose is the same in both preparations. The dose-response curve slopes for acid are identical in the two preparations so, evidently, the vagal innervation must mean more of the same receptors rather than more sensitive ones. The failure of gastrin to stimulate pepsin secretion from denervated mucosa casts doubt on the almost universal belief that gastrin is the secretory hormone for the chief cells. Schofield[3] many years ago showed that, after feeding, Heidenhain pouch motility and pepsin secretion actually fell profoundly.

Vizi *et al.*[3] have advanced strong evidence for an indirect action of gastrin on intestinal smooth muscle. This mechanism seems to be non-nicotinic cholinergic in nature. Might this be so for the action of gastrin on oxyntic cells? As in the intestine ganglionic blockade does not depress the action of pentagastrin, on acid secretion. It does depress pepsin, and AHR602, a muscarinic ganglionic stimulant, augments pentagastrin stimulated acid secretion[4].

The characteristics of cholinergic stimulation of acid and pepsin are different from those of pentagastrin. The latter reaches its peak within 30 min and declines slowly. The former reaches its peak in synchrony with the gastric MMC and declines rapidly to a perigee corresponding to phase I. The peak secretion of acid at the peaks and at the perigee level show dose response relationships which are parallel; the perigee curve is to the right and the secretory maximum is much lower than the peak curve. The same perigee methacholine kinetics are seen after ganglionic blockade which abolishes interdigestive periodicity. The perigee and post-ganglionic block curves, we feel, represent direct action on the oxyntic cells and the peaks the combination of the direct action and phase III facilitation. It is unlikely that ganglionic blocking agents act to block methacholine which is a purely muscarinic drug. Odori and Magee[4] found that AHR 602 in doses which augmented pentagastrin stimulated acid secretion did not affect metacholine or histamine-stimulated secretion, but isoproterenol which is claimed to have a potentiating affect on muscarinic ganglionic activity did[5]. Isoproterenol is a potent inhibitor of gastrin-stimulated secretion[6].

When a purely nicotinic agent (tetramethylammonium) is given acid and pepsin secretion are no longer dependent on or influenced by interdigestive periodicity. A prompt plateau unpunctuated by peaks and depressions is attained.

We conclude that gastrin cannot stimulate pepsin secretion in the absence of the vagi, there is thus no conclusive evidence that the regulation of pepsin secretion is hormonal and that the main action of both gastrin and cholinergic drugs on acid secretion is indirect and neural. Gastrin exhibits some features of muscarinic ganglionic activity and requires vagal innervation for full action. Muscarinic cholinergic agents require recruitment of parietal cells which occurs at phase III of interdigestive peaks and which is nicotinic ganglionic in character. Apart from this cholinomimetic, drugs have a much smaller direct mucarinic action on oxyntic cells.

Methacholine is an agent which is claimed to have a muscarinic ganglionic action, in these experiments only its augmentation by isoproterenol on acid secretion supports this. It must be remembered that the characteristics of peripheral ganglionic transmission have been worked out only in the superior cervical ganglion of the cat and have not been verified in parasympathetic ganglia.

Pepsin secretion seems to be much more straight forward than acid. It is dependent on extrinsic nerves, the vagi, reaches peaks in synchrony with the MMC, is increased substantially even between peaks by cholinomimetic agents but ganglionic blocking agents reduce this and the secretory maximum. Thus it seems we are dealing in the case of cholinomimetics with both a direct action on chief cells and an indirect nicotinic ganglionic one.

References

1. Magee, D. F., Naruse, S. and Pap, A. (1985). Comparison of the action of cholinomimetics and pentagastrin on gastric secretion in dogs. *Br. J. Pharmacol.*, **84**, 347–55
2. Schofield, B. (1959). The inhibition of pepsin output in separated gastric pouches in dogs following feeding and its correlation with motility changes. *Gastroenterology*, **37**, 169–80
3. Vizi, G. E., Bertaccini, C., Impicciatore, M. and Knoll, J. (1973). Evidence that acetylcholine released by gastrin and related polypeptides contributes to their effect on gastrointestinal motility. *Gastroenterol.*, **64**, 268–77
4. Odori, Y. and Magee, D. F. (1969). The action of some agents active at autonomic ganglionic sites on the secretory response of the Heidenhain pouch to various stimuli. *Eur. J. Pharmacol.*, **8**, 221–7

5. de Groat, W. C. and Volle, R. L. (1966). Interactions between catecholamines and ganglionic stimulating agents in sympathetic ganglia. *J. Pharmacol. Exp. Therap.*, **154**, 200–15
6. Magee, D. F. (1976). Adrenergic activity and gastric secretion. *Proc. Soc. Exp. Biol. Med.*, **151**, 659–67

23
Sympathetic neural inhibition of duodenal HCO$_3^-$-secretion in the anaesthetized rat

C. JÖNSON AND L. FÄNDRIKS

INTRODUCTION

The stomach secretes acid and enzymes in order to initiate the digestion of food. Protection against potential autodigestion is essential and involves several mechanisms, e.g. epithelial alkalinization, cell repair, blood flow regulation. In the duodenum, alkaline secretion by the mucosa is considered to be very important in the defence against luminal acid disposed from the stomach. The alkalinity of this secretion is mainly due to epithelial HCO$_3^-$-transport and prostaglandins, hormones and neural mechanisms have been reported to exert regulatory function[1]. Recent reports from our laboratory demonstrate that the sympathetic splanchnic nerves act as an inhibitor on basal and vagally induced duodenal HCO$_3^-$-secretion via an α_2-adrenergic mechanism[2-6]. Exposure of the duodenal mucosa to acid induces an increased epithelial HCO$_3^-$-secretion[1,7]. The present study was undertaken to investigate if a raised sympathetic neural activity, due to a moderate blood loss or direct splanchnic nerve stimulation, interferes with such an acid-induced rise in duodenal HCO$_3^-$-secretion.

METHODS

Experiments were performed on male Sprague–Dawley rats, weighing 260–330 g. The animals were fasted overnight before surgery but had free access to drinking water. Anaesthesia was induced by methohexital (Brietal^R), Lilly Inc.) $25 \, mg \times kg^{-1}$ i.p. and a tracheal cannula was inserted to ensure free airways. The right femoral vein was cannulated for drug infusions and anaesthesia was then maintained with chloralose $50 \, mg \times kg^{-1}$ given as a bolus injection and followed by a continuous infusion at a rate of $25 \, mg \times kg^{-1} \times h^{-1}$. The right femoral artery was cannulated and connected to a pressure transducer for measurements of arterial pressure and heart rate, the latter triggered from the pressure pulse waves. These parameters were recorded on a Grass-polygraph. A slow intra-artrial infusion ($1 \, ml \times h^{-1}$) of $0.3 \, M \, NaHCO_3$, containing 1.7% glucose, was given throughout the experiments to prevent dehydration and acidosis due to the surgical trauma. The left femoral artery was cannulated with a heparinized catheter for later withdrawal of blood. Body temperature was maintained at 38 °C by a heating pad and a heating lamp controlled by a thermostat equipment.

The abdomen was opened by a midline incision and a 1.5 cm segment of the mediodistal duodenum was cannulated *in situ* between two glass tubes connected to a reservoir. The temperature of the reservoir was maintained at 38°C by a water jacket. The perfusate (isotonic NaCl) was recirculated through the duodenal segment by means of a gas lift of 100% N_2. Alkaline secretion into the luminal perfusate was titrated to pH 7.4 by infusion of HCl (made isotonic with NaCl) under automatic control by a pH-stat equipment[7]. The common bile duct was catheterized 5 mm proximal to the papilla of Vater, and bile and pancreatic juice, not under study, was then drained to the outside of the animal. In two groups of animals the splanchnic nerves were cut bilaterally, well proximal to the prevertebral ganglia. In one of these splanchnicotomized groups the distal nerve ends were put on bipolar silver ring electrodes for later nerve stimulations.

Statistical comparison of differences between data were made by use of Newman–Keul's test (between groups) and the Students t-test (within groups). A p-value less than 0.05 was considered significant.

RESULTS

After completion of surgery the animals were left undisturbed for about 1 h in order to stabilize cardiovascular and duodenal functions. The experimental design was then as follows.

Luminal acidification ($n = 5$)

The lumen-perfusing saline was for 5 min changed to 0.01 M HCl made isotonic with NaCl. The acid was then replaced by saline and titration was restarted. This exposure of the duodenal mucosa to HCl raised HCO_3^--secretion by about 60% (from 17 ± 5 to $28 \pm 3 \, \mu mol \times cm^{-1} \times h^{-1}$) (Figures 1 and 2). Mean arterial pressure and heart rate were unaffected by the mucosal acidification procedure.

Luminal acidification and blood loss ($n = 5$)

A modest arterial bleeding of $0.6 \, ml \times 100 \, g$ body weight^{-1}, corresponding to about 10% of the total blood volume[8], is known to raise splanchnic neural discharge[9]. Such a bleeding was performed simultaneously to the acid exposure and in these animals duodenal HCO_3^--secretion did not increase

HCO_3^--secretion (Figures 1 and 2). Mean arterial pressure was transiently lowered from 124 ± 11 to 90 ± 10 mmHg, whereas heart rate was hardly influenced.

Luminal acidification, blood loss and splanchnicotomy (*n* = 5)

In these animals the splanchnic nerves had been cut bilaterally. Arterial pressure was somewhat lower, whereas basal duodenal HCO_3^--secretion was

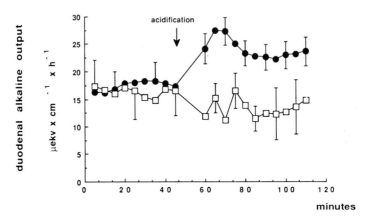

Figure 1 The effect of a 5 min exposure of the duodenal mucosa to 0.01 M HCl on the duodenal alkaline output. One group is treated only with the acid exposure (– ● –) and one group (– □ –) is subjected to a simultaneous 10% blood loss. Values are means ± SEM. The arrow indicates the luminal acid exposure, in (– □ –) together with the arterial bleeding

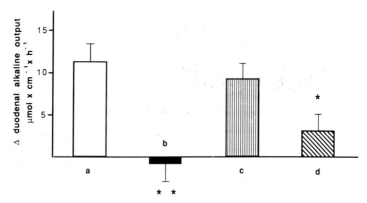

Figure 2 the net change in duodenal HCO_3^--secretion induced by a 5 min exposure of the duodenal mucosa to 0.01 M HCl. Values are means ± SEM of the change in secretion (the highest value after luminal acidification minus the control value prior to the acidification procedure, *n* = 5 for each group). **a** luminal acidification **b** luminal acidification + blood loss; **c** luminal acidification + blood loss + splanchnicotomy; **d** luminal acidification + splanchnicotomy + splanchnic nerve stimulation. Values which differ significantly from the controls (group a) is indicated by asterisks (* = $p < 0.05$, ** = $p < 0.01$)

on a level similar to that in the animals with their splanchnic nerves intact (groups a and b). As in group b, the duodenal acid exposure and the bleeding procedure were performed simultaneously, but in this group of animals the duodenal HCO_3^- secretion increased by about 60% (Figure 2). Mean arterial presure and heart rate responses were similar to those in group b.

Luminal acidification, splanchnicotomy and splanchnic nerve stimulation ($n = 5$)

Bilateral electrical stimulation of the splanchnic nerves (10 Hz, 5 ms, 5 V) started immediately before the 5 min acid-exposure of the duodenal mucosa and was continued throughout the experiment. The splanchnic nerve stimulation increased mean arterial pressure by about 50 mmHg and reduced slightly heart rate. During this nerve stimulation, acid exposure induced a minor rise in duodenal HCO_3^--secretion, markedly reduced compared to the controls (group a) (Figure 2).

DISCUSSION

Recent reports indicate the existence of an autonomic neural regulation of duodenal HCO_3^--secretion in a classical antagonistic fashion[10]: the parasympathetic vagal nerves exert excitatory effects, in part via cholinergic mechanisms[11,12,13]. The sympathetic splanchnic nerves acts mainly inhibitory, via an α_2-adrenergic mechanism, on basal as well as on vagally induced duodenal HCO_3^--secretion in cats and rats[2-6].

Instillation of hydrochloric acid into the lumen of the duodenum increases mucosal HCO_3^--transport. The physiological response is mediated by synthesis of prostaglandins, hormonal factors and by neural mechanisms[1,10]. In the present study, a moderate blood loss, known to increase splanchnic nerve discharge activity[9], inhibited the increase in duodenal HCO_3^--secretion induced by luminal acidification. Furthermore, such a bleeding-induced inhibition of the duodenal HCO_3^--secretory response was absent in splanchnicotomized animals. This suggests that the increased sympathetic nerve activity, in response to bleeding, inhibits the acid-induced rise in duodenal HCO_3^--secretion via the splanchnic nerves. Direct stimulation of the splanchnic nerves also inhibited the acid-induced increase in duodenal HCO_3^--secretion. Consequently, the splanchnic neural inhibition has a peripheral site of action in the intestine, rather than in the CNS. From the present results it is not, however, possible to elucidate the secretory mechanism on which the symathoinhibitory action is exerted. It could be a direct effect on the secreting epithelium or on intramural secretomotor neurons. Furthermore, effects on the intestinal circulation, indirectly influencing epithelial ion-transport, may also be involved.

HCO_3^--secretion by the duodenal mucosa is important in the protection against gastric acid[1]. It is possible that a reduction of the HCO_3^--secretion, due to increased sympathetic activity in connection to, for example, blood loss, physical or mental stress, could make the gastrointestinal mucosa more susceptible to damage by gastric acid.

Acknowledgements

This study was financially supported by the Swedish Medical Research Council (grants 0016 and 2855) and the Gothenburg Medical Society.

References

1. Flemström, G. (1987). Gastric and duodenal mucosal bicarbonate secretion. In Johnson, L.R. (ed.) *Physiology of the Gastrointestinal Tract*, 2nd Edn., pp. 1011–29. (New York: Raven Press)
2. Fändriks, L. (1986). Vagal and splanchnic neural influences on gastric and duodenal bicarbonate secretions. *Acta Physiol. Scand.*, **128** (suppl.), 555
3. Fändriks, L., Jönson, C. and Nylander, O. (1987). Effects of splanchnic nerve stimulation and of clonidine on gastric and duodenal HCO_3^--secretion in the anaesthetized cat. *Acta Physiol. Scand.*, **130**, 251–8
4. Jönson, C. and Fändriks, L. (1987). Bleeding inhibits vagally-induced duodenal HCO_3^--secretion via activation of the splanchnic nerves in anesthetized rats. *Acta Physiol. Scand.*, **130**, 259–64
5. Jönson, C. and Fändriks, L. (1987). Bleeding-induced decrease in duodenal HCO_3^--secretion in the rat is mediated via α_2-adrenoceptors. *Acta Physiol. Scand.*, **130**, 387–91
6. Jönson, C. and Fändriks, L. (1988). Afferent electrical stimulation of mesenteric nerves inhibits duodenal HCO_3^--secretion via a spinal reflex activation of the splanchnic nerves in the rat. *Acta Physiol. Scand.* (In press)
7. Flemström, G., Garner, A., Nylander, O., Hurst, B.C. and Heylings, J.R. (1982). Surface epithelial HCO_3^--transport by mammalian duodenum in vivo. *Am. J. Physiol.*, **243** (*Gastrointest. Liver Physiol.*, **6**), G348–58
8. Lundin, S., Folkow, B. and Rippe, B. (1981). Central blood volume in spontaneously hypertensive rats and Wistar Kyoto normotensive rats. *Acta Physiol. Scand.*, **112**, 257–62
9. Ito, K., Sato, A., Shimamura, K. and Swenson, R.S. (1984). Reflex changes in sympatho-adrenal medullary functions in response to baroreceptor stimulation in anaesthetized rats. *J. Auton. Nerv. Syst.*, **10**, 295–303
10. Fändriks, L., Jönson, C., Nylander, O. and Flemström, G. (1988). Neural influences on gastroduodenal HCO_3^--secretion. In Szabo, S. (ed.) *Ulcer Disease. New Aspects of Pathogenesis and Pharmacology*. (Boston: CRC Press) (In press)
11. Jönson, C., Nylander, O., Flemström, G. and Fändriks, L. (1986). Vagal stimulation of duodenal HCO_3^--secretion in anaesthetized rats. *Acta Physiol. Scand.*, **128**, 65–70
12. Konturek, S.J. and Thor, P. (1986). Relation between duodenal alkaline secretion and motility in fasted and sham-fed dogs. *Am. J. Physiol.*, **251**, (*Gastrointest. Liver Physiol.*, **14**), G591–6
13. Nylander, O., Flemström, G., Delbro, D. and Fändriks, L. (1987). Vagal influence on gastroduodenal HCO_3^--secretion in the cat in vivo. *Am. J. Physiol.*, **252** (*Gastrointest. Liver Physiol.*, **15**), G522–8

24
Participation of cholinergic innervation in the control of human gallbladder emptying

L. GULLO

The role of cholinergic mechanisms in the control of human gallbladder emptying has not been extensively studied. In a recent study we investigated the effect of cholinergic blockade with atropine on cholecystokinin-induced gallbladder emptying in healthy volunteers, by means of real-time ultrasonography[1]. We showed that the intravenous administration of a low dose of atropine (5 μg/kg/h) completely blocked the gallbladder response to submaximal doses of cholecystokinin and partially inhibited (by 52%) the response to a maximal dose. The administration of a higher dose of atropine (15 μg/kg/h) totally abolished gallbladder contraction, even when the maximal dose was given. These results have demonstrated that the response of human gallbladder to cholecystokinin is largely dependent on cholinergic innervation. Our observations have been subsequently confirmed and extended by other investigators, who have showed that direct cholinergic stimulation with bethanecol induces significant gallbladder emptying, and that atropine administration decreases the gallbladder emptying responses to a liquid meal, a solid meal and the infusion of cholecystokinin-octapeptide[2] or cerulein[3]. Thus, there is now much experimental evidence which indicates that, in addition to hormonal mechanisms, neural mechanisms may play an important role in the control of gallbladder emptying in humans.

References

1. (1984). *Digestion*, **29**, 209–13
2. (1985). *Gastroenterology*, **89**, 716–22
3. (1985). *Am. J. Gastroenterol.*, **80**, 1–4

SHORT COMMUNICATION

25
Influence of truncal vagotomy on pancreatic trophism and gastrointestinal hormones

M. BÜCHLER, P. MALFERTHEINER, H. FRIEB,
B. GLASBRENNER AND H. G. BEGER

INTRODUCTION

Truncal vagotomy in rats induces pancreatic hyperplasia, digestive enzyme dissociation and a decreased basal amylase discharge from isolated lobules *in vitro*[1,2,3].

Several reports have dealt with the effects of truncal or selective vagotomy on pancreatic function in humans and various animals[4-10]. It is accepted that truncal vagotomy reduces basal pancreatic secretion in humans and animals, as well as the sensitivity to hormonal secretagogues[4-13].

Besides the well-documented hypergastrinaemia after truncal vagotomy in humans and animals[14,15,16], little is known about gastrointestinal hormone changes and the interrelation between GI hormones and pancreatic trophic adaptation after truncal vagotomy. We therefore determined plasma glucagon, insulin, gastrin and CCK after truncal vagotomy in rats to further elucidate possible mechanisms responsible for exocrine pancreatic adaptation.

MATERIALS AND METHODS

Animals

Forty-two male WKY rats, having an initial body weight of 200–240 g were used in the study. The animals were submitted to surgery under halothane intubation anaesthesia.

Surgical procedure

The rats were randomly divided into three groups.
    Group I: controls (C) (*n* = 12) without gastric surgery but with the

transabdominal implantation of a duodenal tube (silicon, 1.5 mm diameter) surtured to the neck of the animal.

Group II: sham-operated controls (S) ($n = 12$) with gastrotomy and reclosure carefully saving the vagus nerve and with the implantation of a duodenal tube.

Group III: truncal vagotomy (TV) ($n = 19$) was carried out by clearly identifying the anterior and posterior vagal nerves. Afterwards the trunks were resected over a distance of at least 1 cm. In addition, a duodenal tube was placed according to the procedure in the two control groups.

A venous catheter (silicon, 1.5 mm dia.) was placed via the right jugular vein two weeks after surgery.

Diets

The rats were caged individually after surgery. The animals had free access to water and received a standard diet mixture which consisted of 63% carbohydrates, 22% protein and 3% fat with added cellulose, minerals and vitamins (12%). Controlled feeding was initiated on the fourth post-operative day. Calculated per 100 g of body weight, there was no significant difference in the food intake between the different groups.

Test meal and diet stimulation

Eighteen days (median) following the surgical treatment, dietary stimulation was supplied via the duodenal tube. The liquid test meal consisted of 3 ml oil, 2 ml amino acid solution (0.2 g/ml protein 88, Wander GmbH, Osthofen, FRG) and 1 ml glucose (40 g/100 ml). These 6 ml were administered as a bolus within 1 min.

Determination of GI hormones

Blood samples were taken before as well as 5, 15, 30 and 60 min after the meal. Na-EDTA (1.5 mg/ml blood) and aproptinin (Trasylol[R], Bayer AG, Leverkusen, FRG, 10.000 KIU/ml blood) were added to the blood specimens, and the plasma was immediately separated after centrifugation and stored at $-20°C$ until use. Blood glucose was measured with a commercial assay (Glucoquant, Boehringer, Mannheim, FRG), using the hexokinase method[17].

Insulin was determined with a RIA-kit[18] provided by Sorin, Biomedica (Soluggia, Italy).

Glucagon was measured with a radioimmunoassay based on a specific antibody against pancreatic glucagon[19,20]. The antibody was kindly donated by Dr Schusdziarra, München, FRG.

Gastrin was determined with a RIA-technique using an antibody which recognizes G34, G17 and the sequence 8–12 in the gastrin molecule[21,22]. The gastrin determination was kindly carried out by Dr Feurle (Städtisches Krankenhaus, Neuwied, FRG).

Cholecystokinin was analysed with a radioimmunoassay against CCK 8 [23,24,25]. The method of analysis has been extensively described elsewhere[23].

Statistics

The results are expressed as the median with 25 and 75 percentiles, or as median and range. The Wilcoxen test was used for statistical analysis.

RESULTS

Glucose tolerance and insulin

The glucose tolerance after truncal vagotomy was impaired with significantly elevated plasma-glucose values after 15 and 30 minutes compared to the two control groups (Figure 1). Corresponding to the impaired glucose assimilation, the plasma-insulin release was delayed (Figure 2). The total integrated post-prandial insulin release within 60 min was comparable in both the experimental and the control animals (truncal vagotomy: 113.6, 42–285 ng x 60 min; controls: 96.5, 65–161 ng x 60 min. Values are medians and range.)

Pancreatic glucagon

As shown in Figure 3, the plasma-glucagon course, before and after meal stimulation, was comparable in experimental and control animals.

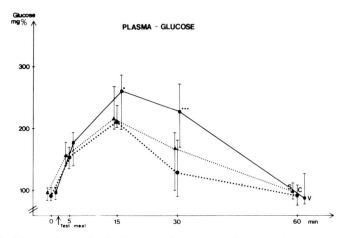

Figure 1 Plasma glucose levels. V = truncal vagotomy, C = controls, S = sham-operated controls. Values are medians and lower and upper quartile. ($*$ = $p < 0.05$, $***$ = $p < 0.001$)

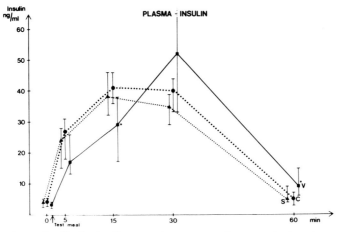

Figure 2 Plasma insulin levels. V = truncal vagotomy, C = controls, S = sham-operated controls. Values are medians and lower and upper quartile. (* = $p < 0.05$)

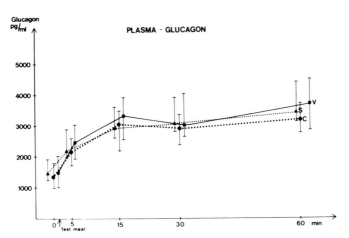

Figure 3 Plasma glucagon levels. V = truncal vagotomy, C = controls, S = sham-operated controls. Values are medians and lower and upper quartile

Gastrin

Depending on the mode of intraduodenal diet infusion, there was no post-prandial increase of plasma gastrin in the two control groups (Figure 4). Following truncal vagotomy, we observed a gastrin peak 5 min after meal stimulation (39% above baseline level). The baseline gastrin levels as well as the four post-prandially elaborated gastrin values were significantly increased in animals after truncal vagotomy (Figure 4).

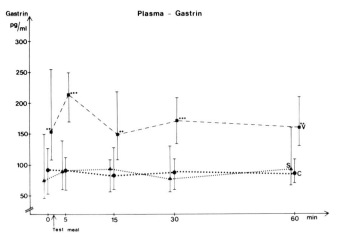

Figure 4 Plasma gastrin levels. V = truncal vagotomy, C = controls, S = sham-operated controls. Values are medians and lower and upper quartile. (** = $p < 0.01$; *** = $p < 0.001$)

Cholecystokinin

According to Figure 5, the baseline and the post-prandial CCK plasma levels were comparable in both experimental and control animals. In the same way, the total integrated post-prandial CCK output was unchanged after truncal vagotomy (truncal vagotomy: 19.2, 14.6–28.5 pg x 60 min; controls 21.4, 9.2–41.5 pg x 60 min. Values are medians and range.)

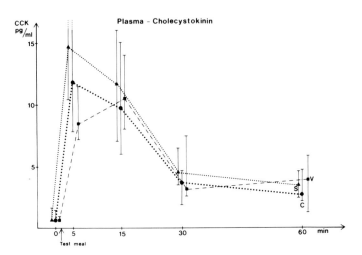

Figure 5 Plasma cholecystokinin levels. V = truncal vagotomy, C = controls, S = sham-operated controls. Values are medians and lower and upper quartile

DISCUSSION

Pancreatic hyperplasia occurs two weeks after truncal vagotomy in rats[3]. It has been supposed that gastric stasis and ectasia induce exocrine pancreatic adaptation after vagisection by means of direct gastropancreatic neural pathways[1,2].

In the present investigation, our interest was directed to the role of gastrointestinal hormones, such as CCK and gastrin, which have been shown to cause exocrine pancreatic growth[26-30]. The pattern of pancreatic adaptation following truncal vagotomy points to a regulatory role of CCK. According to the presented data, CCK appears not to be involved in the trophic adaptation of the exocrine pancreas after truncal vagotomy. In contrast, gastrin, which has been discussed controversially as a pancreatic growth factor, seems to play a role in exocrine pancreatic trophism under conditions of truncal vagotomy. Gastrin plasma values were significantly increased before and after truncal vagotomy in our rat model.

Based on our data, it seems unlikely that insulin or pancreatic glucagon are involved in pancreatic trophism after truncal vagotomy. In addition, it has been shown that pancreatic polypeptide also does not show significant alterations after truncal vagotomy in rats[2], although the post-prandial release of PP is strongly dependent on an intact cholinergic innervation[25,31].

All in all, exocrine pancreatic adaptation following truncal vagotomy in the rat appears to be mediated by at least two factors: direct neural gastropancreatic reflex mechanisms and plasma hypergastrinaemia as a co-factor.

References

1. Tiscornia, O. M., Perec, C. J., Celener, D., DeLehmann, E. S., Caro, L., DePaula, J. and Baratti, C. (1981). Chronic truncal vagotomy: its effect on the weight and function of the rat pancreas. *Mt. Sinai J. Med.*, **48**, 295–304
2. Koop, H., Schwarting, H., Trautman, M., Boerger, H. W., Lankisch, P., Arnold, R. and Creutzfeld, W. (1986). Trophic effect of truncal vagotomy on the rat pancreas. *Digestion*, **33**, 198–205
3. Büchler, M., Malfertheiner, P., Glasbrenner, B. and Beger, H. G. (1987). Pancreatic trophism after truncal vagotomy in rats. *Am. J. Surg.*, **154**, 30–4
4. Dreiling, D. A., Druckerman, L. J. and Hollander, F. (1952). The effect of complete vagisection and vagal stimulation on pancreatic secretion in man. *Gastroenterology*, **20**, 578–86
5. Tankel, H. L. and Hollander, F. (1958). Effect of vagotomy on pancreatic secretion. *Am. J. Physiol.*, **193**, 393–9
6. Moreland, H. J. and Johnson, L. R. (1971). Effect of vagotomy on pancreatic secretion stimulated by endogenous and exogenous secretion. *Gastroenterology*, **60**, 425–31
7. Malagelada, J. R., Go, V. L. W. and Summerskill, W. H. J. (1974). Altered pancreatic and biliary function after vagotomy and pyloroplasty. *Gastroenterology*, **66**, 22–7
8. Debas, H. T., Konturek, S. J. and Grossman, M. J. (1975). Effect of extragastric and truncal vagotomy on pancreatic secretion in the dog. *Am. J. Physiol.*, **228**, 1172–7
9. Lindskov, J., Amtrop, O. and Larsen, H. R. (1976). The effects of highly selective vagotomy on exocrine pancreatic function in man. *Gastroenterology*, **70**, 545–9
10. Anrep, G. (1914). The influence of the vagus on pancreatic secretion. *J. Physiol.*, **49**, 1–9
11. Henriksen, F. W. and Rune, S. J. (1969). Effect of vagotomy on the canine pancreatic secretion after feeding. *Scand. J. Gastroenterol.*, **4**, 435–40
12. Thambugala, R. and Baron, J. H. (1971). Pancreatic secretion after selective and truncal

vagotomy in the dog. *Br. J. Surg.*, **58**, 839–44

13. Mikhailidis, D. P., Foo, Y., Ramdial, L., Kirk, R. M., Rosalki, S. B. and Dandona, P. (1981). Pancreatic exocrine function after truncal and highly selective vagotomy. *J. Clin. Pathol.*, **34**, 963–4

14. Becker, H. D., Arnold, R., Boerger, H. W., Creutzfeld, C., Schafmayer, A. and Creutzfeld, W. (1977). Influence of truncal vagotomy on serum and antral gastrin and G cells. *Gastroenterology*, **72**, 811–14

15. Konturek, S. J., Becker, H. D. and Thompson, J. C. (1974). Effect of vagotomy on hormones stimulating pancreatic secretion. *Arch. Surg.*, **108**, 794

16. Singer, M. V., Niebel, W., Lamners, C., Becher, S., Vesper, J., Hartmann, W., Diemel, J. and Goebell, H. (1981). Effects of truncal vagotomy and antrectomy on bombesin-stimulated pancreatic secretion, release of gastrin and pancreatic polypeptide in the anesthetized dog. *Dig. Dis. Sci.*, **26**, 871–7

17. Deeg, R., Kraemer, W. and Ziegenhorn, J. (1980). Kinetic determination of serum glucose by use of the hexokinase/glucose-6-phosphate dehydrogenase method. *J. Clin. Chem. Chin. Biochem.*, **18**, 49–53

18. Wilson, M. A. and Miles, L. E. M. (eds.) (1977). Radioimmunoassay of Insulin. In *Handbook of Radioimmunoassay*, pp. 275. (New York: M. Decker)

19. Unger, R. H., Eisentraut, A. M., McCall, M. S. and Madison, M. L. (1961). Glucagon antibodies and an immunoassay for glucagon. *J. Clin. Invest.*, **40**, 1280–9

20. Unger, R. H. (1968). Characterisation of the response of circulating GLI to intraduodenal and intravenous administration of glucose. *J. Clin. Invest.*, **47**, 48–65

21. Feurle, G. E., Menzel, J. and Klempa, J. (1983). Contribution of the antrum and duodenum to circulating forms of gastrin in the dog. *Reg. Pept.*, **7**, 127–35

22. Feurle, G. E., Ketterer, H., Becker, H. D. and Creutzfeld, W. (1972). Circadian serum gastrin concentrations in control persons and in patients of ulcer disease. *Scand. J. Gastroenterol.*, **7**, 177–83

23. Schafmayer, A., Werner, M. and Becker, H. D. (1982). Radioimmunological determination of CCK in tissue extracts. *Digestion*, **24**, 146–54

24. Schafmayer, A., Becker, H. D., Werner, M., Foelsch, U. R. and Creuztfeld, W. (1985). Plasma CCK levels in patients with chronic pancreatitis. *Digestion*, **32**, 136–9

25. Foelsch, U. R., Cantor, P., Wilms, H., Schafmayer, A., Becker, H. D. and Creutzfeld, W. (1987). Role of CCK in the negative feedback control of pancreatic enzyme secretion in conscious rats. *Gastroenterology*, **92**, 449–58

26. Dembinski, A. B. and Johnson, L. R. (1980). Stimulation of pancreatic growth by secretin, caerulein and pentagastrin. *Endocrinology*, **16**, 323–8

27. Reber, H. A., Jonson, F., Deveney, K., Montgommery, C. and Way, L. W. (1977). Trophic effects of gastrin on the exocrine pancreas in rats. *J. Surg. Res.*, **22**, 554–60

28. Brants, F. and Morisset, J. (1976). Trophic effects of CCK on pancreatic acinar cells from rats of different ages. *Proc. Soc. Exp. Biol. Med.*, **153**, 523–7

29. Foelsch, U. R., Winkler, K. and Wormsley, K. G. (1978). Influence of repeated administration of CCK and secretin to pancreas of the rat. *Scand. J. Gastroenterol.*, **13**, 663–71

30. Morisset, J. A., Solomon, T. W. and Grossman, M. J. (1979). Effect of secretin and caerulein on pancreatic weight, DNA synthesis and content. *Gastroenterology*, **76**, 1206–11

31. Schwartz, T. W. (1983). Pancreatic polypeptide: a hormone under vagal control. *Gastroenterology*, **85**, 1411–25

26
Effect of thyrotropin-releasing hormone on pancreatic exocrine secretion in the guinea-pig

J. S. DAVISON, L. TREMBLAY AND J. HICKIE

INTRODUCTION

Injection of thyrotropin-releasing hormone (TRH) into the cerebral ventricles or brainstem of several species evokes a generalized excitation of the gastrointestinal tract involving a widespread increase in motility and gastric acid secretion[1-3]. The pathways for these effects are in the vagus nerves and it is generally accepted that most of the effects are due to activation of cholinergic enteric neurons. This is certainly so for gastric acid secretion[3] and gastrointestinal motility[1,2]. We have recently shown[4] that there is no simultaneous activation of enteric inhibitory neurons by comparing TRH-evoked motility with that evoked by electrical stimulation of the vagus nerves in the rat. While such studies have demonstrated some degree of selectivity of the central actions of TRH on vagal neurons, in that only excitatory pathways are activated, they do not exclude the possibility that peripheral, excitatory, non-cholinergic neurons are simultaneously stimulated. In the rabbit colon, there is evidence that the increased rate of transit following intracerebroventricular injection of TRH is due to the vagal activation of non-cholinergic secretomotor neurons[5]. In this study we provide evidence for activation of intrapancreatic, non-cholinergic neurons following intracisternal injection of TRH.

METHODS

Adult guinea-pigs, of either sex, were anaesthetized with urethane (1500 mg/kg i.v.). The pancreatic duct was cannulated for collection of exocrine secretion in lengths of PE tubing and the volume measured. Thereafter, a sample of the secretion was assayed for amylase content using a fluorimetric method described earlier[6]. The animals were placed in a stereotaxic frame in an upright, sitting posture with the head ventrally flexed. A 27-gauge hypodermic needle with polyethylene tubing attached, containing 2.5 μg of TRH in 10 μl saline, was inserted into the cisterna magna. After measuring basal flow for at least 30 min, the TRH was allowed to flow into the cisterna magna by gravity and the pancreatic response followed for a further hour. Drugs such as atropine sulphate (0.1–1.0 mg/kg) or hexamethonium bromide (10 mg/kg) were administered intravenously via an in-dwelling jugular venous catheter. In animals in which vagotomy was performed, the vagi were cut in the neck and basal secretion collected for 30 min, with the animals in a supine position. The animals were then placed in the stereotaxic frame and the intracisternal (i.c.) injection of TRH made immediately. After 30 min, the animals were removed from the frame, placed once again in a supine position and one of the severed vagi lifted on to bipolar silver electrodes and stimulated electrically at 10 V, 0.5 ms, 10 Hz for 5 min. The flow of pancreatic secretion was then followed until it returned to basal levels.

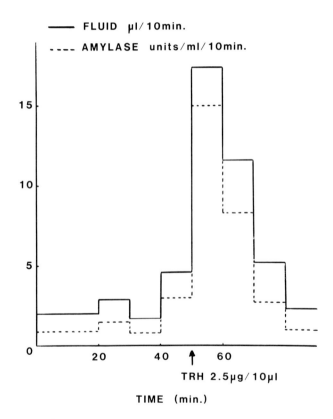

Figure 1 Fluid and amylase release in response to a bolus injection of TRH (2.5 μg in 10 μl of saline) into the cisterna magna of a single anaesthetized guinea-pig. Note the duration of the response and the relationship between fluid output and amylase output

RESULTS

The i.c. injection of 2.5 μg TRH in 10 μl saline evoked a rapid increase of pancreatic flow and amylase output which lasted for approximately 20 min ($n = 6$) (Figure 1). Intravenous atropine (1 mg/kg) produced no reduction in flow and amylase response to i.c. TRH (Figure 2) ($n = 5$), in contrast to the approximately 25% reduction of the response to electrical stimulation of the vagus produced by the same dose of atropine (Figure 1). The response to i.c. TRH was abolished by bilateral cervical vagotomy ($n = 5$) or by i.v. hexamethonium (10 mg/kg) ($n = 5$).

All vagotomized animals responded to electrical stimulation of the vagus with an increase in flow rate and amylase output (Figure 3).

DISCUSSION

The present study shows that centrally acting TRH will activate release of fluid and enzymes from guinea-pig pancreas by stimulation of vagal preganglionic neurons. These neurons are cholinergic since the actions of i.c. TRH are abolished by hexamethonium. The intrapancreatic neurons activated by the preganglionic fibres are, however, largely non-cholinergic. We have shown previously that these are non-adrenergic[6,7] and have provided evidence that they may be VIP-ergic[8].

There is a prevailing holistic view that centrally acting TRH is largely

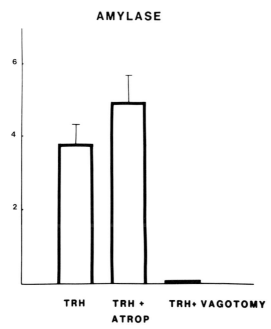

AMYLASE

Figure 2 Amylase release following TRH injection in control, atropinized and vagotomized animals. (Mean values from five experiments)

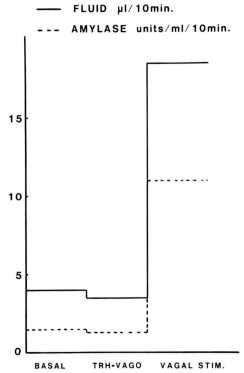

Figure 3 Fluid and amylase release in a single experiment showing the average fluid and amylase output per 10 min calculated from a 30 min collection period. After a basal period, vagotomy was performed followed immediately by an i.c. injection of TRH (2.5 μg in 10 μl of saline); 30 min later the peripheral end of one of the severed vagi was lifted onto bipolar silver electrodes and stimulated at 10 V, 0.5 ms, 10 Hz for 5 min. Note the lack of effect of TRH but the effectiveness of electrical stimulation of the vagus

concerned with the regulation of cholinergic systems. In one sense this might be an accurate summary and is supported by the present finding that the vagal preganglionic fibres activated by i.c. TRH are cholinergic. However, this concept cannot be applied to the peripheral nervous system of the gastrointestinal tract where there are now two clear examples of activation of peripheral non-cholinergic secretomotor pathways by centrally applied TRH. Moreover, in this study, it would appear that the cholinergic intrapancreatic neurons which can be activated by vagal preganglionic fibres[7], were not apparently activated by intracisternal TRH in that atropine did not reduce the response.

In addition, we have recently made some incidental and unpublished observations on gastric motility following i.c. TRH in the rat and have seen several instances of atropine-resistant stimulation of motility following i.c. TRH. We have not studied this systematically but have shown in these same animals that the dose of atropine was sufficient to block the motility response to a supramaximal dose of bethanechol injected intravenously. One possibility we have considered is that, in some animals, there may be an enhanced sympathetic tone that would be inhibited by i.c. TRH, as demonstrated in an earlier neurophysiological study showing a reduction in whole nerve discharge in sympathetic post-ganglionic, nerves following central adminis-tration of TRH[9].

In summary, the concept of TRH being a regulator only of peripheral cholinergic systems is perhaps too simplistic and not particularly helpful in understanding its role in the central regulation of gastrointestinal functions through modulation of the enteric nervous system.

References

1. Lattann, T. R. and Horita, A. (1982). Thyrotropin releasing hormone: centrally mediated effects on gastrointestinal motor activity. *J. Pharmacol. Exp. Therap.*, **222**, 66–70
2. Rogers, R. C. and Hermann, G. E. (1987). Oxytocin, oxytocin antagonist, TRH, and hypothal-amic paraventricular nucleus stimulation effects of gastric motility. *Peptides*, **8**, 505–13
3. Taché, Y. (1988). CNS peptides and regulation of gastric acid secretion. *Annu. Rev. Physiol.*, **50**, 19–39
4. Davison, J. S., Wootton, P. and Hickie, J. (1988). The effects of intracisternal thyrotropin releasing hormone (TRH) on gastroduodenal motility in the rat. *Proc. West. Pharmacol. Soc.*, **31**, 35–7
5. Horita, A., Carino, M. A. and Lai, H. (1986). Pharmacology of thyrotropin-releasing hormone. *Annu. Rev. Pharmacol. Toxicol.*, **26**, 311–32
6. Pearson, G. T., Singh, J., Daoud, M. S., Davison, J. S. and Petersen, O. H. (1981). Control of pancreatic cyclic nucleotide levels and amylase secretion by noncholinergic, nonadrenergic nerves. *J. Biol. Chem.*, **256**, 11025–31
7. Davison, J. S. and Dickson, V. (1984). Vagal nonadrenergic, noncholinergic (NANC) nerves control pancreatic exocrine secretion in the guinea-pig. In Case, R. M., Lingard, J. and Young, J. A. (eds.) *Secretion: Mechanisms and Control*, pp. 225–30. (Manchester: Manchester University Press)
8. Davison, J. S. and Buchan, A. M. J. (1986). VIP-ergic innervation of guinea-pig exocrine pancreas. *Proc. West. Pharmacol. Soc.*, **29**, 467–70
9. Somiya, H. and Tonoue, T. (1984). Neuropeptides as central integrators of autonomic nerve activity: effects of TRH, SRIF, VIP and bombesin on gastric and adrenal nerves. *Reg. Peptides*, **9**, 47–52

27
Pancreatic secretory response to intravenous caerulein and intraduodenal tryptophan before and after stepwise removal of the extrinsic nerves of the pancreas in dogs

M. V. SINGER, W. NIEBEL, H. GOEBELL, J. B. M. J. JANSEN AND C. B. H. W. LAMERS

The relative contributions of the vagus and splanchnic nerves on the one hand, and gastrointestinal hormones (e.g. cholecystokinin, CCK) on the other, as mediators of the pancreatic secretory response to intestinal stimulants, are still incompletely determined. In addition it is not known whether the enteropancreatic, cholinergic, vagovagal reflexes which mediate the early pancreatic enzyme response to intestinal amino acids are only vagovagal and whether they are independent of CCK release.

In two sets of 6 dogs with gastric and pancreatic fistulas, we studied the effect of atropine ($14 \, \text{nmol kg}^{-1}\text{h}^{-1}$ i.v.) on the pancreatic secretory response to intravenous caerulein and to intraduodenal perfusion with tryptophan (both given with a secretin background), before and after stepwise removal of the extrinsic nerves of the pancreas, i.e. coeliac and superior mesenteric ganglionectomy alone or truncal vagotomy alone and truncal vagotomy plus coeliac and superior mesenteric ganglionectomy.

RESULTS

Atropine significantly ($p < 0.05$) depressed the protein output basally and during secretin alone at each stage of innervation. The incremental protein response to caerulein was not altered by the different denervation operations nor by atropine. Truncal vagotomy alone significantly decreased the incremental protein response to low (0.12 and $1.1 \, \text{mmol h}^{-1}$) but not high loads

652

of tryptophan; additional ganglionectomy having no further depressing effect. Atropine significantly reduced the incremental protein response to low loads of tryptophan only in intact innervated animals. Ganglionectomy alone did not alter the incremental protein response to any load of tryptophan. Neither the different surgical procedures nor atropine altered plasma levels of immuno-reactive cholecystokinin (CCK) basally and in response to trypto-phan.

CONCLUSIONS

We conclude that neither the extrinsic nor the intrinsic cholinergic pancreatic nerves modulate the protein response to caerulein. The sympathetic pan-creatic nerves do not mediate the response to tryptophan. The protein response to intraduodenal tryptophan is mediated by long, cholinergic, enteropancreatic reflexes with both afferent and efferent fibres running within the vagus nerves. Release of CCK by intestinal tryptophan is not under cholinergic and splanchnic control.

SHORT COMMUNICATION

28
Central modulation of exocrine pancreatic secretion by opioids and α_2-adrenergic drugs in the rat

C. ROZÉ, J. CHARIOT, J. DE LA TOUR AND C. VAILLE

The cephalic phase of pancreatic secretion is well documented[1], as well as cholinergic and vagal influences on the pancreatic response to intestinal stimulants[2]. However, few data have been published about the effects of centrally administered peptides or neurotransmitters on the control of pancreatic secretion, whereas this point is abundantly documented in the case of gastric secretion[3]. Our group has been involved for several years in the study of central actions of opioids and α_2-adrenergics in the rat, and the purpose of this paper is to summarize our present knowledge in this field.

METHODS

Male Wistar rats were used. They were prepared with pancreatic fistulas in two different ways, allowing either acute or chronic studies, which provide complementary information. In the acute model[4], urethane anaesthesia was used, and pancreatic secretion was collected after stimulation with agents acting either peripherally (secretin, CCK, acetylcholine, vagal electrical stimulation (VES)) or centrally by activating the vagal pathway in the central nervous system (2-deoxy-D-glucose (2DG)). Opiates and adrenergics were usually administered as intravenous (i.v.) or subcutaneous (s.c.) injections. In this model, basal pancreatic secretion is low and the response to exogenous stimulants can be reasonably assigned to the stimulant alone, without potentiation by endogenous factors. The influence of gastric secretion can be eliminated by using pylorus ligation.

In the chronic model[5], the rats were kept in restraint cages, with permanent reintroduction of bile through a Silastic catheter surgically implanted, total derivation of pure pancreatic juice and permanent infusion of the duodenum with a trypsin solution in view of maintaining the trypsin-related enteropancreatic feedback system[6]. A chronic cannula was inserted in the third ventricle of the brain, so that opiates and adrenergics could be administered either in the cerebral ventricles (i.c.v.) or peripherally (i.v. or s.c.). Occasionally, a chronic catheter was inserted in the cisterna magna, allowing intracisternal (i.c.) injections. In this model, basal pancreatic secretion is much higher than in the anaesthetized model, due to a permanent stimulation by endogenous factors comprising especially a large cholinergic contribution[7]. The influence of gastric secretion can be dealt with in this model by using rats with both gastric and pancreatic fistulas, or by using inhibitors of acid secretion.

RESULTS

Opioid agonists

Moderate doses of opiate drugs crossing freely the blood–brain barrier (methadone, morphine, etorphine) all decreased more potently the 2DG- than the SEV-stimulated pancreatic secretion in anaesthetized rats, indicating a main central site of action[8,9]. However, larger doses also displayed some peripheral effects on VES-stimulated pancreatic secretion, indicating that they were also able to depress the release of transmitters from vagal pre- or post-ganglionic fibres[10]. No inhibition of acetylcholine-, secretin- or CCK-stimulated pancreatic secretion was observed, suggesting that no direct effect of opioids could take place on the pancreatic secretory cells.

The opioid peptides β-endorphin, D-Ala-Met-enkephalinamide, dynorphin, were inactive on pancreatic secretion when injected peripherally (i.v.). However, i.c.v. injections of these peptides in nanomolar amounts induced inhibitions of basal pancreatic volume flow, of bicarbonate output, and of total protein output in conscious rats. The peak inhibition was usually observed 40–60 min after the i.c.v. injection, and the output of protein was more decreased (up to 80%, Figure 1) than the output of water and bicarbonate (up to 60%). That this effect was indeed central could be confirmed by using naloxone methylbromide, an opiate antagonist which

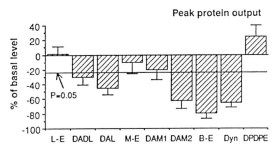

Figure 1 Peak variations of protein output in the pancreatic juice of conscious rats after the intra-cerebroventricular injection of opioid peptides. L-E: Leu-Enkephalin, 45 nmol; DADL: D-Ala-D Leu-Enkephalin 14 nmol, DAL: D-Ala-Leu-Enkephalin 14 nmol; M-E; Met-Enkephalin, 45 nmol; DAM1: D-Ala-Met-Enkephaline, 14 nmol; DAM2: D-Ala-Met-Enkephalinamide, 14 nmol; B-E: β-Endorphin, ovine, 7 nmol; Dyn: Dynorphin 1-13, porcine, 10 nmol; DPDPE: D-Pen(2,5)-Enkephalin, 12 nmol. (Drawn from data in refs 5 and 11 and from unpublished results)

crosses poorly the blood–brain barrier, as compared to naloxone, which crosses freely the blood–brain barrier: the effect of an i.c.v. injection of D-Ala-Met enkephalinamide (14 nmol) was suppressed by naloxone (1 mg/kg, s.c.), but not by naloxone methylbromide (10 mg/kg, s.c.)[11].

Naloxone suppressed the inhibitory action of opioids, whereas α_2 adrenergic antagonists had no effect to prevent this action (Figure 2).

The comparison of the relative potencies of several opioid peptides to inhibit pancreatic secretion after i.c.v. injection has some interest, but these potencies are probably related both to the subtype(s) of opioid receptors accessed by the peptides and to the rate of their metabolic degradation. As an example, an i.c.v. injection of 14 nmol D-Ala-Met enkephalin alone did not significantly decrease pancreatic secretion, whereas it inhibited pancreatic protein output by 80%, an effect lasting for 2 h, when it was associated with inhibitors of peptidases, such as i.c.v. thiorphan (an inhibitor of endopeptidase 24.11, an important enzyme in the degradation of the C-terminal end of enkephalins) and i.c.v. bestatin (an inhibitor of aminopeptidase M, an important enzyme in the degradation of the N-terminal end of enkephalins)[12].

However, the delta specific opioid peptide D-Pen (2, 5)-enkephalin was inactive on pancreatic secretion up to the dose of 12 nmol i.c.v. (Figure 1), even in association with thiorphan and bestatin.

The opiate antagonist naloxone, as well as the peptidase inhibitors thiorphan and bestatin were essentially inactive on pancreatic secretion when injected alone, in the dose range and experimental conditions tested to date.

Adrenergic agonists

The effects of adrenergic agonists and antagonists on pancreatic secretion are complex, and confusing results have been published by several groups using different species and different experimental setups. In the case of α_2 agonists, however, our experimental data show some evidence of central inhibitory effects in rats. The α_2 agonists clonidine[13] and guanabenz[14] inhibited more potently the 2DG- than the VES-stimulated pancreatic

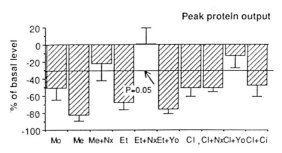

Figure 2 Peak variations of protein output in the pancreatic juice of conscious rats after the subcutaneous injection of opiate and adrenergic agonists and antagonists. Mo: Morphine 5 mg/kg; Me: Methadone 5 mg/kg; Nx: Naloxone 1 mg/kg; Et: Etorphine 3 µg/kg; Yo: Yohimbine 1 mg/kg; Cl: Clonidine 100 µg/kg; Ci: Cimétidine 25 mg/kg. (Drawn from data in refs 9 and 13 and from unpublished results)

secretion in anaesthetized rats. This inhibition was suppressed by α_2 antagonists such as yohimbine (Figure 2) or idazoxan.

Clonidine crosses very readily the blood–brain barrier. When comparing the doses of clonidine inducing 50% of the maximal effect (ED_{50}) on the basal interdigestive secretion of conscious rats after s.c., i.c.v. or i.c. administration, the ED_{50} was similar ($10\,\mu g/kg$ after s.c. or i.c.v. injections (although the slope of the dose-response curves was different). The ED_{50} was, however, about ten times smaller ($0.8\,\mu g/kg$) after i.c. injections, suggesting an effect at the level of the medulla oblongata (the nucleus of tractus solitarius as a target for clonidine in other experimental systems). Moreover, ST91, a clonidine congener crossing poorly the blood–brain barrier, was as potent as clonidine in inhibiting pancreatic secretion after an i.c.v. injection, but far less potent than clonidine after a s.c. injection[15].

Whereas α_2 antagonists inhibited the effects of α_2 adrenergic drugs on pancreatic secretion, naloxone had no effect when associated with these α_2 adrenergics (Figure 2).

CONCLUSION: ACQUISITIONS AND UNRESOLVED ISSUES

Exogenous opiates and opioid peptides can inhibit pancreatic secretion in rats. The peptides are active only after an i.c.v. injection, whereas the opiates are active by both s.c. or i.c.v. routes, as far as they readily cross the blood–brain barrier. The central inhibitions induced by opiates are naloxone sensitive, and they seem to be mediated more by μ than by δ receptors. However, no conclusive detailed study of the opiate receptors involved has been done to date.

Exogenous α_2-adrenergic drugs also inhibit pancreatic secretion in rats, as well as after s.c. and i.c.v. injections, provided they cross readily the blood–brain barrier. The central component of this effect is reversed by α_2 antagonists such as yohimbine or idazoxan. Peripheral effects may also occur, sometimes involving other subtypes of adrenergic receptors.

Two different brain neuronal systems seem to be involved in the effects of opiates and adrenergics on pancreatic secretion, since to date no cross-inhibition has been found between naloxone, yohimbine and their respective agonists. However, more detailed studies might reveal some interferences between these two systems.

Many points remain unknown. The main question is whether these mechanisms are activated in physiological or pathological circumstances, and which are these circumstances. The results obtained after exogenous injections demonstrate that central opiate and α_2 receptors can modulate pancreatic secretion. However, it is doubtful whether appropriate neurons are able to release the adequate peptides or amines near to these receptors, since the antagonists used alone have to date revealed no, or only poor, effects. Most of our results have been obtained in stimulated state in anaesthetized rats, and in basal interdigestive state in conscious rats. More studies using other experimental conditions should help in obtaining more information.

References

1. Anagnostides, A., Chadwick, V. S., Selden, A. C. and Maton, P. N. (1984). Sham feeding and pancreatic secretion. Evidence for direct vagal stimulation of enzyme output. *Gastroenterology*, **87**, 109–14

2. Singer, M. V., Solomon, T. E., Wood, J. and Grossman, M. I. (1980). Latency of pancreatic enzyme response to intestinal stimulants. *Am. J. Physiol.*, **238**, G23–9

3. Taché, Y. (1988). CNS peptides and regulation of gastric acid secretion. *Annu. Rev. Physiol.*, **50**, 19–39

4. Rozé, C., La Tour, J. de, Chariot, J., Souchard, M. and Debray, C. (1975). Technique d'étude de la sécrétion pancréatique externe chez le rat. *Biol. Gastroentérol. (Paris)*, **8**, 291–5

5. Rozé, C., Dubrasquet, M., Chariot, J. and Vaille, C. (1980). Central inhibition of basal pancreatic and gastric secretions by beta-endorphin in rats. *Gastroenterology*, **79**, 659–64

6. Green, G. M. and Lyman, R. L. (1972). Feedback regulation of pancreatic enzyme secretion as a mechanism for trypsin inhibitor-induced hypersecretion in rats. *Proc. Soc. Exp. Biol. Med.*, **140**, 6–12

7. Chariot, J., La Tour, J. de, Anglade, P. and Rozé, C. (1987). Cholinergic mechanisms in the pancreas after extrinsic denervation in the rat. *Am. J. Physiol.*, **252**, G755–61

8. Rozé, C., Chariot, J., La Tour, J. de, Souchard, M., Vaille, C. and Debray, C. (1978). Methadone blockade of 2-deoxyglucose-induced pancreatic secretion in the rat. Evidence for a central site of action. *Gastroenterology*, **74**, 215–20

9. Chariot, J., Appia, F., Vaille, C. and Rozé, C. (1986). Etorphine inhibition of pancreatic exocrine secretion in rats: comparison with methadone. *Eur. J. Pharmacol.*, **121**, 73–81

10. Rozé, C., Dubrasquet, M., Chariot, J. and Vaille, C. (1982). Methadone inhibition of vagally induced pancreatic and gastric secretions in rats: central and peripheral sites of action. *Eur. J. Pharmacol.*, **78**, 271–8

11. Chicau-Chovet, M., Chariot, J. and Rozé, C. (1985). Inhibition centrale de la sécrétion pancréatique externe par le D-ala-2-Metenképhalinamide chez le rat. *Gastroentérol. Clin. Biol.*, **9**, 220–2

12. Chicau-Chovet, M., Chariot, J. and Rozé, C. (1986). Central inhibition of pancreatic and gastric secretions by D-Ala-2 Metenkephalin and peptidase inhibitors (abstr.). *Digestion*, **35**, 12–13

13. Rozé, C., Chariot, J., Appia, F., Pascaud, X. and Vaille, C. (1981). Clonidine inhibition of pancreatic secretion in rats: a possible central site of action. *Eur. J. Pharmacol.*, **76**, 381–90

14. Appia, F., Chariot, J., del Tacca, M. and Rozé, C. (1986). Inhibition of pancreatic secretion by guanabenz in rats (abstr.). *Digestion*, **35**, 5

15. Chariot, J., Appia, F., del Tacca, M., Tsocas, A. and Rozé, C. (1988). Central and peripheral inhibition of exocrine pancreatic secretion by alpha-2 adrenergic agonists in the rat. *Pharmacol. Res. Comm.* (In press)

29
Pancreatic acini desensitization: a response to sustained cholinergic stimulation mechanisms involved

J. MORISSET AND L. LAROSE

Studies were undertaken to characterize and explain the phenomenon of pancreatic acinar cell's desensitization to long and short time exposure to muscarinic agonists. Long-term treatments were performed *in vivo*, those in the short term were done *in vitro*. Desensitization was evaluated from rat dispersed pancreatic acini by measuring amylase release, receptor binding and second messenger production in response to carbamylcholine (C), a muscarinic agonist, caerulein (Cae), a CCK analogue, and secretin (S).

Long-term, chronic bethanechol treatment ($12\,mg\,kg^{-1}$, i.p. for 14 days) caused a four-fold decrease in sensitivity of the acini for amylase release in response to C, the EC_{50} being shifted from 0.69 to $2.9\,\mu M$. Muscarinic receptor concentration evaluated by $[^3H]$-N-methylscopolamine ($[^3H]$-NMS) binding was reduced by 42%. Analysis of C binding revealed that the number of high affinity sites remained constant while their affinity was greatly decreased from 0.24 to $6.1\,\mu M$. The low affinity sites exhibited a slight decrease in affinity from 34 to $150\,\mu M$ and a significant decrease in their number. The observation that amylase release in response to Cae was not affected suggests an homologous densensitization.

Short-term (1 h) exposure of pancreatic acini to increasing concentration of C, (10^{-7}–$10^{-4}\,M$) resulted in a progressive modified subsequent secretory response to this same agonist as evidenced by increased EC_{50} from 0.5 to $4.0\,\mu M$. The phenomenon remained irreversible after 3 h of recovery and was Ca^{2+}-independent. Contrary to what was observed *in vivo*, muscarinic receptor concentration remained unaffected as well as their affinity for C. However, the proportion of the high-affinity sites was decreased, while that of the low affinity increased. The secretory response to Cae again remained unaffected as well as those to the phorbol ester TPA and the Ca^{2+} ionophore A23187. These observations indicate that desensitization does not alter intracellular steps beyond calcium mobilization or protein kinase C activation but modified the classes of the muscarinic receptor. Pre-exposure of pancreatic acini to 0.1 mM C reduced the subsequent secretory response to S by decreasing its efficacy. However, the S-stimulated cAMP production remained normal as well as amylase secretion induced by cholera toxin, forskolin and DBcAMP. Furthermore, the inositol phosphates produced by S were not modified. These data suggest that alteration of the S response cannot be accounted for by changes in the second mesengers production nor to the S receptor.

In conclusion, densensitization of the pancreatic acinar cells to muscarinic agonists results from different alterations of the muscarinic receptors, depending on length of exposure and intensity of the stimulation. The progression goes from receptor down regulation with changes in affinity of both high and low affinity binding sites to changes in proportion in the high and low affinity binding sites. Post-second messenger modifications have also occurred but remained unidentified and may be responsible for the S-reduced secretory response.

Acknowledgements

Supported by MRC of Canada.

30
Nervous control of pancreatic blood supply and secretion (an experimental study)

M. PAPP, G. VARGA, I. DOBRONYI AND E. S. VIZI

INTRODUCTION

It is well established that cholinergic and adrenergic nerves play an important role regulating pancreatic function including blood supply and exocrine secretion.

Although there was no direct evidence that noradrenaline is the primary transmitter responsible for vasoconstriction in pancreaticoduodenal and hepatic arteries, the vessels supplying the pancreas, both noradrenaline[1-2] and sympathetic stimulation[3] had been reported to increase pancreatic vascular resistance. Similarly, hepatic blood supply was shown to be reduced by these treatments[4-5]. The possible direct action of cholinergic nerves on pancreatic and hepatic vascular resistance was not studied until now.

The control of exocrine pancreatic secretion by cholinergic nerves is characterized in detail[6-7]. However, a direct involvement of adrenergic nervous system in the regulation of exocrine secretion has not been clearly elucidated. It has been said that adrenergic stimulation only influences secretion indirectly via alteration of pancreatic blood flow[2]. Direct inhibitory[8] or stimulatory[9] effect has also been suggested.

The purpose of the present study was twofold: (a) to investigate the nervous control of pancreatic blood flow, and (b) to study the nervous regulation of pancreatic enzyme secretion. Studies were carried out with special attention on the interactions between cholinergic and adrenergic effects.

MATERIALS AND METHODS

Isolated hepatic and pancreaticoduodenal arteries

Isolated arteries were dissected from mongrel dogs. Helical strips were set up in an organ bath (5.0 ml) filled with Krebs solution (113 mM NaCl,

4.7 mM KCl, 2.5 mM $CaCl_2$, 1.2 mM KH_2PO_4, 1.2 mM $MgSO_4$, 25 mM $NaHCO_3$ and 11.5 mM glucose). The solution was maintained at 37°C and gassed with 5% CO_2 in oxygen. Preparations were set up under a resting tension of 5 mN and allowed to equilibrate for at least 1 h before experiments. Isometric contractions were recorded. Contractions of the arteries were expressed in millinewtons (mN). Electrical field stimulation (EFS) (1–50 Hz, 1 ms inpulsus length, supramaximal voltage) was applied via two platinium electrodes; one at the top and one at the bottom of the organ bath. Compounds were given directly to the medium in known concentrations.

In some experiments arteries were preloaded with [³H]-noradrenaline and the release of radioactivity (that is the release of noradrenaline) was measured as described in detail previously[10–11].

Superfused rat pancreatic segments

Studies were performed on isolated segments of adult rats (180–220 g)[9]. Male OFA (Sprague–Dawley strain) rats were killed by a blow to the head and the pancreas was quickly removed and placed in a modified Krebs-Henseleit solution of the following composition: NaCl, 103 mM; KCl, 4.7 mM; $CaCl_2$, 2.56 mM; $MgCl_2$, 1.13 mM, $NaHCO_3$, 25 mM; NaH_2PO_4, 1.15 mM;)D-glucose, 2.8 mM; Na pyruvate, 4.9 mM; Na fumarate, 2.7 mM; Na glutamate, 4.9 mM; pH 7.4. The solution was maintained at 37°C and gassed with 5% CO_2 in O_2.

The pancreas was cut into small segments (3–5 mg). A total weight of about 150 mg was placed in a tissue flow chamber of 1 ml capacity, and superfused at a steady rate of 1.4 ml/min with Krebs-Henseleit solution. The first 30 min effluent was discarded. Subsequently, 3 min fractions were examined.

The amylase concentration in the effluent fractions was measured by a spectrophotometric method[12]. The stimulus-evoked amylase release (i.e. that above basal amylase output) was routinely expressed in terms of the peak response in U/min/100 mg tissue. Compounds were added directly to the superfusion solution in known concentrations. EFS was applied as above. Values were given as mean ± SEM. Statistical differences were calculated, using analysis of variance.

RESULTS

Dog hepatic and pancreaticoduodenal arteries

NA produced a concentration-related contraction of the arteries studied (Figure 1). There was no significant difference between the responses for NA obtained after repeated administration and in a cumulative manner. α_1-Adrenoceptor antagonist prazosin inhibited the effect of NA. The mean pA_2 value for prazosin in the hepatic artery was 7.48, and in the pancreaticoduo-denal artery 7.47. The slopes in the Schild plots in both cases were close to unity, indicating that prazosin was acting as a classical competitive antagonist.

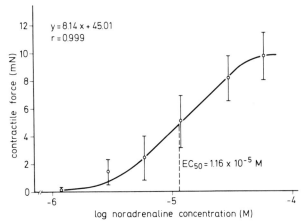

Figure 1 Concentration-response curve of contractions evoked by noradrenaline in isolated pancreaticoduodenal arteries. Isometric contractions were recorded. Contractile force was given in millinewtons (mN). Values are means $\pm$ SEM ($n = 6$)

EFS produced contractions of the isolated arteries (Figure 2) accompanied by tritiated NA release from varicosities. The size of the contraction depended on the frequency of stimulation. Tetrodotoxin (5×10^{-7} M) completely inhibited the contractions elicited by EFS, without affecting the contractions to exogenous NA. Prazosin also inhibited the contractions in response to EFS (Figure 3).

Muscarinic agonist oxotremorine caused a concentration-dependent reduc-

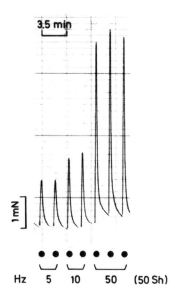

Figure 2 Contractile responses in millinewtons (mN) of an isolated pancreaticoduodenal artery to electrical field stimulation. The number of impulses at 1, 5 and 10 Hz was 50

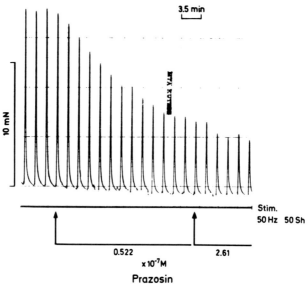

Figure 3 Inhibitory effect of prazosin on contractions of isolated pancreaticoduodenal artery evoked by field stimulation (50 Hz, 50 impulses). The contractile force was given in millinewtons (mN)

tion in size of ESF-induced contraction and NA release (Table 1) without influencing the dose responses to added NA. VIP decreased the responses of the arteries to EFS, although it did not affect the release of NA (Table 1).

Other gastrointestinal peptides (caerulin, CCK-OP, secretin, somatostatin, bovine pancreatic polypeptide, substance P, bombesin, glucagon), in a concentration range of 10^{-10}–10^{-6} M, had no modulatory effect on the basal tension or on EFS- or exogenous NA-evoked contractions of the arterial strips.

Table 1 Inhibitory effect of VIP and oxotremorine on contraction and [^{3}H]noradrenaline release of common hepatic artery in response to electrical field stimulation

	Decrease of contractile force (% previous stimulation)	Decrease of ^{3}H release (% previous stimulation)
Control	1.6 ± 1.3 (10)	1.7 ± 8.1 (5)
VIP, 10^{-6} M	45.5 ± 5.8* (11)	3.4 ± 9.9 (5)
oxotremorine, 10^{-6} M	75.9 ± 5.5* (9)	64.5 ± 9.2* (5)

Values are mean ± SEM; number of observations is shown in parentheses.
Field stimulation was 360 impulses at 2 Hz.
* $p < 0.05$ versus control.

Rat pancreatic segments

Cholinergic agonist urecholine produced concentration-dependent amylase release from the segments. Atropine inhibited the effect of urecholine in competitive manner.

EFS released amylase from the segments. This effect could be inhibited with exogenous atropine by maximum of 80%. Atropine-resistant enzyme discharge in response to EFS could be blocked by β-receptor antagonist propranolol.

NA and β-receptor agonist isoprenaline stimulated amylase release in 10^{-5}–10^{-4} M concentration range (Table 2). The maximal response was only 20% of that which could be elicited by maximal urecholine stimulation.

Lower concentrations (10^{-8}–10^{-7} M) of NA and α_1-adrenoceptor agonist phenylephrine inhibited urecholine evoked amylase release. This effect could be blocked by prazosin (Table 3). The stimulatory effect of urecholine and the β-adrenoceptor agonist isoprenaline was additive (Table 3).

The inhibitory effect of NA on cholinergic stimulation was detectable only during maximal urecholine stimulation. The stimulatory effect of 10^{-4} M urecholine was inhibited by 3×10^{-8} M NA by $23 \pm 4\%$ ($p < 0.05$). NA did not significantly decrease the amylase release evoked by lower concentrations of urecholine.

DISCUSSION

In our experiments direct evidence has been obtained that the neurogenic responses of hepatic and pancreaticoduodenal arteries are mainly due to NA released from axon terminals and this effect is mediated via α_1-adrenoceptors. This is in line with the previous *in vivo* observations that NA causes vasoconstriction within the pancreas[1-2] and decreases hepatic blood flow[4].

The neuroeffector transmission of hepatic and pancreaticoduodenal arteries

Table 2 Concentration-dependent peak amylase response evoked by noradrenaline and isoprenaline in isolated pancreatic segments. Basal amylase release is subtracted

Concentration	Peak amylase response (U/min/100 mg tissue)	
	Noradrenaline	Isoprenaline
10^{-8} M	0.05 ± 0.08	—
10^{-7} M	0.03 ± 0.07	0.12 ± 0.13
10^{-6} M	0.18 ± 0.17	0.09 ± 0.07
10^{-5} M	0.84 ± 0.14	0.66 ± 0.14
10^{-4} M	0.99 ± 0.19	0.90 ± 0.19

Values are mean $\pm$ SEM ($n = 4$—6).

Table 3 Modulation of 10^{-4} M urecholine evoked peak amylase response by noradrenaline, prazosin, phenylephrine, and isoprenaline in isolated pancreatic segments. Data are expressed as ratio to peak amylase response evoked by previous urecholine stimulation

Concentration	Peak amylase response (ratio to control)			
	Noradrenaline	Noradrenaline $+10^{-6}$ M prazosin	Phenylephrine	Isoprenaline
10^{-9} M	0.98	1.04	0.99	—
	± 0.05	± 0.05	± 0.05	
10^{-8} M	0.79*	1.05	0.82*	—
	± 0.08	± 0.06	± 0.06	
10^{-7} M	0.85*	0.93	0.78*	1.02
	± 0.04	± 0.06	± 0.08	± 0.07
10^{-6} M	0.98	1.07	0.82*	1.04
	± 0.05	± 0.04	± 0.07	± 0.06
10^{-5} M	0.97	1.24*	—	1.17*
	± 0.06	± 0.09		± 0.06
10^{-4} M	0.98	1.19*	—	1.21*
	± 0.06	± 0.05		± 0.07

Values are means ± SEM; (n = 4-6);
* $p < 0.05$ vs. control.

is subject to cholinergic presynaptic modulation. Oxotremorine, a powerful muscarinic agonist reduced the neurogenic responses of the arteries without affecting the sensitivity of smooth muscle to exogenous NA, but reducing the release of NA from varicosities.

VIP reduced the responses of the isolated arteries to EFS and exogenous NA but did not affect the release of [^{3}H]-NA from nerve terminals. These findings indicate that the site of action of VIP is post-synaptic and located on the smooth muscle. Our results are consistent with earlier observations that intravenous VIP infusion decreases hepatic arterial blood pressure in dogs[13] and humans[14]. In addition Inoue et al.[15] found that the atrophied pancreas responds in vivo to VIP with increased blood flow but not to administration of secretin.

The other peptides studied (caerulein, CCK-OP, secretin, somatostatin, bovine pancreatic polypeptide, substance P, bombesin, glucagon) failed to affect responses of arteries to both electrical stimulation and administration of NA. Because secretin, caerulein and CCK-OP enhanced the pancreatic blood flow in vivo[16], it seems likely that these hormones exert their vasoactive actions at centrally located sites rather than at the neuroeffector junction.

The significance of cholinergic control of pancreatic enzyme secretion is well established[6-7]. Our results confirm the previous observations that acetylcholine is the main neurotransmitter stimulating exocrine secretion via muscarinic receptors.

The technique of EFS has previously been shown to be a useful tool for studying the nervous pathway controlling pancreatic function[9]. Consistent with the previous investigations, in the present study, EFS-evoked effects were abolished following the blockade of nerve conduction by tetrodotoxin. In agreement with Pearson et al.[9], we found that stimulation of the intrinsic nerves in the rat pancreas evokes an atropine-resistant amylase secretion which could be mimicked by the exogenous application of high concentration of NA or β-adrenergic agonist isoprenaline, and blocked by β-adrenergic antagonist propranolol. We can therefore conclude that adrenergic nerves may stimulate amylase secretion via β-adrenoceptors.

On the other hand, lower concentrations of NA and α_1-adrenergic agonist phenyleprine inhibited urecholine evoked pancreatic enzyme secretion in our experimental conditions. This inhibition could be abolished by α_1-adrenergic antagonist prazosin. This finding confirms the previous *in vivo* observation that pancreatic protein secretion can be inhibited via α_1-adrenoceptors[17]. In addition, our results suggest the inhibitory action of NA is on the acinar cells, since the direct urecholine action was inhibited via a_1-adrenoceptors.

Our observations may explain the previous inconsistent findings[6-7] regarding the adrenergic actions on pancreatic enzyme secretion. According to our observations, adrenergic action can be stimulatory via β-adrenoceptors or inhibitory via α_1-adrenoceptors, depending on the experimental conditions[1]. All other adrenergic actions on pancreatic secretion[6-7] are probably indirect, affecting blood flow or centrally located nervous elements.

In conclusion, both adrenergic and cholinergic nerves are involved in the control of pancreatic enzyme secretion and blood flow. Cholinergic mechanisms look to be more important regulating secretion but their actions can be modulated by adrenergic nerves. Pancreatic blood flow is primarily regulated by adrenergic nerves but their action is subject to cholinergic control.

Acknowledgements

This work was supported by a grant from the Hungarian Academy of Sciences (AKA).

References

1. Richins, C. A. (1953). Effect of sympathetic nerve stimulation on blood flow and secretion in the pancreas of cat. *Am. J. Physiol.*, **173**, 467–70
2. Barlow, T. E., Greenwell, J. R., Harper, A. A. and Scratcherd, T. (1974). The influence of splanchnic nerves on the external secretion, blood flow and electrical conductance of the cat pancreas. *J. Physiol. (Lond.)*, **236**, 421–33
3. Varga, B., Folly, G. and Papp, M. (1974). L'effect de l'excitation electrique du ganglion coelique sur bebit sanguin du pancreas. *Lyon Chir.*, **70**, 168–70
4. Richardson, P. D. I. and Withrington, P. G. (1977). The role of beta-adrenoceptors in the responses of the hepatic arterial vascular bed of the dog to phenylephrine, isoprenaline, noradrenaline and adrenaline. *Br. J. Pharmacol.*, **60**, 239–49
5. Green, H. D., Hall, L. S., Sexton, J. and Deal, C. P. (1959). Autonomic vasomotor responses in the canine hepatic arterial and venous beds. *Am. J. Physiol.*, **196**, 192–202
6. Holst, J. J. (1986). Neural regulation of pancreatic exocrine function. In Go, V. L. W. *et al.* (eds.) *The Exocrine Pancreas: Biology, Pathobiology and Diseases*, pp. 287–300. (New York: Raven Press)
7. Solomon, T. E. (1987). Control of exocrine pancreatic secretion. In Johnson, L. R. *et al.* (eds.) *Physiology of the Gastrointestinal Tract*, 2nd Edn., pp. 1173–207. (New York: Raven Press)
8. Elisha, E. E., Hutson, D. and Scratcherd, T. (1984). The direct inhibition of pancreatic

electrolyte secretion by noradrenaline in the isolated perfused cat pancreas. *J. Physiol. (Lond.)*, **351**, 77–85

9. Pearson, G. T., Singh, J. and Petersen, O. H. (1974). Adrenergic nervous control of cAMP-mediated amylase secretion in the rat pancreas. *Am. J. Physiol.*, **246**, G563–73

10. Varga, G., Papp, M., Harsing, L. G., Toth, I. E., Gaal, Gy., Somogyi, G. T. and Vizi, E. S. (1984). Neuroeffector transmission of the hepatic and pancreatico-duodenal isolated arteries of the dog. *Gastroenterology*, **87**, 1056–63

11. Varga, G., Kiss, J. Z., Papp, M. and Vizi, E. S. (1986). Vasoactive intestinal peptide may participate in the vasodilation of the dog hepatic artery. *Am. J. Physiol.*, **251**, G280–4

12. Bernfeld, P. (1955). Amylases, alpha and beta. In Colowick, S. O. and Kaplan, N. O. (eds.) *Methods in Enzymology*, pp. 149–58. (New York: Academic Press)

13. Thulin, L. (1973). Effects of gastrointestinal peptides on hepatic bile flow and splanchnic circulation. *Acta. Chir. Scand.* (Suppl.), **441**, 1–31

14. Thulin, L., Nyberg, B., Tyden, G. and Sonnefeld, T. (1984). Circulatory effects of VIP in anesthetized man. *Peptides*, **5**, 319–23

15. Inoue, K., Kawano, T., Shima, K., Suzuki, T. K. T., Tobe, T. and Yajima, H. (1981). Relationship between development of fibrosis and hemodynamic changes of the pancreas in dogs. *Gastroenterology*, **81**, 37–47

16. Papp, M., Varga, B. and Folly, G. (1973). Effect of secretin, pancreozymin, histamine and Decholin[R] on canine pancreatic blood flow. *Pflügers Arch.*, **340**, 349–60

17. Mori, J., Satoh, H., Satoh, Y. and Honda, F. (1979). Amines and the rat pancreas: (3) Effects of amines on pancreatic secretion. *Jpn. J. Pharmacol.*, **29**, 923–33

Part III
Enteric Neuroeffector Control

31
Functional changes in opossum oesophagus from experimental obstruction: manometric findings

S. SHIRAZI, K. SCHULZE-DELRIEU, S. NOEL AND H. TUNG

BACKGROUND

Oesophageal obstruction occurs as a complication of peptic oesophageal strictures of tumours or from failure of relaxation of the lower oesophageal sphincter in achalasia. Changes in the function of the oesophagus above the site of the obstruction have been reported in all these conditions, and may be partially reversible[1]. The mechanisms behind these changes have had little study.

We have developed a model of oesohageal obstruction similar to the model of intestinal obstruction used for morphologic studies by some investigators[2]. We used for these studies the American opossum, because its oesophagus is well studied[3], and because the long intra-abdominal segment of the oesophagus lends itself to operative manipulations. In the following we will describe the model and the changes in oesophageal manometry we found after obstruction had become established. We have or will present elsewhere data on the *in vitro* mechanical function of oesophageal smooth muscle and on specific structural changes[4].

METHODS

Six animals were studied. Animals were of either sex and weighed about 1.3 kg when entered into the study. All animals underwent oesophageal manometry using standard methods[3] one day before operation and again 4 weeks after the operation. At the operation, the abdominal segment of the oesophagus was identified and its circumference was measured 2 and 4 cm above the gastro-oesophageal junction. With a tube in the oesophagus to keep its lumen 5 mm open, a gortex band was tied around the oesophagus and fixed to the crura of the diaphragm 2 cm above the LES.

Animals were fed a soft diet *ad libitum.* Most had apparent problems with food intake and gained little weight, if not actually losing. Four weeks following the operation, animals had their oesophagus removed for morphologic or *in vitro* mechanical study.

RESULTS

Morphologic changes

The gortex band produced an inflammatory reaction on the oesophageal surface which led to a progressive narrowing of the oesophageal lumen. The oesophagus above the band became distended, sometimes nearly doubling its circumference (i.e. from about 4 cm pre-operatively to 7.5 cm after the banding, see Table 1). There was no evidence for a change in oesophageal length.

In about half the specimens, the oesophageal mucosa above the band showed diffuse reddening and oedema on gross inspection. Measurements of histologic cross-sections of the oesophageal wall showed an increase in the thickness of the epithelium and of the circular muscle layers; no significant increase could be detected in the other layers of the oesophageal wall. Individual myocytes increased vastly in diameter, and exhibited marked differences in staining (Figure 1).

Oesophageal manometry

The pattern of oesophageal contractions following banding was chaotic. Before banding, more than 90% of dry swallows led to complete peristaltic sequences; after banding less than 20% did so. Contractions were weak or failed altogether at some sites, or they propagated in the retrograde direction or were repetitive (Figure 2).

The position of the LES was unchanged, and its pressures higher after than before banding (Table 2). The percentage of LES relaxation was reduced, but the absolute amplitude of relaxation actually increased.

The amplitude, duration and velocity of oesophageal contractions is given in Table 1. The amplitude of the contractions was significantly reduced 2 and 5 cm above the gastro–oesophageal junction.

DISCUSSION

We have developed a model in which an inflammatory reaction at the outside of the oesophagus leads to obstruction of the oesophageal lumen and distension of the oesophageal body above it. This is accompanied by thickening of some layers of the oesophageal wall and changes in the function of the oesophageal smooth muscle. It is likely that the thickening of the circular oesophageal smooth muscle represents simultaneous increase in cell numbers and increase in cell size, as has been observed in experimental small

Table 1 Morphologic measurement

	Circumference (cm)				Thickness (mm)						
					Mucosa				Circular		
	2 cm	4 cm	6 cm	LES	2 cm	4 cm	6 cm	LES	2 cm	4 cm	6 cm
Control	4.4	4.4	4.1	0.516	0.830	0.610	0.516	0.833	0.193	0.235	0.438
Experimental	6.3	7.5	6.0	1.456	1.088	0.868	1.120	0.616	0.460	0.966	0.840

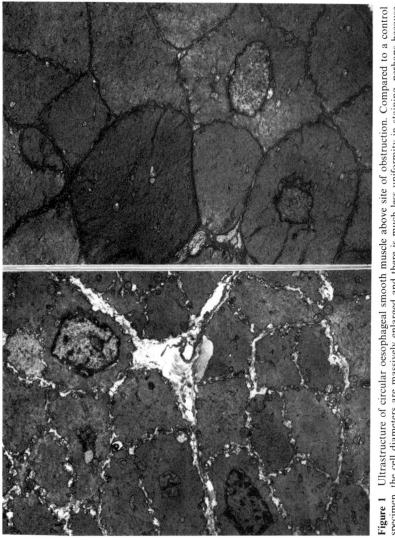

Figure 1 Ultrastructure of circular oesophageal smooth muscle above site of obstruction. Compared to a control specimen, the cell diameters are massively enlarged and there is much less uniformity in staining, perhaps because there are some newly formed cells. The extracellular space is narrow and filled with amorphous ground substance (x 3500)

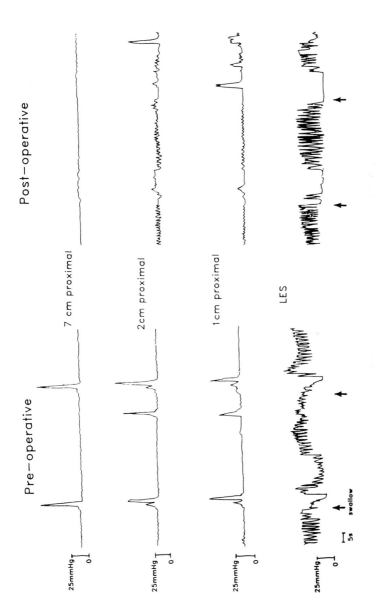

Figure 2 Examples of oesophageal manometry. Pre-operatively,swallows produce consistently sequential contractions throughout the oesophageal body. After the banding, there are weak and repetitive contractions

675

Table 2 Pre-operative and post-operative manometry data

| | LES | | | Oesophageal body | | | |
| | | | | 7 cm | | 2 cm | |
	Position (cm)	Baseline pressure (mmHg)	Percent relaxation	Amplitude (mmHg)	Duration (s)	Amplitude (mmHg)	Duration (s)
Pre-operative	31.14 ± 0.15	31.49 ± 1.61	94.27 ± 1.51	41.12 ± 9.64	4.57 ± 0.66	33.15 ± 5.24	5.13 ± 0.41
Post-operative	31.51 ± 0.21	44.26 ± 1.50	70.22 ± 7.09	12.92 ± 4.18	4.11 ± 0.54	12.40 ± 3.46	5.23 ± 0.38

bowel obstruction in the guinea-pig and rat[2]. In these models of intestinal obstruction, there is also some increase in the size of nerve cell bodies but, overall, the nervous elements do not seem to be able to keep pace with the increase in muscle mass, leading to a relative denervation[2]. To our knowledge, no detailed study has been done of the functional consequences of hypertrophic intestinal smooth muscle.

The manometric changes which followed the operative banding in our model can be summarized as a failure of primary peristalsis to produce consistently LES relaxations and sequential oesophageal contractions. Some of these changes might reflect the inability of the manometric system to sense wall contractions in a distended organ. Others may be mediated by the oesophageal inflammation we observed in the mucosa of some animals. It is known from clinical observations that mucosal inflammation alone can cause oesophageal motor abnormalities[5]. We have observed poor contractions in the oesophageal body in an acute model of oeosphagitis in the opossum[6]. However, in the present study, functional changes did also occur in the absence of grossly visible oesophageal inflammation, so it is doubtful that inflammation was the only mediator of the motor abnormalities.

The manometric findings reported here must be reconciled with data of the *in vitro* mechanical activity of oesophageal smooth muscle in this same model. As reported elsewhere, we have observed an increased spontaneous activity and repetitive mechanical responses to electric stimulation in bands and strips of the oesophageal smooth muscle[4]. In keeping with the apparent muscular hypertrophy, the tension generated by muscle strips from obstructed specimens was considerably higher than that of normal specimens. This implies that the obstruction has led to some lasting functional impairment of the smooth muscle. Some of the features (i.e. impaired LES relaxation) suggest damage of the intrinsic oesophageal nerves. However, this requires more definite testing including dose responses to autonomic drugs and detailed morphologic studies of the myenteric plexus. Also, despite our precautions to keep the band away from the LES, some of the findings may relate to the inflammatory response in its vicinity rather than to damage of neurons reaching it from above.

References

1. Helm, J. F., Dodds, W. J. and Jogan, W. J. (1982). Carcinoma of the cardia masquerading as idiopathic achalasia. **82**, 1082A
2. Gabella, G. (1987). Dynamic aspects of the morphology of the intestinal muscle coat. In Szurszewski, J. H. *Cellular Physiology and Clinical Studies of Gastrointestinal Smooth Muscle*, pp. 5–31. (Amsterdam: Elsevier)
3. Schulze, K., Dodds, W. J. and Christensen, J. (1977). Esophageal manometry in the Opossum. *Am. J. Physiol.*, **233**, E152–9
4. Schulze-Delrieu, K. and Shirazi, S. (1988). Functional denervation of the esophagus from experimental obstruction. *Gastroenterology*, **94**, A414
5. Dodds, W. J., Hogan, W. J., Helm, J. F. and Dent, J. (1981). Pathogenesis of reflux esophagitis. *Gastroenterology*, **71**, 376–94
6. Schulze-Delrieu, K., Custer, T. and Shirazi, S. (1987). Abnormalities of smooth muscle function in experimental esophagitis. *Clin. Res.*, **35**(3), 414A

32
Adrenergic modification of the secretory response to neural stimulation of ground squirrel jejunum *in vitro*

H. V. CAREY

Electrical activation of submucosal neurons in intestines of guinea-pigs, rabbits, mice and humans evokes an increase in chloride secretion that is mediated in part by acetylcholine and in part by non-cholinergic, non-adrenergic neurotransmitters. This study examined the mucosal response to electrical stimulation of the intestinal innervation in the ground squirrel, a seasonal hibernator. Muscle-stripped segments of jejunum in Ussing chambers absorbed sodium ($2.3 \pm 0.4\,\mu\mathrm{Eq.cm}^{-2}.\mathrm{h}^{-1}$) and had a basal chloride flux that was not significantly different from 0 ($1.2 \pm 0.8\,\mu\mathrm{Eq.cm}^{-2}.\mathrm{h}^{-1}$). Basal transmural PD was $+ 1.4 \pm 0.2\,\mathrm{mV}$ (serosa positive); short-circuit current, $1.0 \pm 0.1\,\mu\mathrm{Eq.cm}^{-2}$; tissue conductance, $18.2 \pm 0.9\,\mathrm{mS.cm}^{-2}$. The jejunal innervation was electrically stimulated (7 mA, 10 Hz, 0.5 ms pulse duration) before and after addition of cholinergic and adrenergic antagonists to the serosal bathing solution.

Neural stimulation in the absence of antagonists evoked a significant increase in short-circuit current to $1.9 \pm 0.2\,\mu\mathrm{Eq.cm}^{-2}$ ($p<0.01$, $n = 11$), followed by a fall in current to near or below basal levels during the stimulation period. Short-circuit current rose after the stimulus was terminated. Net Na absorption was unchanged during electrical stimulation ($1.6 \pm 1.0\,\mu\mathrm{Eq.cm}^{-2}.\mathrm{h}^{-1}$, $p>0.05$, $n = 11$), but net Cl secretion increased significantly ($-2.6 \pm 1.1\,\mu\mathrm{Eq.cm}^{-2}.\mathrm{h}^{-1}$, $p<0.05$, $n = 11$). Blockade of muscarinic cholinergic receptors with atropine ($1.0\,\mu\mathrm{M}$) reduced the neurally evoked increase above baseline to 20% of control values. Yohimbine, an α_2-adrenergic receptor antagonist ($0.5\,\mu\mathrm{M}$) added to atropinized tissues partially restored the neurally evoked increase in short-circuit current. Mean short-circuit current during electrical stimulation in non-atropinized tissues was significantly greater during adrenergic blockade.

Thus, neural stimulation of ground squirrel jejunum *in vitro* evokes an increase in chloride secretion as has been shown in other species. Both acetylcholine and non-cholinergic, non-adrenergic transmitters appear to mediate secretion. The findings in ground squirrel intestine contrast with other species, in that the secretory response evoked by neural stimulation is attenuated by simultaneous release of an adrenergic neurotransmitter. This effect may be due to inhibition of secretomotor neurons by norepinephrine acting at α_2-receptors.

Acknowledgements

Supported by NIH DK 38075 and DK38104.

33
Neurotensin and the canine small intestine, motility *in vivo* and *in vitro*, muscle and nerve receptors and sites of degradation

J. E. T. FOX, S. AHMAD, P. KOSTKA, F. CHECLER,
H. D. ALLESCHER, J. P. VINCENT, F. KOSTOLANSKA,
C. Y. KWAN AND E. E. DANIEL

Intra-arterial (i.a.) neurotensin (NT) is ineffective *in vivo* in the quiescence small intestine during anaesthesia (as recorded by circularly oriented serosal strain gauges) while it inhibits phasic activity by release of norepinephrine (10^{-11} mol) and by a direct muscle action (10^{-9} mol). NT given i.a. 20 s before the consistent contractions of i.a. acetylcholine (ACh) at minute intervals produced a delayed increase in ACh response at NT 10^{-11} mol and immediate inhibition at NT 10^{-9} mol. In contrast, *in vitro* in full-thickness, circularly oriented (CM) strips NT increases amplitude and frequency of contractions at 10^{-12} M, inhibits at 10^{-7} M and produces a tonic contraction maximal at 10^{-6} M. Phasic excitation (10^{-11} M) was unchanged by TTX or indomethacin but inhibited reversibly by 5,8,11,14-eicosatetraynoic acid or Ca^{2+}-free incubation, suggesting that phasic activity resulted from release of a lipoxygenase metabolite and was dependent on extracellular Ca^{2+}. Selective dissections to prepare CM strips with and without the deep muscular plexus (DMP) and the myenteric plexus (MP) revealed that the DLP was necessary for the phasic excitation but unnecessary for inhibition and that the MP was unnecessary for either. Thus receptors for NT linked to inhibitory intracellular processes are found in all regions of CM, but those linked to phasic excitation are found on cells near the DLP and *in vivo* excitation by ACh optimizes the participation of these cells. Longitudinal strips (LM) with MP attached respond to NT 10^{-7} M with a TTX-insensitive relaxation.

To study differences between muscle layers and nerves, plasma membrane (PM) vesicles and neural synaptosomes were prepared by differential centrifugation and sucrose gradients from each layer, following dissection of the mucosa-free layers just below the MP. PM purification was followed by measuring 5′nucleotidase enrichment, synaptosomes were identified on the basis of increasing enrichment of nerve specific ^{3}H saxitoxin binding, electron microscopic identification, and for the MP excluded levels of lactate dehydrogenase. Using mono-iodinated Tyr ^{3}HNT as the ligand, specific saturable binding was only measurable in the CM PM and synaptosomes and both exhibited high and low affinity sites. Radiation inactivation studies showed the PM receptor to be 100 000 Daltons and the synaptosomal 200 000 Daltons.

Degradation of NT was studied by incubation of the LM and CM PM vesicles and MP synatosomes with ^{3}HNT and identification of the breakdown products by high-pressure liquid chromatography in the presence of enzyme inhibitors and substrates specific to a range of enzymes. Proline endopeptidase, rat brain soluble metallopeptidase and post-proline dipeptidyl aminopeptidase were present only in the CM while NT-degrading neutral metallopeptidase, endopeptidase 24.11, angiotensin-converting enzyme and unidentified carboxy and aminopeptidases were common to LM and CM PM and to MP synaptosomes. MP synaptosomes degraded NT more rapidly and enzymes were less easily inhibited than PM fractions, which may account for the reduced MP binding. Perfusion of ^{3}HNT through a plasma-free segment *in vivo* showed endopeptidase 24.11 as the principal degrading enzyme.

These results demonstrate a heterogeneous distribution of NT receptors and degrading enzymes in the layers of the canine small intestine which could account for the differences in responses in the various preparations. This heterogeneity may be important for gastrointestinal function.

Acknowledgements

Supported by the MRC of Canada and the CNRS of France.

34
Control of release of vasoactive intestinal polypeptide and substance P from canine small intestine *ex vivo*

H. MANAKA, Y. MANAKA, F. KOSTOLANSKA, E. E. DANIEL AND J. E. T. FOX

The objective of this study was to compare controls over basal and stimulated release of two major neuropeptides of canine small intestine. A preparation with intrinsic nerve supply intact but isolated from the circulation was made and perfused with oxygenated Kreb's Ringer solution at 37°F through the artery at 12 ml/min; the perfusate was collected from the venous outflow and assayed for vasoactive intestinal polypeptide (VIP) and substance P using antisera generously supplied by Professor N. Yanaihara. Circular muscle activity was recorded by strain-gauges. Basal release of VIP was 0.1 pmol/ml and that of substance P was 0.001 pmol/ml, i.e. VIP was released under basal conditions 100 times faster than substance P. Studies of the degradation of VIP and substance P during passage through the gut did not suggest that differential degradation could explain these findings. Basal release of VIP was reduced by at least 80% by tetrodotoxin (TTx) (10^{-6} M), by BHT 920 10^{-7} M, by atropine (3×10^{-5} g/ml), by dynorphine$_{1-13}$ (10^{-7} M) and by metenkephalin (10^{-8} M). TTx, BHT 920, dynorphin and metenkephalin caused phasic and tonic contractions in concentrations which markedly inhibited VIP release. Basal release of VIP was not increased by field stimulation of intrinsic nerves at 5, 10, 20 or 40 Hz, but that of substance P was increased by stimulation at the higher frequencies. Phasic and tonic contractions occurred at all frequencies. TTx inhibited the increased release of substance P by field stimulation.

We conclude that VIP-containing neurons in canine small intestine during anaesthesia are probably spontaneously active, while those containing substance P are not. We suggest that continuous VIP release may exert tonic inhibition of the small intestine in this condition and that agents such as acetylcholine and possibly substance P causing excitation must overcome this inhibition. This high basal release of VIP may help explain the difficulty in demonstrating inhibitory effects of intra-arterial VIP under our conditions. Furthermore, other neuropeptides present in the intrinsic nervous system, such as opiates, may act at or increase motor or transport activity by inhibiting the release of VIP. Turning off of high levels of VIP release in awake animals may play a role in MMC production in the fasting state.

Acknowledgements

Supported by MRC of Canada.

35
The effect of substance P and vasoactive intestinal polypeptide on intestinal contractility and transmural potential difference in the anaesthetized ferret

B. GREENWOOD AND J. S. DAVISON

INTRODUCTION

Our previous studies in the anaesthetized ferret demonstrated that vagal nerve stimulation increased intestinal motility, induced intestinal fluid secretion and caused a rise in transmural potential difference (PD) in the direction of a more negative lumen[1]. Although the vagally induced smooth muscle response was cholinergic, the transmural PD response was in part non-cholinergic[1,2,3]. The aims of the present study were to:

1. investigate the effects of substance P and vasoactive intestinal polypeptide (VIP) on both jejunal contractility and epithelial function, using transmural PD as an indirect marker of electrogenic ion transport across the intestinal tract.
2. Examine whether substance P and/or VIP are possible mediators of the non-cholinergically induced increase in jejunal transmural PD.

Substance P and VIP were selected as likely candidates for the peptides responsible for the atropine-resistant transmural PD response because both substance P[4-8] and VIP[9,10,11] are recognized intestinal secretagogues in many animal species. Furthermore, both peptides are released into the porcine systemic circulation after electrical stimulation of the vagus nerve[12].

METHODS

Experiments were performed on fasted male ferrets (*Mustela Putorius furo*) which were anaesthetized with an intraperitoneal injection of urethane (ethyl carbamate) at a dose of 1.5 g/kg. Throughout the experiment, blood gases were monitored and maintained at physiological values and body temperature was maintained at 38°C. Cannulae positioned within the jugular vein and abdominal aorta, adjacent to the coeliac axis, were used to administer drugs intravenously (i.v.) and intra-arterially (i.a.), respectively.

Measurement of intestinal contractility

To record intestinal contractility in a segment of jejunum, a saline-filled catheter, connected to a pressure transducer, was inserted in the jejunal lumen in order to record intraluminal pressure changes representing intestinal motor activity.

Measurement of transmural potential difference

Transmural PD, an indirect marker of electrogenic ion transport across the intestinal tract, was recorded using two agar salt bridge electrodes; one positioned within the intestinal lumen and the other in contact with the serosal fluid via a wick electrode. The agar salt bridge electrodes were then positioned via calomel half cells to an electrometer and the output displayed on a Beckman or Gould chart recorder.

Experimental protocol

After completion of the surgery, the ferrets were allowed to stabilise for 30 min. After bilateral cervical vagotomy, doses of substance P (0.2–20 μg/kg) or VIP (0.5–50 μg/kg) purchased from Peninsula Laboratories (Belmont, AC, USA) were then administered i.a. Thirty minutes was allowed between injections to ensure that tachyphylaxis did not develop.

RESULTS

The effect of substance P on contractility and transmural PD

Dose-response relationships demonstrated that substance P at doses of between 0.2 and 20 μg/kg administered intra-arterially caused a graded increase in smooth muscle contractility and an increase in transmural PD, in the direction of a more negative lumen (Figure 1). In all subsequent experiments a submaximal dose of substance P was employed.

In the presence of atropine (1 mg/kg i.v.) the substance P-induced contractile response was not altered; however, the rise in transmural PD was significantly inhibited (Figure 1).

In the presence of the neurotoxin tetrodotoxin (5 μg/kg i.a.), the substance P-induced increase in intestinal smooth muscle contractility was not affected. However, the rise in transmural PD was reduced from 3.8 ± 0.5 mV to 0.6 ± 0.1 mV.

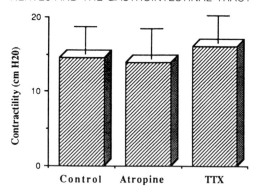

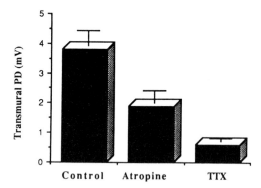

Figure 1 Effect of atropine (1 mg/kg i.v.) and TTX (5 μg/kg i.a.) on the substance P-induced increase in intestinal contractility and rise in transmural PD. Atropine had no effect on the smooth muscle response induced by substance P but significantly inhibited the rise in transmural PD ($p < 0.05$)

Effect of VIP on contractility and transmural PD

After bilateral cervical vagotomy which abolished tone and spontaneous patterns of intestinal motor activity, VIP, without effect on the jejunal smooth muscle, increased transmural PD in the direction of a more negative lumen (Figure 2).

In the presence of cholinergic blockade with atropine (1 mg/kg i.a.) there was no statistically significant effect on the VIP-induced rise in transmural PD (Figure 2).

In the presence of TTX (5 μg/kg i.a.) the VIP-induced rise in transmural PD was not inhibited (Figure 2).

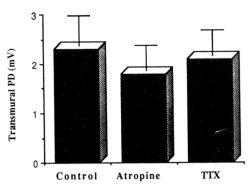

Figure 2 Effect of atropine (1 mg/kg i.v.) on the VIP-induced (5 μg/kg i.a.) increase in transmural PD. In the presence of atropine the rise in transmural PD caused by VIP was not affected

DISCUSSION

In the present series of experiments, intestinal contractility and epithelial function were monitored concurrently in the jejunum of the anaesthetized ferret. The results of the study demonstrate that, after bilateral cervical vagotomy, substance P influenced both aspects of intestinal function: substance P stimulated smooth-muscle activity and increased transmural PD, in the direction of increased lumen negativity. In contrast to the contractile response induced by substance P, VIP had no effect on jejunal smooth muscle activity but, like substance P, VIP increased transmural PD in the direction of a more negative lumen.

The substance P-induced contractile response was not affected by cholinergic blockade with atropine and total neural blockade with TTX. These findings demonstrate that substance P had a direct effect on the jejunal smooth muscle in the ferret. In our quiescent gut preparation, VIP had no effect on jejunal smooth muscle; however, both VIP and substance P increased transmucosal electrogenic ion transport, as monitored by an increase in transmural PD in the direction of increased lumen negativity. Although both peptides increased transmural PD their mechanisms of action differed. Substance P induced a rise in transmural PD that was inhibited by atropine and TTX. However, the VIP-induced increase in transmural PD was the result of a direct effect on the intestinal epithelium, since it was unaffected by atropine or TTX. Since substance P and VIP demonstrate a degree of atropine resistance, both are possible candidates for the non-cholinergically mediated rise in transmural PD induced by electrical stimulation of the cervical vagi in the anaesthetized ferret.

In previous studies[13] we proposed that intestinal motor activity and epithelial transport are linked via either a sequential neural mechanism or synchronously activated parallel neural pathways. In the present study, the absence of a change in jejunal smooth muscle activity, but an increase in transmural PD in the presence of VIP, substantiates the proposal that changes in epithelial transport can occur independently of an alteration in intestinal motor activity.

Acknowledgements

This work was supported by grants from the Medical Research Council of Canada and the National Institute of Health.

References

1. Greenwood, B. and Read, N. W. (1985). Vagal control of fluid transport, transmural potential difference and motility in the ferret jejunum. *Am. J. Physiol.*, **249**, G651–4
2. Greenwood, B. and Davison, J. S. (1985). Role of extrinsic and intrinsic nerves in the relationship between intestinal motility and transmural potential difference in the anesthetized ferret. *Gastroenterology*, **89**, 1286–92
3. Greenwood, B. and Davison, J. S. (1987). Investigation of the vagally induced changes in transmural potential difference in the ferret jejunum in vivo. *J. Auto. Nerv. Syst.*, **19**, 113–18
4. Hubel, K. A., Renquist, K. S. and Sharazi, S. (1984). Neural control of ileal transport. Role of substance P (SP) in rabbit and man. *Gastroenterology*, **86**, 1118
5. Kachur, J. F., Miller, R. J., Field, M. and Rivier, J. (1982). Neurohumoral control of ileal electrolyte transport. II. Neurotensin and substance P. *J. Pharmacol. Exper. Ther.*, **220**, 456–63
6. McFadden, D., Jaffe, B. M. and Zinner, M. J. (1984). Elevated plasma levels of substance P cause jejunal secretion of fluids and electrolytes in the conscious dog. *Gastroenterology*, **86**, 1179
7. Walling, M. W., Brasitus, T. A. and Kimberg, D. V. (1977). Effect of calcitonin and substance P on the transport of Ca, Na and Cl across rat ileum in vitro. *Gastroenterology*, **73**, 89–94
8. Keast, J. R., Furness, J. B. and Costa, M. (1985). Different substance P receptors are found on mucosal epithelial cells and submucous neurones of the guinea pig small intestine. *Naunyn-Schmiedebergs's Arch. Pharmacol.*, **329**, 382–7
9. Cooke, H. J. (1987). Neural and humoral regulation of small intestinal electrolyte transport. In Johnson, L. R. (ed.) *Physiology of the Gastrointestinal Tract*, 2nd Edn., pp. 1307–50. (New York: Raven Press)
10. Cooke, H. J., Carey, H. V. and Walsh, J. (1984). Neural stimulation of intestinal mucosa and the effects of VIP. *Gastroenterology*, **86**, 1053
11. Cooke, H. J., Zafirova, M., Carey, H. V., Walsh, J. H. and Grider, J. (1987). Vasoactive intestinal polypeptide actions on the guinea pig intestinal mucosa during neural stimulation. *Gastroenterology*, **92**, 361–70
12. Fahrenfrug, J., Galbo, H., Holtst, J. J. and Shaffalitzky de Mucdadell, O. B. (1978). Influence of autonomic nervous system on the release of vasoactive intestinal polypeptide from the pordine gastrointestinal tract. *J. Physiol. (Lond.)*, **280**, 405–22
13. Greenwood, B. and Davison, J. S. (1987). The relationship between intestinal motility and secretion. *Am. J. Physiol.*, **252**, G1–7

POSTER ABSTRACT

36
Minimal effects on bowel motor function by 5-HT$_3$-receptors

H. J. LÜBKE, C. WARSKULAT, G. LICHT, T. FRIELING, J. F. ERCKENBRECHT, M. KARAUS, P. ENCK AND M. WIENBECK

The development of new 5-HT$_3$-receptor antagonists (low affinity receptor antagonists) allows for an elucidation of potentially important 5-HT-mechanisms in the gut in health and disease. We, therefore, set out to study the effect of a new 5-HT-receptor antagonist (ICS 205-930) on bowel motor function in healthy volunteers.

METHODS

Ten healthy non-smoking male volunteers (age 18–30 years) were recruited for a prospective randomized, double-blind, cross-over trial comparing ICS 205-930 and placebo. Each subject was investigated for two 7-day periods, separated by an interval of at least 7 days. During the test period they received a defined solid–liquid diet (2500–3000 kcal/d). The trial drugs were administered orally at a dose of 50 mg or identically looking placebo once daily for 7 days. On day 3 the subjects ate a standard breakfast. At the same time they ingested 20 radio-opaque pellets, 100 mg of a blue dye marker and 3.35 g lactulose in 30 ml water. All stools were collected, weighed and X-rayed. Whole gut transit time (gut TT) was determined by the appearance of the dye marker and excretion of 16/20 pellets. Oro-caecal transit time (TT) was defined by a rise in the breath H$_2$ test.

RESULTS

Intersubject variation in stool weight, frequency and transit time was big. ICS tended to have different effects in the upper and lower gut. Whereas TT was accelerated in the former, the latter showed a tendency to be slowed down. In detail ($\bar{x} \pm$ SEM; (*$p < 0.05$, t-test):

	ICS 205-930	Placebo
No. of stools/7 days	6.3 ± 0.7	6.0 ± 0.7
Stool weight (g/d)	111 ± 15	108 ± 9
Gut TT: dye (h)	47.5 ± 7.7	29.9 ± 4.4
Gut TT: Pellets (h)	63.3 ± 8.8	45.0 ± 6.2
Oro-caecal TT (min)	$265 \pm 17^*$	324 ± 27

The drug was well tolerated, no side effects occurred. We conclude that 5-HT$_3$-receptors have minimal effects on gut motor function in normals. A study in patients with gut motor disorders seems warranted.

37
Neural integrity and mast cell proliferation in the sensitized rat small intestine

D. L. VERMILLION AND S. M. COLLINS

Recently we have shown that infection with *Trichinella spiralis* in the rat causes a 20-fold increase in sensitized mast cells in the muscle layers of the proximal jejunum and throughout the small bowel. Subsequent challenge of jejunal muscle with Trichinella antigen causes contraction due to degranulation of mast cells and liberation of 5-HT. In light of a recent report describing a close anatomical relationship between enteric nerves and mast cells[1]. We hypothesized that integrity of enteric nerves may play an important role in the sensitization or proliferation of mast cells in gut muscle. We therefore examined the effects of myenteric plexus ablation on the mast cell-mediated contraction of jejunum from Trichinella-sensitized rats.

Myenteric plexus ablation was induced by serosal application of benzalkonium chloride (BAC) to a limited jejunal segment *in vivo* as described by Fox and Bass[2]. Saline was applied to the serosa of control rats. BAC-treated rats were infected with *T. spiralis* 15 days later, allowed to recover for 55 days and then sacrificed. Isometric tension was recorded from jejunal longitudinal muscle strips *in vitro*. In saline treated rats, field stimulation (40 V, 10 Hz, 0.5 ms) caused muscle contraction and this was abolished by tetrodotoxin. Neural ablation in the BAC-treated segments was evidenced as a lack of a contractile response to field stimulation; the contractile response to field stimulation was preserved in adjacent, non-treated segments proximal and distal to the BAC-treated segment. In tissues from Trichinella-sensitized animals, Trichinella antigen induced contractile responses in the BAC-treated and non-treated adjacent segments. Expressed as a percentage of the carbachol response in each segment, antigen responses were 44% in BAC-treated segments, and 184% and 38% in proximal and distal segments.

Mast cells were increased significantly in the BAC-treated segments of both Trichinella-infected and non-infected rats. Unexpectedly, a significant increase in the numbers of mast cells was also observed in the saline- treated segments compared to non-treated control rats. Tissues from saline- and

BAC-treated segments contracted in response to compound 48/80, a substance that degranulates mast cells, and to rabbit anti-rat IGE. The mast cells in BAC-treated segments from non-infected animals could also be passively sensitized *in vitro* with exposure to serum from Trichinella-infected rats.

The results from this study indicate that: (1) the mast cell mediated contraction of sensitized jejunum does not require the integrity of the myenteric plexus; (2) non-specific irritation of the gut may induce mast cell hyperplasia; and (3) functional innervaton is not necessary for the proliferation of mast cells in the muscle layers of the gut.

Acknowledgements

Supported by MRC Canada.

References

1. Stead *et al.* (1987).
2. Fox and Bass. (1986).

38
Stimulation of intrinsic cholinergic nerves and gastrointestinal motility

J. A. J. SCHUURKES AND J. M. VAN NUETEN

INTRODUCTION

Since the cholinergic system is the driving force of gastrointestinal motility, the first attempts to stimulate GI-motility were performed with direct muscarinic agonists. However, these compounds also affected gastrointestinal secretions as well as muscarinic-receptor mediated processes outside the gastrointestinal tract. This lack of specificity prompted the search for new drugs. Metoclopramide was found to exert motor-stimulating properties; at first mainly contributed to its dopamine-antagonist properties. Indeed, the peripheral dopamine-antagonist, domperidone, was shown to exert gastrokinetic properties. Recently, emphasis was laid on the indirect cholinergic properties of metoclopramide, i.e. stimulation of myenteric cholinergic nerves. To determine the relative contribution of the indirect cholinergic mechanism of action cisapride was developed. Cisapride, while being devoid of dopamine-blocking properties, stimulates motor activity of the oesophagus, stomach, small and large bowel. This stimulation explains the clinical effects of cisapride, i.e. enhanced oesophageal clearance, reduced gastro-oesophageal reflux, accelerated gastric emptying and the reduced transit time through small and large bowel[1]. Of this new class of compounds, cisapride is the first to be approved for clinical use.

The aim of this study is to answer the questions: (1) on what target does cisapride exert its effect? (2) which receptor is involved?

Guinea-pig ileum and colon preparations were chosen as experimental models.

METHODS[2]

The non-terminal ileum and colon ascendens were taken from Pirbright guinea-pigs (350–450 g, fasted overnight) of either sex. Ileal segments, 4.5 cm long, were vertically suspended with a preload of 1 g in 100 ml of Tyrode's solution (37.5 °C), gassed with a mixture of 95% O_2 and 5% CO_2. Contractions were measured isometrically. Transmural excitation was applied over the whole length of the ileum strip by means of two platinum electrodes. The preparation was excited with single rectangular stimuli (1 ms; 0.1 Hz; submaximal current, 80%). Cisapride was administered alone or in the presence of atropine, tetrodotoxin or hexamethonium. On other ileal segments (isotonic recording, 0.75 g preload) the effect of cisapride on cumulatively administered methacholine was compared to the effect of neostigmine. Colonic segments, 4.5 cm long, were vertically suspended with a preload of 2 g in 100 ml of De Jalon solution (37.5°C) and gassed with a mixture of 95% O_2 and 5% CO_2. Contractions were measured isotonically and expressed relative to maximal contractions induced by 3.2×10^{-6} M methacholine (100% contraction = 20 mm). Cisapride was administered alone or in the presence of tetrodotoxin, atropine or their combination.

PHARMACODYNAMICS

Cisapride acts specifically on the muscularis (longitudinal and circular muscle layers with the myenteric plexus in between). It does not enhance gastric or intestinal secretions[1], i.e. it does not act on the mucosa. Cisapride enhances the contractile response of the guinea-pig ileum to submaximal electrical stimulation (Figure 1a). Maximal increase was 35%; EC_{50} value (i.e. the concentration needed to obtain 50% of its maximal effect) was 10^{-8} M. On the colon, cisapride induces a contraction with a maximal response of as much as 40% of the response to methacholine (Figure 1b). The EC_{50} value for this effect was 3×10^{-8} M.

These effects of cisapride could be caused by neurogenic or myogenic, cholinergic or non-cholinergic mechanisms. Several possibilities are indicated in Figure 2.

Ileum

Cisapride has no effect on the non-stimulated ileum. On the electrically stimulated ileum the presence of atropine or tetrodotoxin (5×10^{-7} M) prevents the expression of the effects of cisapride. Thus a non-cholinergic mechanism (Figure 2: 3, 6) as well as a direct effect on smooth muscle cells (Figure 2: 4,6) can be excluded[2].

In contrast to neostigmine, an acetylcholinesterase inhibitor, cisapride does not shift the dose-response curve to methacholine to the left. Cisapride had no effect up to a concentration of 10^{-6} M[2]. This excludes an effect via sensitization (Figure 2: 5) of muscarinic receptors on the smooth muscle cells and an effect on acetylcholinesterase (Figure 2: 7).

The presence of hexamethonium, a blocker of nicotinic ganglionic neuro-transmission does not inhibit the response to cisapride on the electrically stimulated ileum[2]. This excludes an action via ganglionic nicotinergic mechanisms (Figure 2: 2).

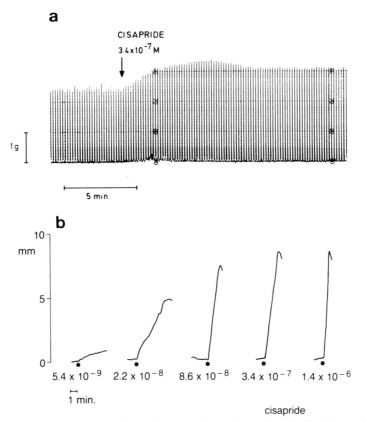

Figure 1   Effect of cisapride on guinea-pig preparations. **a** electrically stimulated ileum; **b** colon ascendens

In conclusion on the guinea-pig ileum cisapride acts via activation of cholinergic end neurons (Figure 2: 1, Figure 3). Our data do not allow a conclusion on whether this effect is mediated via an action on the nerve terminals, on the neuronal cell body or even on an interneuron releasing a non-cholinergic transmitter.

Colon

The presence ot tetrodotoxin (5×10^{-7} M) antagonizes the colonic responses to cisapride by about 50%[2]. Thus, part of its effect is neurogenic; part is myogenic. The presence of atropine (5×10^{-7} M) reduces initial tone (4 mm) and shifts the dose-response curve to the right without depression of the maximal obtainable response[2]. Thus, part of the response is cholinergic, part is non-cholinergic.

The effects of cisapride in the presence of atropine are similar to its effects in the presence of both atropine and tetrodotoxin, indicating that the non-

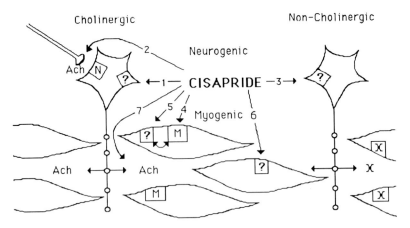

Figure 2 Mechanisms of action for the effects of cisapride on myenteric nerves and smooth muscle cells. The theoretical possibilities 2 to 7, and 2 to 4 could be excluded for the guinea-pig ileum and colon ascendens respectively (for explanation see text; N = nicotinic receptors, ? = unidentified receptor, M = muscarinic receptor, x = receptor for non-cholinergic neuro-transmitter)

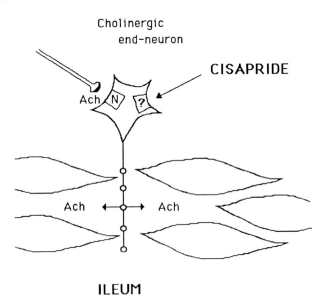

ILEUM

Figure 3 Postulated mechanism of action of cisapride on the electrically stimulated guinea-pig ileum via activation of cholinergic end neurons eventually leading to enhanced release of acetylcholine (for explanation see text; N = nicotinic receptor, ? = unidentified receptor)

cholinergic part of the response to cisapride is non-neurogenic. This excludes possibility 3, Figure 2 for the colon.

The non-cholinergic part of the response can either be neurogenic (as on the ileum) or myogenic. The lack of affinity of cisapride for muscarinic (M_2) receptors and its lack of effect on acetylcholinesterase activity[2] exclude possibilities 4 and 7 (Figure 2) for the colon. Since hexamethonium had no effect on the responses to cisapride, a ganglionic nicotinergic mechanism is also not likely (Figure 2: 2).

In conclusion, part of the response to cisapride on the colon of the guinea-pig is non-cholinergic and non-neurogenic (Figure 4; Figure 2: 6), i.e. a direct effect on smooth muscle cells on non-cholinergic receptors. The other part of the response is cholinergic, mediated either via an indirect effect on cholinergic neurons or via a direct effect on non-cholinergic smooth muscle receptors sensitizing or being sensitized by an effect of acetylcholine on muscarinic receptors (Figures 4; Figures 2: 1,5).

RECEPTOR

The receptors via which cisapride exerts its effect on the guinea-pig ileum cannot be identified with the use of classical pharmacological antagonists for nicotinic, muscarinic (M_2), α- or β-adrenergic, dopaminergic histaminergic, opiate-, GABA- or CCK-receptors or for prostaglandin synthesis.

Cisapride does not interrupt a negative feedback loop of acetylcholine on prejunctional muscarinic-(M_1)-receptors: its effect is not mediated via M_1-receptors[3]. Furthermore, the responses to cisapride are not affected nor

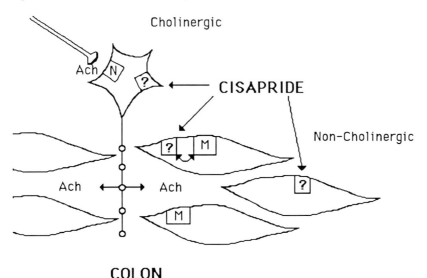

COLON

Figure 4 Postulated mechanism of action of cisapride on the guinea-pig colon ascendens via cholinergic (neurogenic and/or myogenic) and non-cholinergic pathways (for explanation see text; N = nicotinic receptor, ? = unidentified receptor, M = muscarinic receptor)

mimicked by 5-HT$_2$- or 5-HT$_3$-serotonergic antagonists. This indicates that serotonergic receptors are not involved although interference with other not yet classified serotonergic receptors cannot be excluded[4].

As on the ileum, the receptors for cisapride on the colon cannot be identified with classical pharmacological tools. Serotonergic receptors do not seem to be involved since the response cannot be antagonized by serotonergic antagonists (5-HT$_2$-, 5-HT$_3$-receptors) nor by desensitization with serotonin itself. Spasmolytics or Ca^{2+}-entry blockers inhibit the responses to cisapride but also the responses to methacholine, indicating that transmembranal Ca^{2+}-movements are involved in the effects of cisapride. Since analogues of cisapride can inhibit the colonic response to cisapride without having an intrinsic contractile effect and without inhibiting the responses to methacholine, we hypothesize that cisapride may act via specific receptor-mechanisms that as yet cannot be identified[5].

CONCLUSION

Cisapride exerts its motor-stimulating action on the guinea-pig ileum exclusively via activation of cholinergic myenteric neurons. On the colon the major part of the effect is of non-cholinergic, non-neurogenic nature. The receptors via which cisapride exerts its effect cannot yet be identified. The ileal and colonic receptors are located on different structures (neurogenic vs. myogenic) and may be of different nature.

References

1. Johnson, A. G. and Lux, G. (1988). *Progress in the Treatment of Gastrointestinal Motility Disorders: The Role of Cisapride.* (Amsterdam: Excerpta Medica)
2. Schuurkes, J. A. J., Van Nueten, J. M., Van Daele, P. G. H., Reyntjens, A. J. and Janssen, P. A. J. (1985). Motor-stimulating properties of cisapride on isolated gastrointestinal preparations of the guinea pig. *J. Pharmacol. Exp. Ther.*, **234**, 775–83
3. Schuurkes, J. A. J., Van Bergen, P. J. E. and Van Nueten, J. M. (1988). Prejunctional muscarinic (M$_1$)-receptor interactions on guinea-pig ileum: lack of effect of cisapride. *Br. J. Pharmacol.*, **94**, 228–34
4. Pfeuffer-Friederich, I. and Kilbinger, H. (1984). Facilitation and inhibition by 5-hydroxytryptamine and R 51 619 of acetylcholine release from guinea pig myenteric neurons. In Roman, C. (ed.) *Gastrointestinal Motility*, pp. 527–34. (Lancaster: MTP Press)
5. Van Nueten, J. M. and Schuurkes, J. A. J. (1986). Non-cholinergic stimulation of the guinea-pig colon by cisapride. *Gastroenterology*, **90**, 1677

39
Neurokinins and transepithelial transport in the guinea-pig small intestine

R. MATHISON AND J. S. DAVISON

Intestinal electrolyte transport in the small intestine is for the most part regulated by neurotransmitters released from neurons localized to the submucosal plexus[1]. Myenteric, sympathetic and parasympathetic innervations can intervene in regulating the transport processes. Peptides and amines localized to the enteric nerves either enhance secretion (e.g. 5-HT, substance P, VIP, PHI, acetylcholine) or increase absorption (e.g. noradrenaline, somatostatin, NPY). The role of each of these neurotransmitters in regulating epithelial transport is gradually being elucidated[1,2]. We will consider specifically the role of the neurokinins in the guinea-pig, in the form of a mini-review summarizing our own published and unpublished work and that of other laboratories.

NEUROKININS IN THE SMALL INTESTINE

Two genes coding for the neurokinins have been identified[3]: the preprotachykinin A (PPTA) is responsible for the production of substance P (SP) and neurokinin A (NKA), and the PPTB gene codes for NKB. As SP and NKA, but not neurokinin B (NKB), have been identified by RIA and HPLC procedures[4] in the guinea-pig small intestine (GPSI) the PPTA gene is apparently the only one expressed by the enteric neurons. The PPTA encodes for three different mRNAs in rat striatum[5], with each one coding for a different set of gene products: α-mRNA codes uniquely for SP, β-mRNA codes for SP, NKA and neuropeptide K (NPK) and γ-mRNA[6] codes for SP, NKA and neuropeptide-γ (NP-γ). Although the genes for the neurokinins have not been studied in GPSI, circumstantial evidence suggests that the γ-mRNA and β-mRNA are expressed, but not the γ-mRNA. The presence of NPK indicates that β-mRNA is expressed, and as higher concentrations of SP than NKA are found in GPSI the α-mRNA is undoubtedly expressed as well[3]. As NP-γ is not found in GPSI[4], the PPTA gene probably is not processed to give the γ-mRNA product.

The concentrations of SP and NKA are highest in myenteric plexus longitudinal muscle portion, approximately threefold lower in the circular muscle, and tenfold less in the mucosa[4]. The proteolytic inactivation of SP and NKA has been studied[7] with both neurokinins being metabolized by endopeptidase 24.11, and with NKA but not SP being metabolized by bestatin-sensitive endopeptidases. The rate of proteolysis of NKA is nearly twice that of SP, and degradation is 100-fold greater in the epithelial layers than in the smooth muscle layer for both SP and NKA[7]. The absence of NKB in the GPSI is surprising, given that receptors exhibiting a marked selectivity for NKB have been identified[8] on neuronal elements in the guinea-pig ileum.

SP is localized primarily in nerves, although immunoreactive endocrine cells have been noted in intestinal tissues (see 1 for references). The vast majority of the SP-containing nerves that project to the mucosa originate in submucous ganglia[9], with a smaller number arising in the myenteric plexus[10]. Approximately 11% of the submucous plexus neurons contain SP[11]. Both SP and NKA co-localize to vesicular fraction in GPSI, although NPK does not appear to be packaged[3] into granules. Some extrinsic nerves containing SP may project to the transporting epithelia, although the exact proportion is impossible to estimate. Capsaicin treatment, which destroys the primary afferent neurons, does not noticeably modify[1] the pattern of mucosal SP innervation in the guinea-pig.

SUBSTANCE P AND EPITHELIAL TRANSPORT

SP causes an increase in short-circuit current (I_{sc}) in rats, guinea-pigs and rabbits[12,13,14]. The change in I_{sc} is predominantly due to a stimulation of chloride secretion.

Several different techniques have been used positively to identify SP as a neurotransmitter mediating epithelial transport in the guinea-pig small intestine. Desensitization abolishes all but 5% of the effects of exogenous SP in the jejunum, and a SP-antibody inhibited SP action by 85% (Table 1). The responses to electrical field stimulation are also markedly reduced by desensitization and the SP-antibody (Table 1), whereas the actions of an exogenous cholinergic agonist, urecholine, are largely unaffected.

By determining the reduction of the field-stimulated responses in the presence of tetrodotoxin (TTX) the neuronal component in the action of exogenous SP is approximately 89% in the guinea-pig ileum[12,13], and 70% in the jejunum of this species[14] (see Table 1). The atropine-sensitive component in the ileum accounts for 60% of the action of SP in the ileum[13], whereas the cholinergic component of SP action in the jejunum[14] is only 25%. Thus, it would appear that SP exerts a larger influence directly on the epithelial cells in the jejunum than in the ileum and, furthermore, an indirect cholinergic component in the actions of SP is greater in the ileum than in the jejunum. The neurotransmitters mediating the non-cholinergic neuronal

Table 1 Percentage of I_{sc} response remaining consequent to addition of tetrodotoxin (TTX), desensitization with substance P (SP) and addition of a SP-antibody on I_{sc} responses of the guinea-pig jejunal mucosal preparation

	TS	SP	URE
TTX	0.4%	29.4%	94.3%
Desensitization			
− atropine	56.4%	4.7%	90.5%
+ atropine	32.8%	5.3%	90.6%
SP-antibody	44.8%	14.9%	92.4%

The table is a summary of data published by Perdue et al.[14].
Data was calculated from responses obtained with pairs of tissue segments from the same animal; one segment received the treatment described whereas the other was not treated. TS = transmural stimulation; URE = - urecholine

component of SP action (40% in the ileum and some 75% in the jejunum) have not been identified.

The TTX-resistant component of substance P action is antagonized by the SP analogue [arg^1,pro^2,trp^7,Leu^{11}]-SP in the guinea-pig ileum, whereas no significant effect on the TTX-sensitive component of the response is seen with this analogue[13]. These data were interpreted to suggest that the analogue antagonizes the action of SP on epithelial receptors, but not the SP receptors located on submucous neurons.

The actions of neurokinins other than SP have also been examined on the jejunal mucosa of the guinea pig[15]. NKA induced a larger increase in I_{sc} than either SP or NKB (relative activities are NKA = 1.0, SP = 0.63, and NKB = 0.43). The increases in I_{sc} induced by NKA are reduced by 90% with the muscarinic antagonist, atropine, whereas the increases induced by SP and NKB are inhibited by only 45 to 65%, respectively. The neurotoxin, TTX, markedly inhibited the actions of NKA and NKB (by 80–90%), whereas those of SP are reduced to a much lesser extent. These results suggest that NKA acts preferentially on a neuronal neurokinin receptor, whereas SP preferentially activates an epithelial receptor. NKB may be acting as a non-selective agonist on both neuronal and epithelial receptors.

CONCLUSIONS

A combination of immunological, biochemical, pharmacological and physiological approaches for studying neurokinins in the guinea-pig small intestine provides a relatively detailed description of the manner in which these peptides regulate epithelial transport. One interesting feature of the SP response is that the jejunum exhibits a larger proportion of direct epithelial action but a small proportion of acetylcholine mediated actions than the ileum. Further studies are required to characterize the neurokinin receptor subtypes, to identify their localization and to determine why NKA and SP are metabolized at different rates within the mucosa of the intestine. The role of NKB in intestinal transport remains to be elucidated. It also remains to be determined if NKB is actually found in the intestine or if the NK-3 (NKB) receptors are activated by NKB released from extrinsic neurons.

References

1. Keast, J. R. (1987). Mucosal innervation and control of water and ion transport in the intestine. *Rev. Physiol. Biochem. Pharmacol.*, **109**, 1–59
2. Hubel, K. A. (1988). Neural control of intestinal electrolyte transport. In Davison, J. S. and Shaffer, E. A. (eds.) *Gastrointestinal and Hepatic Secretions: Mechanism and Control*, pp. 175–80. (Calgary: University of Calgary Press)
3. Nakanishi, S. (1987). Substance P precursor and kininogen: their structures, gene organizations and regulation. *Physiol. Rev.*, **67**, 1117–42
4. Deacon, C. F., Agoston, D. V., Nau, R. and Conlon, J. M. (1987). Conversion of neuropeptide K to neurokinin A and vesicular colocalization of neurokinin A and substance P in neurons of the guinea pig small intestine. *J. Neurochem.*, **48**, 141–6
5. Krause, J. E., Chirgwin, J. M., Carter, M. S., Xu, Z. S. and Hershey, A. D. (1987). Three rat preprotachykinin mRNAs encode the neuropeptides substance P and neurokinin A. *Proc. Natl. Acad. Sci.*, **84**, 881–5
6. Kage, R., McGregor, G. P., Thim, L. and Conlon, J. M. (1988). Neuropeptide-γ: A peptide isolated from rabbit intestine that is derived from γ-preprotachykinin. *J. Neurochem.*, **50**, 1412–17
7. Nau, R., Schafer, G., Deacon, C. F., Cole, T., Agoston, D. V. and Conlon, J. M. (1986). Proteolytic inactivation of substance P and neurokinin A in the longitudinal muscle layer of the guinea pig small intestine. *J. Neurochem.*, **47**, 856–64
8. Guard, S. and Watson, S. P. (1987). Evidence for neurokinin-3 receptor-mediated tachykinin release in the guinea pig ileum. *European J. Pharmacol.*, **144**, 409–12
9. Keast, J. R., Furness, J. B. and Costa, M. (1984). The origins of peptide and norepinephrine nerves in the mucosa of the guinea pig small intestine. *Gastroenterology*, **86**, 637–44
10. Costa, M., Furness, J. B., Llewellyn-Smith, I. J. and Cuello, A. C. (1981). Projections of substance P-containing neurons within the guinea pig small intestine. *Neuroscience*, **6**, 411–24
11. Furness, J. B., Costa, M., Gibbins, I. L., Llewellyn-Smith, I. J. and Oliver, J. R. (1985). Neurochemically similar myenteric and submucous neurons directly traced to the mucosa of the small intestine. *Cell Tissue Res.*, **241**, 155–63
12. Hubel, K. A., Renquist, K. S. and Shirazi, S. (1984). Neural control of ileal ion transport: role of substance P (SP) in rabbit and man. *Gastroenterology*, **86**, 1118
13. Keast, J. R., Furness, J. B. and Costa, M. (1985). Different substance P receptors are found on mucosal epithelial cells and submucous neurons of the guinea-pig small intestine. *N.S. Arch. Pharmacol.*, **329**, 382–7
14. Perdue, M. H., Galbraith, R. and Davison, J. S. (1987). Evidence for substance P as a functional transmitter in guinea pig intestinal mucosa. *Regulatory Peptides*, **18**, 63–74
15. Mathison, R. and Davison, J. S. (1987). Neurokinins and transepithelial transport in the jejunal mucosa of the guinea pig. *Clin. Invest. Med.*, **10**, B133

40
Sympathetic nerve stimulation decreases the hydraulic conductance of the jejunal mucosa in cats and rats

H. SJÖVALL AND M. HEMLIN

Sympathetic nerve stimulation enhances net fluid absorption from the jejunum in cats and rats. Part of this response is due to an inhibition of electrogenic anion secretion into the lumen. However, a non-electrogenic mechanism also contributes to the sympathetic effect. The aim of the study was to test the hypothesis that sympathetic nerve stimulation promotes net fluid absorption by decreasing the hydraulic conductance of the mucosa, thereby inhibiting passive fluid transport from tissue to lumen.

METHODS

Cat experiments

In five chloralose-anaesthetized cats, two jejunal segments were isolated with intact vascular supply. Net fluid absorption rate in the two segments was continuously registered with a volumetric technique. One segment was perfused with an isotonic Krebs–mannitol solution only, and the other segments with the same solution plus polyethylene glycol (MW 4000), 5 g/l, in order to induce an osmotic passive flux from tissue to lumen. Net fluid absorption rate in the two segments was registered under control conditions and during stimulation of the mesenteric nerves (8 Hz, 5 ms, 10 V).

Rat experiments

Jejunal segments of pentobarbital-anaesthetized rats were mounted in a specially constructed chamber, which allowed continuous measurement of net fluid transport rate (volumetric registration) as well as electrical parameters (potential difference, short-circuit current). The hydraulic conductance (L_p) of the mucosa was determined by registering the changes in net fluid transport rate induced by stepwise changes in hydrostatic pressure on the mucosal side, from $+15$ to $-15\,\text{cm}$ H_2O. L_p was determined in four groups of animals: (a) control animals; (b) during stimulation of the mesenteric nerves; (c) during stimulation of the mesenteric nerves in phentolamine-treated animals and (d) in hexamethonium-pretreated animals.

RESULTS

Cat experiments

In the segments perfused with Krebs–mannitol, mesenteric nerve stimulation had no significant effect on net fluid absorption rate. In the segments where PEG was added to the perfusate, absorption rate was approximately 50% lower than in the other segment, and this difference was abolished by mesenteric nerve stimulation.

Rat experiments

L_p in the extrinsically denervated rat jejunum was $3.6 \pm 0.9\,\mu l \times \text{min}^{-1} \times \text{min}^{-1} \times 100\,\text{cm}^{-2} \times \text{cm}^{-1}\,H_2O$ at positive luminal pressures. At negative luminal presures, L_p increased approximately threefold. At positive luminal pressures, mesenteric nerve stimulation decreased L_p to a value not significantly different from zero, and at negative luminal pressures, nerve stimulation decreased L_p by approximately 50%. The effect of nerve stimulation was attenuated or abolished by phentolamine. Hexamethonium had no significant effect on the measured L_p.

CONCLUSION

The results support that sympathetic nerve stimulation decreases the hydraulic conductance of the jejunal mucosa, via an α-adrenergic mechanism. This effect may explain the non-electrogenic component of the sympathetic absorptive response *in vivo*.

41
Functional and morphological changes during electric field stimulation of rat colon descendens

M. DIENER, P. MESTRES, R. J. BRIDGES AND W. RUMMEL

INTRODUCTION

The mucosa of the rat colon can absorb Na^+ and Cl^- as well as secrete Cl^- into the lumen. The functional state of the epithelium is under the control of the enteric nervous system[1,2]. Intrinsic neurons of the intestine can be excited by electric field stimulation (EFS), resulting in a Cl^- secretion[3,4].

The aim of the present study was to find out, whether the change in the epithelial function after a long-time stimulation was associated with characteristic morphological changes. Two preparations were used: a mucosa–submucosa preparation (MS), containing the submucosal and the mucosal plexus; and a mucosa preparation (M), containing only the mucosal plexus[5,6].

METHODS

The MS-preparation of rat colon descendens was obtained by stripping away the muscularis externa[5]. In addition, for the M-preparation the submucosa was removed by dissection with a glass microscope slide[6]. The tissue was mounted in a modified Ussing chamber and short-circuited by a voltage clamp with compensation for solution and subepithelial resistance[7].

Bipolar rectangular pulses, separated from ground by an isolation unit, were applied in the plane of the tissue by two aluminium foil electrodes[8]. A piece of wet filter paper prevented the contact surface from drying. Stimulus parameters were: frequency, 10 Hz; voltage, 5 V and stimulus duration, 1 ms. Unidirectional fluxes of ^{22}Na and ^{36}Cl were measured in 5 sequential 20 min periods: a first control period; an EFS period; a second control; fluxes after addition of $1.25 \mu M$ tetrodotoxin (TTX); and a last EFS period in the presence of TTX.

For morphological examinations tissues were stimulated for 5 h with an increased frequency (33 Hz), fixed and prepared for electron microscopy. These specimens were compared with control tissue (20 min and 5 h in the chamber without EFS), with a 5 h stimulated tissue after a resting phase of 1 h, and with tissue stimulated for 5 h in the presence of 1.25 μM TTX.

RESULTS

Short-time EFS (stimulation for 20 min) caused an increase in short-circuit current (I_{sc}) in both preparations (Table 1). In the MS-preparation two phases could be distinguished: an early phase, where I_{sc} increased to a peak value; and second stable plateau phase (Figure 1). In the M-preparation only a plateau phase was observed.

Unidirectional flux measurements showed that EFS turned net Cl$^-$ absorption to net Cl$^-$ secretion in the MS-preparation. In contrast, in the M-preparation EFS reduced Na$^+$ and Cl$^-$ absorption to values near zero but did not induce net Cl$^-$ secretion (Table 1).

During long-time stimulation (5 h with an increased frequency) the I_{sc} response to EFS fell to about 20% of the initial response (Figure 1). These preparations were used for morphological studies.

In the stimulated preparations, both in the MS- and in the M-preparation, the area of the Golgi apparatus increased remarkably in the epithelial cells (Figures 2 and 3). The cytoskeleton was strengthened by an increased number of intermediar filaments (Figure 3). These filaments were observed dominantly on the apical pole of the epithelial cells and were often in connection with

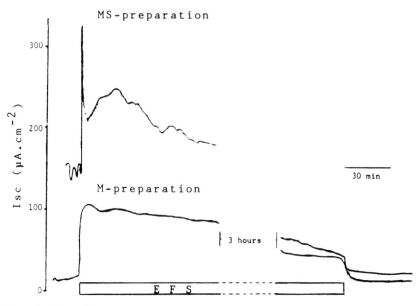

Figure 1   Effect of long-time stimulation on I_{sc}

706

Table 1 Effect of EFS and TTX on unidirectional ion fluxes and I_{sc}

	MS- preparation					M- preparation				
	Control	EFS	Control	TTX	EFS + TTX	Control	EFS	Control	TTX	EFS + TTX
J^{Na}_{ms}	8.3 ± 1.3	6.8 ± 1.2*	9.5 ± 1.3	11.5 ± 1.5*	10.5 ± 1.3	9.1 ± 0.5	6.5 ± 0.4*	8.6 ± 0.4	9.1 ± 0.5	8.0 ± 0.5
J^{Na}_{sm}	4.4 ± 0.4	4.2 ± 0.6	*3.9 ± 0.3*	3.1 ± 0.4*	3.7 ± 0.5	3.9 ± 0.3	4.1 ± 0.3	3.2 ± 0.3	2.9 ± 0.1*	3.1 ± 0.2
J^{Cl}_{ms}	22.8 ± 2.2	17.4 ± 1.7*	22.7 ± 2.1	25.4 ± 2.0*	20.4 ± 2.2	24.3 ± 1.4	20.7 ± 1.4*	23.9 ± 1.8	22.6 ± 1.3	18.8 ± 1.5
J^{Cl}_{sm}	20.3 ± 1.3	26.3 ± 2.4*	17.9 ± 3.1	15.3 ± 1.4*	14.8 ± 1.3	13.5 ± 0.9	20.3 ± 1.3*	12.2 ± 1.1	12.1 ± 0.8	13.6 ± 1.1
I_{sc}	3.4 ± 0.5	6.9 ± 0.6*	2.3 ± 0.5*	0.2 ± 0.1*	0.5 ± 0.1	0.8 ± 0.1	3.9 ± 0.3*	0.6 ± 0.1*	0.4 ± 0.1*	0.8 ± 0.1

$\mu Eq.h^{-1}.cm^{-2}$; $\bar{x} \pm SEM$, * $p < 0.05$ (vs. control 1).

707

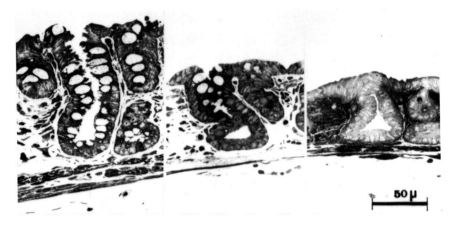

Figure 2 Morphology of epithelial cells in control (left), after 5 h stimulation (middle), and 5 h stimulation with a 1 h resting phase (right)

desmosomes. The foldings of the interdigitations between epithelial cells were more pronounced than in control (Figure 4). The morphological changes did not differ between the MS- and the M-preparation, therefore, only pictures from the MS-preparation are presented.

One hour after termination of stimulation, the observed morphological changes proved to be partially reversible (Figures 2–4). In the preparations, which were stimulated for 5 h in the presence of TTX, these morphological changes did not appear (Figure 5).

DISCUSSION AND CONCLUSIONS

The MS-preparation, consisting of the submucosal and the mucosal plexus, responds to neuronal stimulation with a net chloride secretion. In contrast, the M-preparation, with only the mucosal plexus, responds to EFS with an inhibition of neutral NaCl absorption, suggesting different functions of the mucosal and the submucosal plexus in regulating electrolyte transport[9].

Long-time stimulation of both preparations results in dramatic changes of the morphology of the epithelium (Figure 6). This can be blocked by addition of TTX indicating that the alterations of the epithelial cell structure were neuronally mediated. The increase in the size of the Golgi apparatus and the appearance of intermediar filaments in the cytoskeleton preferentially at the apical region may be related to an increased membrane turnover during intestinal secretion resp. inhibition of absorption.

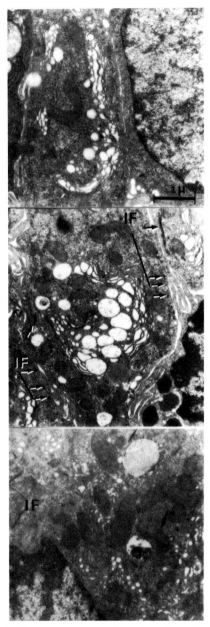

Figure 3 Change in Golgi apparatus and intermediar filaments (IF): control (top), 5 h stimulation (middle) and 5 h stimulation + 1 h recovery (bottom)

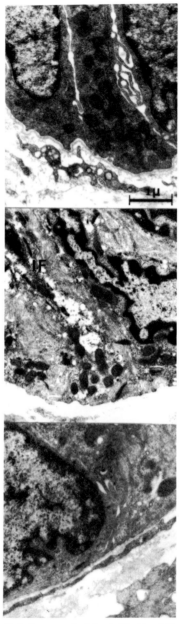

Figure 4 Increase in interdigitations: control (top), 5 h stimulation (middle) and 5 h stimulation + 1 h recovery (bottom)

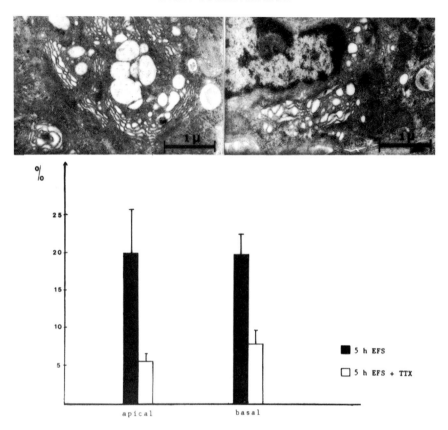

Figure 5 No effects of long-time stimulation are seen in the presence of 1.25 μM TTX. **Left**: control long-time stimulation. **Right**: Long-time stimulation in the presence of 1.25 μM TTX. **Histogram**: percentage area of the Golgi apparatus determined by point-counting stereology. Surface (left) and crypt (right) epithelium. Values are mean ± SD, $n = 34$

Acknowledgement

Supported by DFG, projects Ru 19/49-1 and Di 388/1-2.

References

1. Hubel, K. A. (1985). Intestinal nerve and ion transport: stimuli, reflexes, and responses. *Am. J. Physiol.*, **248**, G261–71
2. Cooke, H. J. (1986). Neurobiology of the intestinal mucosa. *Gastroenterology*, **90**, 1057–81
3. Hubel, K. A. (1978). The effects of electrical field stimulation and tetrodotoxin on ion transport by the isolated rabbit ileum. *J. Clin. Invest.*, **62**, 1039–47
4. Cooke, H. J., Shonnard, K. and Wood, J. D. (1983). Effects of neuronal stimulation on mucosal transport in guinea pig ileum. *Am. J. Physiol.*, **245**, G290–6
5. Andres, H., Bock, R., Bridges, R. J., Rummel, W. and Schreiner, J. (1985). Submucosal plexus and electrolyte transport across rat colonic mucosa. *J. Physiol.*, **364**, 301–12

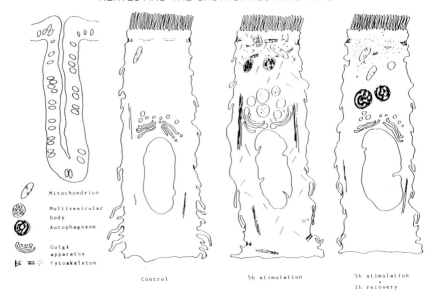

Mitochondrion

Multivesicular body

Autophagosom

Golgi apparatus

Cytoskeleton

Control

5h stimulation

5h stimulation + 1h recovery

Figure 6   Schematic summary of the changes in cell morphology after long-time stimulation

6. Bridges, R. J., Rack, M., Rummel, W. and Schreiner, J. (1986). Mucosal plexus and electrolyte transport across the rat colonic mucosa. *J. Physiol.*, **376**, 531–42
7. Gebhardt, U. (1978). Exakte Kompensation des Lösungswiderstandes bei Anwendung der voltage-clamp Methode an Darmepithelien. Thesis, Universität des Saarlandes, Homburg/-Saar
8. Carey, H. V., Cooke, H. J. and Zafirova, M. (1985). Mucosal responses evoked by stimulation of ganglion cell somas in the submucosal plexus of the guinea-pig ileum. *J. Physiol.*, **364**, 69–79
9. Diener, M., Bridges, R. J., Hubel, K. A. and Rummel, W. (1987). The effects of electric field stimulation on ion transport in rat colon descendens. *Z. Gastroenterologie*, **25**, 383

42
Different neurotransmitters mediate proximal and distal colonic contraction in the rabbit

W. J. SNAPE JR., E. A. MAYER, C. B. KOELBEL AND
J. H. WALSH

INTRODUCTION

Proximal and distal colon have different physiologic functions. The proximal colon is most involved in the conservation of salt and water[1]. The distal colon functions both to store and to eliminate the colonic waste. There are different motility responses in the proximal and distal colon to physiologic and pharmacologic stimuli[2]. It is unclear what role the different responses of colonic smooth muscle versus the enteric plexus play in modulating colonic motility. Previous studies have suggested several differences in the myogenic component in muscle from different regions of the colon. First, there are differences in the numbers of muscarinic receptors present on isolated smooth muscle cells from the proximal and distal colon[3]. Secondly, proximal taenia has increased calcium stores compared to the distal colonic circular smooth muscle[4]. The distal colon responds with increased stress development to exogenous agents compared to the proximal colon[5].

The aim of the present study is to investigate if stimulation of myenteric neurons with electrical field stimulation initiates a different colonic contractile response in muscle taken proximal and distal sites in the rabbit colon. The contribution of different neurotransmitters to these responses will also be investigated.

METHODS

Studies were performed in New Zealand white rabbits which had been anaesthetized with intravenous pentobarbital. A segment of the distal colon 5 cm above the pelvic brim and a segment of proximal colon 3 cm distal to the ileal–colonic junction were excised. The mucosa was immediately removed from the underlying smooth muscle, while the tissue was bathed in carbogenated Krebs solution and maintained at 37°C. Full thickness strips of circular muscle were cut (1.5 cm x 1 mm) and placed in an organ bath. Isometric stress was measured using standard techniques.

All stress was measured at the length of optimal tension (L_o) and was expresed per cross-sectional area. Each drug was diluted in buffer solution and added to the bath to provide the desired molar concentration. Smooth muscle stress development was initiated using electrical field stimulation using 2 mm wide platinum electrodes placed parallel to the muscle strip. The electrical field stimulation was delivered using a supermaximal voltage of 20 V. The pulse duration of 0.9 ms was used since pulse rates of 0.1, 0.5 and 0.9 ms gave similar increases in isometric stress (Figure 1).

The release of neuropeptides during electrical field stimulation was performed after the organ bath and all vials were coated with an organosiline (Prosil 28); 1% bovine serum albumin and 500 units/ml of traysalol were added to the Krebs solution during the electrical field stimulation. The strips were stimulated for 15 minutes using 20 V, 0.9 ms, and 5 Hz as parameters. Peptides concentration were measured using standard radioimmunoassay techniques[6]. Results were expressed as picograms of peptide release normalized to the milligrams net weight of the tissue.

Statistical analysis were performed using Student's t-test for unpaired observations.

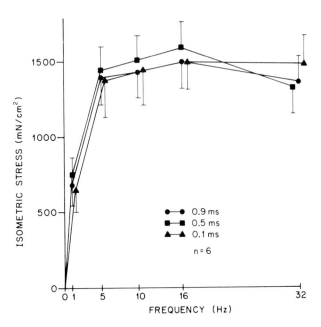

Figure 1 Isometric stress off-contraction development in distal colon using EFS of 20 V and 10 s tracing duration. Different pulse widths are used as the frequency of the pulse is increased

RESULTS

Proximal circular muscle and distal circular muscle responded differently to electrical field stimulation. Proximal circular muscle responded with an on-contraction and without an on-relaxation or off-contraction. In contrast, the distal colonic circular muscle responded with an on-relaxation, an on-contraction and a large off-contraction. The off-contraction had a greater amplitude than the on-contraction.

Increasing concentrations of tetrodotoxin were added to the bath to identify the neural contribution to the response to electrical field stimulation. TTX was a potent inhibitor of all responses, although the effect on distal on-contraction occurred at lower concentrations of TTX than the off-contraction. Figure 2 shows the effect of 3×10^{-6} M TTX on electrical field stimulation of distal muscle. TTX 3×10^{-6} M completely inhibited both the distal on- and off-contraction in distal circular smooth muscle. TTX also inhibited the proximal off-contraction.

Table 1 shows the effect of different neuroreceptor antagonists on electrical field stimulation of the rabbit colon. Atropine inhibited completely the on-contraction in the proximal and distal circular muscle of the colon. However, atropine had no effect on the distal off-contraction. The ganglionic blockade with hexamethonium did not inhibit electrical field stimulation of rabbit colon muscle. Likewise, adrenergic blockade with phentolamine (10^{-6} M) or propranolol(10^{-6} M), opioid blockade with naloxone(10^{-6} M) or serotonergic blockade with methysergide (10^{-6} M) had no effect on electrical field stimulation of colonic muscle.

5-Hydroxytryptamine (serotonin) stimulated a dose-dependent increase in circular muscle contraction of both the proximal and distal circular muscle. Methysergide (10^{-6} M) inhibited this response. The lack of methysergide

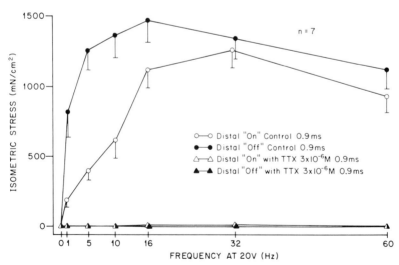

Figure 2 Effect of TTX on on- and off-contraction initiated by EFS (20 V, 0.9 ms, 10 s) of variable frequency in the distal colon

Table 1 Effect of neuroreceptor antagonists on electrical field stimulation of rabbit colon

| | On-contraction | | Off-contraction |
	Proximal	Distal	Distal
TTX (3×10^{-6} M)	+	+	+
Atropine (10^{-6} M)	+	+	NE
Hexamethonium (10^{-6} M)	NE	NE	NE
Phentolamine (10^{-6} M)	NE	NE	NE
Propranolol (10^{-6} M)	NE	NE	NE
Naloxone (10^{-6} M)	NE	NE	NE
Methysergide (10^{-6} M)	NE	NE	NE

NE = no effect

inhibition suggests that a serotonergic nerve is not involved in this response.

Further studies were performed to evaluate the role of the peptide neurotransmitters on the distal off-response. Studies demonstrated that bombesin-like immunoreactivity and substance P-like immunoreactivity increased in the bathing solution after prolonged electrical field stimulation of both the proximal and the distal colonic strips. For this reason, the antagonism of the bombesin and substance P receptors was measured during electrical field stimulation. Bombesin desensitization using 10^{-8} M bombesin inhibited repeat bombesin stimulation (10^{-6} M), but had no effect on inhibiting the off-response in the distal colonic muscle. Substance P desensitization (desensitizing dose = 3×10^{-6} M) inhibited the response to substance P (10^{-8} M $14.3 \pm 3.2\%$) ($p < 0.01$). Spantide (10^{-5} M) and substance P desensitization reduced the off-contraction of distal circular muscle.

DISCUSSION

The present studies suggest that the different physiologic functions of the proximal and distal colon may be mediated by differences in neural connections in these two segments of colon.

Although many neurotransmitters may be present in the myenteric plexus[7], acetylcholine and substance P appear to be the major stimulatory neurotransmitters in the distal colon. Substance P also may have a physiological role in the proximal colon, but acetylcholine appears to be the major stimulatory neurotransmitter in this site. The major difference between the proximal and distal colon may be the presence of inhibitory neurotransmitters: the distal colon has an on-relaxation and an off-contraction. Both these effects could be mediated by the release of an inhibitory neurotransmitter during the neural stimulus.

The relative physiologic importance of the on-contraction and the off-contraction in the distal colon is presently unknown. This mechanism may provide a mechanism for a prolonged contraction. The sole presence of shorter on-contractions in the proximal colon may suggest that short-duration, segmenting contractions are the major form of contractions in the proximal colon. The presence of an off-contraction will allow a long-duration contraction that exists after the neural stimulus has passed. The longer contractions may be responsible for long distance propulsion.

The neurotransmitters that are involved in controlling colonic motility in addition to acetylcholine and substance P are unclear. However, it is apparent that a synapse requiring a nicotinic receptor is unnecessary, once the stimulus has reached the myenteric plexus. Furthermore, the adrenergic, opioid and serotonergic neurons do not appear to play a major role either in inhibition or stimulation of the contractions in this model.

In summary, acetylcholine is the major neurotransmitter responsible for the on-contraction in both the proximal and distal colon. However, substance P is the major mediator of the off-contraction in the distal colon. Although substance P is released in large quantities in the proximal colon of the rabbit, its physiologic function is presently unknown.

Acknowledgements

The authors thank Ms C. Madrigal for secretarial assistance. This study was supported by the National Institutes of Health ROI-DK-31147, the Inflammatory Bowel Disease Center P30-DK-36200 and the National Foundation for Ileitis and Colitis.

References

1. Devroede, G. and Soffie, M. (1973). Colonic absorption in idiopathic constipation. *Gastroenterology*, **64**, 552–61
2. Fink, S. and Friedman, G. (1960). The differential effect of drugs on the proximal and distal colon. *Am. J. Med.*, 534–40
3. Ringer, *M. J., Hyman, P. E., Kao, H. W. and Snape, W. J. Jr.* (1987). [^{3}H]QNB binding and contraction of rabbit colonic smooth muscle cells. *Am. J. Physiol.*, **253**, G656–6
4. Sevy, N. and Snape, W. J. Jr. (1988). Sources of calcium for contraction of distal circular muscle or taenia coli in the rabbit. *Am. J. Physiol.* (In press)
5. Tucker, H. J. and Snape, W. J. Jr. (1979). Cohenn, S.: Comparison of the proximal and distal colonic muscle of the rabbit. *Am. J. Physiol.*, **237**, E383–8
6. Patrono, C., Peskur, B. A. (1987). Radioimmunoassay of gastrointestinal peptides. In *Handbook of Experimental Pharmacology. Radioimmunoassay in Basic and Clinical Pharmacology.* pp. 315–50. (Berlin: Springer Verlag)
7. Johnson, L. R. (ed.) (1987). Histochemistry of the enteric nervous system. In *Physiology of the Gastrointestinal Tract*, pp. 1–40. (New York: Raven Press)

**Part IV
Brain–Gut Interactions**

43
What does the proximal stomach tell the brain?

W. D. BARBER, C. S. YUAN AND T. F. BURKS

INTRODUCTION

The proximal stomach serves as a reservoir concerned with the intake of solids or liquid. This leads to gastric events which have been characterized as receptive relaxation, gastric accommodation and the regulation of intragastric pressure[1]. These events are dependent upon intact vagal input to the caudal brainstem[2]. Studies on the cat have show that the mechanism for gastric accommodation involves 'in-series' tension receptors, served by peripheral processes of primary vagal afferents[3]. The discharge rate of these vagal afferent fibres increases during distension or contraction of the proximal stomach[4-6]. The central processes of these primary vagal afferent fibres have been shown to terminate in the dorsomedial region of the caudal brainstem in nucleus tractus solitarius (NTS) and area postrema[7,8]. Electrophysiological studies have identified neuronal connections between the hypothalamus and NTS, a site receiving gastric vagal input[9].

DISCUSSION

Studies were conducted on cats anaesthetized with chloralose (75 mg/kg) or a mixture of halothane and nitrous oxide supplemented with oxygen. Afferent nerve fibres, serving the proximal stomach, were activated by gastric distension or electrical stimulation to localize and characterize the response of brainstem neurons receiving input from the proximal stomach. These studies identified neurons in NTS which received input from vagal afferent fibres serving mechanoreceptors in the corpus-fundic region of the stomach[10]. Others reported responses in the brainstem of the sheep[11] and the rat to gastric distension[12,13]. Distension of this region of the stomach in the cat caused an excitatory response in 90% of the brainstem units identified while the remaining 10% were inhibitory. These units showed a dynamic and static component in their response to distension of the proximal stomach. The discharge frequency was greater during the distending phase with a decrease in firing rate at sustained levels. The discharge pattern of these brainstem units, which responded to distension of the proximal stomach, was predominantly phasic in character. However, over the period of an hour or more, the activity pattern of some units changed from phasic to tonic discharge patterns modulated by gastric distension. This suggested that sensory receptors, served by vagal afferent fibres which transmitted information to the brainstem, responded to ongoing changes in gastric wall tension. Bilateral vagotomy abolished the response of these units in NTS to gastric distension. We were unable to identify neurons in NTS which responded to distension of the antrum, selected areas of the small or large bowel and rectum.

Local gastric intra-arterial administration of substance P or cholecystokinin (CCK-8) was followed by changes in gastric wall tension of the proximal stomach, which were accompanied by corresponding changes in the activity of neurons in NTS which responded to gastric distension[14,15]. The response of these brainstem units was dependent upon intact vagi. Some neurons in NTS, which responded to distension of the proximal stomach, also showed an increase in activity following local gastric injection of substance P or CCK-8 with no apparent change in gastric wall tension. This suggested that some units in NTS, which received input from vagal afferent fibres that served gastric mechanoreceptors, may also receive input from chemoreceptors. An alternative suggestion may be that these peptides acted upon mechanoreceptors, changing the gain of these sensory receptors.

We recently evaluated the response of brainstem neurons in the central nervous system of the cat, during electrical stimulation of gastric vagal fibres from the proximal stomach and greater splanchnic nerve (submitted for publication). Gastric vagally evoked unitary responses were recorded in NTS and area postrema in the caudal brainstem. The gastric vagally evoked unitary responses consisted of 1–5 spikes. The unitary responses showed a slight variability inthe latency 'jitter' of the response and failed to follow stimulus frequencies above approximately 10 Hz, suggesting that the responses were orthodromic in nature. The mean latency of the gastric vagally evoked brainstem unitary responses was approximately 290 ms, which translated into a conduction velocity of 0.5 m/s or less. This suggested that the reponses were being conducted via C fibres. There was evidence of convergence of input upon single neurons in the brainstem from gastric vagal fibres serving the proximal stomach which travelled in both the dorsal and ventral vagal trunks. Approximately 20% of the gastric vagally evoked unitary responses in NTS also received input from the left greater splanchnic nerve. The splanchnic effect upon the gastric vagally evoked unitary response in NTS was inhibitory in nearly all instances.

Gastric vagally evoked unitary responses were also identified in area postrema. The latency of the response was similar to that observed in NTS. Microstimulation of the area of NTS in which gastric vagally evoked unitary responses were recorded electrophysiologically identified orthodromic and antidromic connections between NTS and area postrema.

Gastric vagally evoked unitary responses were recorded in the hypothalamus in the cat. The unitary responses were histologically localized in the paraventricular, dorsomedial and ventromedial nuclei, and the lateral hypothalamus. The gastric vagally evoked hypothalamic unitary responses were predominantly phasic bursts ranging from a few spikes to short trains. The latency was approximately 370 ms, which translated into a conduction velocity of less than 0.5 m/s. Approximately 20% of the hypothalamic unitary responses which responded to gastric vagal stimulation involved tonically discharging units. The vagal effect upon these tonically active hypothalamic units was inhibitory in the majority of the responses. Some tonically discharging hypothalamic units showed a period of total inhibition of activity ranging from 300 ms to 800 ms, followed by a decrease in tonic activity in response to gastric vagal electrical stimulation. There was also evidence of convergence of input upon single neurons in the hypothalamus from gastric vagal input conveyed in both the dorsal and ventral vagal trunks.

Microstimulation of areas of NTS which responded to electrical stimulation of gastric vagal afferent fibres, serving the proximal stomach, resulted in orthodromic and antidromic responses in neurons in the medial and lateral hypothalamus. The latency of the unitary responses which we observed in the cat was approximately 70 ms and 40 ms respectively for the orthodromic and antidromic responses. Studies in the rat have reported activation of neurons in NTS following microstimulation of the paraventricular nucleus of the hypothalamus[13]. The reciprocal nature of the neuronal connections between caudal brainstem structures and areas in the hypothalamus which receive gastric vagal input from the proximal stomach may have a significant influence on neuronal integrative processes involving food intake.

Distension of the antrum was reported to alter the activity of neurons in the lateral hypothalamus[16]. We have identified neurons in the medial and lateral hypothalamus which were either activated or their ongoing tonic discharge was altered by distension of the corpus-fundic region of the stomach with an intragastric balloon. The distending pressures used were within the physiologic range, less than 15 cm of water. These hypothalamic units responded to gastric distension in a graded manner, an increase in discharge rate with increased intragastric pressure. The majority of the hypothalamic units which responded to gastric distension showed an excitatory response during the distending phase. The response of these hypothalamic neurons, responding to distension of the proximal stomach, was similar to that observed in neurons in NTS.

CONCLUSIONS

These electrophysiological data indicated that there are significant links between the proximal stomach and specific areas of the central nervous system ranging from the caudal brainstem to the hypothalamus in the diencephalon. The caudal brainstem, NTS and adjacent structures, is an obligatory synapse for input from primary vagal afferents serving the proximal stomach. The gastric vagally evoked brainstem unitary responses in NTS were secure with repetitive, predictable responses and showed a concentration of vagal input upon cells in the medial subnucleus of the solitary complex. Areas of NTS which responded to gastric vagal input were reciprocally linked to regions of the medial and lateral hypothalamus which responded to gastric vagal stimulation. These connections suggested that the caudal brainstem received significant input from vagal afferent fibres serving the proximal stomach. The neuronal substrate exists for integration of primary vagal afferent input, in the caudal brainstem, from more rostral regions of the central nervous system in the hypothalamus. There was a significant amount of convergence of input upon single neurons in NTS in the caudal brainstem and in the hypothalamus from gastric vagal afferent fibres serving the proximal stomach which travel in both the dorsal and ventral vagal trunks. Although the precise role of the response of individual neurons evaluated in these studies is not known, the data suggested that these units are positioned to monitor functional events occurring in the proximal stomach such as receptive relaxation, gastric accommodation and regulation of intragastric pressure during the ingestive process.

Acknowledgements

This study was supported by US Public Health Service Grants DK 31804 and DK 35434.

References

1. Kelly, K. A. (1981). Motility of the stomach and gastroduodenal junction. In Johnson, L. R. (ed.) *Physiology of the Gastrointestinal Tract*, pp. 393–410. (New York: Raven Press)
2. Meyer, J. H. (1987). Motility of the stomach and gastrointestinal junction. In Johnson, L. R. (ed.) *Physiology of the Gastrointestinal Tract*, pp. 613–29. (New York: Raven Press)
3. Abrahamsson, H. and Jansson, G. (1973). Vago-vagal gastro-gastric relaxation in the cat. *Acta Physiol. Scand.*, **88**, 289–95
4. Blackshaw, L. A., Grundy, D. and Scratcherd, T. (1987). Vagal afferent discharge from gastric mechanoreceptors during contraction and relaxation of the ferret corpus. *J. Auton. Nerv. Syst.*, **18**, 19–24
5. Iggo, A. (1955). Tension receptors in the stomach and the urinary bladder. *J. Physiol. (Lond.)*, **128**, 593–607
6. Paintal, A. S. (1953). Impulses in vagal afferent fibres from stretch receptors in the stomach and their role in the peripheral mechanism of hunger. *Nature (Lond.)*, **172**, 1194–5
7. Gwyn, D. G., Leslie, R. A. and Hopkins, D. A. (1979). Gastric afferents to the nucleus of the solitary tract in the cat. *Neurosci. Lett.*, **14**, 13–17
8. Kalia, M. and Mesulam, M. M. (1980). Brain stem projections of sensory and motor components of the vagus complex in the cat: II. laryngeal, tracheobronchial, pulmonary, cardiac, and gastrointestinal branches. *J. Comp. Neurol.*, **193**, 467–508
9. Rogers, R. C. and Hermann, G. E. (1985). Gastric-vagal solitary neurons excited by paraventricular nucleus microstimulation. *J. Auton. Nerv. Syst.*, **14**, 351–62
10. Barber, W. D. and Burks, T. F. (1983). Brain stem response to phasic gastric distension. *Am. J. Physiol.*, **245**, G242–8
11. Harding, R. and Leek, B. F. (1973). Central projections of gastric afferent vagal inputs. *J. Physiol. (Lond.)*, **228**, 73–90
12. Ewart, W. R. and Wingate, D. L. (1982). Representation of gastric mechanoreceptor activity in the rat brain. *Scand. J. Gastroenterology*, **17** (suppl. 71), 141–2
13. Rogers, R. C. and Nelson, D. O. (1984). Neurons of the vagal division of the solitary nucleus activated by the paraventricular nucleus of the hypothalamus. *J. Auton. Nerv. Syst.*, **10**, 193–7

14. Barber, W. D. and Burks, T. F. (1987). Brain–gut interactions: brainstem neuronal response to local gastric effects of substance P. *Am. J. Physiol.*, **16**, G369–77
15. Barber, W. D., Stevenson, G. D. and Burks, T. F. (1987). Tachykinins: local gastric effects and brain stem responses. *Am. J. Physiol.*, **252**, G365–73
16. Jeanningros, R. (1984). Modulation of lateral hypothalamic single unit activity by gastric and intestinal distension. *J. Auton. Nerv. Syst.*, **11**, 1–11

.

44
Neural control of initiation and propagation of the retrograde giant contraction asociated with vomiting

I. M. LANG AND S. K. SARNA

INTRODUCTION

Emesis is a complex process involving the co-ordination of different effector systems. It has been hypothesized that this co-ordination is accomplished by specialized neural circuits referred to as pattern generators[1,2]. These central pattern generators control the sequential activation of the effector systems and ensure that these events occur in a stereotypic fashion. The gastrointestinal motor correlates of vomiting comprise one element of this sequence of event[2].

The gastrointestinal motor correlates of vomiting include: (1) a retrograde giant contraction (RGC) which begins at mid small intestine and propagates through the gastric antrum; and (2) a post-RGC series of phasic contractions which occur at all levels of the gastrointestinal tract, but are most prominent in the lower half of the small intestine (Figure 1)[2]. These gastrointestinal motor correlates of vomiting were first recorded over 60 years ago[3], but the neural control of these contractile events has only recently been investigated. This article summarizes recent findings and presents some new information regarding the role of the nervous system in the control of initiation and propagation of the RGC.

CENTRAL NERVOUS SYSTEM

The central nervous system triggers initiation of the RGC because transection of the vagus nerves above the diaphragm[2] or local anaesthesia of both cervical vagi (Figure 2) block the occurrence of all gastrointestinal motor correlates of vomiting without affecting retching or vomitus expulsion. In the sequence of events controlled by the emetic pattern generator, the gastrointestinal events begin before the respiratory events. This sequence

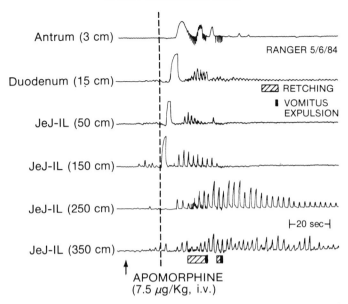

Figure 1 The gastrointestinal motor correlates of vomiting: RGC and post-RGC phasic contractions. Numbers in parentheses indicate distance from the pylorus; the vertical dashed line indicates the time of first observation of the RGC

allows the gastrointestinal motor correlates of vomiting to occur without retching or vomitus expulsion[2,5], and ensures that the RGC always occurs before retching begins[2]. The RGC occurs in a stereotypic fashion, which suggests that it is controlled by pattern generating circuitry. In particular, the RGC always begins at the same site in the small intestine, always propagates through the gastric antrum and always occurs at the same magnitude and duration at each gastrointestinal site[2,4]. These characteristics of the RGC do not depend on the type or intensity of the emetic stimulus[2]. This pattern-generating circuitry may reside in either the central or enteric nervous system. The patterning of the sequential orad activation of the RGC is probably controlled by the CNS because transection of the mesenteric nerves supplying a short segment of the upper jejunum blocked the occurrence of the RGC for a short distance but did not alter the propagation of the RGC across the denervated region[6]. In addition, when these giant contractions were initiated by peripheral mechanisms only, i.e. after intravenous administration of CCK-8, these giant contractions occurred almost simultaneously and did not occur sequentially in an orad direction[4]. This lack of sequential orad propagation implied that this function was normally supplied by pattern generators of the CNS. The anatomical loci of the emetic pattern generator or the motor nuclei controlling initiation of the RGC are unknown.

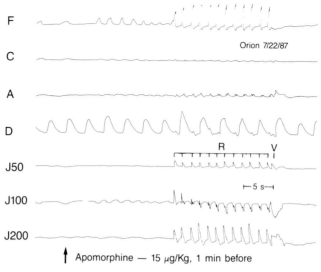

Orion 7/22/87

Figure 2 Blockade of the gastrointestinal motor correlates of vomiting by local anaesthesia of the cervical vagi. Vomiting was activated by apomorphine and the vagus nerves were anaesthetized by injection of bupivacaine into skin loops containing the vagus nerves. These vagal skin loops were formed during a prior surgical procedure. F, fundus; C, corpus; A, antrum; D, duodenum; J, jejunum (numbers after J indicate the distance in cm from the pylorus); R, retching; V, vomiting. The deflections at each retch and vomit are movement artefacts. Note the absence of the RGC or other gastrointestinal motor correlates of vomiting which normally occur before retching and vomiting

PERIPHERAL NEURAL PATHWAYS

The peripheral neural pathway for initiation of the RGC is only partly known. The vagus nerves project all of the efferent fibres controlling initiation of the RGC because supradiaphragmatic vagotomy, but not thoracic sympathectomy and splanchnicectomy, blocked initiation of the gastrointestinal motor correlates of vomiting[2,4]. Transection and reanastomosis of the upper jejunum did not block the occurrence of the RGC at mid-small intestine, therefore the vagal efferent fibres controlling initiation of the RGC do not project long distances along or within the wall of the small intestine[6], rather the mesenteric nerves project these efferent fibres to the small intestine, because transection of the mesenteric nerves blocks the RGC[6]. The route of the vagal efferent fibres from the level of the diaphragm to the mesenteric nerves is unknown.

ENTERIC NERVOUS SYSTEM

Unlike other effector systems involved in emesis, the gastrointestinal musculature is controlled by two complex nervous systems: the central and enteric nervous systems; therefore, some of the pattern-generating neural circuitry controlling the gastrointestinal motor correlates of vomiting may reside in the enteric nervous system. We have found evidence that enteric pattern generators probably determine the nature and magnitude of the RGC at each level of the gastrointestinal tract. Cholecystokinin-octapeptide administered intravenously in relatively high doses was found to activate giant contractions (GC) of the gastrointestinal tract which were similar to RGCs with regard to their magnitude, duration, position in the gastrointestinal tract, myoelectric correlates and initiation in an all-or-none fashion[6]. These CCK-8-induced GCs, however, were probably controlled by the ENS because vagotomy, splanchnicectomy or mesenteric nerve transection[6] did not block these responses.

The enteric nervous system is functionally polarized, in that most of the identified neurons preferentially project aborad[7] and electrical stimulation of a ganglion preferentially activates other ganglia in the aborad direction[8]. This overall aborad projection of the ENS may play a functional role in controlling initiation of the RGC. We found that circumferential transection of the seromuscular layer of the proximal jejunum blocked the occurrence of the RGC for approximately 20 cm aborad of the myotomy but did not affect the RGC as close as 5 cm orad to these transections (Figure 3)[6]. In addition, mesenteric nerve denervation of a 30–60 cm length of jejunum

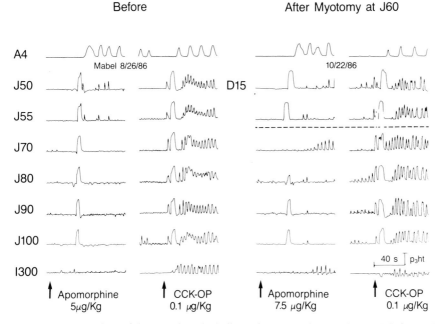

Figure 3 Comparison of the gastrointestinal effects of apomorphine and CCK-OP before and after seromuscular myotomy of the jejunum 60 cm aborad of the pylorus. A, antrum; D, duodenum; J, jejunum; I, ileum (numbers after these letters indicate the distance in cm from the pylorus). P_3ht, peak height of phase III contractions of the migrating motor complex cycle. The dotted line indicates the relative position of the myotomy. Note the blockade of the apomorphine-induced retrograde giant contraction aborad of the myotomy but the lack of effect on CCK-OP-induced responses

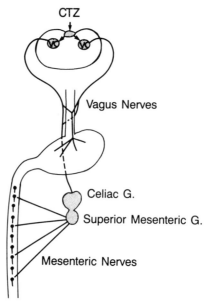

Figure 4 Diagrammatic representation of the neural pathways involved in the initiation and propagation of the retrograde giant contraction. See the text for full description of the role of each element in the pathway

blocked the RGC in the most distal portion of this denervated region only[6].

Transection of the myenteric plexus not only blocked initiation of the RGC but also altered the orad propagation of the RGC. After myotomy the RGC above these cuts began before the RGC below the myotomy ended[6]. The orad RGC, however, did not begin simultaneously with the aboral RGC but occurred only a few seconds earlier than usual[6]. These results suggest that the ENS plays some role in the control of the orad propagation of the RGC. For example, the ENS may function to prevent the premature occurence of RGC's orad to an already propagating RGC.

CONCLUSIONS

The RGC is controlled by pattern generators of the central and enteric nervous systems. The central nervous system triggers initiation of the RGC, controls in large part the orad propagation of the RGC, and co-ordinates the occurrence of the RGC with retching and vomiting. The ENS controls the type and magnitude of the responses at each level of the gastrointestinal tract and participates in the control of the orad propagation of the RGC. The RGC-initiating neural input to one level of the small intestine is propagated aborad by the ENS, and orad propagation of the RGC inhibits the premature occurrence of RGCs at orad sites through the ENS (Figure 4).

Acknowledgements

This research was supported in part by Veterans Administration Research Services Grant 5120-02P (I.M. Lang) and National Institute of Diabetes and Digestive and Kidney Diseases Grant DK32346 (S.K. Sarna).

The secretarial assistance of Mary A. Farrar and the technical assistance of Jeffrey Marvig were greatly appreciated.

References

1. Davis, D. J., Harding, R. K., Leslie, R. A. and Andrews, P. L. R. (1986). The organisation of vomiting as a protective reflex: a commentary. In Davis, C. J., Lake-Bakaar, G. V. and Grahame-Smith, D. G. (eds.) *Nausea and Vomiting: Mechanisms and Treatment*, pp. 65–75 (Berlin: Springer-Verlag)
2. Lang, I. M., Sarna, S. K. and Condon, R. E. (1986). Gastrointestinal motor correlates of vomiting in the dog: quantification and characterization as an independent phenomenon. *Gastroenterology*, **90**, 40–7
3. Alvarez, W. C. (1925). Reverse peristalsis in the bowel, a precursor of vomiting. *J. Am. Med. Assoc.*, **85**, 1051–4
4. Lang, I. M., Marvig, J. and Sarna, S. K. (1988). Comparison of gastrointestinal responses to CCK-8 and associated with vomiting. *Am. J. Physiol.*, **254**, G254–63
5. Ehrlein, H. J. (1981). Inhibition of reverse peristalsis of the intestine by domperidone. *Scand. J. Gastroenterol. Suppl.*, **67**, 199–200
6. Lang, I. M., Marvig, J. and Sarna, S. K. (1987). The role of the enteric nervous system in the initiation and propagation of the gastrointestinal motor correlates of vomiting. *Dig. Dis. Sci.*, **32**, 918
7. Furness, J. B., Costa, M. and Llewellyn-Smith, I. J. (1981). Branching patterns and projections of enteric neurons containing different putative transmitters. *Peptides*, **2**, 119–22
8. Yokoyama, S., Ozaki, T. and Kajitsuka, T. (1977). Excitation conduction in Auerbach's plexus of rabbit small intestine. *Am. J. Physiol.*, **232**, E100–8

45
Permissive regulation of gastrointestinal functions by the vagus nerve

D. GRUNDY

INTRODUCTION

Preganglionic vagal fibres are implicated in the control of many different aspects of gastrointestinal motor and secretory function following the release of both excitatory and inhibitory transmitters from post-ganglionic endings. Thus the vagus is involved in setting the levels of motor and secretory activity appropriate for the post-prandial digestion and subsequent absorption of ingested nutrients[1] and is responsible for the visceral components of emesis[2]. In these respects the extent of vagal influences range from oesophagus to colon and include accessory organs such as the pancreas, liver and gallbladder (Table 1).

The common view of vagal control mechanisms is for specific lines of communication to individual effectors, which are switched on or off by appropriate stimuli emanating either from the gastrointestinal tract itself or from the central nervous system during cephalic responses. However, a question arises because the vagus nerves contain predominantly sensory fibres and in most species fewer than 10% of vagal fibres (out of an approximate total of 30 000 fibres) are efferent[3].

How then are the many vagal influences throughout the gastrointestinal tract and accessory structures achieved through so few efferent fibres? One obvious way is through amplification and distribution of the preganglionic signals by 'command neurons' in the enteric nervous system. On the other hand, the observation that after chronic vagal section there is a return to near normal gastrointestinal functioning indicates that the controlling influences exerted by the vagus are not exclusive. There is considerable overlap between vagal and non-vagal (nervous and hormonal) controls. It is therefore possible that the vagus plays a permissive role in regulating gastrointestinal functions. Such a concept is not new and, indeed, is the principle by which synergism between neural and endocrine control of gastric

Table 1 Summary of gastrointestinal functions influenced by the vagus nerves

Organ	Action
Oesophagus	Peristalsis
LOS	Tone
	Relaxation
Stomach	Corpus relaxation
	Corpus contraction
	Antral contraction
	Acid secretion
	Pepsin secretion
	Mucus secretion
	Mucosal HCO_3^--secretion
	Vasodilation
	Trophic effects
	Gastrin release
	Somatostatin release
Pylorus	Tone
Duodenum	Mucosal HCO_3^--secretion
	Motility
Pancreas	Islet secretion
	Exocrine secretion
	Blood flow
Liver	Bile salt independent choloresis
Gall bladder	Relaxation
	Contraction
Sphincter of Oddi	Inhibition of tone
Jejunum and ileum	Motility
	Electrolyte transport
	Mesenteric blood flow?
Ileocaecal sphincter	Tone
Colon	Motility

and pancreatic secretion is thought to occur[4]. However, such interactions are frequently neglected, as continuing debate over the relative importance of nerves (vagus and otherwise) and hormones indicates[5,6].

In the present paper I have broadened this hypothesis on the basis of two lines of investigation. First, electrophysiological data indicating homogeneity in the vagal efferent supply; and secondly, gastroenterological data showing the importance of vagal tone in setting the level of ongoing gastrointestinal effector activity and its sensitivity to non-vagal regulatory mechanisms.

GASTROINTESTINAL STUDIES

Vagal section or vagal blockade by cooling the nerves to a temperature which prevents impulse conduction results in marked attenuation of gastric, intestinal and colonic contractile activity[7,8,9]. This effect continues after adrenergic receptor blockade or splanchnic nerve section and therefore does not simply reflect the dominance of an unchecked sympathetic supply. Low-frequency electrical stimulation of the peripheral stump of the vagi re-establishes ongoing contractile activity, both in terms of amplitude and discrete patterns of contractions such as seen in the jejunum. Vagal tone, therefore, plays an important role in determining ongoing motor activity. The same is true for pancreatic secretion[10]. Both cholinergic and non-cholinergic mechanisms are involved.

The advantage of vagal cooling over nerve secretion is that it allows observations to be made on restoration of the vagal supply. Interestingly, after just 5 min of vagal blockade there is a transient potentiation of motor and secretory activity immediately after the vagal supply is restored. It is possible that after only short periods without an effective vagal input there is adaptation in the periphery. Indeed, when vagal blockade is maintained for longer periods there can be a partial return of activity.

In addition to these effects on the level of ongoing effector activity vagal section or cooling can also modulate reflexes mediated through non-vagal pathways. The splanchnic nerves, for example, do not influence the ability of the gastric body to accommodate fluid, as indicated by the similar intragastric pressure response to graded distension before and after splanchnic section[11]. However, in the absence of a vagal supply, there is a marked increase in intragastric pressure on cutting the splanchnics. With the vagus intact, therefore, the splanchnics do not contribute to receptive relaxation. When the vagi are cut, the splanchnics help maintain a low intragastric pressure during gastric filling. Vagal tone can therefore suppress reflexes mediated through the sympathetics. In contrast the vagus nerves can augment enteric reflexes. For example, the antral motor response to antral distension is attenuated by bilateral vagotomy or vagal cooling[9]. Although this might ostensibly indicate the involvement of a vagovagal reflex, when vagal tone is artificially restored by low-frequency electrical stimulation the antral response returns. Intra-arterial acetylcholine has a similar effect which is abolished by ganglionic blockade. A tonic preganglionic input to the enteric nervous system is therefore required for full expression of this reflex while an afferent input to the brainstem is not involved.

ELECTROPHYSIOLOGICAL DATA

Vagal tone

The majority of single vagal efferent fibres recorded electrophysiologically in the rat[1,2], ferret[13,14] and dog[15,16] display spontaneous activity which would provide the vagal tone responsible for the results outlined above. This tonic activity consists of a continuous, low-frequency irregular discharge in the absence of any intentional stimulation. From Figure 1 it is apparent that over 95% of efferent fibres discharge spontaneously; most at frequencies between 0.5 and 2 impulses per second. Interspike interval analysis reveals distributions which are either unimodal or pseudo-random and which are modulated by but not dependent on a vagal afferent input to the brainstem[17]. The vagal tone is therefore generated centrally although the absolute level

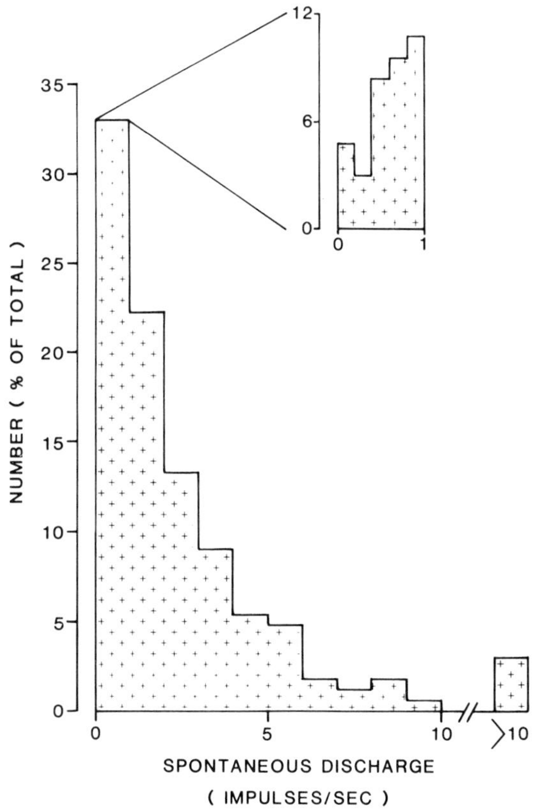

Figure 1   Frequency distribution of spontaneous discharge rates of single vagal efferent fibres recorded in the Urethane anaesthetized ferret. The inset shows discharge rates below 1 impulse per second

of discharge is modified according to the amount of afferent information reaching the vagal motor complex from sensory receptors in the gastrointestinal musculature and mucosa. Cephalic influences also modulate the level of spontaneous discharge[16].

Vagal reflexes

Modulation of vagal efferent discharge by afferent inputs from the gastrointestinal tract forms the basis of vagal reflexes. Given that the extent of the vagal influence on gastrointestinal functions is considerable, it is remarkable that efferent responses fall into only two broad categories: those whose discharge is reduced or completely suppressed; and those which show the opposite response and are excited by afferent stimulation.

Despite variations in thresholds to activation, levels of discharge and the degree to which afferent information converges on individual efferents, the efferent responses generally reflect the amount of excitatory and inhibitory input to the brainstem from different receptor types and from different regions of the gastrointestinal tract. Since the vagus nerves contain two motor pathways to the gastrointestinal tract; the classical cholinergic excitatory pathway and the inhibitory pathway mediating its effect through a non-adrenergic, non-cholinergic post-ganglionic transmitter we proposed that these two pathways are reciprocally modulated[12]. In this way a highly convergent afferent input serves to set levels of discharge in the excitatory and inhibitory pathways that are appropriate to the needs of digestion at any particular moment in time. It is this level of activity that is proposed to set the level of effector activity and moreover determine the sensitivity of the gastrointestinal tract to non-vagal influences. In other words, the vagus may 'gate' reflexes mediated through non-vagal pathways and hormones (Figure 2). In the two extremes one can envisage the 'gates' being either open or closed. However, by regulating the degree to which these are 'ajar' gives the vagus the capacity for fine control of effector responses.

CONCLUSION

The vast majority of vagal efferent fibres are spontaneously active, providing a background vagal tone. The level of vagal tone is adjustable on the basis of afferent inputs from the periphery and descending cephalic influences. Removing this tonic input to the gastrointestinal tract suppresses ongoing secretion and motility and modulates reflexes mediated through non-vagal pathways.

Vagal efferent tone therefore plays a permissive role in the control of gastrointestinal function. This has far-reaching implications for the interpretation of data relevant to the importance of vagal mechanisms in controlling gastrointestinal function because vagal section not only removes the pathway for vagal reflexes but also affects the sensitivity of the gastro-intestinal tract to non-vagal regulatory mechanisms. Some may be attenuated in the absence of a vagal supply while others may only manifest themselves in the absence of ongoing vagal activity.

Modulation of the level of vagal tone provides a means of gating responses mediated through alternative non-vagal pathways and may be the means by which a widespread vagal influence is met by only a small number of vagal

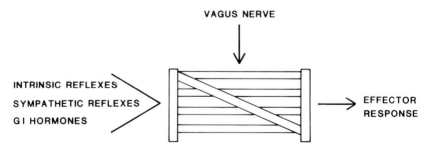

Figure 2 Schematic model for the permissive regulation of gastrointestinal functions by the vagus nerve

efferent fibres.

Since the 'hard-wired' mechanisms controlling gastrointestinal functions are non-vagal, any loss of the vagal input can be effectively overcome by plasticity in the periphery, which returns gastrointestinal functions to near-normal in a relatively short period.

References

1. Hall, K. E., El-Sharkaway, T. Y. and Diamant, N. E. (1986). Vagal control of canine postprandial upper gastrointestinal motility. *Amer. J. Physiol.*, **250**, G501–10
2. Lang, I. M., Sarna, S. K. and Condon, R. E. (1986). Gastrointestinal motor correlates of vomiting in the dog. Quantification and characterization as an independent phenomenon. *Gastroenterol.*, **90**, 40–7
3. Andrews, P. L. R. (1986). Vagal afferent innervation of the gastrointestinal tract. *Prog. in Brain Res.*, **67**, 65–86
4. Grossman, M. I. (1981). Regulation of gastric acid secretion. In Johnson, L. R. (ed.) *Physiology of the Gastrointestinal Tract*, pp. 659–72. (New York: Raven Press)
5. Singer, M. V. (1986). Role of CCK in pancreatic exocrine response to amino-acids and fats. Letter to the editor. *Amer. J. Physiol.*, **250**, G558
6. Stabile, B. and Stubbs, R. S. (1986). Reply. *Amer. J. Physiol.*, **250**, G559
7. Collman, P. I., Grundy, D. and Scratcherd, T. (1983). Vagal influences on the jejunal 'minute rhythm' in the anaesthetized ferret. *J. Physiol.*, **345**, 65–74
8. Collman, P. I., Grundy, D. and Scratcherd, T. (1984). Vagal control of colonic motility in the anaesthetized ferret: evidence for a non-cholinergic excitatory innervation. *J. Physiol.*, **348**, 35–42
9. Grundy, D., Hutson, D. and Scratcherd, T. (1986). A permissive role for the vagus nerves in the genesis of antro-antral reflexes in the anaesthetized ferret. *J. Physiol.*, **381**, 377–84
10. Grundy, D., Hutson, D. and Scratcherd, T. (1983). The response of the pancreas of the anaesthetized cat to secretin before, during and after reversible vagal blockade. *J. Physiol.*, **342**, 517–26
11. Andrews, P. L. R., Grundy, D. and Lawes, I. N. C. (1980). The role of the vagus and splanchnic nerves in the regulation of intragastric pressure in the ferret. *J. Physiol.*, **307**, 401–11
12. Davison, J. S. and Grundy, D. (1978). Modulation of single vagal efferent fibre discharge by gastrointestinal afferents in the rat. *J. Physiol.*, **284**, 69–82
13. Grundy, D., Salih, A. A. and Scratcherd, T. (1981). Modulation of vagal efferent fibre discharge by mechanoreceptors in the stomach, duodenum and colon of the ferret. *J. Physiol.*, **319**, 43–52
14. Blackshaw, L. A., Grundy, D. and Scratcherd, T. (1987). Involvement of gastrointestinal mechano- and intestinal chemoreceptors in vagal reflexes: an electrophysiological study. *J. Auton. Nerv. Syst.*, **18**, 225–34
15. Miolan, J. P. and Roman, C. (1978). Activité des fibres vagales efferentes destinées à la musculature lisse du cardia du chien. *J. Physiol. (Paris)*, **74**, 709–23
16. Miolan, J. P. and Roman, C. (1978). Discharge of efferent vagal fibres supplying gastric antrum: indirect study by nerve suture technique. *Amer. J. Physiol.*, **235**, E366–73
17. Grundy, D. (1988). Vagal control of gastrointestinal function. *Baillière's Clin. Gastroenterol.*, **2**(1), 23–43

46
Comparison of electrical and chemical stimulation of lateral hypothalamus in control of gastric function

H.-S. FENG, J. HAN, J. R. BROBECK AND F. P. BROOKS

We have reported a purely gastric motor response to unilateral electrical stimulation of the lateral hypothalamus (LHA) in anaesthetized cats that is mediated by both vagal trunks and blocked by atropine. Subsequently we have found that bilateral electrolytic lesions in the dorsal motor nucleus (DMV) and nucleus ambiguus were required to block the response. We now compare the effects of microinjection of bicuculline methiodide (1 μg in 200 nl), a GABA antagonist into the LHA with the effects of electrical stimulation. Cats were anaesthetized with chloralose and equipped with a gastric fistula and extraluminal force transducers on the gastric corpus and antrum. Electrical stimulation was applied with a bipolar electrode inserted with a Kopf stereotaxic instrument using coordinates published previously[1]. Drugs were injected through a micropipette. Basal contractions were < 5 G of force. The maximum force of antral contractions during electrical stimulation (1 mA, 10 Hz, and 8 ms pulse duration) was 37.1 ± 1.0 g (12 cats). That with bicuculline was 32.1 ± 1.2 g (8 cats). The difference was statistically significant. Neither stimulus increased acid output. Atropine 1 μg in 200 nl injected into the ipsilateral DMV blocked both antral and corpus contractions induced by electrical stimulation but not those induced by bicuculline. We conclude that chemical, as well as electrical, stimulation of the LHA increase the force of gastric contractions. These results also suggest that the increased force of contractions induced by electrical and GABAergic stimuli in the LHA is mediated by different pathways and neurotransmitters.

References

1. Feng, H.-S., Han, J., Brobeck, J. R. and Brooks, F. P. (1987). *J. Clin. and Invest. Med.*, 140–4

47
Absence of the gastric MMC on cooling blockade of cervical vagus is in part due to unopposed adrenergic inhibition of the stomach

S. A. CHUNG, D. T. VALDEZ AND N. E. DIAMANT

Bilateral cervical cooling blockade of the vagi abolishes the gastric migrating motor complex (MMC) except for the pylorus. One explanation proposes that this finding is due to adrenergic inhibition of the stomach via sympathetic nerves entering the vagi below the level of the blockade. Studies in four chronic dogs were performed to assess this hypothesis.

METHODS

The vagosympathetic nerve trunks were previously isolated in bilateral, cervical skin loops to permit blockade by cooling. Stomach and upper small bowel motor and electrical activity were monitored. Adrenergic blockade was performed by an initial bolus injection of phentolamine (0.3 mg/kg) and propranolol (0.3 mg/kg), and a subsequent continuous intravenous infusion of phentolamine (1.5 mg/kg/h) and propranolol (0.3 mg/kg/h).

RESULTS

Bilateral cervical vagal blockade abolished the gastric MMC, with persistence of phase III of the MMC in the pylorus and upper small bowel. During adrenergic blockade, intermittent gastric contractions were associated with all phases of the intestinal MMC, including phase I. This contractile activity was accentuated during phase III, but never reached the intensity of activity nor demonstrated the typical co-ordination features of the gastric MMC as seen with the vagi intact.

CONCLUSIONS

Absence of the gastric MMC with bilateral cervical cooling blockade appears in part to be due to unopposed sympathetic adrenergic inhibition of the stomach, this inhibition being extrinsic to the cervical vagosympathetic trunks. However, the vagus is the normal, primary pathway for control of the gastric MMC.

48
Rat gastric contractility is increased with elevated intracranial pressure in awake and anaesthetized rats

E. H. LIVINGSTON, E. P. PASARO JR. AND T. R. GARRICK

Central nervous system trauma causing intracranial hypertension is frequently associated with nausea and the development of gastric erosions. Cold restraint induced gastric lesion formation in the rat is associated with increased gastric contractility. We studied the effect of elevated intracranial pressure (ICP) on gastric contractility in anaesthetized (ketamine with acepromazine) and unanaesthetized rats. Male Sprague–Dawley rats were implanted with a gastric strain-gauge force transducer and an intraventricular catheter positioned into the right lateral ventricle. Transducer output was amplified and digitized, and the mean area beneath the contraction curves calculated. Six 15-minute recording periods were obtained: basal, increased ICP and 4 post-treatment. Intracranial pressure was elevated in awake and anaesthetized animals. Anaesthesia without pressure elevation served as a control group. Data are presented as the ratio of the motility index (mean area beneath the individual contraction curves within a recording period) in the experimental versus basal conditions. For anaesthesia controls, the ratio of mean contraction area after induction to those prior to induction is presented.

In 12 studies with 5 conscious rats, elevated ICP caused brief inhibition followed by persistent stimulation of gastric contractions. The forceful con-

Table 1 Interval after ICP returned to baseline

	$ICP = 12\,cm\,H_2O$	$14\,min$	$30\,min$	$45\,min$	$60\,min$
No anaesthesia	1.44	1.8	1.90	1.52	1.20
$\pm$ SE	0.19	0.36	0.32	0.53	0.20
Anaesthesia	0.88	1.16	0.93	2.25	3.00
$\pm$ SE	0.19	0.16	0.28	0.16	0.16

Table 2 Anaesthesia alone

	15 min	30 min	45 min	60 min	75 min
Control	1.23	0.82	1.17	0.96	1.11
±SE	0.38	0.28	0.49	0.37	0.45

tractions usually lasted throughout the observation period. In 4 studies in 3 anaesthetized rats, stimulation was not observed until 30 min after the elevated ICP period. Anaesthesia alone increased the force of contractions; however, when coupled with elevated intracranial pressure, it delayed the onset of forceful contractions which, when they occurred, were stronger than in unanaesthetized animals. Preliminary studies have revealed complete inhibition of the contractile response with vagotomy and dose dependent inhibition with atropine. We conclude that elevated ICP, like cold-water immersion restraint, markedly stimulates gastric contractility. Augmented contractile activity might produce gastric symptoms common in head trauma.

49
Bombesin: medullary and spinal sites of action to inhibit gastric acid secretion in the rat

T. ISHIKAWA, Y. YANG AND Y. TACHÉ

Bombesin injected into the cerebrospinal fluid is more potent than a number of bombesin analogues and unrelated peptides to inhibit gastric acid secretion in rats and dogs. In previous studies, we have localized responsive sites into the paraventricular nucleus[1] and demonstrated that existence of hindbrain sites independent from the hypothalamic sites[2]. In the present study we investigate the medullary and spinal sites of action for bombesin-induced inhibition of gastric acid secretion in rats.

Experiments were done in urethane-anaesthetized rats fasted for 24 h and acutely implanted in the non-glandular part of the stomach with a double cannula. Gastric acid output was measured every 10 min by flushing the stomach with bolus of saline. Peptides or saline were microinjected unilaterally in 100 nl volume using a glass micropipette positioned into different medullary sites according to the coordinates of Paxinos and Watson. The stable TRH analogues RX 77368 (72 pmol) microinjected into the dorsal vagal complex (DVC) induced a long lasting stimulation of gastric acid secretion (TRH: 130 µmol/h vs. saline 10 µmol/h). Bombesin (0.6–6 pmol) injected concomitantly with TRH analogue into the DVC dose dependently suppressed by 35–82% the acid response to TRH. Bombesin (6 pmol) microinjected into the DVC which inhibited by 84% the peak acid response (25 ± 3 µmol/10 min) to TRH analogue, decreased only by 25% the peak response to pentagastrin (10 ± 2 µmol/10 min) whereas intracisternal injection of bombesin (0.6–6 pmol) elicited a dose-related suppression of pentagastrin response by 39–74%. These results suggest that the inhibitory effect of bombesin on acid secretion stimulated by pentagastrin is mediated by other medullary sites. Microinjection of bombesin (0.2–6 pmol) into the nucleus ambiguus dose dependently suppressed by 30–63% the acid response to pentagastrin, whereas injection into the locus coeruleus and central grey were inactive. Other peptides microinjected into the nucleus ambiguus such as corticotropin-releasing factor (62 pmol), and calcitonin gene related peptide

(13 pmol) did not alter the secretory effect of pentagastrin infusion. The inhibitory effect of bombesin microinjected into the nucleus ambiguus is prevented by spinal cord transection at the C_6 level but not by cervical vagotomy. Dose-related inhibition (28–56%) of the pentagastrin response was also obtained following intrathecal (vertebral level T9-10) injection of bombesin (60–300 pmol).

These studies demonstrate that bombesin acts in the dorsal vagal complex to inhibit vagally mediated stimulation of gastric acid secretion. By contrast, the dorsal vagal complex appears less efficient to mediate the inhibitory effect of other non-vagal stimulants such as pentagastrin. The nucleus ambiguus is so far the most sensitive site of action to inhibit pentagastrin stimulated secretion. The spinal cord is also responsive to bombesin, however, the inhibitory effect is less potent than following injection into the cisterna magna or the nucleus ambiguus. These results provide the first evidence of a possible role of the nucleus ambiguus in the regulation of gastric acid secretion as demonstrated by peptide microinjection.

References

1. Ishikawa, T., Yang, Y. and Taché, Y. (1987). *Brain Res.*, **422**, 118
2. Ishikawa, T., Yang, Y. and Taché, Y. (1987). *Am. J. Physiol.*, **15**, G675–84

50
Effect of sham feeding on interdigestive gastroduodenal motility

F. SIELAFF, H. BERNDT AND T. BYTEL

The aim of this study was to evaluate the influence of vagal stimulation on the fasting gastroduodenal motor activity. The interdigestive and post-cibal motility was studied in 18 healthy volunteers aged from 18 to 32 years. Thirty minutes after recording of the second migrating motor complex (MMC) a modified sham feeding (MSF) was performed. One hour later we examined the motility after ingestion of a solid test meal (258 kcal). Pressure activity was recorded using a manometric probe positioned in the antrum, the proximal and distal duodenal as well.

The mean cycle duration of MMC lasted 81.2 ± 29.9 min. (phase 1 = 39.4%; phase 2 = 55.4%; phase 3 = 5.1%). Only 63% of subjects had activity fronts starting in the stomach. The propagation velocity of phase 3 activity from the proximal to distal duodenum was 10.0 ± 2.1 min.

Sham feeding was followed in about two-thirds by increased motor activity in the stomach and duodenum. Six individuals showed a typical antral phase 3 activity and eight had regular MMCs in the duodenum. The appearance of MMC in the distal duodenum after MSF was not connected with the observation of a phase 3 activity in the antrum. In some patients the preparation of MSF alone induced the described changes of motility like an anticipated sham feeding.

We conclude that the vagal activation by MSF modifies the appearance of MMC but it does not induce the phase 3 activity.

51
Central vs. enteric neural control of small intestinal migrating motor complexes

S. K. SARNA, I. M. LANG, J. J. GLEYSTEEN AND
M. F. OTTERSON

In the fasting state the small intestine of most non-ruminant mammals exhibits a migrating motor complex (MMC). This complex is a cyclic group of contractions that usually begins in the proximal duodenum, lasts for about 6–8 min and migrates caudad to the ileocolonic junction at a velocity ranging from 2 to 8 cm/min[1,2]. Concurrent with the start of MMC in the duodenum, the stomach, the lower oesophageal sphincter, the gallbladder and the sphincter of Oddi also show increased motor activity called the cyclic motor activity. The mean cycle length of MMC in dogs and humans is about 100–150 min. The mechanisms of spontaneous initiation and caudad migration of these motor complexes has caught the fancy of many workers in the field over the last two decades. Basically, two mechanisms have been proposed: neural and hormonal. The objective of this paper is to delineate the roles of the central and enteric nervous systems in the regulation of initiation, migration and organization of these motor complexes. The term 'control' here refers to those elements of the nervous system that are essential for the spontaneous initiation and migration of MMC, while the term 'modulation' refers to those elements which are not essential for the above but they may alter the characterstics such as cycle length, velocity of migration and distance of migration. In addition to the neural control, hormonal control of these complexes, mainly by cycling of plasma concentrations of motilin, has also been studied. The reader is referred to other articles for the cause-and-effect relationship between plasma motilin and MMC cycling[1,2].

The central control of MMC implies that there is a specific area of the brain, like the vomiting centre or the defaecation centre, that programmes the cyclic generation of MMC in the duodenum and its caudad migration to the ileum. An essential requirement for this scheme to work is that there should be a neural pathway along which the signals from the CNS are transmitted to the small intestine. If these pathways are interrupted the

MMC should cease to exist. The two likely pathways for the CNS control are the vagus and the splanchnic nerves. Sectioning of either one or both of these nerves does not stop MMC cycling or its caudad migration[4,5,6]. The cycle length after sectioning these nerves may become more variable, but it is not certain if this is a direct effect of the interruption of these pathways or an indirect effect due to functional changes that may occur in the gastrointestinal tract as a result of the absence of complete gut communication with the CNS. Extrinsic denervation of a small segment of the small intestine does not alter the characteristics of MMC in the denervated segment or in the rest of the small intestine[7,8]. These findings suggest that the CNS may not control the initiation and caudad migration of the small intestinal MMC.

Although the input from the CNS may not control the spontaneous MMC, it may affect its characteristics in the fasted and fed states. Labyrinthine stimulation, stress or intercerebroventricular injections of some peptides may induce premature MMCs, disrupt them or initiate MMCs in the post-prandial state[9,11]. The CNS may thus modulate the generation and migration of MMC in the small intestine.

The cyclic motor activity of the stomach may, however, be under an extrinsic neural control. Although vagotomy or splanchnicectomy does not inhibit gastric cyclic motor activity, total extrinsic denervation of the stomach abolishes it[12]. Duodenojejunectomy also inhibits cycling motor activity in the stomach[13]. This suggests that the gastric cyclic motor activity is not an independent oscillator. It depends on an external stimulus to generate cyclic phenomenon. The source of the external signal may be the duodenum.

There are also two schools of thought as to the source of the signal from the duodenum, one that motilin released from the duodenum by the MMC contractions initiates the gastric cyclic motor activity[13] and the other that a neural pathway from the duodenum to the stomach provides the primary stimulus, but motilin may enhance this effect.

Vagal cooling at the cervical level blocks gastric cyclic motor activity. Based on this finding Hall et al.[14] concluded that gastric cyclic motor activity is controlled by the CNS through the vagus nerve. They suggested that the lack of a similar effect after thoracic truncal vagotomy may be because the stomach adapts and an alternate mechanism takes over. Gleysteen et al.[15] reported, however, that vagal cooling at the thoracic level did not block gastric cyclic motor activity. These differences may be explained by the composition of the vagal trunk at the cervical and the thoracic level. First, the vagal trunk at the cervical level has nerve fibres that go to the heart and respiratory systems. Cooling at the cervical level also blocks these fibres, resulting in Horner's syndrome. The reflex actions of these changes in the cardiorespiratory function on the gastrointestinal tract are not known. Additionally, adrenergic and other fibres enter the vagal trunk between the cervical and the thoracic levels. Vagal cooling at the cervical level may block the excitatory vagal input to the stomach and leave the inhibitory input unopposed resulting in the inhibition of cyclic motor activity.

Vagal cooling at the cervical level also reverses post-prandial disruption of MMC cycling in the small intestine. Thoracic truncal vagotomy, on the other hand, has no such effect. It is known that isoproterenol[16] also reverses the post-prandial MMC disruption which suggests a link between cervical vagal cooling and adrenergic dominance.

The enteric neural control of MMC cycling was demonstrated by dividing the small intestine into smaller segments by transections and reanastomoses[17,18]. This procedure did not affect the extrinsic nerves. In the intact small intestine, MMC originated in the proximal duodenum and migrated caudad. After three transections and anastomoses, each smaller segment exhibited independent MMCs up to a period of about 40–60 days (Figure 1). At the end of this period, co-ordination between the segments began to reappear. About 100 days after transections and reanastomoses, the MMCs were co-ordinated along the entire length of the small intestine. In another series of experiments, 2–4 cm long colonic segments were interposed at the transection sites[18]. In this case, the coupling of MMC between segments did not recover up to about 180 days after surgery. These findings suggested that: (1) Each small segment of the small intestine is an independent MMC oscillator; (2) the coupling between these oscillators in the intact small intestine is provided by intrinsic nerves; (2) the intrinsic nerves regenerate with time across a transection and an end-to-end anastomosis; (3) the intrinsic nerves in the small intestine may not regenerate through a foreign neural structure like that of the colon.

The role of intrinsic nerves in the propagation of MMCs was studied by close intra-arterial injections of atropine, hexamethonium and TTX in conscious dogs[19]. Small doses of these antagonists and nerve conduction blockers were injected into a 3–5 cm long segment of the jejunum just before the arrival of phase III activity. Close intra-arterial injection of atropine or hexamethonium blocked the propagation of phase III activity within and beyond the perfused segment (Figure 2). This suggested that both nicotinic and muscarinic receptors are involved in the propagation of MMC. Tetrodotoxin also blocked the MMC in progress, but then with a delay of a few minutes it initiated a new MMC in the perfused segment or distal to it and this MMC migrated caudad. This finding suggested that intrinsic neurons

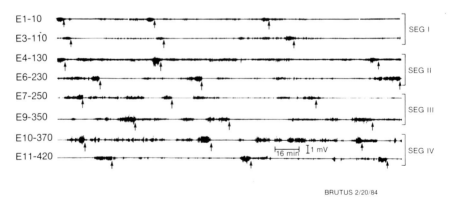

BRUTUS 2/20/84

Figure 1 Independent migrating motor complex cycles occurred in all four segments of the small intestine 112 days after transections and anastomoses. Prior to transections and reanastomoses the MMCs originated in the proximal duodenum and migrated caudad

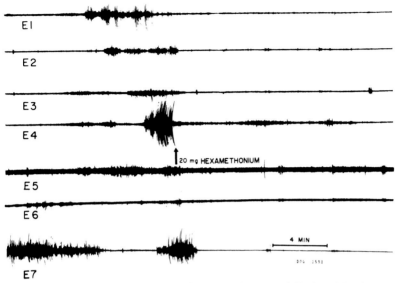

Figure 2 Hexamethonium (20 mg) was perfused close intra-arterially in a jejunal segment perfusing the region between electrodes E4 and E5 just before the beginning of phase III activity at E5. It blocked the migrating myoelectric complex propagation

are essential for MMC propagation. Identical doses of these blockers, given intravenously, had no effect on MMC propagation. Saline injection in the perfused segment also did not block MMC propagation.

The intrinsic and extrinsic nerves also play a role in the organization of the MMC. The onset of phase II activity in the proximal small intestine is closely related to the location of preceding phase III activity in the small intestine[20]. Phase II activity begins in the duodenum when the preceding phase III activity reaches about 80% of the length of the small intestine. The strong contractions during phase III activity may reflexively inhibit contractions at proximal sites to produce phase I activity. The pathway for this inhibition seems to be extrinsic to the intestinal wall. The percentage duration of different phases of the MMC cycle in the duodenum did not change significantly after a single transection and reanastomosis, 60 cm from the pylorus (Table 1).

Strong contractions induced by close intra-arterial injection of neostigmine inhibited the phase III in progress up to 150 cm proximal or distal to the site of injection (Figure 3)[21]. This reflex inhibition of phase III activity was

Table 1 Percentage duration of different phases of duodenal MMC cycle before and after a transection and reanastomosis at 60 cm from the pylorus ($n = 5$)

	Phase I	Phase II	Phase III	Phase IV
Before	69.0 ± 3.0	20.0 ± 3.0	9.0 ± 0.4	$2.0 \pm$
After	77.0 ± 5.0	15.0 ± 2.0	9.0 ± 0.3	$3.0 \pm$

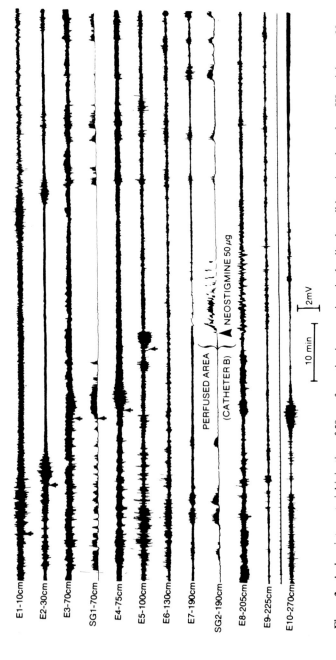

Figure 3 A close intra-arterial injection of 50 μg of neostigmine was given in the distal small intestine when phase III activity was 90 cm proximal to it. The reflex initiated by strong local contractions inhibited phase III activity and stopped its further migration

blocked by injecting atropine, hexamethonium or pirenzepine in a segment located in between the site of stimulation and phase III activity. A transection and reanastomosis between the stimulation site and phase III activity also blocked the reflex inhibition of phase III activity. These findings suggested that the neural pathway for reflex inhibition of phase III activity by large contractions was inside the intestinal wall. This pathway was polysynaptic and contained nicotinic and muscarinic M_1-receptors.

In summary, nerves play an important role in the spontaneous initiation and caudad propagation of small intestinal migrating motor complexes. The enteric nervous system is primarily responsible for the generation and caudad migration of spontaneous MMCs. However, the characteristics of the MMC may be modulated by the CNS. Long polysynaptic intrinsic neural pathways for reflex inhibition of MMC exist within the gut wall. However, the neural pathways to induce phase I activity in the proximal small intestine by the caudad migrating phase III activity may be extrinsic to the small intestine.

Acknowledgements

Supported in part by NIDDK/D grant DK 32346 and VA Merit Review grant 7722-01P.

References

1. Sarna, S. K. (1985). Cyclic motor activity; migrating motor complex. *Gastroenterology*, **89**, 894–913
2. Szurszewski, J. H. (1981). Electrical basis for gastrointestinal motility. In Johnson, L. R. (ed.) *Physiology of the Gastrointestinal Tract*, pp. 1435–66. (New York: Raven Press)
3. Sarna, S., Chey, W. Y., Condon, R. E., Dodds, W. J., Myers, T. and Chang, T. M. (1983). Cause-and-effect relationship between motilin and migrating myoelectric complexes. *Am. J. Physiol.*, **245**, G277–84
4. Weisbrodt, N. W., Copeland, E. M., Moore, E. P., Kearley, R. W. and Johnson, L. R. (1975). Effect of vagotomy on electrical activity of the small intestine of the dog. *Am. J. Physiol.*, **228**, 650–4
5. Marlett, J. A. and Code, C. F. (1979). Effects of celiac and superior mesenteric ganglionectomy on interdigestive myoelectric complex in dogs. *Am. J. Physiol.*, **6**, E432–6
6. Telford, G. L., Go, V. L. W. and Szurszewski, J. H. (1985). Effect of central sympathectomy on gastric and small intestinal myoelectric activity and plasma motilin concentrations in the dog. *Gastroenterology*, **89**, 989–95
7. Sarr, M. G. and Kelly, K. A. (1981). Myoelectric activity of the autotransplanted canine jejunoileum. *Gastroenterology*, **81**, 303–10
8. Bueno, L., Praddaude, F. and Ruckebusch, Y. (1979). Propagation of electrical spiking activity along the small intestine: intrinsic versus extrinsic neural influences. *J. Physiol. (Lond.)*, **292**, 15–26
9. Thompson, D. G., Richelson, E. and Malagelada, J.-R. (1982). Perturbation of gastric emptying and duodenal motility through the central nervous system. *Gastroenterology*, **83**, 1200–6
10. Bueno, L. and Ferre, J.-P. (1982). Central regulation of intestinal motility by somatostatin and cholecystokinin octapeptide. *Science*, **216**, 1427–9
11. McRae, S., Younger, K., Thompson, D. G. and Wingate, D. L. (1982). Sustained mental stress alters human jejunal motor activity. *Gut*, **23**, 404–9
12. Sarna, S. K., Matsumoto, T., Condon, R. E. and Cowles, V. E. (1985). Does stomach have an independent spontaneous cyclic motor activity? *Gastroenterology*, **88** (Abstract), 1571

13. Tanaka, M. and Sarr, M. G. (1987). Total duodenectomy: effect on canine gastrointestinal motility. *J. Surg. Res.*, **42**, 483–93
14. Hall, K. E., El-Sharkawy, T. Y. and Diamant, N. E. (1982). Vagal control of migrating motor complex in the dog. *Am. J. Physiol.*, **243**, G276–84
15. Gleysteen, J. J., Sarna, S. K. and Myrvik, A. L. (1985). Canine cyclic motor activity of stomach and small bowel: the governor is not the vagus. *Gastroenterology*, **88**, 1926–31
16. Yanda, R. and Summers, R. W. (1983). Activity fronts in fed dogs: effect of β-adrenergic agonist. *Am. J. Physiol.*, **245**, G647–50
17. Sarna, S. K., Condon, R. E. and Cowles, V. (1983). The enteric mechanisms of initiation of migrating myoelectric complexes (MMCs) in dogs. *Gastroenterology*, **84**, 814–22
18. Matsumoto, T., Frantzides, C., Sarna, S. K., Condon, R. E. and Cowles, V. E. (1986). Differential sensitivities of morphine and motilin to initiate migrating motor complex in isolated intestinal segments. *Gastroenterology*, **90**, 61–7
19. Sarna, S. K., Stoddard, C., Belbeck, L. and McWade, D. (1981). Intrinsic nervous control of migrating myoelectric complexes. *Am. J. Physiol.*, **241**, G16–23
20. Lang, I. M., Sarna, S. K. and Condon, R. E. (1986). The generation of phases I and II of the migrating myoelectric complex in the dog. *Am. J. Physiol.*, **251**, G201–7
21. Frantzides, C. T., Sarna, S. K., Matsumoto, T., Lang, I. M. and Condon, R. E. (1987). An intrinsic neural pathway for long intestino-intestinal inhibitory reflexes. *Gastroenterology*, **92**, 594–603

52
Stress-induced changes of gastrointestinal transit in the rat

P. ENCK, M. WIENBECK AND J. F. ERCKENBRECHT

Previous investigations of stress effects on gastrointestinal transit in animals have produced conflicting results[1,2,3]. These were due to different stress models used, unphysiological marker techniques, and the lack of recording techniques allowing for multiple measurements in individual animals. We therefore investigated the effects of a novel, and mainly psychological, stress model on gastric emptying, orocaecal transit and colonic transit in rats.

METHODS

Female Wistar rats (c. 200 g) were trained to eat 5 or 15 g of solid food (dry food mixed with water 1:1) within 5 and 30 min, respectively. Gastric emptying was assessed by determining stomach content (percentage of oral intake) after various periods of stress and after rest. Orocaecal transit was measured by breath hydrogen exhalation[4] after the food had been mixed with 1 g of lactose. Colonic transit was measured by the arrival of coloured faeces after infusion of a carmine-red solution into the caecum via a chronically implanted catheter. Stress effects on colonic transit were investigated after i.p. injections of NaCl, naloxone (3 mg/kg b.w.) or propranolol (10 mg/kg b.w.). Faecal pellet output (mean number of pellets/30 min) was controlled under rest and stress. The stressor applied in all experiments was a 'passive avoidance' situation[5] allowing the animal to avoid contact with water at body temperature by sitting on a small platform (Figure 1).

RESULTS

All animals easily learned to consume their daily nutrients within a predefined period. Rats on a restricted feeding schedule maintained their body weight after an initial drop (Figure 2).

Gastric emptying (T/2) showed a significant delay under stress (2.66 h) as

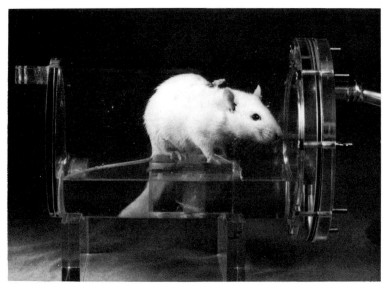

Figure 1 Stress box used for all experiments. The volume of the box is 2500 cc, and it is filled with 500 ml of water at body temperature (30°C). The animals could avoid water contact by climbing onto a plexi glass block (5 x 4 x 3 cm)

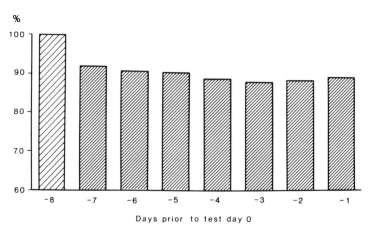

Figure 2 Weight of the animals during the restricted feeding schedule training (day −8 to day 0), expressed as percentage of initial weight at day −8

compared to rest (1.97 h) ($p < 0.05$). Orocaecal transit was 131 min at rest and accelerated to 86 min under stress ($p < 0.05$). Colonic transit significantly ($p < 0.01$) decreased from 13.9 h to 1.25 h (Figure 3).

Faecal pellet output increased from 0.0 at rest to 4.0/30 min under stress. Stress effects on colonic transit could only partly be blocked by either propanolol or naloxone.

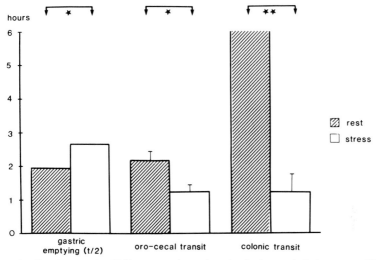

Figure 3 Gastric emptying (T/2), orocaecal transit and colonic transit (in hours, x̄ ± SEM) at rest (left column) and under stress (right column)

DISCUSSION

Stress has differential effects on gastrointestinal transit in rats: it delays gastric emptying but accelerates small bowel transit and colonic transit. These effects are only partly under control of adrenergic pathways or endogenous opioids.

Acknowledgements

Supported by grants En 50/2-1 and Wi 285/5-1 from the Deutsche Forschungsgemeinschaft.

References

1. Gue, M., Fioramonti, J. and Bueno, L. (1987). Disturbance of gastric emptying and intestinal transit induced by acoustic and cold stress in mice. *Am. J. Physiol.*, **253**, G124–8
2. Williams, C. L. Villar, R. G., Peterson, J. M. and Burks, T. F. (1987). Stress-induced changes in intestinal transit in the rat: A model for irritable bowel syndrome. *Gastroenterology*, **94**, 611–21
3. Lenz, H. J., Raedler, A., Greten, H. and Brown, M. R. (1987). CRF initiates biological actions within the brain that are observed in response to stress. *Am. J. Physiol.*, **252**, R34–9
4. Brown, N. J., Rumsey, R. D. E and Read, N. W. (1987). Adaptation of hydrogen analysis to measure stomach to caecum transit time in the rat. *Gut*, **28**, 849–54
5. Mowrer, O. H. (1960). *Learning Theory and Behavior*. (New York: Wiley)

53
CNS opioid influences on intestinal water and electrolyte transport in dogs

M. P. PRIMI AND L. BUENO

There is substantial evidence that opiate agonists develop potent antisecretory action through a direct action on the intestinal mucosa. Endogenous opiates such as enkephalins also exert antisecretory effects at intestinal level but it has been recently postulated that a CNS origin of this activity, or a part of it, cannot be excluded. The present studies were therefore undertaken in the conscious dog in order to evaluate the effects of intracerebroventricular vs. peripheral administration of a stable enkephalin analogue (D-Ala^2, Met^5) enkephalinamide (DALAMIDE) on water and electrolyte transport in the normal and cholera toxin treated intestine and to determine if such effects are related to changes in propulsive activity. These investigations were then extended to other opioid agonists with selective affinity for the classical receptor subtypes to pinpoint the nature of receptors and pathways involved using adrenergic and opiate antagonists. Two groups of six dogs equipped with a 1 m Thiry–Vella (TV) loop of the proximal jejunum and an intracerebroventricular (i.c.v.) cannula were used in these studies. Intestinal transport in the TV loop and concomitant transit time were measured during an infusion (1 ml/min) of an isotonic electrolyte solution alone or containing 0.4 μg/ml of cholera toxin (CT).

In the first series of experiments, basal net water absorption was slightly, but significantly ($p < 0.05$), increased during an i.c.v. infusion of DALAMIDE at 0.5 ng/kg/min, while the secretory effects of cholera toxin were markedly reduced by nearly 75%. Similar effects were observed for Na$^+$ and K$^+$ movement. In contrast, DALAMIDE infused intravenously at a five times higher dose, i.e. 2.5 ng/kg/min did not affect the control and CT-stimulated water and electrolyte movements. The jejunal loop transit times were halved during CT infusion and similar values were observed under DALAMIDE i.c.v. administration.

In the second series of experiments we tested comparatively the effect of selective μ (DAGO), μ and δ (DADLE) and κ (Dynorphin$_{1-13}$) opioid peptide. Similarly to DALAMIDE, DAGO i.c.v. infused at similar dosage (0.5 ng/kg/min) significantly increased the basal net water absorption while DADLE and Dynorphin$_{1-13}$ at similar infusion rate, had no effect. DAGO also markedly reduced by 79.5%, the secretory effects of cholera toxin (0.4 μg/ml). Similar effects were obtained with DALAMIDE and DAGO, when injected i.c.v. as a bolus (100 ng/kg) prior to cholera toxin infusion; they were suppressed after i.v. pretreatment with naltrexone (0.3 mg/kg) but also with propranolol (0.2 mg/kg). In contrast, i.v. phentolamine (0.2 mg/kg) and bilateral truncal vagotomy were unable to block such effects.

These results suggest that (1) Met-Enkephalin and analogues can act centrally to affect intestinal transport of water and electrolytes in dogs and these effects were unrelated to changes in the rate of flow as a consequence of motor alterations; (2) they act probably at central μ receptor and these effects are mediated through central or peripheral β-adrenergic pathways; (3) only μ subtype of opioid receptors seems involved in the CNS control of intestinal secretions.

54
Functional properties of lumbar sympathetic preganglionic neurons regulating motility of hindgut and lower urinary tract

A. BOCZEK-FUNCKE, H.-J. HÄBLER, W. JÄNIG AND
M. MICHAELIS

The distal colon and the urinary bladder receive a dual extrinsic autonomic innervation. The parasympathetic supply that originates mainly in the sacral spinal cord and projects through the pelvic nerves is undoubtedly essential for the regulation of evacuation and continence of both organ systems. The sympathetic preganglionic neurons have their cell bodies in the lumbar spinal cord and project through tne lumbar splanchric nerves; a small part may also project through the distal lumbar sympathetic chain[1]. Electrical stimulation of the lumbar sympathetic outflow leads to relaxation of the colon and contraction of the internal anal sphincter; the trigone and proximal urethra contract, whereas the detrusor may relax after an initial, weak contraction[1,2,3]. The functional significance of this sympathetic outflow for the regulation of continence and evacuation of both organs is still unclear, though there is strong experimental evidence that it exerts powerful inhibition on colonic motility under normal conditions[1,3,4]. Neurophysiological analysis of the discharge patterns of single sympathetic preganglionic neurons projecting to the evacuative organs in the cat shows that each organ system may receive its own sympathetic supply and that these sympathetic supplies are distinct from the sympathetic supply to the blood vessels. The important approach in this analysis was to use the sacral afferent input systems from the pelvic organs as afferent test systems to elicit reflexes in the visceral sympathetic neurons[1,5].

Experiments were performed on chloralose-anaesthetized, paralysed and artificially ventilated cats with intact neuraxis. Activity was recorded from the axons of single preganglionic sympathetic neurons that project in the lumbar splanchnic nerves. A double-chamber rubber balloon was inserted into the colon so that the distal and the more proximal part of this organ could be distended separately. The urinary bladder was distended by small amounts of fluid injected through a urethral catheter. The intracolonic and intravesical pressures were continuously measured. The mucosa of the anal canal was stimulated by mechanical shearing stimuli (see ref. 5 for details).

Three major populations of sympathetic preganglionic neurons that project to the inferior mesenteric ganglion could be discriminated according to their reflex patterns. Neurons of the first group are probably associated with blood vessels and therefore called vasoconstrictor neurons. They behave qualitatively like muscle vasoconstrictor neurons[6] and are strongly influenced by cardiovascular stimuli and weakly by stimuli applied to the pelvic viscera. The second group of neurons is not influenced by cardiovascular stimuli but exhibits distinct reflexes on the visceral stimuli used. These neurons are probably associated with the functions of colon and urinary bladder and are therefore called 'motility-regulating' (MR) neurons. Neurons of the third group do not display any reflexes so far investigated and possibly project to the internal reproductive organs[1].

The MR neurons can further be classified into three subtypes by way of the reflex responses evoked by natural stimulation of the afferents from urinary bladder, colon and anal canal. These three patterns of reflexes are shown in Table 1, Figure 1 illustrates, as an example, the reflex pattern of an MR1 neuron. This type of MR neuron is the most common one: it is excited from the urinary bladder, inhibited from the colon and mostly excited from the anal canal. MR2 neurons are more difficult to detect and exhibit a reflex pattern which is reciprocal to that of the MR1 neurons. Very often these neurons display only either excitation from the colon or inhibition from the urinary bladder. MRA neurons are only excited (or rarely inhibited) from the anal canal.

We propose that MR1 neurons project to the hindgut. This would mean that colon distension abolishes inhibition of colonic motility, allowing the organ to contract, and leads to relaxation of internal anal sphincter. Sacral afferent firing from the urinary bladder which occurs during micturition may increase activity in MR1 neurons, inhibiting in this way colonic motility and activating the internal anal sphincter, thus preventing defaecation. We propose furthermore that the MR2 neurons influence, complementary to the MR1 neurons, the lower urinary tract. This functional interpretation of both types of sympathetic neurons is consistent with the well-known observation that contractions of colon and urinary bladder occur alternatively. MRA

Table 1 Subclassification of lumbar preganglionic motility regulating (MR) neurons

| MR-type (%) | Stimulation of afferents from: | | | Proposed projection to |
	colon	urinary bladder	anal mucosa	
MR1 (55%)	− or ∅	+	Mostly +	Colon
MR2 (29%)	+	− or ∅	Mostly +	Urinary bladder
MRA (12%)	∅	∅	Mostly +	?

+ excitation, − inhibition, ∅ no effect

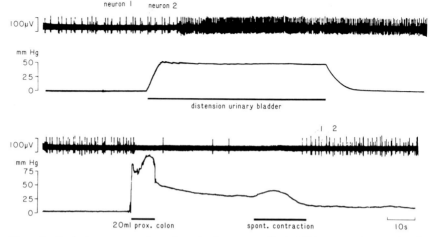

Figure 1 Typical response pattern of two lumbar preganglionic MR1 neurons (neuron 1 and 2) to distension of the urinary bladder and to distension and contraction of the proximal colon in the cat. Both neurons were activated to the first stimulus and inhibited to the second. The neurons projected into the lumbar splanchnic nerves. The activity was recorded from their axons. The cat was anaesthetized with chloralose, artificially ventilated and immobilized with pancuronium bromide

neurons may exert general inhibition on both evacuative organ systems.

The reflex patterns of the MR neurons (MR1, MR2, MRA) are not only found in lumbar preganglionic neurons but also in post-ganglionic neurons that project in the hypogastric nerves[1,7]. This, and the finding that the frequencies of the different types of MR neurons are similar at the pre- and post-ganglionic sites[1] argue that the central messages are faithfully relayed to the target organs. As far as the sympathetic innervation of the colon via the inferior mesenteric ganglion is concerned, it is unclear in which way the post-ganglionic neurons integate preganglionic synaptic activity and synaptic inputs of peripheral origin arising from the enteric plexuses. It is conceivable to assume that both types of synaptic input summate, leading to suprathreshold activation of the post-ganglionic neurons even when both synaptic inputs are subthreshold[8,9].

In summary, we conclude that the reflexes in sympathetic MR1 and MR2 neurons are organized in a reciprocal fashion with respect to the colon and urinary bladder. The same type of reciprocal organization has previously been shown to exist for the sacral parasympathetic outflow[10]. We propose that MR1 neurons are associated with the hindgut and MR2 neurons with the lower urinary tract, both types of neurons conveying multiple viscerovisceral reflexes.

Acknowledgements

Supported by the Deutsche Forschungsgemeinschaft.

References

1. Jänig, W. and McLachlan, E. M. (1987). Organization of lumbar spinal outflow to distal colon and pelvic organs. *Physiol. Rev.*, **67**, 1332–1404
2. Gonella, J., Bouvier, M. and Blanquet, F. (1987). Extrinsic nervous control of motility of small and large intestines and related sphincters. *Physiol. Rev.*, **67**, 902–61
3. Roman, C. and Gonella, J. (1987). Extrinsic control of digestive tract motility. In Johnson, L. R. (ed.) *Physiology of the Gastrointestinal Tract*, 2nd Edn., pp. 507–53. (New York: Raven Press)
4. Hulten, L. (1969). Extrinsic nervous control of colonic motility and blood flow. An experimental study in the cat. *Acta Physiol. Scand.*, **335**(Suppl.), 1–116
5. Bahr, R., Bartel, B., Blumberg, H. and Jänig, W. (1986). Functional characterization of preganglionic neurons projecting in the lumbar splanchnic nerves: neurons regulating motility. *J. Auton. Nerv. Syst.*, **15**, 109–30
6. Jänig, W. (1988). Pre- and postganglionic vasoconstrictor neurons differentiation, types, and discharge properties. *Annu. Rev. Physiol.*, **50**, 525–39
7. Jänig, W., Schmidt, M., Schnitzler, A. and Wesselmann, U. (1987). Functional types of sympathetic post-ganglionic neurones projecting into the hypogastric nerves of the cat. *J. Physiol. (Lond.)*, **390**, 34p
8. Jänig, W. (1988). Integration of gut function by sympathetic reflexes. In Grundy, G. and Read, N. W. (eds.) *Bailliére's Clinical Gastroenterology: Gastrointestinal Neurophysiology*, Vol. 2, No. 1, pp. 45–62. (London: Baillière Tindall)
9. Szurszewski, J. H. (1981). Physiology of mammalian prevertebral ganglia. *Annu. Rev. Physiol.*, **43**, 53–68
10. De Groat, W. C., Nadelhaft, I., Milne, R. J., Booth, A. M., Morgan, C. and Thor, K. (1981). Organization of the sacral parasympathetic reflex pathways to the urinary bladder and large intestine. *J. Auton. Nerv. Syst.*, **3**, 135–60

**Section V
Psychovisceral and Behavioural
Aspects of Gut Function and
Dysfunction**

55
Sham feeding: cephalic-vagal influences on gastric myoelectric activity in humans

R. M. STERN, K. L. KOCH, H. E. CRAWFORD, M. W. VASEY AND W. R. STEWART

The electrogastrogram (EGG) response to the ingestion of food is an increase in amplitude of 3 cpm waves. We hypothesized that sham feeding would stimulate a similar, but perhaps, briefer myoelectric response. Numerous studies have demonstrated the presence of cephalic-vagal gastrointestinal secretory reflexes in humans and lower animals with intact vagi, but few reports of cephalic phase gastric *motor* responses have been found. In the present study sham feeding was used to stimulate cephalic-vagal pathways and electrogastrographic methods were used to measure gastric myoelectric activity.

EGGs were obtained from 47 healthy human subjects before, during and after sham feeding, and before, during and after eating. The subjects chewed and expectorated a hot dog on a roll and later ate a second hot dog. The EGGs obtained from Experiment I ($n = 27$) were handscored and group means compared with a dependent t-test. Amplitude of the 3 cpm waves increased significantly (18.9 mm to 30.3 mm, $p < 0.01$) from before to during sham feeding. However, by 2 min after sham feeding the mean amplitude of the EGG had returned to baseline level. The increase in EGG amplitude from before to during eating was significant (18.6 mm to 26.6 mm, $p < 0.01$), and this increase in activity was still at a level significantly above baseline 3 min post-prandial. Visual inspection of the raw data indicated that, for most subjects, the duration of the post-prandial increase in amplitude of the EGG was approximately 30 min. Experiment II ($n = 20$) was conducted with an identical procedure to Experiment I, but EGGs were computer analysed. Power estimates comprising the frequency band from 2.5–3.5 cpm were averaged and submitted to a repeated measures analysis of variance. The increase in power from before to during sham feeding was significant ($F = 4.44$, $p < 0.05$). The increase in power from before to during eating was significant ($F = 6.36$, $p < 0.02$). As was the case in Experiment I, the increase in power during sham feeding was of brief duration compared to the post-prandial increase. Four vagotomized subjects failed to show any change in their EGG during or immediately after sham feeding.

CONCLUSIONS

Sham feeding in healthy human subjects increases the amplitude of 3 cpm gastric myoelectric activity.

The increase in post-prandial 3 cpm amplitude is prolonged reflecting initial cephalic-vagal activity and subsequent gastric stimulation by luminal contents.

Hand-scored 3 cpm EGG amplitude and computer analysis of 2.5–3.5 cpm EGG power yielded similar results.

The EGG response to sham feeding is a non-invasive method for studying relationships between cephalic-vagal and gastric myoelectric activity in healthy subjects and patients with a variety of gastrointestial disorders.

56
Two sites of action of κ-opioid substances on stress-induced gastric motor inhibition in fasted dogs

L. BUENO, M. GUE, X. PASCAUD AND J. L. JUNIEN

INTRODUCTION

Endogenous opioids are involved in respones to many stressors and exposure to stressful stimuli can produce opiate-like alterations that are reversed by the opiate antagonist naloxone in both rats[1] and humans[2]. Furthermore, some changes in gastrointestinal motility[3] or gastric emptying[4] associated with centrally acting stressful stimuli are reduced by the concomitant infusion of naloxone and adrenergic blockers[5].

It was demonstrated recently that κ-agonists, such as dynorphin, act through specific opioid receptors to inhibit corticotropin releasing factor (CRF) release from the rat hypothalamus[6-8]. On the other hand, Bechara et al.[9], have shown that κ-receptors located outside the blood–brain barrier (especially in the gut) are primarily responsible for mediating the aversive effects of opiates in rats. Consequently, the present study was performed in dogs to evaluate comparatively the effects of centrally and peripherally administration of μ- and κ-opioid agonists on gastric motor inhibition and the associated increase in plasma cortisol level induced by acoustic stress as previously described[10].

MATERIALS AND METHODS

Six adult mongrel dogs weighing 15–18 kg were used for these experiments. Under Halothane (Fluothane U.D.) anaesthesia, three strain-gauge transducers constructed according to a method previously described[11] were sewn on the stomach 15 and 7 cm from the pylorus and on the proximal jejunum 60 cm from the ligament of Treitz. In addition, a stainless steel cannula, 19 mm long, was implanted into the right lateral ventricle of the brain through a hole made on the frontal base 2 mm posterior to the bregma and 5 mm lateral to the sagittal suture.

In four animals, a silicone catheter was also inserted into the jugular vein. At the end of surgery, the free ends of the strain-gauge wires and the catheter were brought subcutaneously to the back of the neck, and the animals were allowed to recover 10–15 days before beginning the experiments. Each day at 17.00, the dogs received a standard meal of 600 g of canned food (Fidèle-Quaker, France).

Gastrointestinal mechanical activity was recorded continuously 23 h per day connecting the strain gauges on a 4-channel Wheatsone bridge amplifier (Vishay, France) connected to a potentiometric recorder (Rikadenki, Japan). Amplitude calibration of each strain gauge was performed before implantation. The experiments were performed at 2-day intervals and 15-h after the last meal.

First series of experiments

40–50 min after the occurrence of a gastric migrating motor complex (MMC), the animals were subjected to music by earphones (80–90 dB) for 1 h according to a procedure previously described[12]. In the animals equipped with jugular catheter, blood samples for plasma cortisol measurements were taken at 15 min intervals from 30 min before vs. 30 min after acoustic stress (AS). AS was preceded (10 min) by intracerebroventricular (i.c.v.) administration of sterilized saline (vehicle) or saline containing various concentrations of dynorphin$^{1-13}$, (Sigma, Laverpillière, France) (10–100 ng/kg), U 50488 (Upjohn, Kalameazoo, MI) (20 ng/kg) and [D-Ala^2, N-Me, P-nitro-Phe^4, Gly^5-ol] enkephalin (Dago, Sigma, France) (20–200 ng/kg). Each treatment was applied without AS as control.

Second series of experiments

AS was performed 30 min after oral administration of ethylketocyclazocine (EKC) (Sterling Winthrop Research Institute, Guildford, UK) and U 50488 at 10 and 100 μg/kg.

Last series of experiments

Ovine CRF (Sigma, France) was injected i.c.v. at a dose of 100 ng/kg, 10 min after previous administration of EKC (50 mg/kg i.c.v.), U 50488 (20 ng/kg i.c.v.), or vehicle.

Motor effects were assessed by measuring the duration of gastric and/or jejunal disruption of the MMC pattern. The values were expressed as mean $\pm$ SE and were compared by analysis of variance and Student's t-test. Plasma cortisol was determined by high performance liquid chromatography according to a method previously described[13].

RESULTS

Influence of i.c.v. administration of κ- vs. μ-agonists

The mechanical activity of the stomach in 14–17 h fasted dogs was characterized by cyclic phases of grouped contractions lasting 28 ± 9 min ($n = 12$) and occurring at 1.5–2 h intervals (Figure 1). This antral contraction, also called migrating motor complex (MMC), was associated with the occurrence of jejunal motor activity, migrating aborally. One hour exposure to AS delayed by 114% the occurrence of the next gastric MMC while the jejunal MMCs were still present at a normal frequency (Figure 1 and Table 1). There was no difference in gastric response in naive and previously tested animals. During AS, plasma cortisol increased significantly ($p < 0.05$) and reached a maximal value 30 min after the beginning of AS (51.8 ± 8.2 ng/ml

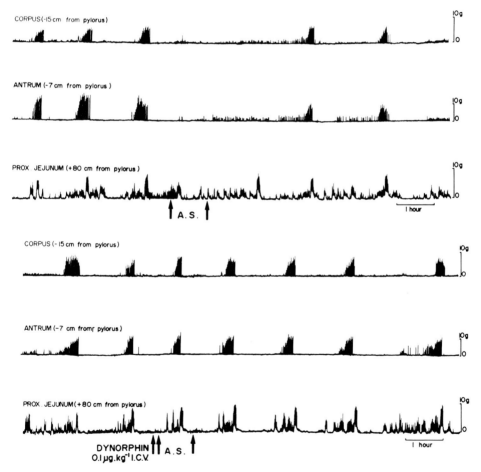

Figure 1 Influence of acoustic stress (AS) and previous intracerebroventricular (i.c.v.) administration of dynorphin$_{1-13}$ on gastrointestinal motility in a fasted dog

Table 1 Comparative influence of dynorphin, EKC, U 50488 and DAGO centrally administered on acoustic stress-induced lengthening of duration of gastric MMC cycle in fasted dogs

	Dose (ng/kg) i.c.v.	Minutes	
		Control	Acoustic stress
Vehicle		76 ± 36	189 ± 46*
Dynorphin$_{1-13}$	10	89 ± 10	146 ± 31*
	20	111 ± 24	88 ± 27†
	100	106 ± 13	101 ± 16
EKC	10	86 ± 17	91 ± 13†
	20	110 ± 31	108 ± 12†
U 50488	20	104 ± 16	105 ± 16†
DAGO	20	108 ± 17	199 ± 44*
	100	111 ± 18	176 ± 29
	200	269 ± 34†	

*†: significantly ($p < 0.05$) different from corresponding control or vehicle values, respectively

vs. 9.6 ± 2.7 ng/ml in control).

Intracerebroventricular administration of dynorphin$_{1-13}$ at a dose of 20 ng/kg 10 min before AS completely abolished the gastric hypomotility induced by AS (Table 1). Similarly, EKC (10 and 20 ng/kg) and U 50488 (20 ng/kg) injected by i.c.v. route suppressed the AS-induced lengthening of the MMC cycle (Table 1). In contrast, DAGO injected centrally (< 200 ng/kg) was unable to block the AS-induced gastric motor changes. Dynorphin$_{1-13}$ injected i.c.v. at doses of 100 ng/kg significantly ($p < 0.01$) reduced by 74.6% the rise in plasma cortisol level associated with AS (Figure 2) while dynorphin had no effect *per se* on plasma cortisol. These effects are reproduced by i.c.v. administration of EKC (10 and 20 ng/kg), but not by central administration of DAGO (100 ng/kg) where plasma cortisol reached 41.1 ± 5.4 ng/ml vs. 36.9 ± 8.1 ng/ml in control conditions (vehicle).

Influence of oral administration of κ- and μ-agonists

Oral administration of U 50488 at a dose of 10 μg/kg abolished the lengthening of the gastric MMC induced by AS. EKC only partially reduced this effect while it has no effect *per se* on gastric and intestinal motility (Table 2).

Influence of EKC and U 50488 on CRF-induced gastric motor inhibition and increase in plasma cortisol

As well as AS, i.c.v. administration of CRF delayed the occurrence of a gastric MMC[14]. Both EKC (50 ng/kg) and U 50488 (20 ng/kg) centrally administered 10 min before i.c.v. administration of oCRF (100 ng/kg) were unable to block the inhibitory effect of CRF on gastric MMC (Table 3).

Table 2 Effects of previous oral (p.o.) administration of ethylketocyclazocine (EKC) and U 50488 on the duration (in minutes) of migrating motor complex (MMC) cycles and their lengthening induced by acoustic stress (mean ± SE, t-test, $p < 0.05$)

	Basal	Acoustic stress Before	Acoustic stress After
Control	77 ± 25	87 ± 13	194 ± 39†
EKC			
10 μg/kg p.o.	92 ± 7	96 ± 11	131 ± 21*†
100 μg/kg p.o.	139 ± 27*	—	—
U 50488 H			
10 μg/kg p.o.	101 ± 20	91 ± 19	102 ± 27*
100 μg/kg p.o.	186 ± 39*	—	—

* significantly different from corresponding control values.
† significantly different from values observed before acoustic stress

i.c.v. Administration of oCRF (100 ng/kg) also increased the plasma cortisol level. The administration of EKC and/or U 50488 had no effect on the hypercortisolemia induced by oCRF.

DISCUSSION

These experiments show that i.c.v. administration of κ but not μ substances act centrally to block the inhibition of gastric motility and plasma cortisol increase induced by AS. Blockade of the AS-induced hypomotility and associated cortisol release by diazepam and muscimol[12] and the similarity with the effects of centrally administered CRF[14], have led us to speculate that CRF release is involved in the central mediation of AS-induced inhibition of gastric motility. It may therefore be postulated that κ-opioid agonist affect the release of CRF; in addition, the lack of effect of κ-agonist centrally administered, on the gastric hypomotility and the associated increase in plasma cortisol level, induced by exogenous CRF, reinforced this hypothesis.

Numerous studies have demonstrated that endogenous peptides are involved in CNS control of pituitary hormones release[15–17]. It has been demonstrated recently that dynorphin an endogenous ligand for κ-receptors[18] and has selective opioid effects on the secretion of anterior pituitary hormones[19] and on feeding behaviour[20,21]. Yajima et al. (1981) have shown, by use of a hypothalamic perfusion system in vitro, that dynorphin$_{1-13}$ reduces the release of CRF from rat hypothalamus.

The similarity between the antagonistic action of dynorphin$_{1-13}$ and EKC on AS-induced gastric motor inhibition and cortisol release suggests the selective involvement of κ-receptors on this model. Furthermore, a local action of κ-opioid agonists is also suspected, by the fact that a blockade of the lengthening of gastric MMC induced by AS is also obtained by oral administration of U 50488, a potent and selective κ agonist which does not develop μ-agonist action in vivo[22]. Absence of complete blockade by EKC could be due to its lower affinity for κ-receptors[23] but also to additional μ_2

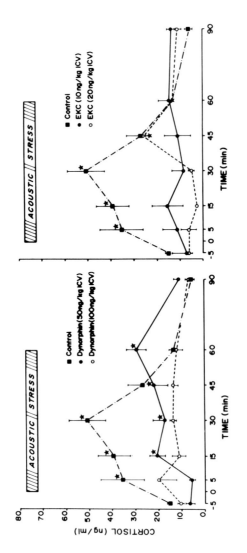

Figure 2 Comparative effects of intracerebroventricular (i.c.v.) administration of dynorphin and ethylketocyclazocine (EKC) on plasma cortisol changes associated with acoustic stress in dogs (mean ± SE, $n = 4$ dogs)
$* p \leqslant 0.05$: (*t*-test), significantly different from control values

Table 3 Comparative influence of EKC and U 50488 centrally administered on ovine CRF-induced inhibition of gastric MMC cycle (duration in minutes) in dogs (mean $\pm$ SE, $n = 6$ dogs)

	Control	Ovine CRF (100 ng/kg i.c.v.)
Vehicle	76 ± 36	213 ± 46*
EKC 50 ng/kg i.c.v.	86 ± 17	192 ± 45*
U 50488 20 ng/kg i.c.v.	104 ± 16	220 ± 38*

* significantly ($p \leqslant 0.05$) different from corresponding control values

and ... antagonistic properties[8,22]. These results are consistent with several studies showing that opiate receptors are present in the gastric and intestinal wall[24,25] particularly in dog, a species presenting nerve cells that contain opiate enkephalin and dynorphin peptide immunoreactive materials in the submucosal plexus, muscularis mucosae and villi of the stomach, pylorus and proximal intestine[26].

Finally, the present work indicates that κ-agonists may exert centrally mediated inhibitory effects on AS-induced gastric motor alterations and cortisol release by inhibiting the CNS release of CRF. It provides evidence of a direct link between peripheral stimulation of opiate receptors located in the gastrointestinal tract and CNS but the level of interaction remains partly unknown and requires further investigations.

Acknowledgements

The authors acknowledge the expert technical assistance of G. Bories and C. del Rio and the secretarial assistance of A. Cortes.

This research was supported by the Institut National de la Recherche Agronomique and by Jouveinal Laboratories.

References

1. Lewis, J. W., Sherman, J. E. and Lieheskind, J. C. (1981). Opioid and non-opioid stress analgesia: assessment of tolerance and cross-tolerance with morphine. *J. Neurosci.*, **1**, 358–63
2. Willer, J. C., Dehen, H. and Cambien, J. (1981). Stress-induced analgesis in humans: endogenous opioids and naloxone-reversible depression of pain reflexes. *Science (Wash. DC)*, **212**, 689–91
3. Stanghellini, V., Malagelada, J. R., Zinsmeister, A. R., Go, V. L. and Kao, P. C. (1983). Stress-induced gastroduodenal motor disturbances in humans: possible humoral mechanisms. *Gastroenterology*, **85**, 83-9
4. Thompson, D. G., Richelson, E. and Malagelada, J. R. (1983). Perturbation of upper gastrointestinal function by cold stress. *Gut*, **24**, 277–81
5. Stanghellini, V., Malagelada, J. R., Zinsmeister, A. R., Go, V. L. M. and Kao, P. C. (1984). Effect of opiate and adrenergic blockers on the gut motor response to centrally acting stimuli (Abstract). *Gastroenterology*, **87**, 1104

6. Yajima, F., Suda, T., Tomori, N., Takashi, S., Nakagami, Y., Ushiyama, T., Demura, H. and Shizume, K. (1986). Effects of opioid peptides on immunoreactive corticotropin releasing factor release from the rat hypothalamus in vitro. *Life Sci.*, **39**, 181–6

7. Plotsky, P. M. (1986). Opioid inhibition of immunoreactive corticotropin-releasing factor secretion into the hypophysial-portal circulation of rats. *Regul. Pept.*, **16**, 235–42

8. Iyengar, S., Kim, H. S. and Wood, P. L. (1986). Kappa opiate agonists modulate the hypothalamic-pituitary-adrenocortical axis in the rat. *J. Pharmacol. Exp. Ther.*, **238**, 429–36

9. Bechara, A. and Van der Kooy, D. (1987). Kappa receptors mediate the peripheral aversive effects of opiates. *Pharmacol. Biochem. Behav.*, **28**(2), 227–33

10. Gue, M., Fioramonti, J., Frexinos, J., Alvinerie, M. and Bueno, L. (1987). Influence of acoustic stress by noise on gastrointestinal motility in dogs. *Dig. Dis. Sci.*, **32**, 1411–17

11. Pascaud, X., Genton, M. J. and Bass, P. (1978). A miniature transducer for recording intestinal motility in unrestrained chronic rats. *Am. J. Physiol.*, **235** (*Endocrinol. Metab. Gastrointest. Physiol.*, **4**), E532–9

12. Gue, M. and Bueno, L. (1986). Diazepam and muscimol blockade of the gastrointestinal motor disturbances induced by acoustic stress in dogs. *Eur. J. Pharmacol.*, **131**, 123–7

13. Alvinerie, M. and Toutain, P. L. Simultaneous determination of corticosterone, hydrocortisone and dexamethasone in dog plasma using high performance liquid chromatography. *J. Pharmacol. Sci.*, **71**, 816–18

14. Bueno, L., Fargeas, M. J., Gue, M., Peeters, T. L., Bormans, V. and Fioramonti, J. (1986). Effects of corticotropin releasing factor on plasma motilin and somatostatin levels and gastrointestinal motility in dogs. *Gastroenterology*, **91**, 884–9

15. Gilbeau, P. M., Almirez, R. G., Holaday, J. W. and Smith, C. G. (1985). Opioid effects on plasma concentrations of luteinizing hormone and prolactin in the adult male rhesus monkey. *J. Clin. Endocrinol. Metab.*, **60**, 299–305

16. Morley, J. E., Willenbring, M. L., Krahn, D. D., Carlson, G. A., Buggs, J. E., Levine, A. S. and Shafer, R. B. (1984). Opioid control of thyroid function. In Delitala, G., Motta, M. and Serio, M. (eds.) *Opioid Modulation of Endocrine Function*, pp. 267–75. (New York: Raven Press)

17. Ropert, J. F., Quigley, M. E. and Yen, S. S. C. (1981). Endogenous opiates modulate pulsatile luteinizing hormone release in humans. *J. Clin. Endocrinol. Metab.*, **52**, 583–7

18. Chavkin, C., James, I. F. and Goldstein, A. (1982). Dynorphin is a specific endogenous ligand of the kappa opioid receptor. *Science* (*Wash. DC*), **215**, 413–15

19. Grossman, A., Gaillard, R. C., McCartney, P., Rees, L. H. and Besser, G. M. (1982). Opiate modulation of the pituitary adrenal axis: effects of stress and circadian rhythm. *Clin. Endocrinol.*, **17**, 279–86

20. Baile, C. A., Keim, D. A., Della-Ferra, M. A. and McLaughlin, C. L. (1981). Opiate antagonists and agonists and feeding in sheep. *Physiol. Behav.*, **26**, 1019–23

21. Jackson, A. and Cooper, S. J. (1986). The involvement of the kappa opiate receptor in the control of food intake in the rat. *Neuropharmacology*, **25**, 653–4

22. Wood, P. L. (1984). Kappa agonist analgesics: evidence for mu^2 and delta opioid receptor antagonism. *Drug. Dev. Res.*, **4**, 429

23. Lahti, R. A., Mickelson, M. M. and Van Voiglanter, P. F. (1985). [^{3}H]-69593 a highly selective ligand for opioid K receptor. *Eur. J. Pharmacol.*, **109**, 281–6

24. Costa, M., Furness, J. B., Gibbins, I. L. and Murphy, R. (1985). Chemical coding and projections of opioid peptide containing neurons in the guinea-pig intestine. *Neurosci. Lett.*, **S19**

25. Schulzberg, M., Hokfelt, T., Nilssen, G., Terenius, L., Rehfeld, J. F., Brown, M., Elde, R., Goldstein, M. and Said, S. (1980). Distribution of peptide and catechol-containing neurones in the gastrointestinal tract of rat and guinea pig: immuno-histochemical studies with antisera to substance-P, vasoactive intestinal polypeptide, enkephalins, somatostatin, gastrin/cholecystokinin, neurotensin and dopamine β-hydroxylase. *Neuroscience*, **5**, 689–93

26. Daniel, E. E., Fox, J. E. T., Allescher, H. D., Ahmad, S. and Kostolanska, F. (1987). Peripheral actions of opiates in canine gastrointestinal tract: actions on nerves and muscles. *Gastroenterol. Clin. Biol.*, **11**, 35–8

57
Cerebral responses after electrical stimulation of the gut: a new approach to the investigation of visceral afferents

T. FRIELING, P. ENCK AND M. WIENBECK

Afferent nervous pathways play an important role in the physiology of the gastrointestinal tract, but methodological difficulties impeded investigation. We used the method of producing cerebral evoked potentials (EPs), by electrical stimulation known from the peripheral nervous system, in order to study visceral afferents from the oesophagus (O) and rectosigmoid colon (R) in 11 and 8 healthy male volunteers, 20–40 years old. The stimulus was applied via a probe containing bipolar Ag/AgCl electrodes which were sucked to the mucosa (O, 20 and 37 cm inc.; R, 20 cm above ano.). Voltage of stimulation (duration, 0.1 ms; frequency, 0.1, 0.2, 0.5, 1 and 3 Hz, random stimulation) was increased, until the volunteers perceived a non-painful sensation. EPs were recorded from the vertex (Cz, 10–20 international system) and forehead (Fz, reference electrode) by EEG-needle electrodes. They were averaged over 20–300 sweeps. Control experiments were done without S and after S of the median and tibial nerves (3 Hz). We evaluated upward (N) and downward (P) deflections of EPs (latencies and amplitudes) (Table 1).

Reproducible EPs were obtained in each volunteer. Amplitudes of EPs were significantly increased with a stimulation frequency of 0.5 and 0.2 Hz compared to 0.5 and 1 Hz. No EPs were recorded without stimulation. Amplitudes of EPs were increased with randomized stimulation and EPs from 37 cm inclusive showed longer latencies (delay: 20 to 35 ms) compared to those from 20 cm inclusive. Stimulation of peripheral nerves showed significantly shorter latencies than those of O and R.

It is concluded that EPs can be recorded from the scalp after electrical stimulation of the digestive tract. These latencies differ depending on the site of stimulation. This technique may be useful in the study of nervous afferent pathways from the gut to the brain in health and disease.

Table 1

| | Latencies (ms) | | | | | N1/P1 | Amplitudes of EPs (μV) | | |
	N1	P1	N2	P2	N3		P1/N2	N2/P2	P2/N3
Oesophagus (0.2 Hz)									
20 cm mean	92.8	162.2	217.2	273.9	388.3	8.2	4.2	5.7	7.7
SD	17.9	19.5	31.7	19.5	28.7	2.7	2.5	3.2	3.4
37 cm mean	125.6	191.1	251.1	311.1	401.7	5.7	4.9	3.8	5.6
SD	35.8	36.8	26.2	25.3	39.0	2.8	2.6	2.0	1.9
Rectosigmoid colon (3 Hz)									
20 cm mean	57.6	72.6	96.5	132.4	152.0	0.7	0.9	0.9	0.7
SD	7.6	8.8	11.7	10.6	10.6	0.2	0.2	0.4	0.2

58
Differential effects of mental stress on interdigestive gastric acid output, pancreatic enzyme output and gastroduodenal motility

G. HOLTMANN, M. V. SINGER, R. KRIEBEL, K. H. STÄCKER AND H. GOEBELL

The aim of the present investigation was to study the acute effects of mental stress, on the gastric and pancreatic secretion and the motility of the upper gastrointestinal (GI) tract. After an overnight fast, 12 healthy volunteers swallowed two multi-lumen tubes which allowed continuous aspiration of gastric and duodenal juices and measuring of motility of the stomach and duodenum. In each study, at least three duodenal phases III of the interdigestive motor complex (IMC) were recorded. Either after the first or the second duodenal phase III (randomized order), a 60 min period of mental stress was begun. Mental stress was induced by an efficiency situation with mental arithmetic and solving anagrams under a financial award.

RESULTS

Mental stress significantly ($p < 0.05$) increased the duration of the IMC (interval between two duodenal phases III) by 51% (87 ± 11 vs. 132 ± 18 min, mean $\pm$ SEM, $n = 12$). During mental stress and the following 30 min resting period, gastric acid output significantly increased by about 30% compared to controls. Duodenal flow rate was not altered during the actual stress period but significantly decreased by more than 73% in the following 30 min resting period. Outputs of pancreatic enzymes (trypsin, chymotrypsin, lipase) were unchanged but duodenal enzyme concentrations significantly increased during mental stress. Cardiovascular parameters (mean arterial blood pressure, heart rate) significantly increased during the stress period.

Table 1 Gastric and pancreatic responses to stress

Time periods (min)		Stress		Rest
		0–30	30 –60	60–90
Gastric acid output	Control	1.5 ± 0.5	1.6 ± 0.5	1.9 ± 0.8
(mmol/30 min)	Stress	1.1 ± 0.6	2.1 ± 0.7*	2.6 ± 0.9
Duodonal flow rate	Co ntrol	23 ± 8.5	30 ± 10	40 ± 11
(ml/30 min)	Stress	26 ± 7.5	28 ± 8.9	15 ± 6.4*
Chymotrypsin- conc.	Control	3.6 ± 0.5	3.7 ± 0.9	5.4 ± 0.8
(U/ml)	Stress	3.9 ± 0.4	5.7 ± 0.9*	5.5 ± 0.6

(x ± SEM, $n = 12$, * $p < 0.05$ vs. control)

CONCLUSIONS

We conclude that acute mental stress has different effects on the stomach, pancreas and the upper GI motility. It causes an increase of interdigestive gastric output but prolongs the length of the IMC. Some of the effects of mental stress are not limited to the stress period itself. Whereas the mechanisms of action are incompletely understood, this controlled study clearly demonstrates that central nervous activity induced by mental stress causes alterations of the motility and secretion of the upper GI tract.

59
Neural–gut interactions in disease

**M. CAMILLERI, J.-R. MALAGELADA, R. D. FEALEY,
A. J. CAMERON AND E. P. DIMAGNO**

Although the effects of psychologic and other forms of stress on gut function have been extensively evaluated in recent years, the interaction between the gut and its extrinsic neural control is probably best exemplified by the effects of various neurologic diseases on gastrointestinal motility.

METHODS

We assessed upper gut motility by means of a pneumohydraulic perfusion system with an 8 or 12 lumen manometric assembly. At least three manometric ports were positioned in the proximal small bowel. Studies included 3 h fasting and 2 h after ingestion of a standard solid–liquid 511 calorie meal. Cervical cord transection patients were asymptomatic and specifically recruited for assessment of motility in this condition. The other patients were referred for evaluation of unexplained nausea, vomiting or upper abdominal pain. The effects of the following disorders on upper gut motility were assessed since they exemplified different anatomic levels of disease of the nervous system: posterior fossa tumours ($n = 12$), cervical cord transection ($n = 5$), autonomic neuropathy due to diabetes and amyloidosis ($n = 40$), and pandysautonomia ($n = 5$).

RESULTS

Tumours of the medulla oblongata unassociated with other cranial nerve signs result in antral hypomotility, and disorders in the propagation velocity of the interdigestive migrating motor complex (IMC). Cervical cord transections result in a disorganization of the antral component of the IMC. Post-ganglionic sympathetic lesions, with or without cholinergic involvement, that are due to autonomic neuropathies or pandysautonomia, typically result in antral hypomotility (fasting and post-prandially); unco-ordinated intestinal burst-like activity with tonic changes in baseline pressure during fasting; and failure of the meal to suppress IMC-like activity or to induce a fed pattern.

CONCLUSIONS

Upper gut dysmotility in neurologic diseases demonstrates the importance of neural–gut interactions.

Disturbances of peripheral neural pathways result in more marked derangements of gastric and small bowel motility than those due to brainstem or cervical cord lesions.

The finding of similar manometric features in patients with unexplained nausea and vomiting necessitates careful assessment of the neurologic system to exclude disease at any level of the axis between the brain and the gut.

60
Irritable bowel syndrome: irritability of bowel, of mind, of both or of none? A critical review

G. STACHER

IRRITABILITY OF BOWEL?

The name 'irritable bowel syndrome' (IBS) suggests that the syndrome is, at least in part, determined by a specific 'irritability' of the bowel. However, such an irritability has neither been defined nor is there any good evidence that the bowel of IBS patients as a group or of a circumscript subpopulation with the syndrome is, in fact more irritable than the bowel of asymptomatic individuals. Already early studies carried out to test the contractile responses of the colon to 'irritant' stimuli, such as an emotive interview, the ingestion of a meal and the administration of neostigmine, were unable to detect a difference between patients with the IBS and healthy controls[1,2]. A report that patients with IBS of the spastic colon type exhibited a considerable hyperactivity in the resting state and, characteristically, displayed much more colonic activity after neostigmine administration than did normal controls[3] was contradicted by the results of later investigations[4-6]. Several reports suggested that IBS patients characteristically had an increased activity at the three cycles per minute frequency of colonic myoelectric slow waves in the resting state[7-10], and a prolonged increase in colonic motor activity at that frequency after eating[9]. These findings, however, could not be confirmed and other authors were unable to detect such a higher incidence of the three minute frequency component or a specific response to a meal[4].

It has also been reported that IBS patients had significantly more contractile colonic activity during the night than healthy controls[11]. However, since sleep is associated with a greatly reduced colonic motility[12,13], the higher activity in the patients might have simply reflected that they slept less well than their more fortunate 'controls'. A study on small intestinal motor activity over prolonged periods revealed no differences in nocturnal motility between IBS patients and healthy individuals[14].

Kumar and Wingate[15] reported, under the somewhat sensational heading

'Paroxysmal enteric dysrhythmia (otherwise known as the IBS)', that in IBS patients subjected to a long period of intermittent mental stress, they had observed either a total abolition of the activity fronts of the migrating motor complex at the duodenojejunal flexure or a paroxysmal, irregular contractile activity, which occurred spontaneously or evoked by stress and was associated, in some patients, with IBS symptoms. The specificity of such features for patients with the IBS, however, has still to be confirmed. Other authors reported that, in patients with 'functional abdominal pain', the pattern of jejunal motor activity was not different from that in healthy controls and that the occurrence of pain bore no relationship to the recorded motility[16].

A characteristic of IBS patients with diarrhoea was proposed to be the presence of regular groups of aborally propagated contractions, occurring at intervals of 1–2 minutes[14,17,18]. However, this activity, which has been described earlier as minute rhythm[19] or peristaltic rush[20,21] and to occur also during the normal MMC, may constitute a pattern specific of patients with diarrhoea not only with but without the IBS.

A series of authors proposed a hypersensitivity to pain to be characteristic of patients with the IBS. Ritchie[22] reported that in 78% of 60 IBS patients the sensibility to pain induced by the inflation of a balloon in the pelvic colon was greatly increased in relation to gut wall tension. He hypothesized that this was due to some sort of surface hyperalgesia of the colonic mucosa, analogous to that which may be caused by pain substances in the skin. Others expressed the view that the level of pain perception in the IBS was the same as in healthy subjects. There would, however, be a difference in the tendency to report pain; in other words, the IBS patient would be more likely to say, 'Yes, that's painful'[23].

Kullmann and Fielding[24] reported the distensibility of the rectum to be significantly lower in IBS patients than in controls for both sensation threshold and maximal tolerable volume. They felt that this was possibly due to an increased awareness of contents in the rectum brought about by subjective stress. Similarly, it was found that the degrees of rectal distension required to elicit a desire to defaecate and to cause discomfort were significantly lower in IBS patients than in healthy controls[25]. This rectal hypersensitivity, however, was reported to return to normal once the IBS symptoms disappeared, which suggests that it is a reaction to the symptoms rather than a constitutional abnormality[24]. Moreover, Latimer et al.[26] found that IBS patients, psychologically disturbed patients without bowel symptoms, and healthy subjects did not differ in their self-ratings of pain induced by the inflation of a balloon in the rectosigmoid and that the proportion of individuals experiencing pain in the three groups did not differ significantly. Findings that many patients with IBS exhibited exceedingly high and largely fluctuating resting pressures in the upper anal canal[27] are still waiting for confirmation.

In conclusion, the available data cannot be viewed as providing evidence for the existence of a specific irritability of the bowel to external or internal stimuli or of characteristic patterns of colonic or small intestinal motor activity in patients with the IBS.

IRRITABILITY OF MIND?

There is a long tradition to link the symptoms of the IBS to emotional disturbances, psychological abnormalities or psychiatric disease, but it has also been suggested that the patient with IBS is distinguished from the healthy person only in the kind or degree of stress which is needed to evoke symptoms[28]. 'Irregular nervous manifestations, hysterical often or of hysterical type' were felt to be very common in patients suffering from the syndrome[29], who were also described as nervous, neurasthenic and hypochondriacal[30], to have a neurotic personality structure[30,31], or to be of marked emotional instability[33]. Some authors reported a high prevalence of hysteria and depression in patients with the syndrome[34,35], and that IBS patients who had predominantly diarrhoea, but not those who had predominantly pain, were significantly more anxious and neurotic than general medical patients[36]. In a recent survey on 14 102 middle-aged men and women it was found that symptoms of bloating, rumbling and cramping abdominal pain were much more strongly associated with symptoms of depression, sleeping difficulties and problems of coping than with lifestyle, dietary and social variables together[37].

A series of studies were aimed at identifying psychological characteristics of patients with the IBS. It was reported that 17 patients, as compared with a group of 20 healthy subjects, showed significantly elevated levels of anxiety, interpersonal sensitivity, depression, hostility and somatization of affect, but that there was no correlation between the amount of psychopathology and either severity of symptoms or colonic motility[38]. However, to demonstrate that a sample from a particular illness population differs on certain psychological factors from a control sample is in no sense to demonstrate the aetiological significance of those factors. Moreover, the significance of such differences is questioned by the fact that many IBS patients have suffered for years from unpleasant symptoms and have undergone many clinical investigations only to be told that nothing is wrong, certainly can be sufficient to make them mildly neurotic. Others found no differences in the level of anxiety and in somatization of anxiety between IBS patients and patients hospitalized for other medical reasons, and suspected that elevated anxiety levels found in earlier studies had reflected hospitalization or worry regarding the nature of the patients' illness before this. This notion was supported by the findings of a study[40] which led to the conclusion that figures for the frequency of psychoneurosis in small, possibly atypical hospital-based groups cannot safely be applied to the silent majority who do not bring their symptoms to a doctor: persons experiencing psychological distress are more likely to seek care for comparable symptoms than those without.

Similar conclusions were drawn from a survey of 566 healthy people[41]. Of that group, 86 individuals had bowel dysfunction compatible with the IBS, the majority of whom, i.e. 62%, had never been to a doctor for their complaints. Although those who consulted physicians were more likely to report abdominal pain than those who did not, behavioural influences rather than pain were felt to have led to their seeking health care. A more recent study investigated the contribution health care-seeking behaviours might have on symptomatic and psychological features of the condition[42]. It was found that certain psychosocial features, such as abnormal personality patterns, greater illness behaviours and lower positive stressful life event scores, characterized IBS patients and discriminated them from individuals with IBS who had not sought medical treatment and from healthy controls; whereas the two latter groups did not differ from each other. Thus, these data support the notion that psychosocial or purely social[43] factors determine what patients with the IBS will see physicians. For patients with a psychiatric or psychologic disorder, IBS symptoms may as well serve only as a pretext for their seeking of help.

However, IBS patients seeking health care must not necessarily show increased psychopathology. A study on patients with the IBS attending an outpatient clinic for their complaints and on blood donors who had symptoms indicative of the IBS but had not reported them, showed that patients of both groups did not exhibit more anxiety, depression, obsessive compulsion and interpersonal sensitivity than healthy controls[44]. One study[45] suggested that higher anxiety and obsession, as well as a greater tendency to internalized hostility, of IBS patients may be best explained as consequences of diagnostic uncertainty rather than as causing their illness: IBS patients frequently feared that their condition may be both grave and incurable. A recent report[46] indicated that in patients with medical disorders such as IBS, inflammatory bowel disease and non-gastrointestinal cancer, traditional psychiatric instruments overdiagnosed depression, histrionic personality, as well as anxiety, and that the proper psychiatric diagnosis in most of these patients should be Adjustment Disorder.

Taken together, the available data do not speak in favour of specific associations between the IBS and psychological abnormalities, psychiatric disease, or a heightened mental irritability.

CONCLUSION

For the time being, there is no evidence that the IBS in fact is characterized by a specific irritability of the bowel, of the mind or of both. Thus, the term IBS reflects unproven hypotheses and therefore has to be viewed as misguiding and creating confusion. It should be abandoned for terms simply describing the symptoms for which the patients seek health care, i.e. painful constipation, painful diarrhoea or deranged bowel habits with pain.

References

1. Almy, T. P., Hinkle, L. E., Berle, B. and Kern, F. (1949). Alterations in colonic function in man under stress. III. Experimental production of sigmoid spasm in patients with spastic constipation. *Gastroenterology*, **12**, 437–49
2. Wangel, A. G. and Deller, D. J. (1965). Intestinal motility in man. III. Mechanisms of constipation and diarrhea with particular reference to the irritable colon syndrome. *Gastroenterology*, **48**, 69–84
3. Chaudhary, N. A. and Truelove, S. C. (1961). Human colonic motility: a comparative study

of normal subjects, patients with ulcerative colitis, and patients with the irritable bowel syndrome. III. Effects of emotions. *Gastroenterology*, **40**, 27–36

4. Sarna, S., Latimer, P., Campbell, D. and Waterfall, W. E. (1982). Effect of stress, meal and neostigmine on rectosigmoid electrical control activity (ECA) in normals and in irritable bowel syndrome patients. *Dig. Dis. Sci.*, **27**, 582–91
5. Baldi, F., Corinaldesi, R., Ferrarini, F., Cassan, M., Brunetti, G. and Barbara, L. (1983). Manometry of the sigmoid colon in the irritable bowel syndrome (IBS). In Labò, G. and Bortolotti, M. (eds.) *Gastrointestinal Motility*, pp. 229–33. (Verona: Cortina International)
6. Cumming, J., Kelly, M. J. and Smith, C. L. (1983). The significance of propulsive, retropulsive, and segmenting contractions of the colon and rectum in the irritable bowel syndrome. *Gut*, **24**, A368
7. Snape, W. J. Jr., Carlson, G. M. and Cohen, S. (1976). Colonic myoelectric activity in the irritable bowel syndrome. *Gastroenterology*, **70**, 326–39
8. Snape, W. J. Jr., Carlson, G. M., Matarazzo, S. A. and Cohen, S. (1977). Evidence that abnormal myoelectrical activity produces colonic motor dysfunction in the irritable bowel syndrome. *Gastroenterology*, **72**, 383–7
9. Sullivan, M. A., Cohen, S. and Snape, W. J. Jr. (1978). Colonic myoelectrical activity in irritable-bowel syndrome. *N. Engl. J. Med.*, **298**, 878–83
10. Taylor, I., Darby, C. and Hammond, P. (1978). Comparison of rectosigmoid myoelectrical activity in the irritable colon syndrome during relapses and remissions. *Gut*, **19**, 923–9
11. Reynolds, J. R., Clark, A. G. and Hardcastle, J. D. (1986). 24 hour colonic motor activity in patients with the irritable bowel syndrome. *Gastroenterology*, **90**, 1602
12. Stacher, G. and Fink, G. (1973). Die Motilität des Verdauungstraktes im Schlaf. In Jovanović/, U. J. (ed.) *The Nature of Sleep*, pp. 59–62 (Stuttgart: Gustav Fischer Verlag)
13. Reynolds, J. R., Clark, A. G., Evans, D. F. and Hardcastle, J. D. (1985). Diurnal variations of colonic motility in man. *Gastroenterology*, **88**, 1554
14. Kellow, J. E., Gill, R. C. and Wingate, D. L. (1987). Proximal gut motor activity in irritable bowel syndrome (IBS) patients at home and at work (abstr.). *Gastroenterology*, **92**, 1463
15. Kumar, D. and Wingate, D. L. (1985). The irritable bowel syndrome: paroxysmal motor disorder. *Lancet*, **2**, 973–7
16. Kingham, J. G., Bown, R., Colson, R. and Clark, M. L. (1984). Jejunal motility in patients with functional abdominal pain. *Gut*, **25**, 375–80
17. Kellow, J. E. and Phillips, S. F. (1987). Altered small bowel motility in irritable bowel syndrome is correlated with symptoms. *Gastroenterology*, **92**, 1885–93
18. Read, N. W. (1985). The mechanism of diarrhoea in the irritable bowel syndrome. In Read, N. W. (ed.) *Irritable Bowel Syndrome*, pp. 173–84 (London: Grune & Stratton)
19. Fleckenstein, P. (1977). Migrating electrical spike activity in the fasting human small intestine. *Am. J. Dig. Dis.*, **22**, 769–75
20. Golenhofen, K. (1976). Spontaneous activity and functional classification of mammalian smooth muscle. In Bülbring, E. and Shuba, M. F. (eds.) *Physiology of Smooth Muscle*, pp. 91–7 (New York: Raven Press)
21. Fleckenstein, P. and Øigaard, A. (1978). Electrical spike activity in the human small intestine. A multiple electrode study of fasting diurnal variations. *Am. J. Dig. Dis.*, **23**, 776–80
22. Ritchie, J. A. (1973). Pain from distension of the pelvic colon by inflating a balloon in the irritable colon syndrome. *Gut*, **14**, 125–35
23. Drossman, D. A. and Sandler, R. S. (1985). Irritable bowel syndrome: the role of psychosocial factors. In Read, N. W. (ed.) *Irritable Bowel Syndrome*, pp. 67–78 (London: Grune & Stratton)
24. Kullmann, G. and Fielding, J. F. (1981). Rectal distensibility in the irritable bowel syndrome. *Ir. Med. J.*, **74**, 140–2
25. Sun, W. M. and Read, N. W. (1988). Anorectal manometry and rectal sensation in patients with the IBS. *Gastroenterology*, **94**, A450
26. Latimer, P., Campbell, D., Latimer, M., Sarna, S., Daniel, E. and Waterfall, W. (1979). Irritable bowel syndrome: a test of the colonic hyperalgesia hypothesis. *J. Behav. Med.*, **2**, 285–95
27. Devroede, G. (1985). Mechanisms of constipation. In Read, N. W. (ed.) *Irritable Bowel Syndrome*, pp. 127–39 (London: Grune & Stratton)
28. Almy, T. P. (1957). What is the 'irritable colon'? *Am. J. Dig. Dis.*, **2**, 93–7

29. Da Costa, J. M. (1871). Membranous enteritis. *Am. J. Med. Sci.*, **62**, 321–38
30. Hale White, W. (1905). A study of 60 cases with membranous colitis. *Lancet*, **2**, 1229–35
31. Hurst, A. F. (1919). *Constipation and Allied Intestinal Disorders*, 2nd Edn. (London: Frowde)
32. Palmer, R. L., Stonehill, E., Crisp, A. H., Waller, S. L. and Misiewicz, J. J. (1974). Psychological characteristics of patients with the irritable bowel syndrome. *Postgrad. Med. J.*, **50**, 416–19
33. Bockus, H. L., Bank, J. and Wilkinson, S. A. (1928). Neurogenic mucous colitis. *Trans. Am. Gastroenterol. Assoc.*, **31**, 277–97
34. Hislop, I. G. (1971). Psychological significance of the irritable colon syndrome. *Gut*, **12**, 452–7
35. Young, S. J., Alpers, D. H., Norland, C. C. and Woodruff, R. A. (1976). Psychiatric illness and the irritable bowel syndrome. Practical implications for the primary physician. *Gastroenterology*, **70**, 162–6
36. Esler, M. D. and Goulston, K. J. (1973). Levels of anxiety in colonic disorder. *N. Engl. J. Med.*, **288**, 16–20
37. Johnsen, R., Jacobsen, B. K. and Førde, O. H. (1986). Associations between symptoms of irritable colon and psychological and social conditions and lifestyle. *Br. Med. J.*, **292**, 1633–5
38. Whitehead, W. E., Engel, B. T. and Schuster, M. M. (1980). Irritable bowel syndrome. Physiological and psychological differences between diarrhea-predominant and constipation-predominant patients. *Dig. Dis. Sci.*, **25**, 404–13
39. Ryan, W. A., Kelly, M. G. and Fielding, J. F. (1983). Personality and the irritable bowel syndrome. *Ir. Med. J.*, **76**, 140–1
40. Welch, G. W., Stace, N. H. and Pomare, E. W. (1984). Specificity of psychological profiles of irritable bowel syndrome patients. *Aust. N.Z. J. Med.*, **14**, 101–4
41. Sandler, R. S., Drossman, D. A., Nathan, H. P. and McKee, D. C. (1984). Symptom complaints and health care seeking behavior in subjects with bowel dysfunction. *Gastroenterology*, **87**, 314–18
42. Drossman, D. A., McKee, D. C., Sandler, R. S., Mitchell, C. M., Lowman, B. C., Burger, A. L. and Cramer, E. M. (1987). Psychosocial factors in irritable bowel syndrome: a multivariate study (abstr). *Gastroenterology*, **92**, 1374
43. Talley, N. J., Phillips, S. F., Melton, L. J., Bruce, B., Hench, V. S. and Zinsmeister, A. R. (1988). A controlled study of psychosocial factors in presenters and nonpresenters with functional bowel disease (FBD). *Gastroenterology*, **94**, A454
44. Welch, G. W., Hillman, L. C. and Pomare, E. W. (1985). Psychoneurotic symptomatology in the irritable bowel syndrome: a study of reporters and non-reporters. *Br. Med. J.*, **291**, 1382–4
45. Kumar, D., Pfeffer, J. and Wingate, D. L. (1986). Are irritable bowel syndrome (IBS) patients truly neurotic — or just anxious? (abstr). *Gastroenterology*, **90**, 1505
46. Kovnat-Adler, K., Turner, R., Roemer, R., Malmud, E., Krevsky, B. and Fisher, R. S. (1987). Misleading psychiatric diagnoses in patients with GI disorders (abstr). *Gastroenterology*, **92**, 1481

61
Food-induced hypotension in human subjects with impaired autonomic nervous function: pathophysiological changes and therapeutic strategies

C. J. MATHIAS, R. BANNISTER, S. R. BLOOM, P. CORTELLI, D. F. DA COSTA, J. S. KOONER, S. RAIMBACH AND S. WOOD

INTRODUCTION

It is now recognized that food ingestion is a powerful stimulus, not only to the gastrointestinal tract but to a range of physiological systems which involve the neuroendocrine, cardiovascular and autonomic nervous systems. The interactions between these systems are difficult to determine in normal humans and much information has been gained from studying patients with autonomic lesions, some of whom exhibit pronounced changes after food ingestion. In this review we describe recent evidence on the pathophysiological mechanisms accounting for post-prandial hypotension and concentrate on patients with chronic autonomic failure, in whom these changes are of clinical importance as food ingestion considerably enhances postural hypotension.

PATIENTS

The patients in whom these studies have been performed belonged to the primary or idiopathic variety of chronic autonomic failure, in whom detailed investigations did not provide clues towards the precise aetiology of their lesions[1]. There were two major groups with this disorder: patients with pure autonomic failure with lesions affecting only the autonomic nervous system and those with multiple system atrophy or the Shy–Drager Syndrome who had additional neurological abnormalities involving the basal ganglia and/or the cerebellum and pyramidal tracts. The disorder in these patients was characterized by severe orthostatic hypotension and a series of physiological, pharmacological and biochemical tests[2] confirmed sympathetic failure, often with associated impairment of cardiac parasympathetic function. The changes in blood pressure after food were similar in both groups and the results were therefore combined for the purpose of this review. In all our studies measurements were made with the patients lying flat, so as to exclude the effects of head-up posture on the cardiovascular system.

HAEMODYNAMIC CHANGES FOLLOWING FOOD INGESTION

In the autonomic failure patients, ingestion of a standard meal consisting of toast, butter, marmalade, eggs and orange juice (66 g of carbohydrate, 22 g of fat and 18 g of protein; 530 kcals) resulted in a marked fall in blood pessure (Figure 1) which occurred within 15 min, reached its lowest level after about 60 min and remained below baseline levels 3 h after food ingestion. There were minimal changes in heart rate, consistent with a cardiac vagal lesion, and there were no changes in either the forearm muscle or cutaneous circulation.

This differed markedly from the response in normal subjects, studied under

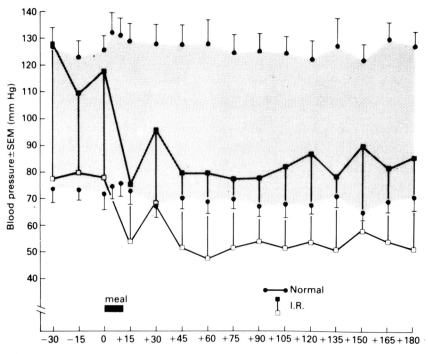

Figure 1 Supine systolic and diastolic blood pressure before and after a standard meal in normal subjects (stippled area with $\pm$ SEM) and in a patient with pure autonomic failure (IR, continuous lines). Blood pressure does not change in normal subjects. In the patient there is a rapid fall in blood pressure to levels as low as 80/50 mmHg, which remain low even in the supine position over the 3 h observation period (from ref. 3)

identical circumstances, in whom blood pressure did not fall. In the normal subjects there was an elevation in heart rate, together with a rise in both stroke volume and cardiac output. There were no changes in cutaneous bloodflow but forearm bloodflow fell, with a rise in forearm vascular resistance, indicative of active constriction in vessels supplying skeletal muscle. In the normal subjects there was a fall in calculated peripheral vascular resistance, suggestive of dilatation in certain vascular territories. Dilatation did not occur in the periphery in either muscle or skin and it was likely, as observed by others[4], that this was secondary to the large increase in superior mesenteric artery bloodflow which occurs soon after food ingestion.

In the normal subjects, therefore, blood pressure after food ingestion was maintained by a series of adjustments, partially neurogenically mediated with a probable humoral component, which occurred in cardiac output and the skeletal muscle circulation. The fall in blood pressure in our autonomic failure patients after a meal, in the absence of these changes, suggests that the sympathetic nervous system was largely responsible for the compensatory changes in normal humans, although there may have been an associated humoral component.

EFFECTS OF DIFFERENT FOOD COMPONENTS

To determine the cardiovascular effects of different food components patients were studied after carbohydrate, protein or fat, in similar volumes and matched so as to provide an identical caloric load. Carbohydrate was administered as glucose in a solution of $1 \, g/kg$ bodyweight. After glucose there was a rapid and substantial fall in blood pressure, and the temporal profile of the hypotensive response was similar to that after a mixed meal (Figure 2). Although there were no changes observed in the haematocrit or plasma osmolality this solution of glucose may have exerted osmotic effects intralumenally thus reducing plasma volume. We therefore studied the same patients after an iso-osmotic solution of the carbohydrate xylose. Xylose is similar in taste and actively absorbed like glucose, but undergoes minimal metabolism and does not raise glucose and insulin levels as it is an inert carbohydrate. After xylose there was a smaller and less prolonged fall in blood pressure (Figure 3) with a small rise in the haemotocrit. The major actions of glucose in lowering blood pressure therefore appeared to be independent of its osmotic effects and may have been secondary to the stimulation of insulin and other pancreatico-gastrointestinal peptides.

Protein given as whey protein (Maxipro) caused only a small and transient fall in blood pressure. Lipid, given as Prosperol, caused a smaller fall in blood pressure which recovered earlier than after glucose alone. Carbohydrate was therefore the most potent food component in lowering blood pressure, followed by lipid, with protein having minimal effects.

GASTRIC EMPTYING AND POST-PRANDIAL HYPOTENSION

Following food ingestion, other factors, in addition to a lack of appropriate corrective sympathetic reflexes, may have contributed to the fall in blood

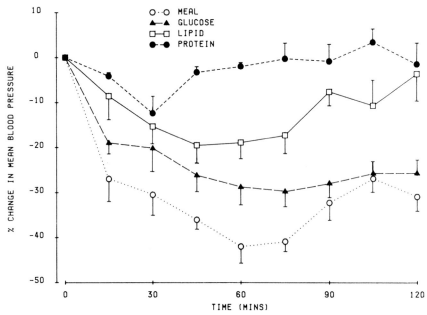

Figure 2 Percentage change in mean blood pressure in 6 patients with autonomic failure given either a standard mixed meal or an iso-caloric and isovolumic solution of carbohydrate (glucose 1 g/kg bodyweight), lipid (Prosperol 0.95 ml/kg) or protein (Maxipro 1 g/kg) alone. Vertical bars indicate $\pm$ SEM (from ref. 5)

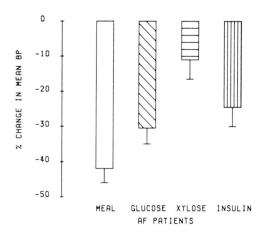

Figure 3 Percentage change in mean blood pressure (BP) in a group of patients with chronic autonomic failure when studied after a mixed meal, oral glucose, oral xylose or after 0.15 units/kg of a bolus injection of insulin. Part of the fall in blood pressure after glucose may be due to its osmotic effects, as seen after xylose

pressure. Patients with autonomic failure often have vagal impairment, which is known to affect the heart and may involve the gut, thus causing abnormal motility. The 'dumping syndrome' may occur after vagotomy and gastric drainage procedures, resulting in abnormal gastric motility, and a similar situation may have been present in our patients. The 'dumping syndrome' is attributed to hyperosmotic solutions rapidly entering the jejunum, resulting in intralumenal accumulation of fluid, which causes a contraction of the plasma volume, as indicated by a rise in the haemotocrit[6]. This results in weakness, perspiration, tachycardia with palpitations and, occasionally, a modest fall in blood pressure, even in patients with an assumed intact sympathetic nervous system. This is indicative of an autonomic response to the reduced plasma volume. We did not observe a rise in the haemotocrit or plasma osmolality in our patients with autonomic failure after food, making it less likely that such a sequence of events was responsible. These assessments are, however, indirect and relatively insensitive, and small changes in plasma volume, sufficient to cause significant haemodynamic effects in our patients with abnormal corrective reflexes, may have occurred. Other factors to consider include excessive secretion of various glands in response to food and abnormal fluid and electrolyte shifts within the gut, which are known to be influenced by adrenergic nerve activity[7].

To investigate gastric motility we used technetium-labelled bran followed by a mixed meal given in the sitting position, with scinti-scanning to determine the rate of gastric emptying. Many of the patients with autonomic failure had increased gastric emptying when compared to normal subjects. However, post-prandial hypotension occurred in patients with normal emptying and even in patients with gastroparesis. It seems unlikely that enhanced gastric emptying is the primary factor responsible for the hypotension, but its role in contributing to hypotension in some patients needs to be further evaluated.

CHANGES IN PANCREATICO–GUT HORMONES AND THEIR POTENTIAL ROLE IN POST-PRANDIAL HYPOTENSION

Ingestion of food results in the release of pancreatic and gastrointestinal hormones, some of which are known to have vasodilatatory effects. These effects may be enhanced in patients with autonomic failure, who are highly sensitive to the blood pressure lowering effects of a variety of vasodilator agents[2,8]. A range of hormones, which included gastrin, motilin, pancreatic polypeptide, somatostatin, insulin, enteroglucagon, vasoactive intestinal polypeptide, cholecystokinin and neurotensin, was measured before and after a standard mixed meal in our patients. The majority of hormones had a normal profile, except for three: enteroglucagon, pancreatic polypeptide and neurotensin; each of which rose to a greater extent in the patients. The first two are not known to have vasodilatatory or negative cardiac inotropic effects and are unlikely to have been responsible for the hypotension. Neurotensin, however, is a vasodilator[9] and may have been contributory. All our measurements were made in a peripheral vein, so there may have

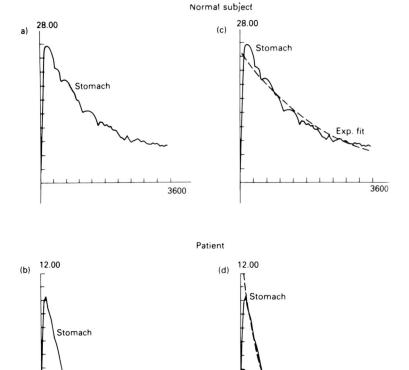

Figure 4 Gastric emptying curves in (a) a normal subject and (b) a patient with autonomic failure. Integrated counts are indicated on the vertical axis and time in seconds on the horizontal axis. A computer exponential (Exp.) fit is indicated. In the autonomic failure patient there is rapid emptying initially (Exp. I) with a later slower phase (Exp. II) (from ref. 3)

been significant differences in other potent vasodilators, such as vaso-active intestinal polypeptide within the splanchnic bed, where most of the vascular changes accounting for post-prandial hypotension probably occur. The precise role of individual peptides in the hypotensive response is difficult to assess without the availability of selective antagonists, unless more direct invasive assessment of their release, with the inherent ensuing difficulties, are employed.

The role of insulin in the observed responses was of interest for a variety of reasons. In the oral glucose and xylose studies the former caused a considerably greater fall in blood pressure, which may have been linked to its effect on insulin release. Furthermore, previous studies in patients who were tetraplegic due to a cervical spinal cord transection and who also have sympathetic dysfunction[10] had confirmed an hypotensive effect of insulin[11].

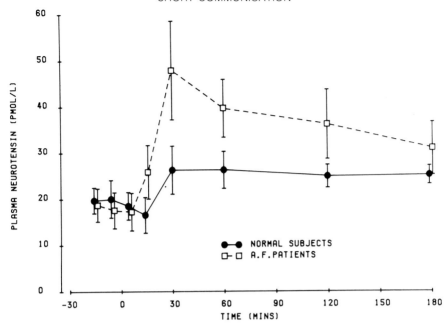

Figure 5 Plasma levels of neurotensin in normal subjects (continuous line) and autonomic failure patients (interrupted line) before and after a standard meal ingested at time 0. There is a significantly greater response in the autonomic failure patients (from ref. 3)

In our autonomic failure patients, an intravenous bolus of 0.15 units/kg of insulin lowered blood pressure within 5 min, with a 20% reduction after 20 min which occurred before the onset of hypoglycaemia[12].

Hypoglycaemia is a potent stimulus to peptide and hormone release and the effects of insulin were therefore studied in the presence of a glucose clamp to prevent such changes. In these studies three incremental dose infusion rates of insulin progressively lowered blood pressure while euglycaemia was maintained[13]. In the insulin-euglycaemia studies there were no changes in the vasculature of the skin or skeletal muscle and no fall in cardiac output, making it likely that the effects of insulin were predominantly occurring within the splanchnic region. Our studies therefore indicate that insulin may play a major role in post-prandial hypotension.

EFFECT OF THE PEPTIDE RELEASE INHIBITOR, SMS 201-995 (OCTREOTIDE)

To determine further the role of peptides in post-prandial hypotension we studied the effects of the somatostatin analogue SMS 201-995 (Octreotide) which in normal subjects (in a dose of 50 µg s.c.) prevents the release of a range of pancretico–gut peptides following food or glucose ingestion. A similar dose in autonomic failure patients followed by a glucose challenge (1 g/kg bodyweight) half an hour later, prevented the hypotension which occurred in the placebo phase of the study (Figure 6). The glucose-induced rise in levels of neurotensin, vasoactive intestinal polypeptide and insulin were all suppressed by SMS 201-995[14]. No changes were observed in the cutaneous and skeletal muscle circulation in the periphery and in cardiac function, suggestive of changes largely with the splanchnic territory. It is likely therefore that SMS 201-995 prevented the action of those peptides responsible for post-prandial hypotension, which probably have major effects either directly or indirectly on the large splanchnic vascular bed.

THERAPEUTIC STRATEGIES

A number of approaches to prevent post-prandial hypotension have been previously tried[15]: Indomethacin was used on the basis that it would block formation of vasodilatatory prostaglandin production, but without success; Propranolol may have enhanced the depressor effect, while antihistaminics such as diphenhydramine and cimetidine were ineffective. The vasopressor agent dihydroergotamine, although successful in reducing postural hypotension, did not prevent post-prandial hypotension[16]. It may be that none of these substances block the release of those peptides which are responsible for the hypotension and have significant effects on the splanchnic circulation. Our studies with the somatostatin analogue SMS 201-995 indicate that such an approach may be beneficial in preventing food-induced hypotension, as also demonstrated in limited short-term studies in patients with other

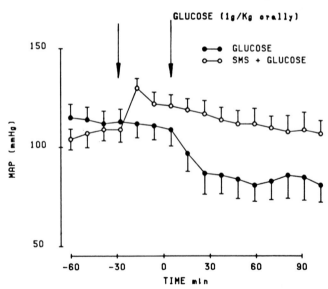

Figure 6 Levels of mean arterial blood pressure (MAP) in 7 patients with chronic autonomic failure after oral glucose given after pretreatment with either placebo (open circles) or the somatostatin analogue SMS 201-995 (Octreotide) 50 μg s.c. (filled circles), given at −30 (first arrow). After placebo, glucose caused a substantial fall in blood pressure; this was reversed by pre-treatment with SMS 201-995

autonomic disorders[17]. SMS 201-995 needs to be administered subcutaneously and availability of orally active analogues is awaited. Other agents such as caffeine (200 mg orally) has been reported to be effective[16,18] although the mechanism by which it prevents post-prandial hypotension is unclear.

Alternative approaches could be aimed primarily at reversing or preventing the major pathophysiological changes which we have defined. Altering carbohydrate intake with spacing of meals, the use of less readily digested carbohydrates or the use of substances such as guar gum, which slow glucose absorption, may prevent surges of insulin and other peptides and thus be beneficial. Reduction in gastric motility may be of benefit in some patients. The use of selective peptide antagonists should, however, be a major step forward in our determining more precisely the role of different peptides released during food ingestion. At present, the use of analogues of somatostatin appear to be the most promising approach to reducing post-prandial hypotension, which contributes to morbidity in many patients with autonomic failure.

Acknowledgements

CJM thanks the Wellcome Trust, the Brain Research Trust and the Medical Research Council for their support. The gastric-emptying studies were performed in collaboration with the Department of Clinical Physics at St. Mary's Hospital.

References

1. Mathias, C. J. (1987). Autonomic dysfunction. *Br. J. Hosp. Med.*, **38**, 238–43
2. Bannister, R. and Mathias, C. J. (1988). Testing autonomic reflexes. In Bannister, R. (ed.) *Autonomic Failure. A Textbook of Clinical Disorders of the Autonomic Nervous System*, 2nd Edn., pp. 289–307. (Oxford: Oxford University Press)
3. Mathias, C. J., da Costa, D. F. and Bannister, R. (1988). Post cibal hypotension in autonomic disorders. In Bannister, R. (ed.) *Autonomic Failure. A Textbook of Clinical Disorders of the Autonomic Nervous System*, 2nd Edn., pp. 367–80. (Oxford: Oxford University Press)
4. Qamar, M. I. and Read, A. E. (1986). The effect of feeding and sham feeding on the superior mesenteric artery bloodflow in man. *J. Physiol. (Lond.)*, **377**, 399P
5. Mathias, C. J., da Costa, D. F., Fosbraey, P., McIntosh, C. and Bannister, R. (1988). Factors contributing to food induced hypotension in patients with autonomic dysfunction. In Vanhoutte, P. N. (ed.) *Proceedings of the 4th International Symposium on Vasodilatation*. (New York: Raven Press) (In press)
6. Roberts, R. E., Randall, H. T. and Farr, H. W. (1954). Cardiovascular and blood volume alterations resulting from intra-jejunal administration of hypotonic solutions to gastrectomized patients. The relationship of these changes to the dumping syndrome. *Ann. Surg.*, **140**, 631–40
7. Sjovall, H., Jodal, M. and Lundgren, O. (1987). Sympathetic control of intestinal fluid and electrolyte transport. *News Physiol. Sci.*, **2**, 214–17
8. Mathias, C. J., Mathews, W. B. and Spalding, J. M. K. (1977). Postural changes in plasma renin activity and response to vaso-active drugs in a case of Shy Drager Syndrome. *J. Neurol. Neurosurg. Psyciatr.*, **40**, 138–43
9. Carraway, R. and Leeman, S. (1973). Isolation of a new hypotensive peptide, neurotensin from hypothalamus. *J. Biol. Chem.*, **248**, 6854–61
10. Mathias, C. J. and Frankel, H. L. (1988). Cardiovascular control in spinal man. *Annu. Rev.*

Physiol., **50**, 577–92

11. Mathias, C.J., Frankel, H.L., Turner, R.L. and Christensen, N.J. (1979). Physiological responses to insulin hypoglycaemia in spinal man. *Paraplegia,* **17**, 319–26

12. Mathias, C.J., da Costa, D.F., Fosbraey, P., Christensen, N.J. and Bannister, R. (1987). Hypotensive and sedative effects of insulin in autonomic failure. *Br. Med. J.,* **295**, 161–3

13. Bannister, R., da Costa, D.F., Kooner, J.S., MacDonald, I.A. and Mathias, C.J. (1987). Insulin induced hypotension in autonomic failure in euglycaemia in man. *J. Physiol. (Lond.),* **382**, 36P

14. Mathias, C.J., Raimbach, S.J., Cortelli, P., Kooner, J.S. and Bannister, R. (1988). The somatostatin analogue SMS 201-995 inhibits peptide release and prevents glucose-induced hypotension in autonomic failure. *J. Neurol.,* **235** (suppl.), S74–75

15. Robertson, D., Wade, D. and Robertson, S.M. (1981). Post prandial alterations in cardiovascular haemodynamics in autonomic dysfunctional states. *Am. J. Cardiol.,* **48**, 1048–52

16. Hoeldtke, R.D., Cavanaugh, S.T., Hughes, J.D. and Polansky, M. (1986). Treatment of orthostatic hypotension with dihydroergotamine and caffeine. *Ann. Int. Med.,* **105**, 168–73

17. Hoeldtke, R.D., O-Dorisio, T.M. and Boden, G. (1986). Treatment of autonomic neuropathy with a somatostatin analogue SMS 201-995. *Lancet,* **11**, 602–5

18. Onrot, J., Goldberg, R., Biaggioni, I., Hollister, A.S., Kincaid, D. and Robertson, D. (1985). Haemodynamic and humoral effects of caffeine in autonomic failure. Therapeutic implications for post-prandial hypotension. *N. Engl. J. Med.,* **313**, 549–54

62
Peripheral transduction mechanism in visceral pain perception of irritable bowel patients

R. HOELZL, L.-P. ERASMUS, M. KRATZMAIR

Increased visceral pain sensitivity has been reported repeatedly to be a psychophysiological marker of irritable bowel syndrome (IBS) since Ritchie's study[1]. However, stable association with clinical symptomatology and identification of underlying pathophysiological mechanisms are still lacking, because nociceptive thresholds can be lowered by peripheral visceral, as well as central or psychological, factors. A possible peripheral cause of lowered pain thresholds is increased tonus or wall tension. It would result in steeper slope of the transduction characteristic for distension stimuli. In consequence, pain threshold is reached at lower levels of distension. Symptomatic sub-groups, in which this mechanism is responsible for abdominal pain symptoms, should be differentiated by lowered pain thresholds to graded distension as well as higher bowel tonus and/or increased tonic response to colonic distension.

To answer this question, the present study compared visceral pain sensitivity and tonic pressure response to graded distension of three subgroups of IBS patients with frequent pain reports and defined by predominant bowel symptoms (constipation, 15; diarrhoea, 16; alternating, 15; organic causes and lactase deficiency excluded) with each other and 9 healthy controls. Stimuli were applied through a new rectosigmoidal probe, which allows quantification of tonic pressure responses of the sigmoid colon to distension unconfounded by balloon characteristics.

Levels of distension tolerated until first pain report differentiated clearly between IBS and control groups with lower thresholds in IBS patients. Individual comparisons of subgroups, however, showed that this was due only to patients with diarrhoea-predominant and alternating symptoms. Constipated patients did not differ from controls. Tonic pressure responses produced a complementary pattern: They were lowest for controls and constipated patients, while groups with diarrhoea-predominant and alternating symptomatology, in accordance with their higher pain sensitivity, had steeper rises in pressure (Friedman and U-Tests, 5% throughout).

For these subgroups of IBS, then, altered peripheral transduction of distending stimuli through increased wall tension seems to be a parsimonious explanation of their pain symptoms. Changes in afferent information processing at higher stages, that is, in visceral pain perception *per se*, 'instrumental' pain behaviour, etc., need not be assumed. In fact, there may be peripheral reasons of tonic pressure response changes found. If, however, psychological factors are involved in altered visceral pain perception of diarrhoeic subgroups of IBS, they should be expected to operate through changes in efferent commands controlling smooth muscle tonus and its consequences on peripheral signal transduction, rather than through changes in afferent signal transmission or processing. A different mechanism must be working in constipated subjects.

The basic mechanism of tonus-dependent transduction of distending stimuli was verified meanwhile in two analogue experiments with healthy subjects[2].

References

1. Ritchie, J. (1973). Pain from distension of the pelvic colon by inflating a balloon in the irritable colon syndrome. *Gut*, **14**, 125–32
2. Kratzmair, M., Erasmus, L.-P., Hartl, L. and Hölz, R. (1987). Influence of stimulus parameters on the perception of colonic distension. *Psychophysiology*, **24**, 597

63
The illness behaviour model of irritable bowel syndrome: experimental support

S. M. MCHUGH, K. KERSEY AND N. E. DIAMANT

Irritable bowel syndrome (IBS) has variously been conceptualized as a psychiatric, psychophysiological or pathophysiological disorder and, more recently, according to an illness behaviour (IB) perspective. Following the IB model, we hypothesized that IBS patients would differ from healthy control (HC) subjects not seeking medical attention on the basis of cognitive, affective and social measures, in addition to their somatic complaints. Forty-six IBS subjects (males = 8.45 ± 15 years; females = 28.39 ± 28 y) were compared to 48 healthy young controls (males = 25.28 ± 5y; females = 23.21 ± = 2 yrs) using questionnaires measuring gastrointestinal and general somatic symptoms, affective state (depression and trait anxiety), somatization tendencies, introspectiveness, social supports, health practices and beliefs, and cognitive measures such as self-efficacy. The questionnaire items or scores for which the IBS and HC subjects differed were subjected to a factor analysis which showed that four factors accounted for 60% of the variance (V) between the groups.

Factor I (31% V) was very highly correlated with self-efficacy estimations of confidence and avoidance of toileting in work, recreational and social circumstances. Factor II (17%) was most strongly correlated with the typical gastrointestinal symptoms of IBS but also included fatigue, bowel and general health worries and was weakly to moderately strongly correlated with anxiety, depression and somatization measures. Factor III (7%) correlated with further self-efficacy estimations for travel by various modes and Factor IV (5%) with an anxiety measure.

CONCLUSIONS

These data are consistent with an illness behaviour model. Psychological measures accounted for more of the variance between IBS and HC subjects than do their bowel and somatic symptoms. The results indicate that more investigation should be devoted to these areas.

Index